Pharmaceutical Calculations

15th EDITION

Preface

The 15th edition of *Pharmaceutical Calculations* marks the introduction of Professor Shelly Stockton as co-author. Professor Stockton's experience in pharmacy practice and her expertise in teaching pharmaceutics and pharmacy calculations are reflected in her substantial contributions to this textbook. Combined with the many progressive changes recommended by a select review team of pharmacy students, practitioners, and educators, this new edition maintains the standard for today's academic and basic practice requirements in the subject area of pharmaceutical calculations.

Each chapter has been thoroughly revised with the focus directed toward providing basic pharmaceutical calculations along with supporting explanations of the pharmaceutical or clinical purpose underpinning each type of calculation. Hundreds of new problems have been added to include many current products encountered in pharmacy practice. Relevance is further demonstrated by the inclusion of select product labels directly linked to example problems. New in this edition are *Authors' Extra Points* that provide brief explanations of select underlying subjects, as: *pharmacopeias*, *electronic prescriptions*, *drug names*, and the *regulation of pharmacy compounding*. A section on equianalgesic dosing for narcotic analgesics has been added to Chapter 10 along with dosing tables related to the subject.

All of the valued features of the previous edition have been retained and enhanced, including the following: in-chapter *example problems* with step-by-step solutions; end-of-chapter *practice problems* with answers; *Case-in-Point* features that provide clinical or pharmaceutical case studies; *Calculations Capsules* that provide boxed summaries of chapter calculations; *CalcQuiz* sections that provide a limited number of *un*solved problems, useful as homework, quiz, or assessment exercises; and, the *Comprehensive Review Problems* at the end of the book that provide multipart solved problems for student use as a final self-assessment.

Throughout its history, this textbook has served as a valuable resource in meeting the instructional needs of pharmacy students in the area of pharmaceutical calculations. This new edition is expected to continue to meet that need.

Acknowledgments

The author gratefully acknowledges the contributions to this revision by the following persons: Tom Schoenbachler, for insights into contemporary community pharmacy practice; Deborah Elder, for contributions in the area of pharmacy compounding; Ken Duke, for problems in the area of nuclear pharmacy; Warren Beach, for some Case-in-Point calculations; Flynn Warren, for a host of problems including many relating to institutional pharmacy practice; Michael Ansel and Catherine Chuter, for information on the verification and data processing of electronic prescriptions; Les Ramos and Margaret Ramos, for their input in various areas of clinical calculations; Hardeep Saluja and Sarai Flynn for contributions to the chapter on bioavailability and pharmacokinetics; Patra Kositchaiwat and Ryan Varghese for their input in the area of electrolyte solution calculations; and Loyd V. Allen, Jr. for his continued courtesy in allowing use of formulas published in the *International Journal of Pharmaceutical Compounding*.

Gratitude is expressed to the following reviewers, whose experience was drawn upon during the planning process and whose thoughtful analysis and constructive comments led to many of the changes in this revision: Stacy Cairns, Kimberly Daugherty, David Dubins, Heather Gegenhuber, Nancy Kleiman, William Kolling, Kimberly Nguyen, and Tien Phan.

Particular thanks are offered to Tari Broderick, Senior Acquisitions Editor, and Stephanie Roulias, Product Development Editor, for their support and guidance during the revision process and to the other exceptional people at Wolters Kluwer Health | Lippincott Williams & Wilkins for their work in the design, preparation, and production of this revision. Finally, special appreciation is extended to Tom Conville for his expertise in copyediting and assistance in resource development.

Howard C. Ansel
Athens, Georgia

Shelly J. Stockton
Weatherford, Oklahoma

Contents

Introduction

Scope of Pharmaceutical Calculations

The use of calculations in pharmacy is varied and broad-based. It encompasses calculations performed by pharmacists in traditional as well as in specialized practice settings and within operational and research areas in industry, academia, and government. In the broad context, the scope of pharmaceutical calculations includes computations related to:

- chemical and physical properties of drug substances and pharmaceutical ingredients;
- biological activity and rates of drug absorption, bodily distribution, metabolism, and excretion (pharmacokinetics);
- statistical data from basic research and clinical drug studies;
- pharmaceutical product development and formulation;
- prescriptions and medication orders including drug dosage, dosage regimens, and patient adherence to medication treatment plans;
- pharmacoeconomics; and other areas.

For each of these areas, there is a unique body of knowledge. Some areas are foundational, whereas others are more specialized, constituting a distinct field of study. This textbook is foundational, providing the basic underpinnings of calculations applicable to pharmacy practice in community, institutional, and industrial settings.

In community pharmacies, pharmacists receive, fill, and dispense *prescriptions* and provide relevant drug information to ensure their safe and effective use. Prescriptions may call for *prefabricated* pharmaceutical products manufactured in industry, or, they may call for individual components to be weighed or measured by the pharmacist and *compounded* into a finished product. In hospitals and other institutional settings, *medication orders* are entered into a patient's medical chart, becoming part of the electronic medical record.

In the preparation of pharmaceuticals, both medicinal and nonmedicinal materials are used. The medicinal components (*active therapeutic ingredients or ATIs*) provide the benefit desired. The nonmedicinal ingredients (*pharmaceutical excipients*) are included in a formulation to produce the desired pharmaceutical qualities, as physical form, chemical and physical stability, rate of drug release, appearance, and taste, when desired.

Whether a pharmaceutical product is produced in the industrial setting or prepared in a community or institutional pharmacy, pharmacists engage in calculations to achieve standards of quality. The difference is one of scale. In pharmacies, relatively small quantities of medications are prepared and dispensed for specific patients. In industry, *large-scale* production is designed to meet the requirements of pharmacies and their patients on a national and even international basis. The latter may involve the production of hundreds of thousands of dosage units of a specific drug product during a single production cycle. The preparation of the various dosage forms and drug delivery systems (defined in Appendix B), containing carefully calculated, measured, verified, and labeled quantities of ingredients, enables accurate dosage administration.

A Step-Wise Approach toward Pharmaceutical Calculations

Success in performing pharmaceutical calculations is based on:

- An understanding of the purpose or goal of the problem
- An assessment of the arithmetic process required to reach the goal
- An implementation of the correct arithmetic manipulations

For many pharmacy students, particularly those without pharmacy experience, difficulty arises when the purpose or goal of a problem is not completely understood. The background information provided in each chapter is intended to assist the student in understanding the purpose of each area of calculations. Additionally, the following steps are suggested in addressing the calculation problems in this textbook as well as those encountered in pharmacy practice.

STEP 1. Take the time necessary to carefully read and thoughtfully consider the problem *prior to* engaging in computations. An understanding of the purpose or goal of the problem and the types of calculations that are required will provide the needed direction and confidence.

STEP 2. Estimate the dimension of the answer in both quantity and units of measure (e.g., milligrams) to satisfy the requirements of the problem. A section in Chapter 1 provides techniques for *estimation.*

STEP 3. Perform the necessary calculations using the appropriate method both for efficiency and understanding. For some, this might require a step-wise approach, whereas others may be capable of combining several arithmetic steps into one. Mathematical equations should be used only after the underlying principles of the equation are understood.

STEP 4. Before assuming that an answer is correct, the problem should be read again and all calculations checked. In pharmacy practice, pharmacists are encouraged to have a professional colleague check all calculations prior to completing and dispensing a prescription or medication order. Further, if the process involves components to be weighed or measured, these procedures should be double-checked as well.

STEP 5. Finally, consider the *reasonableness* of the answer in terms of the numerical value, including the proper position of a decimal point, and the units of measure.

1

Fundamentals of Pharmaceutical Calculations

OBJECTIVES

Upon successful completion of this chapter, the student will be able to:

- Demonstrate the use of *percent* in pharmaceutical calculations.
- Apply the method of *ratio and proportion* in problem solving.
- Apply the method of *dimensional analysis* in problem solving.
- Demonstrate an understanding of significant figures.
- Apply and validate the method of *estimation* in pharmaceutical calculations.

Pharmaceutical calculations is the area of study that applies the basic principles of mathematics to the preparation and efficacious use of pharmaceutical preparations. It includes calculations from initial product formulation through clinical administration and outcomes assessment.

Mathematically, pharmacy students beginning use of this textbook are well prepared. The basic units of measurement and problem-solving methods have been previously learned and are familiar. The newness lies in the terminology used and in the understanding of the pharmaceutical/clinical purpose and goal of each computation. *Of vital importance is an appreciation of the need for accuracy, as each calculation must be understood to be directly applicable to the health outcomes and safety of patients.*

This initial chapter introduces some basic aspects and methods of pharmaceutical calculations.

Units of Measurement

Pharmacy and all other health professions utilize the ***International Systems of Units (SI)***, commonly referred to as the ***metric system.*** This familiar system, with its base units (*meter, liter, kilogram*) and corresponding subdivisions, is presented in detail in Chapter 2. Pharmaceutical calculations often require the accurate conversion of quantities from a given or calculated unit to another (e.g., *milligrams* to *micrograms*). Proficiency in operating within this system is fundamental to the practice of pharmacy.

Two other systems of measurement are presented in *Appendix A*. The *avoirdupois system* is the common system of commerce, which has not fully been replaced in the United States by the International System of Units. Many product designations are *dual scale;* that is, equivalent SI and common system measures. It is in the common system that goods are packaged and sold by the ounce, pound, pint, quart, and gallon or linearly measured by the inch, foot, yard, and mile. The *apothecaries' system of measurement* is the traditional system of pharmaceutical measurement, which is now largely of historic significance. *Intersystem conversion* remains an exercise in pharmaceutical calculations and is a component of Appendix A.

Percent

The term ***percent*** and its corresponding sign, %, mean "in a hundred." So, *50 percent* (*50%*) means 50 parts in each one hundred of the same item.

In pharmacy, percent most often is used to: (a) define the concentration or strength of a pharmaceutical preparation (e.g., a 10% ointment), (b) describe the accuracy of a method or procedure (e.g., a 5% error in a measurement or weighing), and (c) quantify a parameter in a clinical study (e.g., 15% of subjects exhibited a particular effect). Calculations relating to subject area (a) are presented in Chapter 6, and those of subject area (b) are presented in Chapter 3.

The following examples demonstrate the use of percent to define a clinical result.

(1) *During a clinical study involving 2430 subjects, 2% of the subjects developed a headache. How many patients experienced this adverse effect?*

NOTE: In performing a pharmaceutical calculation, a given percent may be used directly (as when using a calculator), or it may be converted to a ratio or decimal fraction (e.g., 2% = 2/100 = 0.02).

$$2430 \times 2\% = 48.6 \text{ or } \mathbf{48\ patients,}$$

$$\text{or, } 2430 \times 2/100 = 48.6 \text{ or } \mathbf{48\ patients,}$$

$$\text{or, } 2430 \times 0.02 = 48.6 \text{ or } \mathbf{48\ patients.}$$

(2) *During a clinical study, 48 out of a total of 2430 patients developed a headache. Calculate the percent of patients who experienced this adverse effect.*

$$\frac{48}{2430} \times 100\% = 1.975 \text{ or } \approx \mathbf{2\%}$$

PRACTICE PROBLEMS

1. In a clinical study of niacin as a lipid-altering agent, 60% of the 90 patients in the study group developed flushing. Calculate the number of patients having this reaction.
2. In a clinical study of divalproex sodium (DEPAKOTE) in patients prone to migraine headaches, nausea occurred in 62 of 202 patients whereas the use of a placebo resulted in nausea in 8 of 81 patients. Compare these data in terms of percent of subjects reporting nausea in each study group.
3. If a clinical study of a new drug demonstrated that the drug met the effectiveness criteria in 646 patients of the 942 patients enrolled in the study, express these results as a decimal fraction and as a percent.
4. Ritonavir (NORVIR) oral solution contains, in addition to ritonavir, 43.2% alcohol and 26.57% propylene glycol. Calculate the quantities of each of these two ingredients in a 240-mL bottle of the oral solution.
5. If a 60-gram tube of an ointment contains 2.5 grams of active ingredient, calculate the percent concentration of active ingredient in the ointment.
6. The literature for a pharmaceutical product states that 26 patients of the 2103 enrolled in a clinical study reported headache after taking the product. Calculate (a) the decimal fraction and (b) the percentage of patients reporting this adverse response.

Ratio and Proportion

Ratio

The relative amount of two quantities (one to the other), is called their ***ratio***. A ratio resembles a common fraction except in the manner in which it is presented. For example, the fraction ½ may be expressed as the ratio, 1:2, and is not read as "one half," but rather as "one is to two." Rules governing common fractions apply to ratios. For example, if the two terms of a ratio are either multiplied or divided by the same number, the value remains unchanged. The *value* is the quotient of the first term divided by the second term. For instance, the value of the ratio 20:4 is 5. If the ratio is multiplied by 4, becoming 80:16, or divided by 4, becoming 5:1, the value remains 5. When two ratios have the same value, they are termed ***equivalent ratios,*** as is the case with the ratios 20:4, 80:16, and 5:1.

As described next, equivalent ratios provide the basis for problem solving by the *ratio and proportion* method.

Proportion

A ***proportion*** is the expression of the equality of two ratios. It may be written in any one of three standard forms:

$$(1)\quad a:b=c:d$$

$$(2)\quad a:b::c:d$$

$$(3)\quad \frac{a}{b}=\frac{c}{d}$$

Each of these expressions is read: *a is to b as c is to d*, and *a* and *d* are called the *extremes* (meaning "outer members") and *b* and *c* the *means* ("middle members").

In any proportion, *the product of the extremes is equal to the product of the means.* This principle allows us to find the missing term of any proportion when the other three terms are known. If the missing term is a *mean*, it will be *the product of the extremes divided by the given mean*, and if it is an *extreme*, it will be *the product of the means divided by the given extreme.* Using this information, we may derive the following fractional equations:

$$\text{If } \frac{a}{b}=\frac{c}{d}, \text{ then}$$

$$a=\frac{bc}{d},\ b=\frac{ad}{c},\ c=\frac{ad}{b},\ \text{and } d=\frac{bc}{a}.$$

In a proportion that is properly set up, the position of the unknown term does not matter. However, some persons prefer to place the unknown term in the fourth position—that is, in the denominator of the second ratio. *It important to label the units in each position (e.g., mL, mg) to ensure the proper relationship between the ratios of a proportion.*

The application of ratio and proportion enables the solution to many of the pharmaceutical calculation problems in this text and in pharmacy practice.

(1) *If 3 tablets contain 975 milligrams of aspirin, how many milligrams should be contained in 12 tablets?*

$$\frac{3\text{ (tablets)}}{12\text{ (tablets)}}=\frac{975\text{ (milligrams)}}{\text{x (milligrams)}}$$

$$\text{x (milligrams)}=\frac{12\text{ (tablets)}\times 975\text{ (milligrams)}}{3\text{ (tablets)}}=\textbf{3900 milligrams}$$

(2) *If 3 tablets contain 975 milligrams of aspirin, how many tablets should contain 3900 milligrams?*

$$\frac{3\ \text{(tablets)}}{x\ \text{(tablets)}} = \frac{975\ \text{(milligrams)}}{3900\ \text{(milligrams)}}$$

$$x\ \text{(tablets)} = \frac{3\ \text{(tablets)} \times 3900\ \text{(milligrams)}}{975\ \text{(milligrams)}} = \textbf{12 tablets}$$

(3) *If 12 tablets contain 3900 milligrams of aspirin, how many milligrams should 3 tablets contain?*

$$\frac{12\ \text{(tablets)}}{3\ \text{(tablets)}} = \frac{3900\ \text{(milligrams)}}{x\ \text{(milligrams)}}$$

$$x\ \text{(milligrams)} = \frac{3\ \text{(tablets)} \times 3900\ \text{(milligrams)}}{12\ \text{(tablets)}} = \textbf{975 milligrams}$$

(4) *If 12 tablets contain 3900 milligrams of aspirin, how many tablets should contain 975 milligrams?*

$$\frac{12\ \text{(tablets)}}{x\ \text{(tablets)}} = \frac{3900\ \text{(milligrams)}}{975\ \text{(milligrams)}}$$

$$x\ \text{(tablets)} = \frac{12\ \text{(tablets)} \times 975\ \text{(milligrams)}}{3900\ \text{(milligrams)}} = \textbf{3 tablets}$$

Proportions need not contain whole numbers. If common or decimal fractions are supplied in the data, they may be included in the proportion without changing the method. For ease of calculation, it is recommended that common fractions be converted to decimal fractions prior to setting up the proportion.

(5) *If 30 milliliters (mL) represent 1/6 of the volume of a prescription, how many milliliters will represent ¼ of the volume?*

$$\tfrac{1}{6} = 0.167 \text{ and } \tfrac{1}{4} = 0.25$$

$$\frac{0.167\ \text{(volume)}}{0.25\ \text{(volume)}} = \frac{30\ \text{(mL)}}{x\ \text{(mL)}}$$

$$x = 44.91 \text{ or} \approx \textbf{45 mL}$$

CALCULATIONS CAPSULE

Ratio and Proportion

- A *ratio* expresses the relative magnitude of two like quantities (e.g., 1:2, expressed as "1 to 2.")
- A proportion expresses the equality of two ratios (e.g., 1:2 = 2:4).
- The four terms of a proportion are stated as:

$$a : b = c : d,\ \text{or},\ a : b :: c : d,\ \text{or}\ \frac{a}{b} = \frac{c}{d}$$

  and expressed as "*a* is to *b* as *c* is to *d*."
- Given three of the four terms of a proportion, the value of the fourth, or missing, term may be calculated by cross multiplication and solution.
- The ratio-and-proportion method is a useful tool in solving many pharmaceutical calculation problems

Dimensional Analysis

When performing pharmaceutical calculations, some students prefer to use a method termed ***dimensional analysis*** (also known as ***factor analysis***, ***factor-label method***, or ***unit-factor method***). This method involves the logical sequencing and placement of a series of ratios (termed ***factors***) into an equation. The ratios are prepared from the given data as well as from selected *conversion factors* and contain both arithmetic quantities and their units of measurement. Some terms are inverted (to their reciprocals) to permit the cancellation of like units in the numerator(s) and denominator(s) and leave only the desired terms of the answer. One advantage of using dimensional analysis is the consolidation of several arithmetic steps into a single equation.

In solving problems by dimensional analysis, the student unfamiliar with the process should consider the following steps[1,2]:

STEP 1. Identify the wanted unit of the answer (e.g., mL, mg, etc.) and place it at the beginning of the equation. Some persons prefer to place a question mark next to it.

STEP 2. Identify the given quantity(ies) and its (their) unit(s) of measurement.

STEP 3. Identify the conversion factor(s) that is (are) needed for the "unit path" to arrive at the arithmetic answer in the unit wanted.

STEP 4. Set up the ratios such that the cancellation of the units of measurement in the numerators and denominators will retain only the wanted unit as identified in *Step 1*.

STEP 5. Perform the arithmetic computation by multiplying the numerators, multiplying the denominators, and dividing the product of the numerators by the product of the denominators.

The general scheme shown here and in the "Calculations Capsule: Dimensional Analysis" may be helpful in using the method.

		Unit Path			
	Given Quantity	Conversion Factor as Needed	Conversion Factor as Needed	Conversion Computation	Wanted Quantity and Unit
___ (Wanted Unit) =					=

Example Calculations Using Dimensional Analysis

(1) *How many fluidounces (fl. oz.) are there in 2.5 liters (L)?*

STEP 1. The wanted unit for the answer is *fluidounces*.

STEP 2. The given quantity is *2.5 L*.

STEP 3. The conversion factors needed are those that will take us from liters to fluidounces.

As the student will later learn, these conversion factors are as follows:
1 liter = 1000 mL (to convert the given 2.5 L to milliliters)
1 fluidounce = 29.57 mL (to convert milliliters to fluidounces)

STEP 4. Set up the ratios in the unit path

		Unit Path			
	Given Quantity	Conversion Factor as Needed	Conversion Factor as Needed	Conversion Computation	Wanted Quantity and Unit
fl.oz. (Wanted Unit) =	2.5 L	1000 mL	1 fl. oz.		=
		1 L	29.57 mL		

NOTE: The unit path is set up such that all units of measurement will cancel out except for the unit wanted in the answer, *fluidounces*, which is placed in the numerator.

STEP 5. Perform the computation:

Unit Path

	Given Quantity	Conversion Factor as Needed	Conversion Factor as Needed	Conversion Computation		Wanted Quantity and Unit
fl.oz. (Wanted Unit) =	2.5 ~~L~~	1000 ~~mL~~	1 fl. oz.	2.5 × 1000 × 1	= 2500	= 84.55 fl. oz.
		1 ~~L~~	29.57 ~~mL~~	1 × 29.57	29.57	

or

$$2.5\,\cancel{L} \times \frac{1000\,\cancel{mL}}{1\,\cancel{L}} \times \frac{1\ \text{fl. oz.}}{29.57\,\cancel{mL}} = \frac{2.5 \times 1000 \times 1}{1 \times 29.57} = \frac{2500}{29.57} = \mathbf{84.55\ fl.\ oz.}$$

NOTE: The student may wish to see the problem solved by ratio and proportion:

STEP 1.

$$\frac{1\,(\text{L})}{2.5\,(\text{L})} = \frac{1000\,(\text{mL})}{x\,(\text{mL})};\ x = \mathbf{2500\ mL}$$

STEP 2.

$$\frac{29.57\,(\text{mL})}{2500\,(\text{mL})} = \frac{1(\text{fl. oz.})}{x\,(\text{fl. oz.})}$$

$$x = \mathbf{84.55\ fl.\ oz.}$$

CALCULATIONS CAPSULE

Dimensional Analysis

- An alternative method to ratio and proportion in solving pharmaceutical calculation problems.
- The method involves the logical sequencing and placement of a series of ratios to consolidate multiple arithmetic steps into a single equation.
- By applying select conversion factors in the equation—some as reciprocals—unwanted units of measure cancel out, leaving the arithmetic result and desired unit.
- Dimensional analysis scheme:

Unit Path

	Given Quantity	Conversion Factor as Needed	Conversion Factor as Needed	Conversion Computation	Wanted Quantity and Unit
___ (Wanted Unit) =					=

(2) *A medication order calls for 1000 milliliters of a dextrose intravenous infusion to be administered over an 8-hour period. Using an intravenous administration set that delivers 10 drops/milliliter, how many drops per minute should be delivered to the patient?*
Solving by dimensional analysis:

$$8 \text{ hours} = 480 \text{ minutes (min)}$$

$$\underset{\cdot}{?} \text{ drops} = 1000 \cancel{\text{mL}} \times \frac{10 \text{ drops}}{1 \cancel{\text{mL}}} \times \frac{1}{480 \text{ min}} = 20.8 \text{ or } \mathbf{21 \text{ drops per minute}}$$

NOTE: "drops" was placed in the numerator and "minutes" in the denominator to arrive at the answer in the desired term, *drops per minute.*
The student may wish to see this problem solved by ratio and proportion:
Step 1.

$$\frac{480 \text{ (min)}}{1 \text{ (min)}} = \frac{1000 \text{ (mL)}}{x \text{ (mL)}}; \ x = \mathbf{2.08 \text{ mL}}$$

Step 2.

$$\frac{1 \text{ (mL)}}{2.08 \text{ (mL)}} = \frac{10 \text{ (drops)}}{x \text{ (drops)}}; \ x = 2.08 \text{ mL or } \mathbf{21 \text{ drops per minute}}$$

The following problem is often used to demonstrate the process of dimensional analysis.

(3) *Calculate the number of seconds in a day.*

$$\underset{\cdot}{?} \text{ s} = 1 \cancel{\text{day}} \times \frac{24 \cancel{\text{h}}}{1 \cancel{\text{day}}} \times \frac{60 \cancel{\text{min}}}{1 \cancel{\text{h}}} \times \frac{60 \cancel{\text{s}}}{1 \cancel{\text{min}}} = 1 \times \frac{24 \times 60 \times 60}{1 \times 1 \times 1} = \mathbf{86{,}400 \text{ s}}$$

CASE IN POINT 1.1 A pharmacist consults with a parent on the use of a cough syrup for her 5-year-old child. The nonprescription cough syrup contains, in each 5-mL (milliliters), 10 mg (milligrams) of dextromethorphan HBr, a cough suppressant, and 100 mg of guaifenesin, an expectorant. The package label indicates that the dose for a child 2 to 6 years of age is 1/4 of the adult dose of two teaspoonfuls. The pharmacist suggests using an oral syringe calibrated in 0.25-mL units for dosing. If a standard teaspoonful is equivalent to 5 mL, (a) how many milliliters should be administered to the child, and (b) how many milligrams of each of the two therapeutic ingredients would be administered per child's dose?

PRACTICE PROBLEMS

1. If an insulin injection contains 100 units of insulin in each milliliter, how many milliliters should be injected to receive 40 units of insulin?
2. An injection contains 2 mg of medication in each milliliter (mL). If a physician prescribes a dose of 0.5 mg to be administered to a hospital patient three times daily, how many milliliters of injection will be required over a 5-day period?
3. In a clinical study, a drug produced drowsiness in 30 of the 1500 patients studied. How many patients of a certain pharmacy could expect similar effects, based on a patient count of 100?
4. A formula for 1250 tablets contains 6.25 grams of diazepam. How many grams of diazepam should be used in preparing 550 tablets?
5. If 100 capsules contain 400 mg of an active ingredient, how many milligrams of the ingredient will 48 capsules contain?
6. Each tablet of TYLENOL WITH CODEINE contains 30 mg of codeine phosphate and 300 mg of acetaminophen. By taking 2 tablets daily for a week, how many milligrams of each drug would the patient take?
7. A cough syrup contains 10 mg of dextromethorphan hydrobromide per 5 mL. How many milligrams of the drug are contained in a 120-mL container of the syrup?
8. If an intravenous fluid is adjusted to deliver 15 mg of medication to a patient per hour, how many milligrams of medication are delivered per half minute?
9. The biotechnology drug filgrastim (NEUPOGEN) is available in syringes containing 480 micrograms (mcg) of filgrastim per 0.8 mL. How many micrograms of the drug would be administered by each 0.5 mL injection?
10. An oral solution contains, in each milliliter, 80 mg of lopinavir and 20 mg of ritonavir. How many milligrams of each drug would be contained in a calculated dose of 0.4 mL?
11. Aripiprazole (ABILIFY) injection is available in single-dose vials containing 9.75 mg of aripiprazole in each 1.3 mL of injection. Calculate the volume of injection that would provide a dose of 5.25 mg of aripiprazole.
12. Acyclovir (ZOVIRAX) suspension contains 200 mg of acyclovir in each 5 mL. How many milligrams of acyclovir are contained in a pint (473 mL) of suspension?
13. A metered dose inhaler contains 225 mg of metaproterenol sulfate, which is sufficient for 100 inhalations. How many micrograms (mcg) of metaproterenol sulfate would be administered with each inhalation if there are 1000 micrograms in each milligram?
14. A pediatric vitamin drug product contains the equivalent of 0.25 mg of fluoride ion in each milliliter. How many milligrams of fluoride ion would be provided by a dropper that delivers 0.6 mL?
15. If a pediatric vitamin contains 1500 units of vitamin A per milliliter of solution, how many units of vitamin A would be administered to a child given 2 drops of the solution from a dropper calibrated to deliver 20 drops per milliliter of solution?
16. An elixir contains 25 mg of drug in each 5 mL. How many milligrams of the drug would be used in preparing 4000 mL of the elixir?
17. An elixir of ferrous sulfate contains 220 mg of ferrous sulfate in each 5 mL. If each milligram of ferrous sulfate contains the equivalent of 0.2 mg of elemental iron, how many milligrams of elemental iron would be represented in each 5 mL of the elixir?
18. An estradiol transdermal patch is available in various patch sizes. The patch size is closely proportional to the amount of drug contained in the patch. If the patch

containing 0.025 mg of estradiol is 6.5 cm^2 in size, calculate the approximate size of the patch containing 0.1 mg of estradiol.

19. If an ophthalmic solution contains 1 mg of dexamethasone phosphate in each milliliter of solution, how many milligrams of dexamethasone phosphate would be contained in 2 drops if the eyedropper used delivered 20 drops per milliliter?
20. A 15-mL package of nasal spray delivers 20 sprays per milliliter of solution, with each spray containing 1.5 mg of drug. (a) How many total sprays will the package deliver? (b) How many milligrams of drug are contained in the 15-mL package of the spray?
21. A penicillin V potassium preparation provides 400,000 units of activity in each 250-mg tablet. How many total units of activity would a patient receive from taking 4 tablets a day for 10 days?
22. If a 5-g packet of a potassium supplement provides 20 milliequivalents of potassium ion and 3.34 milliequivalents of chloride ion, (a) how many grams of the powder would provide 6 milliequivalents of potassium ion, and (b) how many milliequivalents of chloride ion would be provided by this amount of powder?
23. If a potassium chloride elixir contains 20 milliequivalents of potassium ion in each 15 mL of elixir, how many milliliters will provide 25 milliequivalents of potassium ion to the patient?
24. The blood serum concentration of the antibacterial drug ciprofloxacin increases proportionately with the dose of drug administered. If a 250-mg dose of the drug results in a serum concentration of 1.2 micrograms of drug per milliliter of serum, how many micrograms of drug would be expected per milliliter of serum following a dose of 500 mg of drug?
25. The dosage of the drug thiabendazole (MINTEZOL) is determined in direct proportion to a patient's weight. If the dose of the drug for a patient weighing 150 pounds is 1.5 grams, what would be the dose for a patient weighing 110 pounds?
26. If 0.5 mL of a mumps virus vaccine contains 5000 units of antigen, how many units would be present in each milliliter if the 0.5 mL of vaccine was diluted to 2 mL with water for injection?
27. A sample of Oriental ginseng contains 0.4 mg of active constituents in each 100 mg of powdered plant. How many milligrams of active constituents would be present in 15 mg of powdered plant?

NOTE: *Solve problems 28 to 32 by dimensional analysis, using the following equivalencies as needed:*

1 gram (g) = 1000 milligrams (mg)
1 mg = 1000 micrograms (mcg)
1 kilogram (kg) = 2.2 pounds (lb)

28. If 120 mL of a syrup contains 1.2 g of rimantadine HCl, and if a 2.5-mL dose of the syrup is administered, how many milligrams of rimantadine HCl would be given?
29. How many milliliters of an injection containing 0.25 mg of drug in each milliliter should be administered to provide a dose of 10 mcg?
30. An injection intended for pediatric use contains 100 mcg of digoxin per milliliter. What volume of injection should be administered to provide a dose of 0.04 mg?
31. A patient is to receive 2 mg of drug from an injection labeled to contain 150 mcg/mL. Calculate the milliliters of injection to administer.
32. The dose of a drug is 0.05 mg for each kilogram of a patient's weight. The drug is available as an oral liquid containing 50 mcg/0.1 mL. Calculate the dose of the oral liquid, in milliliters, for a patient who weighs 132 lb.

Alligation

Alligation is an arithmetic method of solving problems relating mixtures of components of different strengths. There are two types of alligation: ***alligation medial*** and ***alligation alternate***.

Alligation medial may be used to determine the strength of a common ingredient in a mixture of two or more preparations. For example, if a pharmacist mixed together known volumes of two or more solutions containing known amounts of a common ingredient, the strength of that ingredient in the resulting mixture can be determined by alligation medial.

Alligation alternate may be used to determine the proportion or quantities of two or more components to combine in order to prepare a mixture of a desired strength. For example, if a pharmacist wished to prepare a solution of a specified strength by combining two or more other solutions of differing concentrations of the same ingredient, the proportion or volumes of each solution to use may be determined by alligation alternate.

Alligation medial and alligation alternate may be used as options in solving a number of pharmaceutical calculations problems. The methods and problem examples are presented in Chapter 15.

Significant Figures

When we *count* objects accurately, *every* figure in the numeral expressing the total number of objects must be taken at its face value. Such figures may be said to be *absolute*. When we record a *measurement*, the last figure to the right must be taken to be an *approximation*, an admission that the limit of possible precision or of necessary accuracy has been reached and that any further figures to the right would not be significant—that is, either meaningless or, for a given purpose, needless.

A denominate number, like 325 *grams*, is interpreted as follows: The 3 means *300 grams*, neither more nor less, and the 2 means *exactly 20 grams more;* but the final 5 means *approximately 5 grams more*, that is, *5 grams plus or minus some fraction of a gram*. Whether this fraction is, for a given purpose, negligible depends on how precisely the quantity was (or is to be) weighed.

Significant figures, then, are consecutive figures that express the value of a denominate number accurately enough for a given purpose. The accuracy varies with the number of significant figures, which are all absolute in value except the last, and this is properly called *uncertain*.

Whether *zero* is significant, however, depends on its position or on known facts about a given number. The interpretation of *zero* may be summed up as follows:

(1) Any zero between digits is significant.

(2) Initial zeros to the left of the first digit are never significant; they are included merely to show the location of the decimal point and thus give place value to the digits that follow.

(3) One or more final zeros to the right of the decimal point may be taken to be significant.

Examples:

Assuming that the following numbers are all denominate:

(1) In *12.5*, there are *three* significant figures; in *1.256*, *four* significant figures; and in *102.56*, *five* significant figures.

(2) In *0.5*, there is *one* significant figure. The digit *5* tells us how many *tenths* we have. The nonsignificant *0* simply calls attention to the decimal point.

(3) In *0.05*, there is still only *one* significant figure, as there is in *0.005*.

(4) In *0.65*, there are *two* significant figures, and likewise *two* in *0.065* and *0.0065*.
(5) In *0.0605*, there are *three* significant figures. The first *0* calls attention to the decimal point, the second *0* shows the number of places to the right of the decimal point occupied by the remaining figures, and the third *0* significantly contributes to the value of the number. In *0.06050*, there are *four* significant figures, because the final *0* also contributes to the value of the number. [*It should be noted, however, that in pharmacy practice "trailing zeros" are not retained as a result of a calculation as they may lead to misinterpretation and error.*]

CALCULATIONS CAPSULE

Significant Figures

- Digits other than zero are significant.
- A zero between digits is significant.
- Zeros used only to show the location of the decimal point are not significant.
- The *United States Pharmacopeia* states that in performing pharmaceutical calculations, all figures are to be utilized until the calculations are completed and then only the significant figures retained in the final result.[3]

One of the factors determining the degree of approximation to perfect measurement is the precision of the instrument used. It would be incorrect to claim that 7. *76 milliliters* had been measured in a graduate calibrated in units of *1 milliliter*, or that *25.562 grams* had been weighed on a balance sensitive to 0.01 gram.

We must clearly distinguish *significant figures* from *decimal places.* When recording a measurement, the number of decimal places we include indicates *the degree of precision with which the measurement has been made*, whereas the number of significant figures retained indicates *the degree of accuracy* that is sufficient for a given purpose.

Sometimes we are asked to record a value "correct to (so many) decimal places." We should never confuse this familiar expression with the expression "correct to (so many) significant figures." For example, if the value *27.625918* is rounded to *five decimal places*, it is written *27.62592*; but when this value is rounded to *five significant figures*, it is written *27.626*.

Rules for Rounding

(1) When rounding a measurement, retain as many figures as will give only one *uncertain* figure. For example, in using a ruler calibrated only in full centimeter units, it would be correct to record a measurement of 11.3 centimeters but not 11.32 centimeters, because the 3 (tenths) is uncertain and no figure should follow it.
(2) When eliminating superfluous figures following a calculation, add 1 to the last figure retained in a calculation if it is 5 or more. For example, 2.43 may be rounded off to 2.4, but 2.46 should be rounded off to 2.5.
(3) When adding or subtracting *approximate* numbers, include only as many decimal places as are in the number with the *fewest* decimal places. For example, when adding 162.4 grams + 0.489 gram + 0.1875 gram + 120.78 grams, the sum is 283.8565 grams, but the rounded sum is 283.9 grams. However, when an instrument has the capability to weigh precisely all the quantities in such a calculation, rounding may be deemed inappropriate.

In this regard, *there is an assumption made in pharmaceutical calculations that all measurements in the filling of a prescription or in compounding a formula are performed with equal precision by the pharmacist.* Thus, for example, if the quantities 5.5 grams, 0.01 gram, and 0.005 gram are specified in a formula, they may be added as if they are precise weights, with a sum of 5.515 grams.

(4) When multiplying or dividing two approximate numbers, retain no more significant figures than the number having the fewest significant figures. For example, if multiplying 1.6437 grams by 0.26, the answer may be rounded from the calculated 0.427362 gram to 0.43 gram.

(5) When multiplying or dividing an approximate number by an absolute number, the result should be rounded to the same number of significant figures as in the approximate number. Thus, if 1.54 milligrams is multiplied by 96, the product, 243.84 milligrams, may be rounded to 244 milligrams, or to three significant figures.

(6) Oftentimes, logic plays a role. For example, when a calculation is performed to determine the *number of doses* available from a medication or the *number of drops* to be administered to a patient, it is both logical and practical to express the answer in whole units.

PRACTICE PROBLEMS

1. State the number of significant figures in each of the *italicized* quantities:
   (a) One fluidounce equals *29.57* milliliters.
   (b) One liter equals *1000* milliliters.
   (c) One inch equals *2.54* centimeters.
   (d) The chemical costs *$1.05* per pound.
   (e) One gram equals *1,000,000* micrograms.
   (f) One microgram equals *0.001* milligram.
2. Round each of the following to three significant figures:
   (a) 32.75
   (b) 200.39
   (c) 0.03629
   (d) 21.635
   (e) 0.00944
3. Round each of the following to three decimal places:
   (a) 0.00083
   (b) 34.79502
   (c) 0.00494
   (d) 6.12963
4. If a mixture of seven ingredients contains the following approximate weights, what can you validly record as the approximate total combined weight of the ingredients?
   26.83 grams, 275.3 grams, 2.752 grams, 4.04 grams, 5.197 grams, 16.64 grams, and 0.085 gram.
5. Perform the following computations, and retain only significant figures in the results:
   (a) 6.39 – 0.008
   (b) 7.01 – 6.0
   (c) 5.0 × 48.3 grams
   (d) 24 × 0.25 gram
   (e) 56.824 ÷ 0.0905
   (f) 250 ÷ 1.109

Estimation

It is important for pharmacy students and pharmacists to recognize the *reasonableness* of the result of a calculation. By performing an *estimation* of the answer *prior* to calculation, the approximate result may be predetermined. This helps assure the correct dimension of the answer including the critical placement of a decimal point.

The technique of estimation is demonstrated by the examples that follow. Rounding of numbers is a component of this process.

Add the following numbers: 7428, 3652, 1327, 4605, 2791, and 4490.

Estimation:

The figures in the thousands column add up to 21,000, and with each number on the average contributing 500 more, or every pair 1000 more, we get 21,000 + 3000 = 24,000, *estimated answer* (actual answer, 24,293).

In *multiplication*, the product of the two leftmost digits plus a sufficient number of *zeros* to give the right place value serves as a fair estimate. The number of *zeros* supplied must equal the total number of all discarded figures to the left of the decimal point. Approximation to the correct answer is closer if the discarded figures are used to round the value of those retained.

Multiply 612 by 413.

Estimation:

$4 \times 6 = 24$, and because we discarded four figures, we must supply four zeros, giving 240,000, *estimated answer* (actual answer, 252,756).

In division, the given numbers may be rounded off to convenient approximations, but again, care is needed to preserve the correct place values.

Divide 2456 by 5.91.

Estimation:

The numbers may be rounded off to 2400 and 6. We may divide 24 by 6 mentally, but we must remember the two zeros substituted for the given 56 in 2456. The estimated answer is 400 (actual answer, 416).

PRACTICE PROBLEMS

1. Estimate the sums:

(a)	(b)	(c)
5641	3298	$75.82
2177	368	37.92
294	5192	14.69
8266	627	45.98
3503	4835	28.91
		49.87

2. Estimate the products:
   (a) $42 \times 39 =$
   (b) $596 \times 204 =$
   (c) $8431 \times 9760 =$
   (d) $0.0726 \times 6951 =$
   (e) $6.1 \times 67.39 =$
3. Estimate the quotients:
   (a) $171 \div 19 =$
   (b) $184 \div 2300 =$
   (c) $98{,}000 \div 49 =$
   (d) $1.0745 \div 500 =$
   (e) $458.4 \div 8 =$

CALCQUIZ

1.A. Digoxin (LANOXIN) pediatric elixir contains 0.05 mg (milligram) of digoxin in each milliliter (mL) of elixir. If there are 1000 μg (micrograms) in each milligram, how many micrograms of digoxin would be delivered in each dose of 0.6 mL?

1.B. A probiotic colon health product contains, in each capsule, 3 billion viable cells of *Lactobacillus acidophilus* and *Bifidobacterium longum*. Express, by exponential notation, the number of viable cells in a container of 30 capsules.

1.C. A liquid dietary supplement is packaged in 10-mL dropper containers to deliver 2000 international units of vitamin D_3 in each drop (0.027 mL). Calculate the number of drops delivered per milliliter.

1.D. The drug pramlintide (SYMLIN) is an antihyperglycemic agent for use in patients with diabetes treated with insulin. A 5-mL vial contains 600 μg of pramlintide per milliliter. A 0.05-mL dose measures 5 insulin units on the syringe used for injection and provides 30 μg of pramlintide. Calculate the number of micrograms of pramlintide and the corresponding measurement of insulin units on the syringe with the administration of 0.075 mL of injection.

1.E. A physician prescribed mometasone furoate monohydrate (NASONEX) nasal spray for a patient, with directions to administer two sprays into each nostril once daily. If each spray contains 50 μg of drug and the container can deliver a total of 120 sprays, how many micrograms of drug would the patient receive daily, and how many days of use will the prescription last the patient?

ANSWERS TO "CASE IN POINT" AND PRACTICE PROBLEMS

Case in Point 1.1

1 teaspoonful = 5 mL

Adult dose = 2 teaspoonfuls = 10 mL

(a) Child's dose = 1/4 × 10 mL (2 teaspoonfuls) = 2.5 mL

(b) $\underline{?}\text{ mg dextromethorphan HBr} = \dfrac{10\text{ mg} \times 2.5\text{ mL}}{5\text{ mL}} = 5\text{ mg dextromethorphan HBr}$

and

$$\underline{?}\text{ mg guaifenesin} = \frac{100\text{ mg} \times 2.5\text{ mL}}{5\text{ mL}} = 50\text{ mg guaifenesin}$$

Proof of calculations: child's dose is ¼ of adult dose:

Child's calculated dose of cough syrup/adult dose = 2.5 mL/10 mL = ¼ √

Child's calculated dose of dextromethorphan HBr/adult dose = 5 mg/20 mg = ¼ √

Child's calculated dose of guaifenesin/adult dose = 50 mg/200 mg = ¼ √

Percent

1. 54 patients
2. 30.7% DEPAKOTE subjects
   9.9% placebo subjects
3. 0.69 or 69%
4. 103.68 mL alcohol
   63.77 mL propylene glycol
5. 4.17%
6. 0.012 or 1.2% of patients

Ratio, Proportion, and Dimensional Analysis

1. 0.4 mL insulin injection
2. 3.75 mL
3. 2 patients
4. 2.75 g diazepam
5. 192 mg
6. 420 mg codeine phosphate
   4200 mg acetaminophen
7. 240 mg dextromethorphan hydrobromide
8. 0.125 mg
9. 300 mcg filgrastim
10. 32 mg lopinavir and 8 mg ritonavir
11. 0.7 mL aripiprazole injection
12. 18,920 mg acyclovir
13. 2250 mcg metaproterenol sulfate
14. 0.15 mg fluoride ion
15. 150 units vitamin A
16. 20,000 mg
17. 44 mg elemental iron
18. 26 cm^2
19. 0.1 mg dexamethasone phosphate
20. (a) 300 sprays
    (b) 450 mg
21. 16,000,000 units
22. (a) 1.5 g
    (b) 1 milliequivalent chloride ion
23. 18.75 mL
24. 2.4 mcg ciprofloxacin
25. 1.1 g thiabendazole
26. 2500 units antigen
27. 0.06 mg
28. 25 mg rimantadine HCl
29. 0.04 mL injection
30. 0.4 mL injection
31. 13.3 mL injection
32. 6 mL oral liquid

Significant Figures

1. (a) four
   (b) four
   (c) three
   (d) three
   (e) seven
   (f) one
2. (a) 32.8
   (b) 200
   (c) 0.0363
   (d) 21.6
   (e) 0.00944
3. (a) 0.001
   (b) 34.795
   (c) 0.005
   (d) 6.130
4. 330.8 g
5. (a) 6.38
   (b) 1.0
   (c) 240 g
   (d) 6.0 g
   (e) 628
   (f) 225

Estimation

1. (a) 20,500 *(19,881)*
   (b) 14,500 *(14,320)*
   (c) $240.00 *($253.19)*
2. (a) 40 × 40 = 1600 *(1638)*
   (b) 600 × 200 = 120,000 *(121,584)*
   (c) 8000 × 10,000 = 80,000,000 *(82,286,560)*
   (d) (7 × 70) = 490 *(504.6426)*
   (e) 6 × 70 = 420 *(411.079)*
3. (a) 170 ÷ 20 = 8.5 *(9.0)*
   (b) 180 ÷ 2000 = 0.09 *(0.08)*
   (c) 9800 ÷ 5 = 1960 *(2000)*
   (d) 0.01 ÷ 5 = 0.002 *(0.002149)*
   (e) 460 ÷ 8 = 57.5 *(57.3)*

References

1. Dimensional Analysis–Tripod.com. Available at: http://susanp3.tripod.com/snurse/id28.htm. Accessed October 16, 2015.
2. Craig GP. *Clinical Calculations Made Easy*. 4th Ed. Baltimore, MD: Lippincott Williams & Wilkins, 2008.
3. The United States Pharmacopeial Convention. *United States Pharmacopeia 32 National Formulary* 27. Rockville, MD: The United States Pharmacopeial Convention, 2009;1:675.

2

International System of Units

OBJECTIVES

Upon successful completion of this chapter, the student will be able to:

- Demonstrate an understanding of the International System of Units.
- Convert measures within the International System of Units.
- Convert measures between the International System of Units and other systems of measure used in pharmacy.
- Apply the International System of Units in pharmaceutical calculations.

The ***International System of Units*** (*SI*), formerly called the ***metric system***, is the internationally recognized decimal system of weights and measures. The system was formulated in France in the late 18th century. Over the years, effort has been made in the United States to transition from use of the common systems of weights and measures (e.g., pounds, feet, gallons) to the international system. Today, the pharmaceutical research and manufacturing industry, the *United States Pharmacopeia–National Formulary*,[a] and all the health professions reflect conversion to the SI system. The advantages include the simplicity of the decimal system, the clarity provided by the base units and prefixes, and the ease of scientific and professional communications provided through the use of a universally accepted system.

The base units of the SI are the *meter* (for length), the *kilogram* (for weight), and the *liter* (for volume).[b] Subdivisions and multiples of these base units, their relative values, and their corresponding prefixes are shown in Table 2.1.

Guidelines for the Correct Use of the SI

The following are select guidelines for the correct use of the SI from the U.S. Metric Association, with additional considerations relevant to the practice of pharmacy[1,2]:

- Unit names and symbols are not capitalized except when used at the beginning of a sentence or in headings. However, the symbol for liter (L, l) may be capitalized or not. *For example*, for four grams, use 4 g and *not* 4 G; for 4 millimeters, use 4 mm and *not* 4 MM; but, for 4 liters, 4 L or 4 l are acceptable.
- In the United States, the decimal marker (or decimal point) is placed on the line with the number; however, in some countries, a comma or a raised dot is used, *for example*, 4.5 mL (United States) and 4,5 mL or 4·5 mL (non-United States).

[a]The *United States Pharmacopeia—National Formulary* (USP–NF) establishes standards for the quality, purity, and strength of prescription and nonprescription medicines. These standards, which are recognized and used by over 140 countries, are published in printed volumes and electronically. *The Authors' Extra Point at the end of this chapter further describes the USP–NF and other national, regional, and international pharmacopeias.*

[b]Although not included in this text, the SI includes measures of force, viscosity, electricity, luminance, and many others in a variety of disciplines.

Table 2.1 • PREFIXES AND RELATIVE VALUES OF THE INTERNATIONAL SYSTEM (SI)

Prefix	Meaning
Subdivisions	
atto-	one-quintillionth (10^{-18}) of the basic unit
femto-	one-quadrillionth (10^{-15}) of the basic unit
pico-	one-trillionth (10^{-12}) of the basic unit
nano-	one-billionth (10^{-9}) of the basic unit
micro-	one-millionth (10^{-6}) of the basic unit
milli-	one-thousandth (10^{-3}) of the basic unit
centi-	one-hundredth (10^{-2}) of the basic unit
deci-	one-tenth (10^{-1}) of the basic unit
Multiples	
deca-	10 times the basic unit
hecto-	100 times (10^{2}) the basic unit
kilo-	1000 times (10^{3}) the basic unit
myria-	10,000 times (10^{4}) the basic unit
mega-	1 million times (10^{6}) the basic unit
giga-	1 billion times (10^{9}) the basic unit
tera-	1 trillion times (10^{12}) the basic unit
peta-	1 quadrillion times (10^{15}) the basic unit
exa-	1 quintillion times (10^{18}) the basic unit

- Periods are not used following SI symbols except at the end of a sentence, *for example*, 4 mL and 4 g, *not* 4 mL. and 4 g.
- A compound unit that is a ratio or quotient of two units is indicated by a solidus (/) or a negative exponent, *for example*, 5 mL/h or 5 $mL{\cdot}h^{-1}$.
- Symbols should not be combined with spelled-out terms in the same expression, *for example*, 3 mg/mL, *not* 3 mg/milliliter.
- Plurals of unit names, when spelled out, have an added "s." Symbols for units, however, are the same in singular and plural, *for example*, 5 milliliters or 5 mL, *not* 5 mLs.
- Two symbols exist for microgram: *mcg* (often used in pharmacy practice) and μg (SI).
- The symbol for square meter is m^2; for cubic centimeter, cm^3; and so forth. In pharmacy practice, a cubic centimeter (cm^3) is considered equivalent to a milliliter.[2] The symbol "cc," for cubic centimeter, is *not* an accepted SI symbol.
- Decimal fractions are used, not common fractions, *for example*, 5.25 g, *not* 5¼ g.
- A zero always should be placed in front of a leading decimal point to prevent medication errors caused by *uncertain* decimal points, *for example*, 0.5 g, *not* .5 g. ***It is critically important for pharmacists to recognize that a misplaced or misread decimal point can lead to an error in calculation of a minimum of one-tenth or 10 times the desired quantity.***
- To prevent misreadings and medication errors, "trailing" zeros *should not* be placed following a whole number on prescriptions and medication orders, *for example*, 5 mg, *not* 5.0 mg. However, in some tables (such as those of the SI in this chapter), pharmaceutical formulas, and quantitative results, trailing zeros often are used to indicate exactness to a specific number of decimal places.
- In selecting symbols of unit dimensions, the choice generally is based on selecting the unit that will result in a numeric value between 1 and 1000, *for example*, 500 g, *rather than* 0.5 kg; 1.96 kg, *rather than* 1960 g; and 750 mL, *rather than* 0.75 L.

Special Considerations of the SI in Pharmacy

Although some remnants of the common systems of measurement (see Appendix A) in pharmacy remain, the use of the SI is nearly total. The system is used to manufacture and label pharmaceutical products (Fig. 2.1); write, fill, and compound prescriptions and institutional medication orders; dose patients; express clinical laboratory test results; and communicate both verbally and through scientific and professional literature.

In the large-scale manufacture of dosage forms, pharmaceutical ingredients are measured in kilogram and kiloliter quantities. In the community and institutional pharmacy, compounding and dispensing in milligram, gram, and milliliter quantities are more common. Drug doses are typically administered in milligram or microgram amounts and prepared in solid dosage forms, such as tablets or capsules, or in a stated volume of a liquid preparation, such as an oral solution (e.g., 30 mg/5 mL) or injection (e.g., 2 mg/mL). Doses for certain drugs are calculated on the basis of body weight and expressed as mg/kg, meaning a certain number of *milligrams of drug per kilogram of body weight*. Clinical laboratory values are in metric units and expressed, for example, as mg/dL, meaning *milligrams of drug per deciliter of body fluid* (such as blood).

Particle Size and Nanotechnology

Drug particle size has long been an important consideration in pharmaceutical technology. Through the milling and reduction of drug materials to micron size, the surface area of particles is increased (Fig. 2.2) and pharmaceutical and clinical benefits often accrue. These benefits may include the following[3]:

- Increased aqueous dissolution rates for poorly soluble substances
- Improved bioavailability, with increased rates of absorption of orally administered drugs
- Lower oral dosage possibilities with enhanced drug absorption
- Expanded formulation options in the preparation of stable and predictable pharmaceutical suspensions and colloidal dispersions for all routes of administration, including oral, parenteral, respiratory, ophthalmic, and nasal.

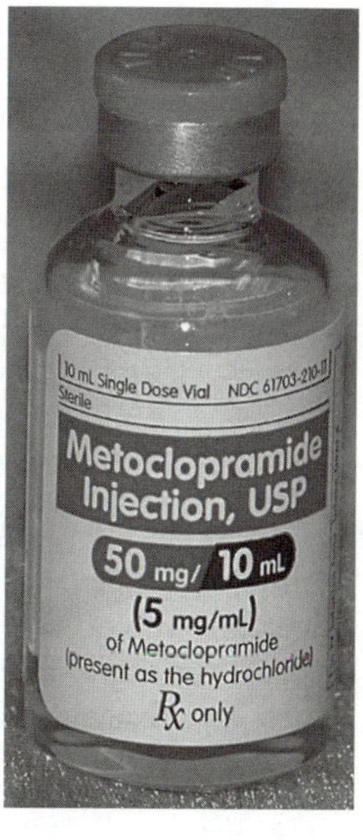

FIGURE 2.1 • Example of a pharmaceutical product with the label indicating the strength and quantity (50 mg/10 mL) in SI or metric units. *(Reprinted with permission from Lacher BE. Pharmaceutical Calculations for the Pharmacy Technician. Philadelphia, PA: Lippincott Williams & Wilkins; 2007.)*

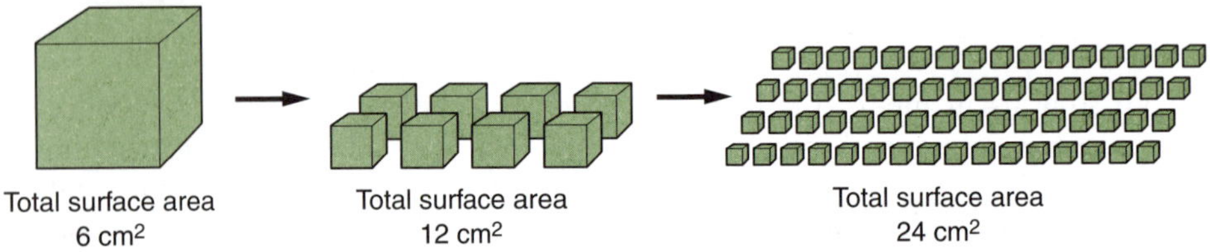

FIGURE 2.2 • Depiction of increased surface area by particle size reduction. *(Adapted from company literature, Nanocrystal, Elan Drug Delivery, Inc.)*

An area of technology with great potential is nanotechnology. ***Nanotechnology*** centers on the understanding and control of matter between approximately 1 and 100 nanometers (nm) in size, referred to as the ***nanoscale*** range.[4] For perspective, a nanometer is one-billionth of a meter; about 25,400,000 nm equals 1 inch; the helix of DNA has a diameter of about 2 nm; and a typical bond between two atoms is about 0.15 nm.[5] Nanotechnology has applications for many potential products, including those that integrate chemistry, the biological sciences, medicine, and computer technology.

Measure of Length

The meter is the primary unit of length in the SI.

The **table of metric length:**

1 kilometer (km)	=	1,000,000 meters
1 hectometer (hm)	=	100,000 meters
1 decameter (dam)	=	10,000 meters
1 meter (m)		
1 decimeter (dm)	=	0.100 meter
1 centimeter (cm)	=	0.010 meter
1 millimeter (mm)	=	0.001 meter
1 micrometer (μm)	=	0.000,001 meter
1 nanometer (nm)	=	0.000,000,001 meter

The table may also be written:

1 meter = 0.001 kilometer
0.01 hectometer
0.1 decameter
10 decimeters
100 centimeters
1000 millimeters
1,000,000 micrometers
1,000,000,000 nanometers

Examples of the use of linear measurement in pharmacy include the dimensions of transdermal skin patches, expressed in cm^2; the use of a patient's height and weight in calculating the doses of certain drugs; and the clinical reference to the size of a patient's physical structure, as a tumor, usually measured in mm or cm. As a point of reference, 1 inch is equivalent to 2.54 centimeters or 25.4 millimeters (Fig. 2.3).

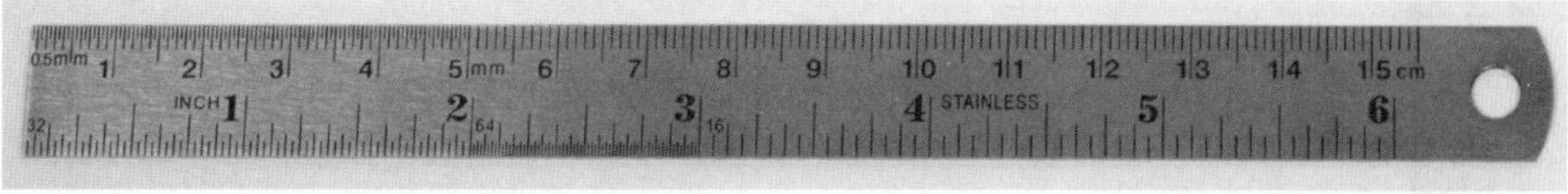

FIGURE 2.3 • Ruler calibrated in millimeter, centimeter, and inch units. *(Courtesy of Schlenker Enterprise, Ltd.)*

Another application of linear measurement is in *distance exercise*, undertaken as a component of maintaining good health status. These programs are typically measured by both time and distance in miles or kilometers, the relationship of which is demonstrated in Table 2.2.

Measure of Volume

The *liter* is the primary unit of volume. It represents the volume of the cube of one-tenth of a meter, that is, of 1 dm^3.

The **table of metric volume:**

1 kiloliter (kL)	=	1000,000 liters
1 hectoliter (hL)	=	100,000 liters
1 decaliter (daL)	=	10,000 liters
1 liter (L)		
1 deciliter (dL)	=	0.100 liter
1 centiliter (cL)	=	0.010 liter
1 milliliter (mL)	=	0.001 liter
1 microliter (μL)	=	0.000,001 liter

This table may also be written:

1 liter = 0.001 kiloliter
0.010 hectoliter
0.100 decaliter
10 deciliters
100 centiliters
1000 milliliters
1,000,000 microliters

Although not precisely equivalent, the milliliter is so nearly the same volume as the cubic centimeter (cm^3, cc), the *United States Pharmacopeia–National Formulary* states: "One milliliter (mL) is used herein as the equivalent of 1 cubic centimeter (cc)."[2]

Measurement of volume is commonplace for the pharmacist in preparing and dispensing liquid medications and for the patient in measuring dosage. Examples of pharmaceutical graduates for measuring volume are shown in Figure 2.4.

Table 2.2 • **DEMONSTRATIONS OF LINEAR RELATIONSHIPS**

	Feet	Yards	Miles	Meters	Kilometers
1 mile	5280	1760	1	1609.3	1.6093
1 kilometer	3280.8	1093.6	0.62137	1000	1

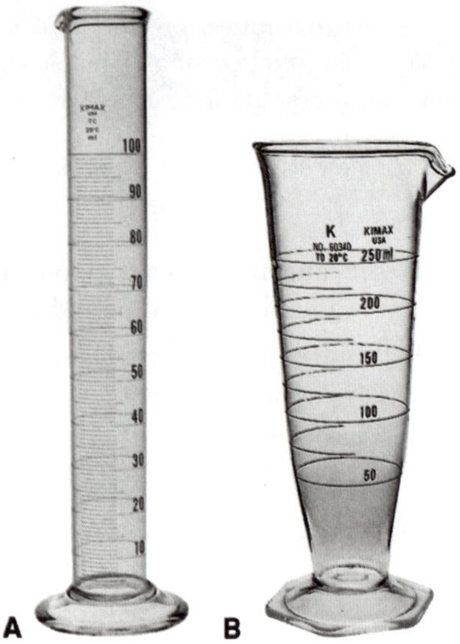

FIGURE 2.4 • Examples of metric-scale cylindrical **(A)** and conical pharmaceutical graduates **(B)**. *(Courtesy of Kimble/Kontes Glass.)*

Measure of Weight

The primary unit of weight in the SI is the *gram*, which is the weight of 1 cm^3 of water at 4°C, its temperature of greatest density. **For practical purposes, 1 cm^3 of water ≈ 1 mL ≈ 1 g of weight.**

The **table of metric weight:**

1 kilogram (kg)	=	1,000,000 grams
1 hectogram (hg)	=	100,000 grams
1 dekagram (dag)	=	10,000 grams
1 gram (g)		
1 decigram (dg)	=	0.100 gram
1 centigram (cg)	=	0.010 gram
1 milligram (mg)	=	0.001 gram
1 microgram (μg or mcg)	=	0.000,001 gram
1 nanogram (ng)	=	0.000,000,001 gram
1 picogram (pg)	=	0.000,000,000,001 gram
1 femtogram (fg)	=	0.000,000,000,000,001 gram

This table may also be written:

1 gram = 0.001 kilogram
0.010 hectogram
0.100 decagram
10 decigrams
100 centigrams
1000 milligrams
1,000,000 micrograms
1,000,000,000 nanograms
1,000,000,000,000 picograms
1,000,000,000,000,000 femtograms

The weighing of components in the manufacture of a pharmaceutical product and in the compounding of a prescription or medication order is a usual function of a pharmacist. And, since most therapeutic agents are solid substances (i.e., powders), their doses are determined and expressed in units of weight, most often in milligrams. An example of a metric set of weights is shown in Chapter 3.

Prescription Writing Style Using the SI

Prescriptions written in the SI use Arabic numerals *before* the abbreviations for the denominations (e.g., 6 g). Quantities of weight are usually written as grams and *decimals* of a gram, and volumes as milliliters and *decimals* of a milliliter:

℞	Dextromethorphan HBr	320 mg
	Guaifenesin	3.2 g
	Cherry syrup, to make	240 mL

Fundamental Computations

Reducing SI Units to Lower or Higher Denominations by Using a Unit Position Scale

The metric system is based on the decimal system; therefore, conversion from one denomination to another can be done simply by moving the decimal point as demonstrated in Figure 2.5.

To change a metric denomination to the next smaller denomination, move the decimal point one place to the right.

To change a metric denomination to the next larger denomination, move the decimal point one place to the left.

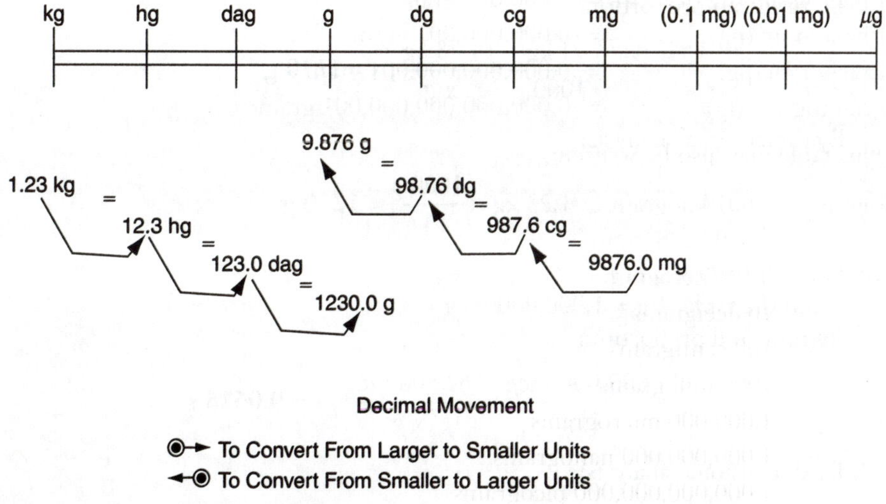

FIGURE 2.5 • Position scale of units of weight.

(1) *Reduce 1.23 kilograms to grams.*

$$1.23 \text{ kg} = \mathbf{1230\ g}$$

(2) *Reduce 9876 milligrams to grams.*

$$9876 \text{ mg} = \mathbf{9.876\ g}$$

In the first example, 1.23 kg is to be converted to grams. On the scale, the gram position is three decimal positions from the kilogram position. Thus, the decimal point is moved three places toward the right. In the second example, the conversion from milligrams also requires the movement of the decimal point three places, but this time to the left.

(3) *Reduce 85 micrometers to centimeters.*

$$85\ \mu\text{m} = 0.085 \text{ mm} = \mathbf{0.0085\ cm}$$

(4) *Reduce 2.525 liters to microliters.*

$$2.525 \text{ L} = 2525 \text{ mL} = \mathbf{2{,}525{,}000\ \mu L}$$

The 3-Decimal Point Shift

In pharmacy practice, and health care in general, the denominations most used differ by 1000 or by a factor of 3 decimal places. Thus, on the decimal scale (Fig. 2.5), a 3-place decimal point shift, left to right or right to left, will yield most commonly used denominations.

<u>3-Place Shift for Common Weight Denominations:</u>
kilograms (kg) _ _ _ grams (g) _ _ _ milligrams (mg) _ _ _ micrograms (mcg)

<u>3-Place Shift for Common Volume Denominations:</u>
liters (L) _ _ _ milliliters (mL)

Reducing SI Units to Lower or Higher Denominations by Ratio and Proportion or by Dimensional Analysis

(5) *Reduce 1.23 kilograms to grams.*
From the table: 1 kg = 1000 g
By ratio and proportion:

$$\frac{1 \text{ kg}}{1000 \text{ g}} = \frac{1.23 \text{ kg}}{\text{x g}};\ \text{x} = \mathbf{1230\ g}$$

By dimensional analysis:

$$1.23 \text{ kg} \times \frac{1000 \text{ g}}{1 \text{ kg}} = \mathbf{1230\ g}$$

(6) *Reduce 62,500 mcg to g.*
From the table: 1 g = 1,000,000 mcg
By ratio and proportion:

$$\frac{1{,}000{,}000 \text{ mcg}}{1 \text{ g}} = \frac{62{,}500 \text{ mcg}}{\text{x g}};\ \text{x} = \mathbf{0.0625\ g}$$

By dimensional analysis:

$$62{,}500 \text{ mcg} \times \frac{1 \text{ g}}{1{,}000{,}000 \text{ mcg}} = \mathbf{0.0625\ g}$$

CALCULATIONS CAPSULE

International System of Units (SI)

- The SI or decimal system of measurement is used in the practice of pharmacy and throughout the pharmaceutical industry.
- The primary SI units for calculating mass or weight (gram), volume (liter), and length (meter) are used along with prefixes to indicate multiples or subdivisions of the primary units.
- To change an SI denomination to the next *smaller* denomination, the decimal point is moved one place to the right:

gram(g) > decigram(dg > centigram(cg > milligram(mg)

5.555g = 55.55 dg = 555.5 cg = 5555 mg

Each value is equivalent.

- To change an SI denomination to the next *larger* denomination, the decimal point is moved one place to the left:

kilogram(kg) > hectogram(hg) > dekagram(dag) > gram(g)

5.555 kg = 55.55 hg = 555.5 dag = 5555 g

Each value is equivalent.

- A unit position scale (e.g., see Fig. 2.5), ratio and proportion, or dimensional analysis may be used to change denominations.
- Only numbers of the same *denomination* may be added to or subtracted from one another.

Recognizing Equivalent Expressions

On occasion, it may be necessary to recognize, or prove by calculation, equivalent expressions. For example, a given quantity expressed in terms of "mg/100 mL" is equivalent to "mg/dL."

Practice problems (#47 to #50) at the conclusion of this chapter provide exercises to determine equivalent expressions.

Addition and Subtraction

To add or subtract quantities in the SI, reduce them to a *common denomination*, preferably a base unit, and arrange their denominate numbers for addition or subtraction as ordinary decimals.

(1) *Add 1 kg, 250 mg, and 7.5 g. Express the total in grams.*

1 kg	=	1000. g
250 mg	=	0.25 g
7.5 g	=	7.5 g
		1007.75 g or **1008 g**

(2) *Add 4 L, 375 mL, and 0.75 L. Express the total in milliliters.*

$$\begin{array}{lcr} 4\text{ L} & = & 4000\text{ mL} \\ 375\text{ mL} & = & 375\text{ mL} \\ 0.75\text{ L} & = & 750\text{ mL} \\ \hline & & \mathbf{5125\ mL} \end{array}$$

(3) *A capsule contains the following amounts of medicinal substances: 0.075 g, 20 mg, 0.0005 g, 4 mg, and 500 mg. What is the total weight of the substances in the capsule?*

$$\begin{array}{lcl} 0.075\text{ g} & = & 0.075\text{ g} \\ 20\text{ mg} & = & 0.02\text{ g} \\ 0.0005\text{ g} & = & 0.0005\text{ g} \\ 4\text{ mg} & = & 0.004\text{ g} \\ 500\ \mu\text{g} & = & 0.0005\text{ g} \\ \hline & & 0.1000\text{ g or } \mathbf{100\ mg} \end{array}$$

(4) *Subtract 2.5 mg from 4.85 g.*

$$\begin{array}{lcl} 4.85\text{ g} & = & 4.85\text{ g} \\ 2.5\text{ mg} & = & -0.0025\text{ g} \\ \hline & & 4.8475\text{ g or } \mathbf{4.848\ g} \end{array}$$

(5) *A prescription calls for 0.06 g of one ingredient, 2.5 mg of another, and enough of a third to make 0.5 g. How many milligrams of the third ingredient should be used?*

$$\begin{array}{lcl} \text{1st ingredient: } 0.06\text{ g} & = & 0.06\text{ g} \\ \text{2nd ingredient: } 2.5\text{ mg} & = & 0.0025\text{ g} \\ \hline & & 0.0625\text{ g} \end{array}$$

$$\begin{array}{ll} \text{Total weight:} & 0.5\text{ g} \\ \text{Weight of 1st and 2nd:} & -0.0625\text{ g} \\ \hline \text{Weight of 3rd:} & 0.4375\text{ g or } \mathbf{437.5\ mg} \end{array}$$

Multiplication and Division

Because every measurement in the SI is expressed in a single given denomination, problems involving multiplication and division are solved by the methods used for any decimal numbers.

(1) *Multiply 820 mL by 12.5 and express the result in liters.*

$$820\text{ mL} \times 12.5 = 10250\text{ mL} = \mathbf{10.25\ L}$$

(2) *Divide 0.465 g by 15 and express the result in milligrams.*

$$0.465\text{ g} \div 15 = 0.031\text{ g} = \mathbf{31\ mg}$$

CASE IN POINT 2.1 A nurse telephones a pharmacy regarding the proper quantity of an injection to administer to a pediatric patient from a 1-mL vial containing 0.1 mg of digoxin. The attending physician had prescribed a dose of 25 mcg. How many milliliters should be the pharmacist's response?

Relation of the SI to Other Systems of Measurement

In addition to the International System of Units, the pharmacy student should be aware of two other systems of measurement: the ***avoirdupois*** and ***apothecaries'*** systems. The avoirdupois system, widely used in the United States in measuring body weight and in selling goods by the ounce or pound, is slowly giving way to the international system. The apothecaries' system, once the predominant pharmacist's system of volumetric and weight measure, has also largely been replaced by the SI. The pharmacist must still appreciate the relationship between the various systems of measurement, however, and deal effectively with them as the need arises.

The avoirdupois and apothecaries' systems of measurement, including all necessary equivalents and methods for intersystem conversion, are presented in Appendix A. The example equivalents presented in Table 2.3 are useful in gaining perspective and in solving certain problems in the text—for example, when there is need to convert fluid ounces to milliliters or kilograms to pounds. These equivalents should be committed to memory.

> When quantities in units of the apothecaries' or avoirdupois systems of measurement (see Appendix A) are encountered, it is suggested that they be converted to equivalent quantities in SI units and the required calculation then solved in the usual manner.

Example Problems

(1) *An injection contains 5 mg of drug in each 10-mL vial. If the dose of the drug for a patient is determined to be 150 μg, how many milliliters should be administered?*

$$150\ \mu g \times \frac{10\ \text{mL}}{5\ \text{mg}} \times \frac{1\ \text{mg}}{1000\ \mu g} = \mathbf{0.3\ mL}$$

Table 2.3 • SOME USEFUL EQUIVALENTS

Equivalents of length		
1 inch	=	2.54 cm
1 meter (m)	=	39.37 in
Equivalents of volume		
1 fluid ounce (fl. oz.)	=	29.57 mL
1 pint (16 fl. oz.)	=	473 mL
1 quart (32 fl. oz.)	=	946 mL
1 gallon, United States (128 fl. oz.)	=	3785 mL
1 gallon, United Kingdom	=	4545 mL
Equivalents of weight		
1 pound (lb, avoirdupois)	=	454 g
1 ounce (oz, avoirdupois)	=	28.35 g
1 kilogram (kg)	=	2.2 lb

(2) *A patient is determined to have a total serum cholesterol level of 240 mg/dL. What is the equivalent value in mg/100 mL?*

1 dL = 100 mL; thus, 240 mg/dL = **240 mg/100 mL**

(3) *The dose of a drug is 0.5 mg/kg of body weight/day. What is the equivalent dose in μg/lb/day?*

0.5 mg = 500 μg
1 kg = 2.2 lb

Thus, 0.5 mg/kg/day = 500 μg/2.2 lb/day = **227.3 μg/lb/day**

(4) *An oral suspension contains 1.5 g of the therapeutic agent in a pint of the suspension. Calculate the quantity of therapeutic agent, in milligrams, present in each 5-mL dose.*

$$? \text{ mg} = 5 \text{ mL} \times \frac{1.5 \text{ g}}{1 \text{ pt}} \times \frac{1000 \text{ mg}}{1 \text{ g}} \times \frac{1 \text{ pt}}{473 \text{ mL}} = 15.86 \text{ or } \mathbf{15.9 \text{ mg}}$$

Or, by ratio and proportion:

1.5 g = 1500 mg
1 pint = 473 mL

$$\frac{1500 \text{ mg}}{473 \text{ mL}} = \frac{x \text{ mg}}{5 \text{ mL}}; \ x = 15.86 \text{ or } \mathbf{15.9 \text{ mg}}$$

CASE IN POINT 2.2 A hospital pharmacist is asked to prepare an intravenous infusion of dopamine. Based on the patient's weight, the pharmacist calculates a dose of 500 mcg/min for continuous infusion. The concentration of a premixed dopamine infusion is 400 mg/250 mL. What is the concentration of the infusion on a mcg/mL basis? How many milligrams of dopamine is the patient to receive in the first hour of treatment? How long will the infusion last?

PRACTICE PROBLEMS

1. What is the weight, in milligrams, of 100 tablets, each containing 20 mcg of a therapeutic agent?
2. Add 7.25 L and 875 cL. Reduce the result to milliliters.
3. Add 0.0025 kg, 1750 mg, 2.25 g, and 825,000 μg, and express the answer in grams.
4. Reduce 1.256 g to micrograms, to milligrams, and to kilograms.
5. Are the terms mcg/mL and mg/L equivalent or not equivalent?
6. A low-strength aspirin tablet contains 81 mg of aspirin per tablet. How many tablets may a manufacturer prepare from 0.5 kg of aspirin?
7. Adhesive tape made from fabric has a tensile strength of not less than 20.41 kg/2.54 cm of width. Reduce these quantities to grams and millimeters.
8. In a clinical study, the drug methotrexate produced a blood level of 6.6 μg of methotrexate in each milliliter of blood (6.6 μg/mL). Express the methotrexate blood level in terms of mg/dL.

9. An inhalation aerosol contains 225 mg of metaproterenol sulfate, which is sufficient for 300 inhalations. How many micrograms of metaproterenol sulfate would be contained in each inhalation?
10. TRIPHASIL-28 birth control tablets are taken sequentially, 1 tablet per day for 28 days, with the tablets containing the following:
Phase 1—6 tablets, each containing 0.05 mg levonorgestrel and 0.03 mg ethinyl estradiol
Phase 2—5 tablets, each containing 0.075 mg levonorgestrel and 0.04 mg ethinyl estradiol
Phase 3—10 tablets, each containing 0.125 mg levonorgestrel and 0.03 mg ethinyl estradiol; then, 7 inert tablets (no drug).
How many total milligrams each of levonorgestrel and ethinyl estradiol are taken during the 28-day period?
11. COLCRYS scored tablets each contain 0.6 mg of colchicine. How many micrograms of colchicine would a patient take by administering one-half tablet?
12. The following clinical laboratory data are within normal values for an adult. Convert each value to mcg/mL:
(a) Ammonia, 30 mcg/dL
(b) Folate, 18 pg/mL
(c) Serum creatinine, 1.0 mg/dL
(d) Prostate-specific antigen (PSA), 3 ng/mL
(e) Cholesterol, total, 150 mg/dL
13. The package insert for DONNATAL EXTENTABS indicates the amount of phenobarbital present in each tablet, in milligrams and in the equivalent weight (3/4 grains) in the apothecary system. Refer to Appendix A and calculate the milligrams of phenobarbital present in each tablet.
14. Levothyroxine sodium tablets (SYNTHROID) are available in 12 different strengths ranging from 25 to 300 μg. Express this range in milligrams.
15. Norgestrel and ethinyl estradiol tablets are available containing 0.5 mg of norgestrel and 50 μg of ethinyl estradiol. How many grams of each ingredient would be used in making 10,000 tablets?
16. Approximately 0.02% of a 100-mg dose of the drug miglitol (GLYSET) has been shown to appear in human breast milk. Calculate the quantity of drug detected, in milligrams, following a single dose.
17. How many grams of digoxin (LANOXIN) would be required to make 25,000 tablets each containing 250 mcg of digoxin?
18. Adalimumab (HUMIRA), a recombinant human monoclonal antibody, is available in a prefilled syringe containing 40 mg/0.8 mL of injection. Calculate the concentration of drug on a mg/mL basis.
19. If an injectable solution contains 25 μg of a drug substance in each 0.5 mL, how many milliliters would be required to provide a patient with 0.25 mg of the drug substance?
20. A patient is instructed to take one 50 μg tablet of pergolide mesylate (PERMAX) a day for the first two days of treatment; 150 μg/day on the third, fourth, and fifth days of treatment; 250 μg/day on the sixth, seventh, and eighth days; and 350 μg on the ninth day and return to the physician for assessment. During this treatment period, how many milligrams of drug were taken?
21. Treatment with the drug carvedilol for heart failure is initiated with a dose of 3.125 mg twice daily and then increased every two weeks with twice daily doses of

6.25 mg, 12.5 mg, and 25 mg. How many of each of these tablet strengths should be dispensed for this protocol?

22. Digoxin (LANOXIN) is available for parenteral pediatric use in a concentration of 0.05 mg/mL. How many milliliters would provide a dose of 40 μg?
23. ROXANOL oral solution contains 0.6 g of morphine sulfate in each 30-mL bottle affixed with a calibrated dropper. Calculate (a) the concentration of morphine sulfate on a mg/mL basis and (b) the milligrams of morphine sulfate delivered by a 0.6-mL dose.
24. The starting dose of sodium oxybate oral solution (XYREM) is 4.5 g/night divided into two equal doses and administered 2.5 to 4 hours apart. How many milliliters of the oral solution containing sodium oxybate, 500 mg/mL, should be administered in each divided dose?
25. An intravenous solution contains 500 μg of a drug substance in each milliliter. How many milligrams of the drug would a patient receive from the intravenous infusion of a liter of the solution?
26. If an intravenous solution containing 123 mg of a drug substance in each 250-mL bottle is to be administered at the rate of 200 μg of drug per minute, how many milliliters of the solution would be given per hour?
27. An oral inhalation (DULERA) to treat asthma provides, in each inhalation, 100 μg of mometasone furoate and 5 μg of formoterol fumarate. The recommended dose is "two inhalations twice daily (morning and evening)." Calculate the quantity of each drug inhaled daily and express the answers in milligrams.
28. An injection contains 50 mcg/0.5 mL of drug. How many μL of the injection should be administered to deliver 0.04 mg of drug?
29. An injection containing 7.5 mg of leuprolide acetate is administered to a patient weighing 25 kg. Calculate the dose on a mcg/lb basis if 1 kg = 2.2 lb.
30. A gas chromatograph column measures 1.8 m in length and 3 mm in internal diameter. Convert these measurements to inches.
31. A prefilled syringe contains 20 mg of drug in 2 mL of solution. How many micrograms of drug would be administered by an injection of 0.5 mL of the solution?
32. A vial contains 80 mg of drug in 2 mL of injection. How many milliliters of the injection should be administered to obtain 0.02 g of drug?
33. One-half liter of solution for intravenous infusion contains 2 g of drug. How many milliliters of the solution would contain 0.5 mg of drug?
34. A 125-mL container of amoxicillin contains 600 mg/5 mL. How many milliliters would be used to administer 400 mg of amoxicillin?
35. An effervescent tablet has the following formula:

Acetaminophen	325 mg
Calcium carbonate	280 mg
Citric acid	900 mg
Potassium bicarbonate	300 mg
Sodium bicarbonate	465 mg

(a) Calculate the total weight, in grams, of the ingredients in each tablet.
(b) How many tablets could be made with a supply of 5 kg of acetaminophen?

36. A new analytic instrument is capable of detecting picogram quantities of a chemical substance. How many times more capable is this instrument than one that can detect nanogram quantities of the same chemical?
37. The rate of drug delivered to the skin by fentanyl transdermal patches is directly proportional to the dimension of the patch. If a patch size of 5.25 cm^2 delivers

12 mcg/hour of fentanyl, calculate the delivery rate of drug expected from a 31.5-cm^2 patch.

38. If an albuterol inhaler contains 18 mg of albuterol, how many inhalation doses can be delivered if each inhalation dose contains 90 μg?
39. Acetaminophen, in amounts greater than 4 g per day, has been associated with liver toxicity. What is the maximum number of 500-mg tablets of acetaminophen that a person may take daily and not reach the toxic level?
40. A lung tumor measuring 2.1 cm was detected in a patient. What are the equivalent dimensions in millimeters and in inches?
41. The recommended dose for a brand of nicotine patch is one 21-mg dose per day for 6 weeks, followed by 14 mg per day for 2 weeks, and then 7 mg per day for 2 more weeks. What total quantity, in grams, would a patient receive during this course of treatment?
42. A medical device is sterilized by gamma radiation at 2.5 megarads (Mrad). Express the equivalent quantity in rads.
43. A round transdermal patch measures 4.3 cm in diameter. Convert this dimension to inches and millimeters.
44. A solution for direct IV bolus injection contains 125 mg of drug in each 25 mL of injection. What is the concentration of drug in terms of μg/μL?
45. The total number of human genomic characters is 3.5 billion. Express this quantity numerically without using a decimal point.
46. Conjugated estrogen tablets (PREMARIN) are available in strengths of 0.3 mg, 0.45 mg, 0.625 mg, 0.9 mg, and 1.25 mg. If patient "A" took one tablet daily of the lowest dose and patient "B" took one tablet daily of the highest dose, what is the difference in the total quantities taken between patients "A" and "B" over a period of 30 days?
    (a) 2.85 mg
    (b) 2850 mcg
    (c) 2.85 cg
    (d) 2.85 dg
47. Teratogenic studies of insulin glargine were undertaken in rats at doses up to 0.36 mg/kg/day. This is equivalent to which of the following?
    (a) 360 cg/lb/day
    (b) 792 mcg/lb/day
    (c) 360 mg/lb/day
    (d) 163.6 mcg/lb/day
48. Pharmacy students, traveling to attend a national pharmacy meeting, were on an airplane with an average air speed of 414 miles per hour. Which is the closest equivalent air speed?
    (a) 6 mi/min
    (b) 257 km/h
    (c) 666 km/h
    (d) 180 m/s
49. The product of biotechnology, filgrastim (NEUPOGEN), is available in vials containing 0.3 mg of drug in each milliliter. Which choice is equivalent in concentration?
    (a) 0.03 mg/0.1 dL
    (b) 300 mcg/0.01 dL
    (c) 3 mcg/0.01 cL
    (d) 300 mcg/10 cL

50. In a clinical study of finasteride (PROSCAR), a single oral dose of 5 mg resulted in an average blood concentration of 37 ng of drug per milliliter (37 ng/mL) of blood plasma. This is equivalent to which of the following?
    (a) 37,000 mcg/mL
    (b) 0.037 mcg/mL
    (c) 0.000037 mg/cL
    (d) 0.0037 mcg/dL

CALCQUIZ

2.A. A health news story that received widespread attention in recent years involved the successful premature birth of octuplets. The eight babies ranged in weight from 1 lb 8 oz to 3 lb 4 oz. Using the equivalents for the avoirdupois system given in this chapter, calculate the babies' range in weight, in grams and in kilograms.

2.B. Levothyroxine sodium tablets are available in 11 different strengths, ranging from 0.025 mg to 200 μg. Calculate the difference, in micrograms, between these two strengths.

2.C. An inhalation aerosol contains 0.03 g of albuterol sulfate per canister and is labeled to deliver 200 full inhalations. If each inhalation contains 108 μg of albuterol sulfate, how many milligrams of drug would remain in the canister?

2.D. A 0.5-mL container of an investigational ophthalmic solution contains a drug in a concentration of 0.01 mg/mL. How many micrograms of drug would be administered in a 50-μL drop?

2.E. A long-acting formulation of leuprolide acetate requires injection only once every 3 months. Clinical studies revealed that 4 hours following a single injection, the mean blood plasma level of leuprolide was 36.3 ng/mL and dropped over the next month to a steady level of 23.9 ng/mL. Express the difference between these the two values in μg/dL.

ANSWERS TO "CASE IN POINT" AND PRACTICE PROBLEMS

Case in Point 2.1

$$0.1 \text{ mg/mL} = 100 \text{ mcg/mL}$$

$$25 \text{ mcg} \times \frac{1 \text{ mL}}{100 \text{ mcg}} = 1/4 \text{ mL}$$

or 0.25 mL

Case in Point 2.2

Concentration of infusion, mcg/mL:

$$\frac{400 \text{ mg}}{250 \text{ mL}} = \frac{400{,}000 \text{ mcg}}{250 \text{ mL}}$$
$$= 1600 \text{ mcg/mL}$$

mg, dopamine, first hour:

$$\frac{500\text{ mcg}}{1\text{ min}} \times \frac{60\text{ min}}{1\text{ h}} \times \frac{1\text{ mg}}{1000\text{ mcg}}$$
$$= 30\text{ mg/h}$$

Infusion duration:

$$400\text{ mg} \times \frac{1\text{ min}}{500\text{ mcg}} \times \frac{1000\text{ mcg}}{1\text{ mg}}$$
$$= 800\text{ min} = 13\text{ h, }20\text{ min}$$

Practice Problems

1. This is a bit of a trick question. The weight of the *therapeutic agent* in the 100 tablets may easily be calculated as 2 mg; however, the question asks for the *weight of the 100 tablets*, which cannot be calculated without the known weight of *all* of the tablets' components, both therapeutic and nontherapeutic (as tablet fillers, binders, etc.) or by actually weighing the tablets.
2. 16,000 mL
3. 7.325 g
4. 1,256,000 mcg
   1256 mg
   0.001256 kg
5. Equivalent
6. 6,172 aspirin tablets
7. 20,410 g/25.4 mm
8. 0.66 mg/dL
9. 750 mcg metaproterenol sulfate
10. 1.925 mg levonorgestrel
    0.68 mg ethinyl estradiol
11. 300 mcg colchicine
12. (a) Ammonia, 0.3 mcg/mL
    (b) Folate, 0.000018 mcg/mL
    (c) Serum creatinine, 10 mcg/mL
    (d) Prostate-specific antigen (PSA), 0.003 mcg/mL
    (e) Cholesterol, 1500 mcg/mL
13. 48.75 mg phenobarbital
14. 0.025 to 0.3 mg levothyroxine sodium
15. 5 g norgestrel
    0.5 g ethinyl estradiol
16. 0.02 mg miglitol
17. 6.25 g digoxin
18. 50 mg/mL
19. 5 mL
20. 1.65 mg pergolide mesylate
21. 28 carvedilol tablets of each strength
22. 0.8 mL
23. (a) 20 mg/mL morphine sulfate
    (b) 12 mg morphine sulfate
24. 4.5 mL oxybate oral solution
25. 500 mg
26. 24.39 mL
27. 0.4 mg mometasone furoate and 0.02 mg formoterol fumarate
28. 400 μL
29. 136.4 mcg/lb
30. 70.866 or 70.9 inches
    0.118 or 0.12 inches
31. 5000 mcg
32. 0.5 mL
33. 0.125 mL
34. 3.33 mL
35. (a) 2.27 g
    (b) 15,384 tablets
36. 1000 times
37. 72 mcg/h
38. 200 doses
39. 8 tablets
40. 21 mm and 0.83 inches.
41. 1.176 g nicotine
42. 2,500,000 rads
43. 1.69 inches and 43 mm
44. 5 μg/μL
45. 3,500,000,000 or 35×10^8
46. (c) 2.85 cg
47. (d) 163.6 mcg/lb/day
48. (c) 666 km/h
49. (b) 300 mcg/0.01 dL
50. (b) 0.037 mcg/mL

AUTHORS' EXTRA POINT

PHARMACOPEIAS

The *United States Pharmacopeia* and the *National Formulary* (USP-NF) is a combination of two books of standards, designated under the U.S. Federal Food, Drug, and Cosmetics Act as the official compendia for drugs marketed in the United States.[a,b] The *United States Pharmacopeia (USP)* contains monographs for drug substances, dosage forms, compounded preparations, and dietary supplements whereas *National Formulary (NF)* contains monographs for pharmaceutical excipients. The combined volume is published annually in hard copy and online with the standards under continual revision through the issuance of supplements, bulletins, and announcements.

The USP-NF is published by the *United States Pharmaceutical Convention*, comprised of representatives of over 400 member organizations representing academic institutions, health practitioners, scientific associations, consumer groups, manufacturers, governmental bodies, and other interested groups. The established standards are enforced in the United States under the authority of the federal Food and Drug Administration.

Although the USP-NF standards are used in more than 140 countries, there are a number of other pharmacopeias published around the world. Among the countries issuing national pharmacopeias are Argentina, Brazil, China, Egypt, France, Germany, India, Indonesia, Japan, Mexico, Philippines, Russia, Spain, Switzerland, and the United Kingdom (*British Pharmacopoeia*). In addition, there are regional pharmacopeias, namely, the *European Pharmacopoeia* and the *African Pharmacopoeia*. And internationally, there is *The International Pharmacopoeia*, published by the World Health Organization.[c]

Canada, under its "Food and Drugs Act," utilizes a number of pharmacopeias, including the *USP-NF, European Pharmacopoeia (Ph.Eur), Pharmacopée française (Ph.F),* the *British Pharmacopoeia (BP), and The International Pharmacopoeia (Ph. Int.).*

[a] http://www.usp.org/usp-nf

[b] The term "pharmacopeia" comes from the Greek *pharmakon*, meaning "drug," and *poiein*, meaning "make," the combination indicating any recipe, formula, or standard required to make a drug or drug product.

[c] http://www.who.int/medicines/publications/pharmacopoeia/WHOPSMQSM2006_2_IndexPharmacopoeiasUpdated.pdf

References

1. U.S. Metric Association. Correct SI-metric usage. Available at: http://lamar.colostate.edu/~hillger/correct.htm. Accessed July 11, 2014.
2. *United States Pharmacopeia 32 National Formulary* 27. Vol. 1. Rockville, MD: United States Pharmacopeial Convention, 2009; 9.
3. Junghanns J-UAH, Müller H. Nanocrystal technology, drug delivery and clinical applications. *International Journal of Nanomedicine* 2008;3(3):295–310. Available at: http://www.ncbi.nlm.nih.gov/pmc/articles/PMC2626933/. Accessed April 11, 2014.
4. National Nanotechnology Initiative. *What is nanotechnology*. Available at: http://www.nano.gov/html/facts/whatIsNano/html. Accessed March 6, 2011.
5. Seeman NC. Nanotechnology and the double helix. *Scientific American* 2004;290:64–75.

3

Pharmaceutical Measurement

OBJECTIVES

Upon successful completion of this chapter, the student will be able to:

- Describe instruments for volumetric measurement and characterize their differences in application and accuracy.
- Describe the correct procedure when using a pharmaceutical balance.
- Define *sensitivity requirement* and apply it in calculations.
- Perform calculations by the aliquot method.
- Demonstrate an understanding of *percentage of error* in pharmaceutical measurement.

Pharmaceutical measurement is an important part of pharmacy practice. It is employed in community and institutional pharmacies, in pharmaceutical research, in the development and manufacture of pharmaceuticals, in chemical and product analysis, and in quality control. This chapter focuses on the equipment and methods used in the accurate measurement of therapeutic and pharmaceutical materials in the community and institutional practice of pharmacy.

The expertise of pharmacists in accurately weighing and measuring materials is a historical and unique skill, acquired through professional education and training. Moreover, this capability is an *expectation* of other health professionals and the patient community being served. It is not an overstatement to say that *patients' lives depend on it.*

The role of the pharmacist in providing pharmaceutical care includes the ability and responsibility to ***compound***—that is, to accurately weigh, measure volume, and combine individual therapeutic and pharmaceutical components in the formulation and preparation of prescriptions and medication orders.

Measurement of Volume

Common instruments for the pharmaceutical measurement of volume range from micropipettes and burettes used in analytic procedures to large, industrial-size calibrated vessels. The selection of measuring instrument should be based on the level of precision required. In pharmacy practice, the most common instruments for measuring volume are cylindric and conical (cone-shaped) graduates (Fig. 3.1). For the measurement of small volumes, however, the pharmacist often uses a calibrated syringe or, when required, a pipette.

Whereas cylindric graduates are calibrated in SI or metric units, conical graduates are usually dual scale, that is, calibrated in both metric and apothecary units of volume. Both glass and plastic graduates are commercially available in a number of capacities, ranging from 5 to 1000 mL and greater.

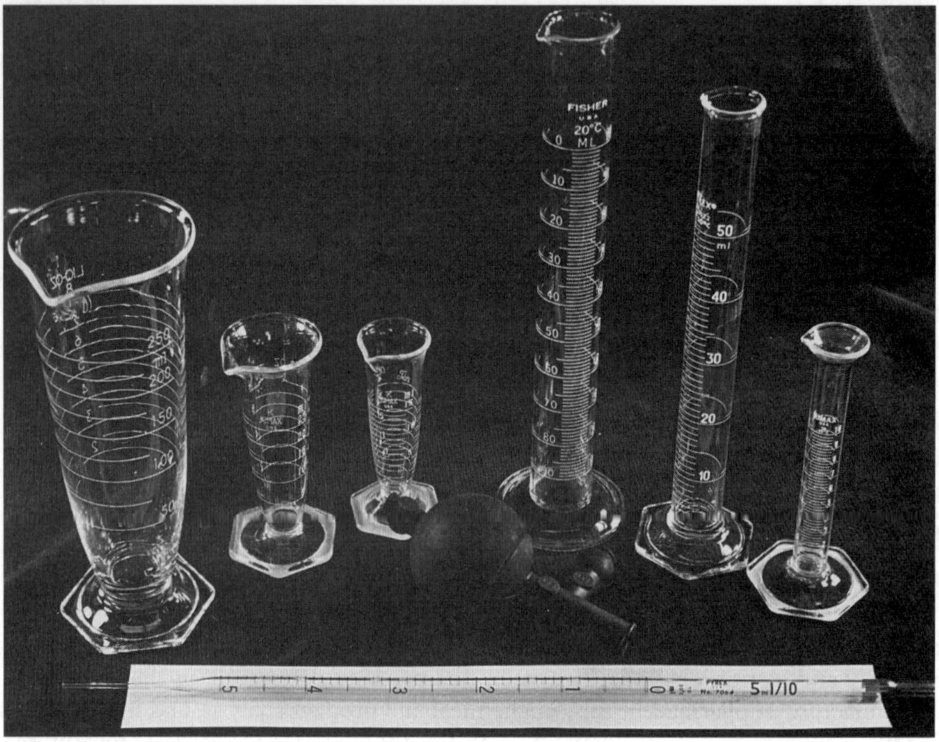

FIGURE 3.1 • Examples of conical and cylindric graduates, a pipette, and a pipette-filling bulb for volumetric measurement.

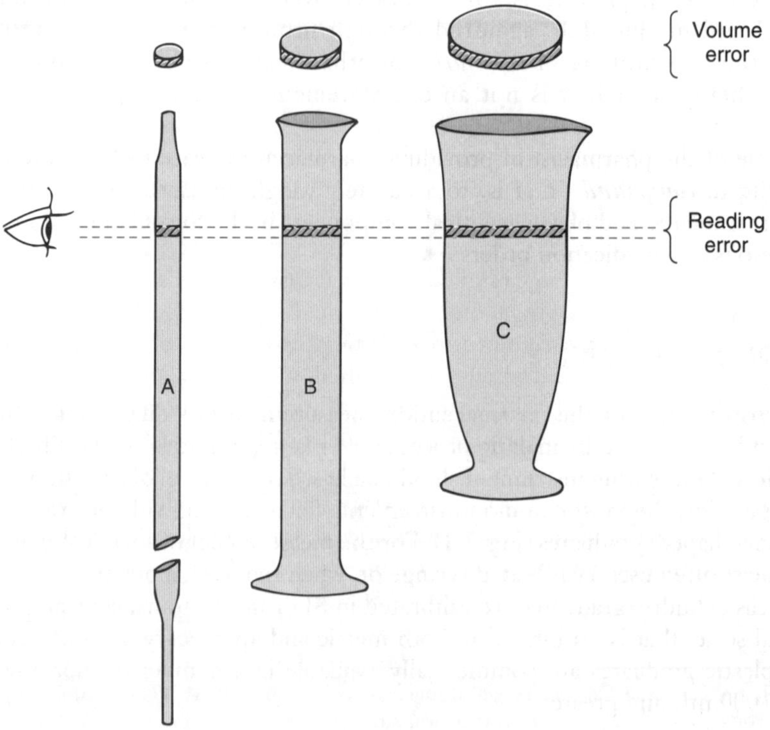

FIGURE 3.2 • Volume error differentials due to instrument diameters. **(A)** Volumetric pipette; **(B)** cylindric graduate; and **(C)** conical graduate.

As a general rule, it is best to select the graduate with a capacity equal to or just exceeding the volume to be measured. Measurement of small volumes in large graduates increases the potential for error. The design of a volumetric apparatus is an important factor in measurement accuracy; the narrower the bore or chamber, the lesser the error in reading the meniscus and the more accurate the measurement (Fig. 3.2). According to the *United States Pharmacopeia*, a deviation of ±1 mm in the reading of the meniscus when using a 100-mL cylindrical graduate results in an error of approximately 0.5 mL and 1.8 mL at the 100-mL mark when using a 125-mL conical graduate.[1]

It is essential for the pharmacist to select the proper type and capacity of instrument for volumetric measure and to carefully observe the meniscus at eye level to achieve the desired measurement.

Measurement of Weight

There is a wide range of weights, balances, and scales available for pharmaceutical measurement. The proper selection depends upon the particular task at hand. Standard prescription balances and highly sensitive electronic balances generally suffice in traditional pharmaceutical compounding, whereas large-capacity scales are used in the industrial manufacture of pharmaceutical products. Whichever instrument is used, however, it must meet established standards for sensitivity, accuracy, and capacity.

A differentiation may be made between a *scale* and a *balance*. A *scale* measures a single object's weight (think of a bathroom scale). A scale reading will differ if the gravity is different, that is, less at higher elevations and greater at sea level. A *balance* uses a lever and fulcrum, or a pivoting point, to compare the masses of two different objects. A weight of known mass is used to measure the substance being weighed. A balance is more precise than a scale. *Analytical balances* are characterized by a precision/capacity ratio of 1/500,000 or better and a readability of 0.1 mg or better. *Microbalances* have readabilities as low as 0.001 mg, and *ultramicrobalances* have readabilities as low as 0.0001 mg.[a]

Some terminology associated with balances and scales is presented in Table 3.1.

Class A prescription balances (Fig. 3.3) are designed for the weighing of medicinal or pharmaceutical substances required in the filling of prescriptions or in small-scale compounding. Some prescription balances have a weighbeam and rider, and others a dial, to add up to 1 g of weight. As required, additional external weights may be added to the right-hand balance pan. The material to be weighed is placed on the left-hand pan. Powder papers are added to each pan before any additions, and the balance is leveled by leveling feet or balancing screws. Weighings are performed through the careful portion-wise (by spatula) addition and removal of the material being weighed, with the balance being *arrested* (pans locked in place by the control knob) during each addition and removal of material and *un*arrested with the lid closed for determinations of balance rest points. When the unarrested pans neither ascend nor descend, and the index plate shows the needle is in the center, the material and balance weights are considered equivalent. The student may wish to refer to other sources, such as the *United States Pharmacopeia*, for more detailed information on the proper use and testing of the prescription balance.[1]

[a]Balances of all types are available from several manufacturers including OHAUS Corporation (http://us.ohaus.com/us/en/home/products.aspx), Sartorius Corporation (http://www.sartorius.us/us/products/laboratory/laboratory-balances/), and A&D Weighing (http://www.andonline.com/weighing/).

Table 3.1 • SOME TERMINOLOGY ASSOCIATED WITH BALANCES AND SCALES[a]

Term	Meaning
Accuracy	The degree of agreement between the value displayed on a balance and the true value of the quantity measured.
Calibration	Adjusting a measuring device to a reference point or standard unit of measure. Calibration is critical to accuracy, and although most balances are calibrated during manufacture, calibration should be verified at installation and performed periodically to maintain accuracy. Some balances are self-calibrating.
Capacity	The maximum weight measurable by the balance or scale.
Load	The weight applied to the receiving balance or scale.
Precision	The degree of agreement between repeated measurements of the same quantity.
Readability	The smallest fraction of a division to which a balance or scale can be read.
Sensitivity requirement	The load (weight) that will cause a change of one division on the index plate on a balance.
Stability	The degree of constancy of measurement of an instrument when subject to variation in external factors such as time, temperature, and supply voltage.

[a]Sources: http://www.scalesonline.com/t/ScaleTerminology and http://www.ohaus.com/us/en/home/support/glossary.aspx

Minimally, a Class A prescription balance should be used in all prescription compounding procedures. Balances of this type have a ***sensitivity requirement (SR)*** of 6 mg or less with no load and with a load of 10 g in each pan. *To avoid errors of greater than 5% when using this balance, the pharmacist should not weigh less than 120 mg of material (i.e., a 5% error in a weighing of 120 mg = 6 mg).* Most commercially available Class A balances have a maximum capacity of 120 g.

The term ***sensitivity requirement*** is defined as the load that will cause a change of one division on the index plate of the balance. It may be determined by the following procedure:

(1) Level the balance.
(2) Determine the rest point of the balance.
(3) Determine the smallest weight that causes the rest point to shift one division on the index plate.

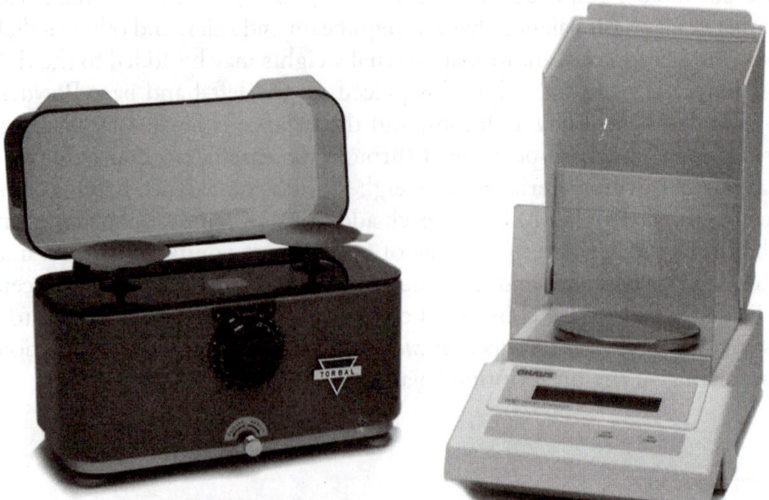

FIGURE 3.3 • Torbal torsion balance and Ohaus electronic balance. *(Courtesy of Torbal and Ohaus.)*

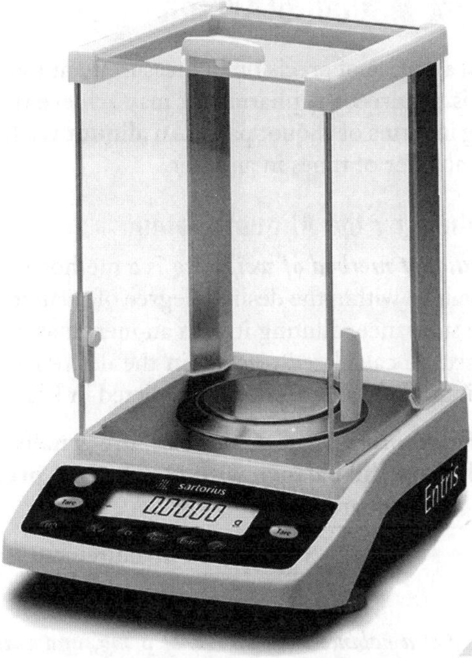

FIGURE 3.4 • Sartorius BasicLite analytical balance. *(Courtesy of Sartorius Corporation.)*

For greater accuracy than a Class A prescription balance allows, many pharmacies utilize high-precision electronic analytical balances to weigh very small quantities (Fig. 3.4). Many of these balances are capable of weighing accurately 0.1 mg, are self-calibrating, and are equipped with convenient digital readout features. The usual maximum capacities for balances of this precision range from about 60 to 210 g depending upon the model. A set of metric weights that may be used to weigh materials on a prescription balance and/or used to calibrate an analytical balance is shown in Figure 3.5.

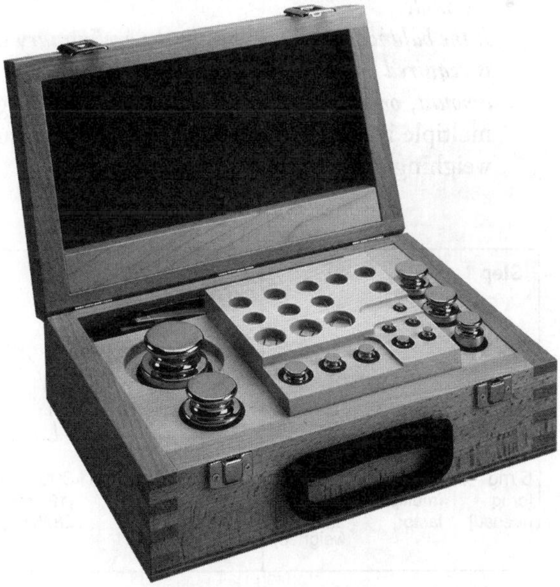

FIGURE 3.5 • Set of metric weights. *(Courtesy of Mettler-Toledo, Inc.)*

Aliquot Method of Weighing and Measuring

When a degree of precision in measurement that is beyond the capacity of the instrument at hand is required, the pharmacist may achieve the desired precision by calculating and measuring in terms of aliquot parts. An **aliquot** is a fraction, portion, or part that is contained an exact number of times in another.

Weighing by the Aliquot Method

The ***aliquot method of weighing*** is a method by which small quantities of a substance may be obtained within the desired degree of accuracy by weighing a larger-than-needed portion of the substance, diluting it with an inert material, and then weighing a portion (aliquot) of the mixture calculated to contain the desired amount of the needed substance. A stepwise description of the procedure is depicted in Figure 3.6 and is described as follows:

Preliminary Step. **Calculate the smallest quantity of a substance that can be weighed on the balance with the desired precision.**

The equation used:

$$\frac{100\% \times \text{Sensitivity Requirement (mg)}}{\text{Acceptable Error (\%)}} = \text{Smallest Quantity (mg)}$$

On a balance with an SR of 6 mg, and with an acceptable error of no greater than 5%, a quantity of not less than 120 mg must be weighed.

$$\frac{100\% \times 6\text{ mg}}{5\%} = 120\text{ mg}$$

STEP 1. **Select a multiple of the desired quantity that can be weighed with the required precision.**

- If the quantity of a required substance is *less than* the minimum weighable amount, select a "multiple" of the required quantity that will yield an amount equal to or greater than the minimum weighable amount. (A larger-than-necessary multiple may be used to exceed the minimum accuracy desired.)
- *Example:*
  *If the balance in the example in the preliminary step is used, and if 5 mg of a drug substance is required on a prescription, then a quantity at least **25 times** (the multiple) the desired amount, or 125 mg (5 mg × 25), must be weighed for the desired accuracy.* (If a larger multiple is used, say 30, and 150 mg of the substance is weighed [5 mg × 30], then a weighing error of only 4% would result.)

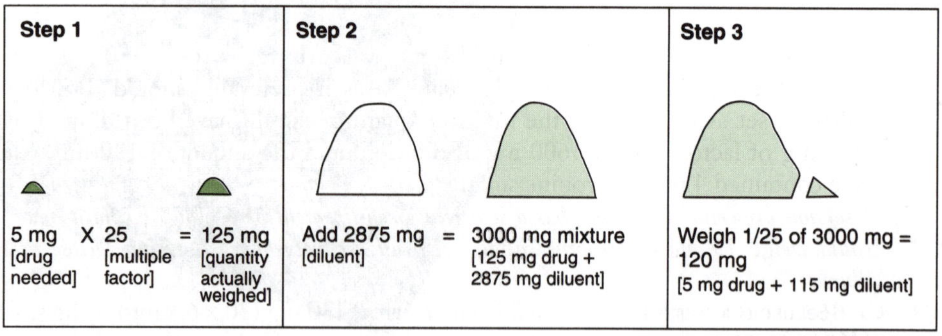

FIGURE 3.6 • Depiction of the aliquot method of weighing using the example described in the text.

STEP 2. Dilute the multiple quantity with an inert substance.

- *The amount of inert diluent* to use is determined by the fact that the aliquot portion of the drug–diluent mixture weighed in *Step 3* must be equal to or greater than the minimum weighable quantity previously determined.
- By multiplying the amount of the aliquot portion to weigh in *Step 3* by the multiple selected in *Step 1*, the total quantity of the mixture to prepare is determined.
- *Example:*

  According to the preliminary step, 120 mg or more must be weighed for the desired accuracy. If we decide on 120 mg for the aliquot portion in Step 3, and multiply it by the multiple selected in Step 1 (i.e., 25), we arrive at 3000 mg for the total quantity of the drug–diluent mixture to prepare. Subtracting the 125 mg of drug weighed in Step 1, we must add 2875 mg of diluent to prepare the 3000 mg of drug–diluent mixture.

STEP 3. Weigh the aliquot portion of the dilution that contains the desired quantity.

- Since ***25 times*** the needed amount of drug substance was weighed (*Step 1*), an aliquot part equal to 1/25 of the 3000-mg drug–diluent mixture, or 120 mg, will contain the required quantity of drug substance.
- *Proof:* $\frac{1}{25} \times 125$ mg (drug substance weighed in *Step 1*) = 5 mg

  $\frac{1}{25} \times 2875$ mg (diluent weighed in *Step 2*) = $\underline{115 \text{ mg}}$

  120 mg aliquot part

Example Problems

(1) *A torsion prescription balance has a sensitivity requirement of 6 mg. Explain how you would weigh 4 mg of atropine sulfate with an accuracy of ±5%, using lactose as the diluent.*

Because 6 mg is the potential balance error, 120 mg is the smallest amount that should be weighed to achieve the required precision.

If 120 mg, or **30** times the desired amount of atropine sulfate, is chosen as the multiple quantity to be weighed in *Step 1*, and if 150 mg is set as the aliquot to be weighed in *Step 3*, then:

1. Weigh **30** × 4 mg 120 mg of atropine sulfate
2. Dilute with <u>4380</u> mg of lactose
   to make 4500 mg of dilution
3. Weigh 1/30 of dilution, or 150 mg of dilution, which will contain 4 mg of atropine sulfate

Proof:

$$\frac{4500 \text{ mg (dilution)}}{150 \text{ mg (dilution)}} = \frac{120 \text{ mg (atropine sulfate)}}{x \text{ mg (atropine sulfate)}}$$

$$= \mathbf{4\ mg}$$

In this example, the weight of the aliquot was arbitrarily set as 150 mg, which exceeds the weight of the multiple quantity, as it preferably should. If 120 mg had been set as the aliquot, the multiple quantity should have been diluted with 3480 mg of lactose to get 3600 mg of dilution, and the aliquot of 120 mg would have contained 4 mg of atropine sulfate.

(2) *A torsion prescription balance has a sensitivity requirement of 6.5 mg. Explain how you would weigh 15 mg of atropine sulfate with an accuracy of ±5%, using lactose as the diluent.*

Because 6.5 mg is the potential balance error, 130 mg (20 × 6.5 mg) is the smallest amount that should be weighed to achieve the required accuracy.

If **10** is chosen as the multiple, and if 130 mg is set as the weight of the aliquot, then:

1. Weigh **10** × 15 mg 150 mg of atropine sulfate
2. Dilute with 1150 mg of lactose
   to make 1300 mg of dilution
3. Weigh $\frac{1}{10}$ of dilution, or 130 mg, which will contain **15 mg** of atropine sulfate

> ***NOTE: It is important for the student to recognize that answers to aliquot calculations may vary, but still be correct, depending upon the multiple factors arbitrarily chosen for use.***

Measuring Volume by the Aliquot Method

The aliquot method of measuring volume, which is identical in principle to the aliquot method of weighing, may be used when relatively small volumes must be measured with great precision:

STEP 1. Select a multiple of the desired quantity that can be measured with the required precision.
STEP 2. Dilute the multiple quantity with a compatible diluent (usually a solvent for the liquid to be measured) to an amount evenly divisible by the multiple selected.
STEP 3. Measure the aliquot of the dilution that contains the quantity originally desired.

Example Problems

(1) *A formula calls for 0.5 mL of hydrochloric acid. Using a 10-mL graduate calibrated from 2 to 10 mL in 1-mL divisions, explain how you would obtain the desired quantity of hydrochloric acid by the aliquot method.*

If **4** is chosen as the multiple, and if 2 mL is set as the volume of the aliquot, then:

1. Measure **4** × 0.5 mL 2 mL of the acid
2. Dilute with 6 mL of water
   to make 8 mL of dilution
3. Measure $\frac{1}{4}$ of dilution, or 2 mL of dilution, which will contain **0.5 mL** of hydrochloric acid.

(2) *A prescription calls for 0.2 mL of clove oil. Using a 5-mL graduate calibrated in units of 0.5 mL, how would you obtain the required amount of clove oil using the aliquot method and alcohol as the diluent?*

If **5** is chosen as the multiple, then:

1. Measure **5** × 0.2 mL 1 mL of clove oil
2. Dilute with 4 mL of alcohol
   to make 5 mL of dilution
3. Measure $\frac{1}{5}$ of the dilution, or 1 mL, which contains **0.2 mL** of clove oil.

Least Weighable Quantity Method of Weighing

This method may be used as an alternative to the aliquot method of weighing to obtain small quantities of a drug substance.

After determining the quantity of drug substance that is desired and the smallest quantity that can be weighed on the balance with the desired degree of accuracy, the procedure is as follows:

STEP 1. Weigh an amount of the drug substance that is *equal to or greater than* the least weighable quantity.

STEP 2. Dilute the drug substance with a calculated quantity of inert diluent such that a predetermined quantity of the drug–diluent mixture will contain the desired quantity of the drug.

If 20 mg of a drug substance is needed to fill a prescription, explain how you would obtain this amount of drug with an accuracy of ±5% using a balance with an SR of 6 mg. Use lactose as the diluent.

In this problem, 20 mg is the amount of drug substance needed. The least weighable quantity would be 120 mg. The amount of drug substance to be weighed, therefore, must be equal to or greater than 120 mg. In solving the problem, 120 mg of drug substance is weighed. In calculating the amount of diluent to use, a predetermined quantity of drug–diluent mixture must be selected to contain the desired 20 mg of drug substance. The quantity selected must be greater than 120 mg because the drug–diluent mixture must be obtained accurately through weighing on the balance. An amount of 150 mg may be arbitrarily selected. The total amount of diluent to use may then be determined through the calculation of the following proportion:

$$\frac{\text{20 mg (drug needed for ℞)}}{\text{150 mg (drug–diluent mixture to use in ℞)}} = \frac{\text{120 mg (total drug substance weighed)}}{\text{x mg (total amount of drug–diluent mixture prepared)}}$$

x = 900 mg of the drug–diluent mixture to prepare

Hence, 900 mg − 120 mg = **780 mg** of diluent (lactose) to use

It should be noted that in this procedure, each weighing, including that of the drug substance, the diluent, and the drug–diluent mixture, must be determined to be equal to or greater than the least weighable quantity as determined for the balance used and accuracy desired.

CALCULATIONS CAPSULE

Weighing Accuracy

- The sensitivity requirement (SR) of a balance must be known or determined. An SR of 6 mg is usual.
- An error in weighing of ±5% or less is acceptable.
- The smallest quantity that should be weighed on a prescription balance is determined by the equation:

$$\frac{100\% \times \text{Sensitivity Requirement (mg)}}{\text{Acceptable Error (\%)}} = \text{Smallest Quantity (mg)}$$

  That quantity is usually about 120 mg.
- To weigh smaller quantities, an electronic balance or the aliquot method of weighing should be used.

Percentage of Error

Because measurements in the community pharmacy are never *absolutely* accurate, it is important for the pharmacist to recognize the limitations of the instruments used and the magnitude of the errors that may be incurred. When a pharmacist measures a volume of liquid or weighs a material, two quantities become important: (1) the *apparent* weight or volume measured and (2) the possible excess or deficiency in the actual quantity obtained.

Percentage of error may be defined as *the maximum potential error multiplied by 100 and divided by the quantity desired.* The calculation may be formulated as follows:

$$\frac{\text{Error} \times 100\%}{\text{Quantity desired}} = \text{Percentage of error}$$

Calculating Percentage of Error in Volumetric Measurement

The percentage of error in a measurement of volume may be calculated from the above equation, relating the volume in error (determined through devices of greater precision) to the volume desired (or apparently measured).

Using a graduated cylinder, a pharmacist measured 30 mL of a liquid. On subsequent examination, using a narrow-gauge burette, it was determined that the pharmacist had actually measured 32 mL. What was the percentage of error in the original measurement?

$$32 \text{ mL} - 30 \text{ mL} = 2 \text{ mL, the volume of error}$$

$$\frac{2 \text{ mL} \times 100\%}{30 \text{ mL}} = \mathbf{6.7\%}$$

Calculating Percentage of Error in Weighing

The various scales and balances used in pharmaceutical weighing have ascribed to them different degrees of precision. As described previously in this chapter, knowledge of the *sensitivity requirement* of the balance being used is critical in weighing to a specified degree of accuracy. The sensitivity requirement of a balance may be used to determine the percentage of error in a given weighing.

(1) *When the maximum potential error is ±4 mg in a total of 100 mg, what is the percentage of error?*

$$\frac{4 \text{ mg} \times 100\%}{100 \text{ mg}} = \mathbf{4\%}$$

(2) *A prescription calls for 800 mg of a substance. After weighing this amount on a balance, the pharmacist decides to check by weighing it again on a more sensitive balance, which registers only 750 mg. Because the first weighing was 50 mg short of the desired amount, what was the percentage of error?*

$$\frac{50 \text{ mg} \times 100\%}{800 \text{ mg}} = \mathbf{6.25\%}$$

Examples of Measurement Applications in Pharmaceutical Compounding

The following are examples of the calculations applied in weighing and measuring in the compounding of pharmaceutical formulas or medication orders. Many additional problems are found in Chapter 17, *Selected Calculations in Contemporary Compounding.*

(1)[2]

Misoprostol	400 μg
Polyethylene oxide	200 mg
Hydroxypropyl methylcellulose	15 g

Compounding Instructions:

(1) Accurately weigh each of the ingredients.
(2) Place the misoprostol in a mixing vessel, and add the polyethylene oxide in equal portions until thoroughly blended.
(3) Add the hydroxypropyl methylcellulose in portions until all ingredients are thoroughly blended.
(4) Label and dispense.
   (a) *Would a torsion prescription balance allow the accurate direct weighing of each ingredient? Explain.*
   (b) *Explain how the misoprostol might be accurately obtained using a torsion prescription balance and the aliquot method of weighing.*
   (c) *How many misoprostol tablets, each containing 0.2 mg, could be used in compounding this order? How would they be combined?*

Answers:

(a) Not for the misoprostol. The least weighable quantity using a torsion balance is 120 mg (with an SR of 6 mg and an acceptable error of ±5%), and the misoprostol required is 400 μg or 0.4 mg. An analytical balance could be used.
(b) The pharmacist could weigh 300 times the required amount of misoprostol, 120 mg (300 × 0.4 mg = 120 mg); then, mix that with 35,880 mg of polyethylene oxide to make 36,000 mg of mixture from which a 120-mg aliquot portion could be taken to provide the 0.4 mg of misoprostol (and 119.6 mg of polyethylene oxide). However, this would be very wasteful of the ingredients, so the better option is provided by (c).
(c) Two misoprostol tablets each containing 0.2 mg (200 μg) would provide the 400 μg required. The tablets would be pulverized using a mortar and pestle and the other ingredients combined in portions as described in the compounding instructions as stated above.

(2)[2]

Fentanyl citrate	2.5 mg
Methylparaben	10 mg
Propylparaben	10 mg
Propylene glycol	0.2 mL
Normal saline solution	10 mL

Compounding Instructions:

(1) Accurately weigh and measure each of the ingredients.
(2) Dissolve the methylparaben and the propylparaben in the polyethylene glycol.

(3) Dissolve the fentanyl citrate in the normal saline solution.
(4) Slowly add the solution of the parabens to the fentanyl citrate solution and mix well.
(5) Sterilize by filtering through a sterile 0.2-μm filter into a sterile metered spray bottle.
(6) Label and dispense.
 (a) *What type of balance should be used to weigh the fentanyl citrate and the parabens?*
 (b) *What are the best options in measuring the propylene glycol?*

Answers:

(a) An analytical balance should be used.
(b) A graduated pipette or a graduated syringe.

CASE IN POINT 3.1 A pharmacist is asked to compound the following formula for the preparation of 100 capsules[3]:

Estriol	200 mg
Estrone	25 mg
Estradiol	25 mg
Methocel E4M	10 g
Lactose	23.75 g

Using a balance that has an SR of 6 mg, the aliquot method of weighing, lactose as the diluent, and an error in weighing of 4% show, by calculations, how the correct quantity of estrone can be obtained to accurately compound the formula.

CASE IN POINT 3.2 A physician prescribed 25 4-mg capsules of a drug for a special needs patient, knowing that the dose prescribed was considered "subtherapeutic." The lowest strength commercially available tablets contain 25 mg.

The pharmacist decided to select the minimum required number of 25-mg tablets (4 tablets), reduce them to a powder with a mortar and pestle, weigh the powder (280 mg), and continue the process using the aliquot method. She called upon her pharmacy student intern to calculate (a) the minimum quantity of lactose (diluent) to use in preparing the crushed tablet–diluent mixture and (b) the quantity of the mixture to use to fill each capsule.

The prescription balance had an SR of 6 mg, and a weighing error of 5% was acceptable.

Show your calculations for (a) and (b), and (c) prove that your answer to (b) is correct by demonstrating that each capsule would indeed contain 4 mg of drug.

PRACTICE PROBLEMS

Calculations of Aliquot Parts by Weighing

1. A prescription calls for 50 mg of chlorpheniramine maleate. Using a prescription balance with a sensitivity requirement of 6 mg, explain how you would obtain the required amount of chlorpheniramine maleate with an error not greater than 5%.
2. A prescription balance has a sensitivity requirement of 0.006 g. Explain how you would weigh 0.012 g of a drug with an error not greater than 5%, using lactose as the diluent.
3. A torsion prescription balance has a sensitivity requirement of 4 mg. Explain how you would weigh 5 mg of hydromorphone hydrochloride with an error not greater than 5%. Use lactose as the diluent.
4. A torsion prescription balance has a sensitivity requirement of 0.004 g. Explain how you would weigh 0.008 g of a substance with an error not greater than 5%.
5. A prescription balance has a sensitivity requirement of 6.5 mg. Explain how you would weigh 20 mg of a substance with an error not greater than 2%.

Calculations of Aliquot Parts by Measuring Volume

6. ℞

Sodium citrate	5 g
Tartar emetic	0.015 g
Cherry syrup ad	120 mL

Using a balance with a sensitivity of 4 mg, an acceptable weighing error of 5% and cherry syrup as the solvent for tartar emetic, how could you obtain the correct quantity of tartar emetic to fill the prescription?

7. A formula calls for 0.6 mL of a coloring solution. Using a 10-mL graduate calibrated from 2 to 10 mL in 1-mL units, how could you obtain the desired quantity of the coloring solution by the aliquot method? Use water as the diluent.
8. Using a 10-mL graduate calibrated in 1-mL units, explain how you would measure 1.25 mL of a dye solution by the aliquot method. Use water as the diluent.
9. The formula for 100 mL of pentobarbital sodium elixir calls for 0.75 mL of orange oil. Using alcohol as a diluent and a 10-mL graduate calibrated in 1-mL units, how could you obtain the desired quantity of orange oil?

Calculations of Percentage of Error

10. A pharmacist attempts to weigh 120 mg of codeine sulfate on a balance with a sensitivity requirement of 6 mg. Calculate the maximum potential error in terms of percentage.
11. In compounding a prescription, a pharmacist weighed 0.05 g of a substance on a balance insensitive to quantities smaller than 0.004 g. What was the maximum potential error in terms of percentage?
12. A pharmacist weighed 475 mg of a substance on a balance of dubious accuracy. When checked on a balance of high accuracy, the weight was found to be 445 mg. Calculate the percentage of error in the first weighing.

13. A 10-mL graduate weighs 42.745 g. When 5 mL of distilled water is measured in it, the combined weight of the graduate and water is 47.675 g. By definition, 5 mL of water should weigh 5 g. Calculate the weight of the measured water and express any deviation from 5 g as percentage of error.
14. A graduate weighs 35.825 g. When 10 mL of water is measured in it, the weight of the graduate and water is 45.835 g. Calculate the weight of the water, and express any deviation from 10 g as percentage of error.
15. A pharmacist attempts to weigh 0.375 g of morphine sulfate on a balance of dubious accuracy. When checked on a highly accurate balance, the weight is found to be 0.400 g. Calculate the percentage of error in the first weighing.

Measurement Applications in Compounding

16.[4]

Carvedilol	100 mg
Water, purified	10 mL
Ora-Blend SF suspension	90 mL

Compounding Instructions:

(1) Weigh carvedilol.
(2) Grind carvedilol powder in a mortar with the purified water until a smooth paste results.
(3) Add the Ora-Blend SF (sugar-free) suspension slowly with mixing in the mortar until a smooth, uniform suspension results.
(4) Pour into amber glass bottle for labeling and dispensing.
   (a) *Describe the type of balance to best use to weigh the carvedilol.*
   (b) *If a torsion prescription balance is used to weigh the carvedilol, describe the aliquot method that may be used.*
   (c) *If 12.5-mg carvedilol tablets are used as the source of the drug, describe the compounding procedure to use.*

CALCQUIZ

3.A. A pharmacist receives a prescription for ear drops, calling for 0.05 mL of glacial acetic acid, 2 mL of glycerin, and 8 mL of purified water. Using a 10-mL graduated cylinder calibrated in 0.5-mL units, explain how the required quantity of glacial acetic acid could be obtained.

3.B. A pharmacist quizzes a pharmacy intern on the aliquot method in the preparation of 12 capsules each to contain 80 mg of morphine sulfate and 3.2 mg of naltrexone hydrochloride. Lactose is to be used as a diluent, a prescription balance with a sensitivity of 6 mg is proposed, and a 4% error is acceptable. Provide the relevant calculations.

3.C. The aliquot method was used to obtain 8 mg of a drug with a prescription balance having a sensitivity of 6 mg. A weighing error of 5% was accepted. If 140 mg of the drug was weighed, added to 2.1 g of lactose, and 120 mg of the mixture used to provide the required quantity of drug, were the calculations correct or incorrect?

3.D. In preparing a zinc oxide ointment, 28.35 g of zinc oxide was used rather than the correct quantity, 31.1 g. What percentage error was incurred?

ANSWERS TO "CASE IN POINT" AND PRACTICE PROBLEMS

Case in Point 3.1

The smallest quantity that should be weighed on the balance:

$$\frac{100\% \times 6\text{ mg}}{4\%} = 150\text{ mg}$$

Quantity desired (estrone): 25 mg
Multiple factor selected: 6
Aliquot portion selected: 150 mg

Estrone (25 × 6)	150 mg
Lactose	750 mg
Aliquot mixture	900 mg
Aliquot portion (900 mg ÷ 6)	150 mg of mixture will provide 25 mg estrone

Case in Point 3.2

The smallest quantity that should be weighed on the balance:

$$\frac{100\% \times 6\text{ mg}}{5\%} = 120\text{ mg}$$

(a) Quantity of mixture required to prepare 25 capsules each containing the weighable quantity of 120 mg:

120 mg × 25 (capsules) = 3000 mg

Quantity of lactose required equals the quantity of mixture required less the weight of the crushed tablets:

300 mg − 280 mg = 2720 mg or 2.72 g of lactose required

(b) Quantity of mixture to fill each capsule:

3000 mg ÷ 25 (capsules) = 120 mg

(c) Proof of 4 mg of drug per capsule:
Amount of drug in mixture:

25 mg (per tablet) × 4 (tablets) = 100 mg

Amount of drug per capsule:

100 mg ÷ 25 (capsules) = 4 mg

or,

$$\frac{100\text{ mg }(\textit{drug})}{3000\text{ mg }(\textit{mixture})} = \frac{x}{120\text{ mg }(\textit{mixture})}$$

$$= 4\text{ mg}$$

Practice Problems

Aliquot Parts by Weighing

1. Weigh	150 mg chlorpheniramine maleate
Dilute with	450 mg lactose
to make	600 mg mixture
Weigh/use	200 mg mixture
2. Weigh	120 mg drug
Dilute with	1380 mg inert powder
to make	1500 mg mixture
Weigh/use	150 mg mixture
3. Weigh	80 mg hydromorphone hydrochloride
Dilute with	1520 mg lactose
to make	1600 mg mixture
Weigh/use	100 mg mixture
4. Weigh	160 mg substance
Dilute with	3840 mg inert powder
to make	4000 mg mixture
Weigh/use	200 mg mixture
5. Weigh	400 mg substance
Dilute with	7600 mg inert powder
to make	8000 mg mixture
Weigh/use	400 mg mixture

Aliquot Parts by Measuring Volume

6. Weigh	90 mg tartar emetic
Dilute to	12 mL cherry syrup
Measure/use	2 mL mixture
7. Measure	3 mL coloring agent
Dilute to	10 mL water
Measure/use	2 mL solution
8. Measure	5 mL dye
Dilute to	8 mL water
Measure/use	2 mL solution
9. Measure	3 mL orange oil
Dilute to	8 mL alcohol
Measure/use	2 mL solution

Percentage of Error

10. 5%
11. 8%
12. 6.32%
13. 1.4%
14. 0.1%
15. 6.67%

16. (a) An analytical balance
    (b) Weigh 200 mg carvedilol and mix with 20 mL of purified water. Measure 10 mL of the mixture to provide 100 mg of carvedilol.
    (c) Eight 12.5-mg carvedilol tablets may be pulverized in a mortar with the purified water and a portion of Ora-Blend SF suspension, as needed, until smooth. The remaining portion of the suspension vehicle may then be added and blended until a uniform product results.

References

1. Prescription balances and volumetric apparatus. *United States Pharmacopeia 32 National Formulary* 27. Rockville, MD: United States Pharmacopeial Convention, 2009;1:691–692.
2. Young L, Allen LV Jr, eds. *The Art, Science, and Technology of Pharmaceutical Compounding*. 2nd Ed. Washington, DC: American Pharmaceutical Association; 2002.
3. Hormone replacement therapy. *Secundum Artem* 8(1):4. Available at: http://www.paddocklabs.com. Accessed June 6, 2012.
4. Pharmaceutical Service Division, Ministry of Health Malaysia. *Extemporaneous Formulary*. Putrajaya, Malaysia. Available at: http://www.moh-extemporaneous-formulary-2011.pdf. Accessed April 15, 2014.

4

Interpretation of Prescriptions and Medication Orders

OBJECTIVES

Upon successful completion of this chapter, the student will be able to:

- Demonstrate an understanding of the format and components of traditional prescriptions and e-prescriptions.
- Demonstrate an understanding of the format and components of a typical institutional medication order.
- Interpret common abbreviations and symbols used on prescriptions and medication orders and apply them correctly in pharmaceutical calculations.
- Apply calculations to indicate medication adherence.

By definition, a ***prescription*** is an order for medication issued by a physician, dentist, or other properly licensed medical practitioner. A prescription designates a specific medication and dosage to be prepared and dispensed by a pharmacist and administered to a particular patient.

A prescription may be written on preprinted prescription forms (traditional prescriptions) or transmitted to a pharmacy by computer (e-prescription), telephone, or facsimile (FAX). As shown in Figure 4.1, a typical preprinted prescription form contains the traditional symbol ℞ (meaning "recipe," "take thou," or "you take"), name, address, telephone number, and other pertinent information regarding the prescriber. Blank areas are used by the prescriber to provide patient information, the medication desired, and directions for use. A prescription written by a veterinarian generally includes the animal species and/or the pet's name and the name of the owner.

In hospitals and other institutions, the forms are somewhat different and are referred to as ***medication orders***. A medication order may be written (paper) or transmitted electronically. A typical paper medication order sheet is shown in Figure 4.2.

A prescription or medication order for an infant, child, or an elderly person may include the age, weight, and/or body surface area (BSA) of the patient. This information is applicable in dose calculation (as discussed in Chapter 8). An example of a prescription for a pediatric patient is shown in Figure 4.3.

A prescription may call for a prefabricated dosage form (e.g., tablet) or it may call for multiple components and require *compounding* by a pharmacist.[a] A medication may

[a]The *extemporaneous compounding* of prescriptions is an activity for which pharmacists are uniquely qualified by virtue of their education, training, and experience. "Traditional" *pharmacy compounding* involves the mixing, packaging, labeling, and dispensing of a medication upon receipt of a prescription or medication order for a specific patient. *Extended compounding* activities involve the outsourcing of compounded medications to other health care providers. *Pharmaceutical manufacturing* is the large-scale production of product for the marketplace. A distinction between these different activities is provided by legislation, guidelines, and regulations of state boards of pharmacy and the federal Food and Drug Administration.[1,2]

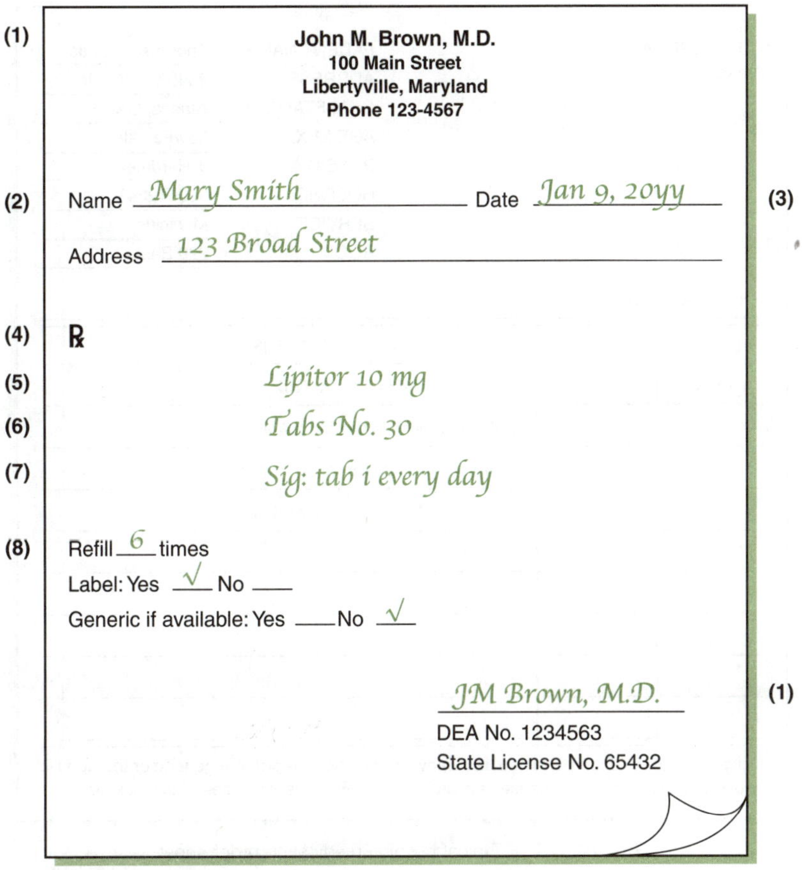
(1) John M. Brown, M.D.
100 Main Street
Libertyville, Maryland
Phone 123-4567

(2) Name Mary Smith Date Jan 9, 20yy (3)
Address 123 Broad Street

(4) ℞
(5) Lipitor 10 mg
(6) Tabs No. 30
(7) Sig: tab i every day

(8) Refill 6 times
Label: Yes √ No
Generic if available: Yes No √

JM Brown, M.D. (1)
DEA No. 1234563
State License No. 65432

FIGURE 4.1 • Components of a typical prescription. Parts labeled are as follows:
(1) Prescriber information and signature.
(2) Patient information.
(3) Date prescription was written.
(4) ℞ symbol (the Superscription), meaning "take thou," "you take," or "recipe."
(5) Medication prescribed (the Inscription).
(6) Dispensing instructions to the pharmacist (the Subscription).
(7) Directions to the patient (the Signa).
(8) Special instructions. It is important to note that for any Medicaid or Medicare prescription and according to individual state laws, a handwritten language by the prescriber, such as "Brand necessary," may be required to disallow generic substitution.
NOTE: When filling the prescription, the pharmacist adds a prescription number for identification.

be prescribed by its brand name or by the nonproprietary (*generic*) name.[b] In some cases, the product selection may be affected by pharmacy regulations and/or by provider–payer options.

Prescriptions requiring compounding include the name and quantities of each ingredient, the form into which they are to be prepared (e.g., syrup, capsules), and directions for patient use. Definitions and descriptions of dosage forms and drug delivery systems are presented in Appendix B.

[b]A brief overview of the designation of nonproprietary and brand names may be found in *Authors' Extra Point A* at the end of this chapter.

CITY HOSPITAL
Athens, GA 30600

PATIENT NAME:	Thompson, Linda
ADDRESS:	2345 Oak Circle
CITY, STATE:	Athens, GA
AGE/SEX:	35y/Female
PHYSICIAN:	J. Hardmer
HOSP.NO:	900612345
SERVICE:	Medicine
ROOM:	220 East

PHYSICIAN'S ORDER

DATE	TIME	ORDERS
02/01/yy	1200	1. Propranolol 40 mg po QID
		2. Furosemide 20 mg po q AM
		3. Flurazepam 30 mg at HS prn sleep
		4. D 5 W + 20 mEq KCl/L at 84 mL/hr
		Hardmer, MD

Unless "No substitution permitted" is clearly written after the order, a generic or therapeutic equivalent drug may be dispensed according to the Formulary policies of this hospital.

FIGURE 4.2 • Typical hospital medication order sheet.

Mary M. Brown, M.D.
Pediatric Clinic
110 Main Street
Libertyville, Maryland
Phone 456-1234

Name *Suzie Smith* Age *5* Weight *39.4* lb

Address *123 Broad Street* Date *Jan 9, 20yy*

℞ *Omnicef Oral Suspension*
125 mg/5 mL
Disp. 100 mL
Give 14 mg/kg/day x 10 days

Sig: ____ *tsp q 12 h*

Refill *0* times
Label: Yes *√* No ___
Generic if available: Yes ___ No *√*

Mary Brown, M.D.
DEA No. MB5555555
State License No. 23456

FIGURE 4.3 • Example of a prescription for a pediatric patient.

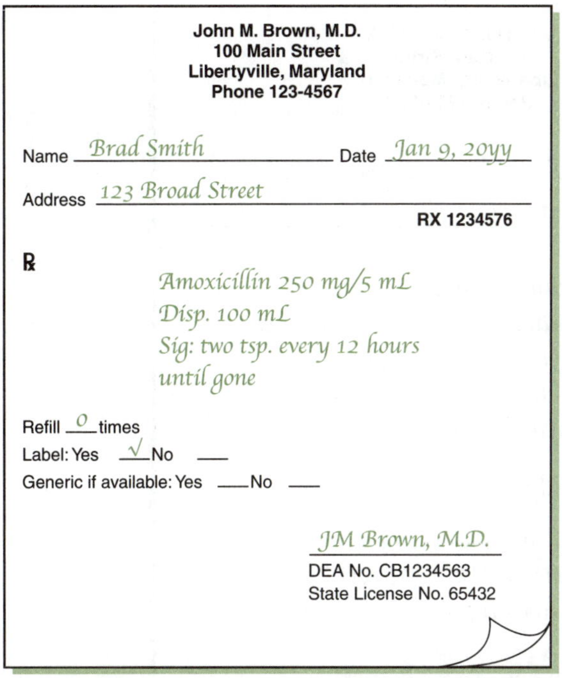

A

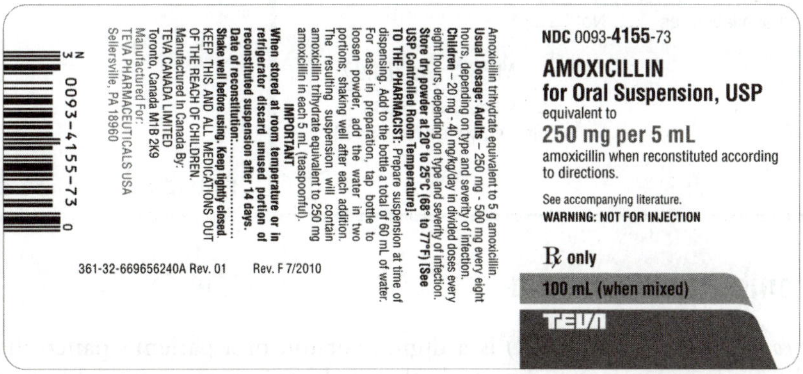

B

FIGURE 4.4 • **A.** Example of a prescription written for a generic drug. **B.** Label of product which may be used by a pharmacist in filling the prescription called for in Figure 4.4A. *(Source: http://dailymed.nlm.nih.gov/dailymed/about.cfm. Courtesy of Teva Pharmaceuticals.)*

Examples are shown for prescriptions calling for trade name products (Figs. 4.1 and 4.3), a generic drug (Fig. 4.4A), and compounding (Fig. 4.5). Figure 4.4B shows the label of a product that may be used by the pharmacist in filling the medication order as prescribed in Figure 4.4A.

Tamper-Resistant Prescription Pads

To prevent the unauthorized copying, modification, or counterfeiting of prescriptions, ***tamper-resistant prescription pads*** have been developed. The tamper-resistant qualities of these prescription forms are accomplished through the use of security paper, erase-resistant paper, thermochromatic ink (which results in the appearance of the word "VOID" on photocopies), and/or imbedded holograms.

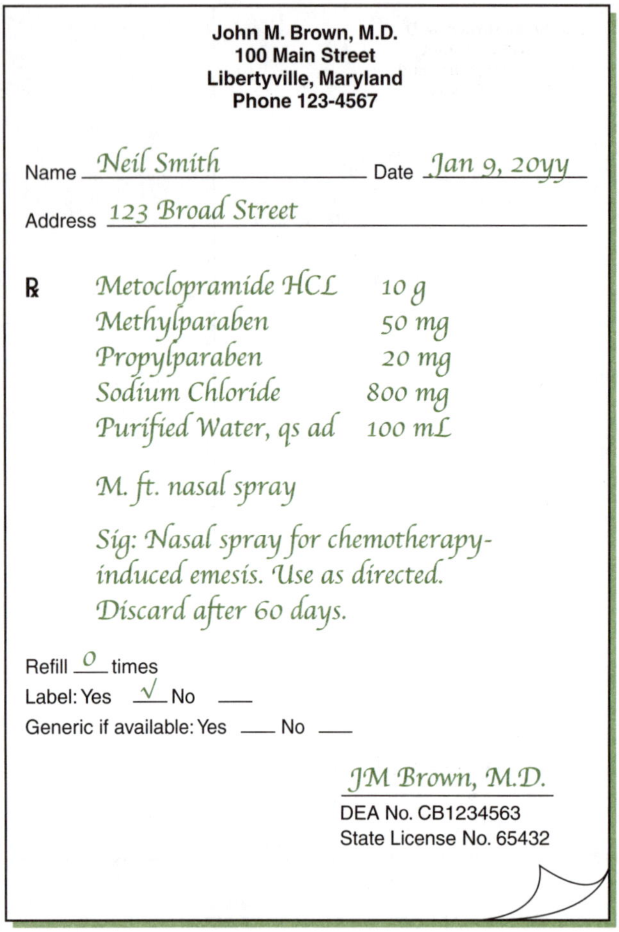

John M. Brown, M.D.
100 Main Street
Libertyville, Maryland
Phone 123-4567

Name Neil Smith Date Jan 9, 20yy

Address 123 Broad Street

℞	Metoclopramide HCL	10 g
	Methylparaben	50 mg
	Propylparaben	20 mg
	Sodium Chloride	800 mg
	Purified Water, qs ad	100 mL

M. ft. nasal spray

Sig: Nasal spray for chemotherapy-induced emesis. Use as directed. Discard after 60 days.

Refill 0 times
Label: Yes √ No __
Generic if available: Yes __ No __

JM Brown, M.D.
DEA No. CB1234563
State License No. 65432

FIGURE 4.5 • Example of a prescription requiring compounding.

Electronic Health Record

An *electronic health record* (EHR) is a digital version of a patient's paper chart. EHRs are real-time, patient-centered records that make information available instantly and securely to authorized users. An EHR can contain a patient's medical history, diagnoses, medications, treatment plans, immunization dates, allergies, radiology images, and laboratory and test results. Integrated electronic health information systems allow doctors, nurses, pharmacists, and other health care providers to appropriately access and securely share a patient's vital medical information electronically—with the intent of improving the speed, quality, safety, and cost of patient care. In the hospital and in other institutional settings, these systems include *computerized physician order entry* (CPOE) by which a physician can order medications and provide other instructions for a patient's care.

e-Prescribing/e-Prescriptions

Electronic prescribing (e-prescribing) is the computer-to-computer transfer of prescription information between authorized prescribers, pharmacies, intermediaries, and payers under nationally accepted standards.[3] In the inpatient or outpatient setting, a medication order for

Table 4.1 • SOME E-PRESCRIBING OPERATIONAL FUNCTIONS WITHIN ELECTRONIC HEALTH RECORD (EHR) SOFTWARE PROGRAMS

View Medication History
Update Medication History
Order Prescription During Patient Visit

- Select Diagnosis Associated with the Prescription
- Review Patient Coverage Information
- Select Medication & Dosage
- Enter Sig (Directions for Medication Use)
- Review Clinical Decision Support Information & Alerts
- Patient Medication Education Information Available
- Search for and Select Patient's Preferred Pharmacy
- Submit Prescription Electronically

Approve Prescription Requests/Renewals

a patient is entered into an automated data entry system as a personal computer or a handheld device loaded with ***e-prescribing*** software and sent to a pharmacy as an ***e-prescription***. Some e-prescribing operational functions within EHR software programs are displayed in Table 4.1. When an e-prescription is received in the pharmacy, it is printed out as the illustration shown in Figure 4.6.

XYZ PHARMACY SYSTEM
Electronically Transmitted to Smith Pharmacy
1234 Broad Street
Anytown, State, Zip

Date: 10/20/20yy
Rx # 9876543 ID # 11223344

Patient Information
Last Name: Jones
First Name: Mary
DOB: 10/18/YY Phone: (XXX)-888-7777
Sex: F
Address: 567 King Street
Anytown, State, Zip

Drug, SIG, and Refill Information
Drug Name: Gabapentin
Strength: 100 mg
Quantity: 60 Dose Form: capsules
SIG: Take 1 capsule at bedtime
Refills: 6
Label: yes

Prescriber Information
Last Name: Brown
First Name: James M
Address: 100 Main Street
Anytown, State, Zip
DEA: CB1234XXX
NPI: 9876543XXX

FIGURE 4.6 • Illustration of an electronically transmitted prescription as received by a pharmacy. (DEA, Drug Enforcement Administration; NPI, National Provider Identifier.)

Among the advantages cited for *e-prescriptions* over traditional paper prescriptions are reduced errors due to prescription legibility, concurrent software screens for drug allergies and drug interactions, integrated information exchange between health care providers, reduced incidence of altered or forged prescriptions, efficiency for both prescriber and pharmacist, and convenience to the patient, whose prescription would likely be ready for pickup upon arrival at the pharmacy.[4,5]

Additional e-prescribing images are displayed in *Authors' Extra Point B* at the end of this chapter.

Hospital and Other Institutional Medication Order Forms

As noted previously, a typical *paper medication order form* used in the hospital setting is shown in Figure 4.2. In addition, other forms may be used within a hospital by specialized units such as infectious disease, cardiac care, pediatrics, obstetrics, orthopedics, and others.[6] Drug-specific forms also may be used, as for heparin dosing, electrolyte infusions, and morphine sulfate in patient-controlled anesthesia. An example of the latter is shown in Figure 4.7.

Other types of patient care facilities, such as outpatient clinics, intermediate- and long-term care facilities (Fig. 4.8), cancer treatment centers, and others, utilize institution-specific forms for medication orders.

City Hospital

Patient Controlled Anesthesia (PCA) Orders

MORPHINE SULFATE INJECTION, 1 mg/mL

Patient Information (Label)

Physician:

Date: Time:

1. Mode (check) ☐PCA ☐Continuous ☐PCA & Continuous

			DOSING GUIDELINES
2. PCA Dose	= ________	mL (mg)	1 mL (1 mg)
3. Period between Injections	= ________	minutes	10 minutes
4. Basal (Continuous) Rate	= ________	mL (mg)/hr	1 mL (1 mg)/hr
5. One-Hour Limit	= ________	mL (mg)	7 mL (7 mg)
6. Initial Loading Dose	= ________	mL (mg)	2-5 mL (2-5 mg)

7. Additional Instructions:

Physician's Signature ____________________________

FIGURE 4.7 • Example of a hospital form for prescribing a specific drug treatment: patient-controlled anesthesia. *(Adapted from* www.hospital-forms.com. *Ref.*[6]*)*

MEDICATION ORDER FORM CITY NURSING HOME *Physician's Orders*					
Attending Physician:			Order Number: (preprinted)		
Resident's Name:				Room Number:	
DRUG	QUANTITY	DOSE AND ROUTE	FREQUENCY	DIAGNOSIS	ADMINISTRATION TIMES
1.					____AM ____PM ____AM ____PM
2.					____AM ____PM ____AM ____PM
3.					____AM ____PM ____AM ____PM
4.					____AM ____PM ____AM ____PM
Physician's Signature:				Time/Date Ordered:	
Signature of Nurse Receiving Order:				Time/Date Ordered:	
Ordered from Pharmacy, Time/Date:				Received from Pharmacy, Time/Date:	

FIGURE 4.8 • Example of a nursing home medication order form.

Paper medication forms in most health care institutions have been largely replaced by *computerized physician order entry* (CPOE) as a part of the transition to EHR systems (EHRs).

Military Time

Military time is used not only in the military but in civilian life as well, such as in hospitals, law enforcement, and emergency services. Its use provides an unambiguous expression of time. In health care institutions, military time may be used to record the time of a patient's admission, when a medication was administered, the time of surgery, and so forth.

Table 4.2 compares the expressions of military time and regular time. Military time is verbalized, as for example, "twenty-three hundred hours." Colons may be used to separate hours and minutes, as 1331 or 13:31 hours (31 minutes past 1 o'clock in the afternoon), and when desired seconds, as 1331:42 or 13:31:42.

Form of Compounded Prescriptions

The quantities of ingredients designated on prescriptions to be compounded are written using SI metric units as illustrated in the examples below.

In prescription writing, the decimal point may be replaced by a vertical line to designate whole or decimal fractions of grams or milliliters. If the designations "g" or "mL" are absent, as in the second illustration, they are presumed. Unless otherwise noted, solid materials are presumed to be grams and liquids, milliliters.

Table 4.2 • COMPARATIVE EXPRESSIONS OF REGULAR AND MILITARY TIME

Regular Time	Military Time	Regular Time	Military Time
Midnight	0000	Noon	1200
1:00 AM	0100	1:00 PM	1300
2:00 AM	0200	2:00 PM	1400
3:00 AM	0300	3:00 PM	1500
4:00 AM	0400	4:00 PM	1600
5:00 AM	0500	5:00 PM	1700
6:00 AM	0600	6:00 PM	1800
7:00 AM	0700	7:00 PM	1900
8:00 AM	0800	8:00 PM	2000
9:00 AM	0900	9:00 PM	2100
10:00 AM	1000	10:00 PM	2200
11:00 AM	1100	11:00 PM	2300

Illustration of prescriptions written in SI metric units:

℞	Acetylsalicylic acid	4 g
	Phenacetin	0.8 g
	Codeine sulfate	0.5 g
	Mix and make capsules no. 20	
	Sig. one capsule every 4 hours	

℞	Dextromethorphan	0	18
	Guaifenesin syrup	1	2
	Alcohol	2	1
	Flavored syrup ad	60	
	Sig. 5 mL as needed for cough		

Prescription and Medication Order Accuracy and Verification

It is the responsibility of the pharmacist to ensure that each prescription and medication order received is correct in its form and content, is appropriate for the patient being treated, and is subsequently filled, labeled, dispensed, and administered accurately. In essence, each medication should be:

- Therapeutically appropriate for the patient
- Prescribed at the correct dose
- Dispensed in the correct strength and dosage form
- Correctly labeled with complete instructions for the patient or caregiver
- For the patient in a hospital or other health care facility, each medication must be administered to the correct patient, at the correct time, and by the correct rate and route of administration

Medication verification is the term used when there is a process in place to assure the above bullet points. It is performed initially through the careful reading, filling (including calculations), checking, and dispensing of the prescription or medication order. The process often is enhanced by technologies, as the computer matching of a drug package bar code with the prescription order and/or by matching the drug's bar code to a patient's coded wrist band in a patient care facility (termed *bedside medication verification*).

Errors and Omissions

To ensure such accuracy, the pharmacist is obliged to review each prescription (both traditional and e-prescription) and medication order in a step-by-step manner to detect errors and omissions. *If there is any question regarding a prescription or medication order, the pharmacist must seek clarification from the prescriber.*

Among the items that the pharmacist should check for the correct reading and interpretation of a prescription or medication order are as follows:

- Prescriber information, including address and telephone number, Drug Enforcement Administration (DEA) number (for authority to prescribe schedule drugs including narcotics), state license number and/or the National Provider Identifier (NPI), an identification number for participating health care providers, and signature
- Date of the order and its currency to the request for filling
- Patient identification information and, if pertinent to dose determination, the patient's age, weight, and/or other parameters
- Drug prescribed, including dose, preparation strength, dosage form, and quantity
- Clarity of any abbreviations, symbols, and/or units of measure
- Clarity and completeness of directions for use by the patient or caregiver
- Refill and/or generic substitution authorization
- Need for special labeling, such as expiration date, conditions for storage, and foods and/or other medications not to take concomitantly
- A listing of the ingredients and quantities for orders to be compounded

Once the prescription or medication order is filled and the label prepared, before dispensing, the pharmacist should make certain of the following:

- The filled prescription or medication order contains the correct drug, strength, dosage form, and quantity. Placing a medication's indication (use) on the prescription label has been shown to be of benefit in understanding of the use of their medication for some patients, particularly older patients and those taking multiple medications.[7] The bar coding of pharmaceutical products used in hospital settings is required by the federal Food and Drug Administration (FDA) as an added protection to ensure accurate product dispensing and administration (Fig. 4.9).
- The pharmacy-imprinted serial number on the label matches that on the order.
- The label has the name of the correct patient and physician; the correct drug name, quantity, and strength; the name or initials of the pharmacist who filled the order; and the number of refills remaining. Additional label information and/or auxiliary labels may be required.

It is important that the instructions for use by the patient be clearly understood. This may require that the pharmacist add words of clarity to the labeled instructions. For example, instead of "Take two tablets daily," the directions might indicate whether the two tablets are to be taken at once or at separate and specified times. In addition, if the patient or caregiver has difficulty with the language, verbal reinforcement may be required.

Refer to the prescription shown in Figure 4.4A to identify any errors and/or omissions in the following prescription label.

Main Street Pharmacy
150 Main Street
Libertyville, Maryland
Phone 456-1432

℞ 1234576	Jan 10, 20yy
Brad Smith	Dr. J. M. Brown
Take 2 teaspoonfuls every 12 hours.	
Ampicillin 250 mg/5 mL	100 mL
Refills: 0	Pharmacist: AB

Error: Drug name incorrect.
Omission: Directions incomplete.

NOTE*:* There would be a serious question of whether the patient received the correct medication.

Additional examples of errors and omissions are presented in the practice problems at the end of the chapter.

Use of Roman Numerals on Prescriptions

Roman numerals commonly are used in prescription writing to designate *quantities*, as the (1) quantity of medication to be dispensed and/or (2) quantity of medication to be taken by the patient per dose.

The student may recall the eight letters of fixed values used in the Roman system:

ss	=	½	L or l	=	50
i or j	=	1	C or c	=	100
V or v	=	5	D or d	=	500
X or x	=	10	M or m	=	1000

The student also may recall that the following rules apply in the use of Roman numerals:

(1) A letter repeated once or more repeats its value (e.g., xx = 20; xxx = 30).
(2) One or more letters placed *after* a letter of greater value *increases* the value of the greater letter (e.g., vi = 6; xij = 12; lx = 60).
(3) A letter placed *before* a letter of greater value *decreases* the value of the greater letter (e.g., iv = 4; xl = 40).
(4) Use the simplest choice among the possible options. For instance, to indicate the number 60, "lx" would be preferred over "xxxxxx."

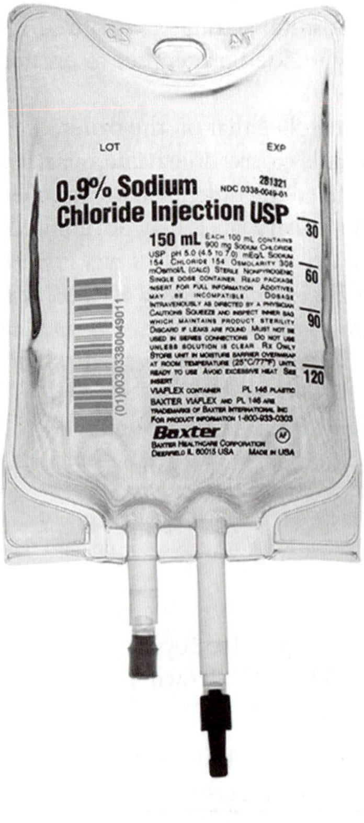

FIGURE 4.9 • Example of a product bar code used on pharmaceuticals for positive drug identification to reduce medication errors. *(Courtesy of Baxter Healthcare Corporation.)*

Capital or lowercase letters may be used. Dotting the lowercase "i" or placement of a horizontal line above the "i" with the dot atop serves to avoid misinterpretation. A "j" may be used as the final "i" in a sequence (e.g., viij). Additional examples are:

iv = 4	xl = 40	cdxl = 440	cmxcix = 999
viii = 8	xc = 90	lxxii = 72	MCDXCII = 1492
xii = 12	cl = 150	cxxvi = 126	mdclxvi = 1666
xxiv = 24	lxiv = 64	lxxxiv = 84	mm = 2000

When Roman numerals are used, the tradition of placing the numerals after the term or symbol generally is followed (e.g., capsules no. xxiv; fluid ounces xij).

Use of Abbreviations and Symbols

Although reduced by the transition to e-prescribing, the use of abbreviations remains on prescriptions and medication orders. Many prescription abbreviations are derived from the Latin through its historical use in medicine and pharmacy, whereas others have evolved through prescribers' use of writing shortcuts. A list of some of these abbreviations is presented in Table 4.3. Unfortunately, medication errors can result from the misuse, misinterpretation, and illegible writing of abbreviations and through the use of *ad hoc*, or made-up, abbreviations. The use of a controlled vocabulary, a reduction in the use of abbreviations, care in the writing of decimal points, and the proper use of leading and terminal zeros have been urged to help reduce medication errors.[8–10]

Among the specific recommendations to help reduce medication errors arising from poorly written, illegible, or misinterpreted prescriptions and medication orders are the following[8–10]:

- *A whole number should be shown without a decimal point and without a terminal zero (e.g., express 4 milligrams as 4 mg and not as 4.0 mg).*
- *A quantity smaller than one should be shown with a zero preceding the decimal point (e.g., express two tenths of a milligram as 0.2 mg and not as .2 mg).*
- *Leave a space between a number and the unit (e.g., 10 mg and not 10mg).*
- *Use whole numbers when possible and not equivalent decimal fractions (e.g., use 100 mg and not 0.1 g).*
- *Use the full names of drugs and not abbreviations (e.g., use phenobarbital and not PB).*
- *Use USP designations for units of measure (e.g., for grams, use g and not Gm or gms; for milligrams, use mg and not mgs or mgm).*
- *Spell out "units" (e.g., use 100 units and not 100 u or 100 U since an illegible U may be misread as a zero, resulting in a 10-fold error, i.e., 1000). The abbreviation I.U., which stands for "International Units," should also be spelled out so it is not interpreted as I.V., meaning "intravenous."*
- *Certain abbreviations that could be mistaken for other abbreviations should be written out (e.g., write "right eye" or "left eye" rather than use o.d. or o.l., and spell out "right ear" and "left ear" rather than use a.d. or a.l.).*
- *Spell out "every day," rather than use q.d.; "every other day," rather than q.o.d; "four times a day," rather than q.i.d; and "three times a week," rather than t.i.w. to avoid misinterpretation.*
- *Avoid using d for "day" or "dose" because of the profound difference between terms, as in mg/kg/day versus mg/kg/dose.*
- *Integrate capital or "tall man" letters to distinguish between "look-alike" drug names, such as AggraSTAT and AggreNOX, hydrOXYZINE and hydrALAZINE, and DIGoxin and DESoxyn.*
- *Amplify the prescriber's directions on the prescription label when needed for clarity (e.g., use "Swallow one (1) capsule with water in the morning" rather than "one cap in a.m.").*

Table 4.3 • SELECTED ABBREVIATIONS, ACRONYMS, AND SYMBOLS USED IN PRESCRIPTIONS AND MEDICATION ORDERS[a–c]

Abbreviation (Latin Origin[d])	Meaning
Prescription-Filling Directions	
aa. (*ana*)	of each
ad (*ad*)	up to; to make
disp. (*dispensatur*)	dispense
div. (*dividatur*)	divide
d.t.d. (*dentur tales doses*)	give of such doses
ft (*fiat*)	make
M. (*mice*)	mix
No. (*numero*)	number
non rep. or NR (*non repatatur*)	do not repeat
q.s. (*quantum sufficit*)	a sufficient quantity
q.s. ad (*quantum sufficiat ad*)	a sufficient quantity to make
Sig. (*Signa*)	write (directions on label)
Quantities and Measurement	
BSA	body surface area
cm^3	cubic centimeter or milliliter (mL)
f or fl (*fluidus*)	fluid
flʒ or fʒ[e]	fluid dram
fl℥ss or f℥*ss*[e]	half-fluid ounce
g	gram
gal	gallon
gtt (*gutta*)	drop
I.U. or IU[b]	international unit(s)
lb (*libra*)	pound
kg	kilogram
L	liter
m^2 or M^2	square meter
mcg	microgram
mEq	milliequivalent
mg	milligram
mg/kg	milligrams (of drug) per kilogram (of body weight)
mg/m^2	milligrams (of drug) per square meter (of body surface area)
mIU or milli-IU	thousandth of an international unit
MIU[b]	million international units
mL	milliliter
mL/h	milliliters (of drug administered) per hour (as through intravenous administration)
mOsm or mOsmol	milliosmoles
oz.	ounce
pt.	pint
qt.	quart
ss or $\overline{ss}$ (*semissem*)	one-half
tbsp.	tablespoonful
tsp.	teaspoonful
Signa/Patient Instructions	
a.c. (*ante cibos*)	before meals
ad lib. (*ad libitum*)	at pleasure, freely
admin	administer
am (*ante meridiem*)	morning
aq. (*aqua*)	water
ATC	around the clock
b.i.d. (*bis in die*)	twice a day
c or $\bar{c}$ (*cum*)	with
d (*die*)	day
dil. (*dilutus*)	dilute
et	and
h. or hr. (*hora*)	hour
h.s. (*hora somni*)	at bedtime
i.c. (*inter cibos*)	between meals
min. (*minutum*)	minute
m&n	morning and night
N&V	nausea and vomiting
noct. (*nocte*)	night
NPO (*non per os*)	nothing by mouth
p.c. (*post cibos*)	after meals
pm (*post meridiem*)	afternoon; evening
p.o. (*per os*)	by mouth (orally)
p.r.n. (*pro re nata*)	as needed
q (*quaque*)	every
qAM	every morning
q4h, q8h, etc.	every (*number*) hours
q.i.d. (*quarter in die*)	four times a day
rep. (*repetatur*)	repeat
s (*sine*)	without
s.i.d. (*semel in die*)	once a day
s.o.s. (*si opus sit*)	if there is need; as needed
stat. (*stamin*)	immediately
t.i.d. (*ter in die*)	three times a day
ut dict. (*ut dictum*)	as directed
wk.	week
Medications	
APAP	acetaminophen
ASA	aspirin
AZT	zidovudine
EES	erythromycin ethylsuccinate
HC	hydrocortisone
HCTZ	hydrochlorothiazide
MTX	methotrexate
NSAID	nonsteroidal anti-inflammatory drug
NTG	nitroglycerin
Clinical	
Afib	atrial fibrillation
ADR	adverse drug reaction

Table 4.3 • SELECTED ABBREVIATIONS, ACRONYMS, AND SYMBOLS USED IN PRESCRIPTIONS AND MEDICATION ORDERS[a–c] *(Continued)*

Abbreviation (Latin Origin[d])	Meaning
BM	bowel movement
BP	blood pressure
BS	blood sugar
CAD	coronary artery disease
CHD	coronary heart disease
CHF	congestive heart failure
COPD	chronic obstructive pulmonary disease
GERD	gastrointestinal reflux disease
CRF	chronic renal failure
CV	cardiovascular
ENT	ears, nose, and throat
GI	gastrointestinal
GFR	glomerular filtration rate
GU	genitourinary
HA	headache
HBP	heart rate
HR	high blood pressure
HRT	hormone replacement therapy
HT or HTN	hypertension
IOP	intraocular pressure
MI	myocardial ischemia/infarction
OA	osteoarthritis
Pt	patient
QL	quality of life
RA	rheumatoid arthritis
SOB	shortness of breath
TPN	total parenteral nutrition
UA	urine analysis
URI	upper respiratory infection
UTI	urinary tract infection
Dosage Forms/Vehicles	
amp.	ampul
cap.	capsule
D5LR	dextrose 5% in lactated Ringer's
D5NS	dextrose 5% in normal saline (0.9% sodium chloride)
D5W	dextrose 5% in water
D10W	dextrose 10% in water
elix.	elixir
inj.	injection
NS	normal saline
½NS	half-strength normal saline
oint or ungt. (*unguentum*)	ointment
pulv. (*pulvis*)	powder
RL, R/L or LR	Ringer's lactate or lactated Ringer's
sol. (*solutio*)	solution
supp. (*suppositorium*)	suppository
susp.	suspension
syr. (*syrupus*)	syrup
tab. (*tabletta*)	tablet
Routes/Location of Administration	
a.d. (*auris dextro*)	right ear
a.s. (*auris sinistro*)	left ear
a.u. (*auris utro*)	each ear (both)
CIVI	continuous (24 hours) intravenous infusion
ID	intradermal
inj	injection
IM	intramuscular
IT	intrathecal
IV	intravenous
IVB	intravenous bolus
IV drip	intravenous infusion
IVP	intravenous push
IVPB	intravenous piggyback
NGT	nasogastric tube
o.d. (*oculo dextro*)	right eye
o.s. (*oculo sinistro*)	left eye
o.u. (*oculo utro*)	each eye (both)
p.o. or PO (*per os*)	by mouth
rect. (or *pro recto*)	rectal or rectum
SL	sublingual
SubQ or SC	subcutaneously
Top.	topically
V or PV (*pro vagina*)	vaginally

[a]The abbreviations set in **boldface type** are considered most likely to appear on prescriptions. It is suggested that these be learned first.

[b]In practice, periods and/or capital letters may or may not be used with the abbreviations. Some abbreviations, acronyms, and symbols have medication error risks associated with their use. Therefore, the Institute for Safe Medication Practices (ISMP) and the Joint Commission on Accreditation of Healthcare Organizations (JCAHO) have issued a list of items prohibited from use and others considered for prohibition (see text).[8] These designated items are not included in Table 4.3, with the exception of *hs, I.U., MIU, subQ, AZT,* and *HCTZ,* which are included for instructional purpose due to their remaining use in practice.

[c]A database of acronyms and abbreviations related to Food and Drug Administration (FDA) may be found at http://www.fda.gov/AboutFDA/FDAAcronymsAbbreviations/ucm070296.htm.

[d]Muldoon HC. *Pharmaceutical Latin.* 4th Ed. New York: John Wiley & Sons, 1952.

[e]A fluid dram (flʒ) is 1/8th of a fluid ounce (29.57 mL) or ≈3.69 mL; however, when the dram symbol is written in the *signa* portion of a prescription, the prescriber may intend the interpretation to be "teaspoonful." Similarly, when a half-ounce symbol (f℥*ss*) is indicated in the *signa*, a "tablespoon" or 15 mL may be intended.

The Institute for Safe Medication Practices (ISMP) regularly publishes a list of abbreviations, symbols, and dose designations that it recommends for consideration for discontinuance of use.[9]

The portions of the prescription presenting directions to the pharmacist (the Subscription) and the directions to the patient (the Signa) commonly contain abbreviated forms of English or Latin terms as well as Arabic and Roman numerals. The correct interpretation of these abbreviations and prescription notations plays an important part in pharmaceutical calculations and thus in the accurate filling and dispensing of medication.

Although described fully in Chapter 7, it should be noted here that when appearing in the Signa, the symbol ʒi, *5 mL*, and the abbreviation *tsp.* are each taken to mean "one teaspoonful," and the symbol ℥ *ss*, *15 mL*, and the abbreviation *tbsp.* are each taken to mean "one tablespoonful."

> AUTHORS' NOTE: some abbreviations used in this chapter may appear only infrequently in practice and are included here for instructional purposes.

Examples of prescription directions to the pharmacist:

(a) *M. ft. ung.*
Mix and make an ointment.

(b) *Ft. sup. no xii*
Make 12 suppositories.

(c) *M. ft. cap. d.t.d. no. xxiv*
Mix and make capsules. Give 24 such doses.

Examples of prescription directions to the patient:

(a) *Caps. i. q.i.d. p.c. et h.s.*
Take one (1) capsule four (4) times a day after each meal and at bedtime.

(b) *gtt. ii rt. eye every a.m.*
Instill two (2) drops in the right eye every morning.

(c) *tab. ii stat tab. 1 q. 6 h. × 7 d.*
Take two (2) tablets immediately, then take one (1) tablet every 6 hours for 7 days.

CASE IN POINT 4.1 A pharmacist received the following prescription, which requires the correct interpretation of abbreviations prior to engaging in calculations, compounding, labeling, and dispensing.

℞	Lisinopril	
	Hydrochlorothiazide aa.	10 mg
	Calcium phosphate	40 mg
	Lactose q.s. ad	300 mg
	M.ft. cap. i D.T.D. # 30	
	Sig: cap. i AM a.c.	

(a) How many milligrams each of lisinopril and hydrochlorothiazide are required to fill the prescription?

(b) What is the weight of lactose required?

(c) Translate the label directions to the patient.

Medication Scheduling, Medication Adherence, and Medication Disposal

Medication scheduling may be defined as the frequency (i.e., times per day) and duration (i.e., length of treatment) of a drug's prescribed or recommended use. Some medications, because of their physical, chemical, or biological characteristics or their dosage formulations, may be taken just once daily for optimum benefit, whereas other drug products must be taken two, three, four, or more times daily for the desired effect. Frequency of medication scheduling is also influenced by the patient's physical condition and the nature and severity of the illness or condition being treated. Some conditions, such as indigestion, may require a single dose of medication for correction. Other conditions, such as a systemic infection, may require multiple daily, around-the-clock dosing for 10 days or more. Long-term maintenance therapy for conditions such as diabetes and high blood pressure may require daily dosing for life.

For optimum benefit of the medications prescribed, it is incumbent on the patient to adhere to the prescribed dosage regimen.

Medication adherence (formerly referred to as *compliance*) indicates a patient's following of the instructions for taking the medication prescribed, including the correct dose, dosing frequency, and duration of treatment. ***Medication nonadherence*** is a patient's failure to adhere or comply with the instructions.

Patient nonadherence may result from a number of factors, including unclear or misunderstood directions, undesired side effects of the drug that discourage use, lack of patient confidence in the drug and/or prescriber, discontinued use because the patient feels better or worse, economic reasons based on the cost of the medication, absence of patient counseling and understanding of the need for and means of compliance, confusion over taking multiple medications, and other factors. Frequently, patients forget whether they have taken their medications. Special compliance aids are available to assist patients in their proper scheduling of medications. These devices include medication calendars, reminder charts, special containers, and smartphone apps.

Patient nonadherence is not entirely the problem of ambulatory or noninstitutionalized patients. Patients in hospitals, nursing homes, and other inpatient settings are generally more compliant because of the efforts of health care personnel who are assigned the responsibility of issuing and administering medication on a prescribed schedule. Even in these settings, however, a scheduled dose of medication may be omitted or administered incorrectly or in an untimely fashion because of human error or oversight.

The consequences of patient nonadherence may include worsening of the condition, the requirement of additional and perhaps more expensive and extensive treatment methods or surgical procedures, otherwise unnecessary hospitalization, and increased total health care cost. Students interested in additional information on medication adherence are referred to other sources of information.[11–13]

Medication nonadherence has been measured in a number of ways, including by biological sample (i.e., determining medication blood levels), patient surveys, monitoring the on-time refilling of prescriptions, examining prescription drug claim (insurance) data, and by other means.

Consider the following illustrations.

(1) ℞ Hydrochlorothiazide 50 mg
Tablets No. XC
Sig. i q AM for HBP

If the prescription was filled initially on April 15, on about what date should the patient return to have the prescription refilled?

Answer: 90 tablets, taken 1 per day, should last 90 days, or approximately 3 months, and the patient should return to the pharmacy on or shortly before July 15 of the same year.

(2) ℞ Penicillin V Potassium Oral Solution 125 mg/5 mL
Disp. ______ mL
Sig. 5 mL q 6 h ATC × 10 d

How many milliliters of medicine should be dispensed?

Answer: 5 mL times 4 (doses per day) equals 20 mL times 10 (days) equals 200 mL.

A pharmacist may calculate a patient's percent compliance rate as follows:

$$\% \text{ Compliance rate} = \frac{\text{Number of days supply of medication}}{\text{Number of days since last Rx refill}} \times 100$$

(3) *What is the percent compliance rate if a patient received a 30-day supply of medicine and returned in 45 days for a refill?*

$$\% \text{ Compliance rate} = \frac{30 \text{ days}}{45 \text{ days}} \times 100 = \mathbf{66.6\%}$$

In determining the patient's actual (rather than apparent) compliance rate, it is important to determine if the patient had available and used extra days' dosage from some previous filling of the prescription.

Medication disposal is an important consideration for safety and environmental concerns. Medications that are no longer used or out of date may be disposed of by the following methods: (a) "take back" programs for disposal by pharmacies; (b) mixing medications with kitty litter, coffee grounds, or other such materials and disposing along with household trash; and (c) flushing medications down the drain for specific drugs as approved by the FDA.[14]

CASE IN POINT 4.2 A 72-year-old male who is diabetic is admitted to the emergency room with shortness of breath and general weakness. Tests reveal anemia, hypotension, atrial fibrillation, and coronary artery blockage. During 2 weeks of hospitalization, the patient receives intravenous infusions, oral medications, and blood transfusions; four cardiovascular stents are inserted; and the patient is discharged with the following prescriptions:

Clopidogrel bisulfate (PLAVIX) tablets, 75 mg, 1 tab q.d.
Pioglitazone hydrochloride (ACTOS) tablets, 15 mg, 1 tab q.d.
Pantoprazole sodium (PROTONIX) tablets, 40 mg, 1 tab b.i.d.
Simvastatin (ZOCOR) tablets 40 mg, 1 tab q.d. h.s.
HUMULIN 70/30, inject 35 units q.d. am and 45 units q.d. pm
Carvedilol (COREG) tablets, 3.125 mg 1 tab b.i.d. × 2 wk; then 6.25 mg 1 tab b.i.d.
Amiodarone hydrochloride (CORDARONE) tablets, 200 mg, 2 tabs b.i.d. × 7 d; then 1 tab b.i.d. × 7 d; then 1 tab q.d.
Duloxetine hydrochloride (CYMBALTA) capsules, 30 mg, 1 cap q.d. × 7 d; then 1 cap b.i.d.

(a) How many total tablets and capsules would the patient initially be taking daily?
(b) If HUMULIN contains 100 units per milliliter, how many milliliters would be administered each morning and each evening?
(c) How many CORDARONE tablets would constitute a 30-day supply?
(d) If 60 CYMBALTA capsules were initially dispensed and the patient requested a refill after 17 days, is *medication nonadherence* and thus the patient's well-being a reasonable concern? Show calculations.

PRACTICE PROBLEMS

Authors' Note: some abbreviations used in these practice problems may appear only infrequently in practice and are included here for instructional purposes.

1. Interpret each of the following *Subscriptions* (directions to the pharmacist) taken from prescriptions:
   (a) Disp. supp. rect. no. xii
   (b) M. ft. iso. sol. Disp. 120 mL
   (c) M. et div. in pulv. no. xl
   (d) DTD vi. Non rep.
   (e) M. et ft. ung. Disp. 10 g
   (f) M. et ft. caps. DTD xlviii
   (g) M. et ft. susp. 1 g/tbsp. Disp. 60 mL
   (h) Ft. cap. #1. DTD no.xxxvi N.R.
   (i) M. et ft. pulv. DTD #C
   (j) M. et ft. I.V. inj.
   (k) Label: hydrocortisone, 20 mg tabs
2. Interpret each of the following *Signas* (directions to the patient) taken from prescriptions:
   (a) Gtt. ii each eye q. 4 h. p.r.n. pain.
   (b) Tbsp. i in ⅓ gl. aq. q. 6 h
   (c) Appl. am & pm for pain prn.
   (d) Gtt. iv right ear m. & n.
   (e) Tsp. i ex aq. q. 4 or 5 h. p.r.n. pain
   (f) Appl. ung. left eye ad lib.
   (g) Caps i c aq. h.s. N.R.
   (h) Gtt. v each ear 3 × d. s.o.s.
   (i) Tab. i sublingually, rep. p.r.n.
   (j) Instill gtt. ii each eye of neonate
   (k) Dil. c = vol. aq. and use as gargle q. 5 h
   (l) Cap. ii 1 h. prior to departure, then cap. i after 12 h
   (m) Tab i p.r.n. SOB
   (n) Tab i qAM HBP
   (o) Tab ii q 6 h ATC UTI
   (p) ʒii 4 × d p.c. & h.s.
   (q) ℥ss a.c. t.i.d.
   (r) Add crushed tablet to pet's food s.i.d.
3. Interpret each of the following taken from medication orders:
   (a) AMBIEN 10 mg p.o. qhs × 5 d
   (b) 1000 mL D5W q. 8 h. IV c 20 mEq KC1 to every third bottle
   (c) Admin. prochlorperazine 10 mg IM q. 3 h. prn N&V
   (d) Minocycline HCl susp. 1 tsp p.o. q.i.d. DC after 5 d
   (e) Propranolol HCl 10 mg p.o. t.i.d. a.c. & h.s.
   (f) NPH U-100 insulin 40 units subc every day am
   (g) Cefamandole nafate 250 mg IM q12h
   (h) Potassium chloride 15 mEq p.o. b.i.d. p.c.
   (i) Vincristine sulfate 1 mg/m^2 pt. BSA
   (j) Flurazepam 30 mg at HS prn sleep
   (k) D5W + 20 mEq KCl/L at 84 mL/h
   (l) 2.5 g/kg/day amino acids TPN
   (m) Epoetin alfa (PROCRIT) stat. 150 units/kg subQ. 3 × wk. × 3–4 wks

(n) MTX 2.5 mg tab t.i.d. 1 ×/wk
(o) HCTZ tabs 12.5 mg q.d. am

4. (a) If a 10-mL vial of insulin contains 100 units of insulin per milliliter, and a patient is to administer 20 units daily, how many days will the product last the patient? (b) If the patient returned to the pharmacy in exactly 7 weeks for another vial of insulin, was the patient compliant as indicated by the percent compliance rate?
5. A prescription is to be taken as follows: 1 tablet q.i.d. the first day; 1 tablet t.i.d. the second day; 1 tablet b.i.d. × 5 d; and 1 tablet q.d. thereafter. How many tablets should be dispensed to equal a 30-day supply?
6. In preparing the prescription in Figure 4.3, the pharmacist calculated and labeled the dose as "1 teaspoonful every 12 hours." Is this correct or in error?
7. Refer to Figure 4.1 and identify any errors or omissions in the following prescription label:

> Patient: Mary Smith Dr. JM Brown
> Date: Jan 9, 20yy
> Take 1 capsule every day in the morning
> Refills: 5

8. Refer to Figure 4.4A and identify any errors or omissions in the following prescription label:

> Patient: Brad Smith Dr. JM Brown
> Date: Jan 9, 20yy
> Take two (2) teaspoonfuls every twelve (12) hours until all of the medicine is gone
> Amoxicillin 250 mL/5 mL
> Refills: 0

9. Refer to Figure 4.5 and identify any errors or omissions in the following prescription label:

> Patient: Brad Smith Dr. JM Brown
> Date: Jan 9, 20yy
> Nasal spray for chemotherapy-induced emesis. Use as directed. Discard after 60 days.
> Metoclopramide HCl
> 10 g/100 mL Nasal Spray
> Refills: 0

10. Refer to Figure 4.2 and identify any errors or omissions in a transcribed order for the first three drugs in the medication order:
(a) Propranolol, 40 mg orally every day
(b) Flutamide, 20 mg orally every morning
(c) Flurazepam, 30 mg at bedtime as needed for sleep
11. Refer to Figure 4.6 and identify any errors in the following prescription label:

> Patient: Mary Jones Dr. JM Brown
> Date: Oct 20, 20yy
> Swallow one (1) capsule at bedtime.
> Gabapentin 100 mg
> 10 g/100 mL Nasal Spray
> Rx: 9876543 Refills: 6

12. In a clinical study of drug–drug interactions, the following drugs were coadministered:
    Ritonavir: 600 mg b.i.d. p.o. × 7 d
    Theophylline: 3 mg/kg q8h × 7 d
    Translate the directions
13. Translate "10 mIU/mL."
14. The package insert for interferon alpha-2b states the dose based on body surface area (BSA) for the treatment of hepatitis B as *3 MIU/m² TIW for the first week of therapy followed by dose escalation to 6 MIU/m² TIW (maximum of 10 MIU/m² TIW) administered subcutaneously for a total duration of 16 to 24 weeks.* Translate the portion which states "*6 MIU/m² TIW.*"
15. Translate "simvastatin 20 mg q.p.m."
16. Interpret the following from the literature: "*lopinavir/ritonavir 400 mg/100 mg b.i.d + efavirenz 600 mg q.d.*"
17. Using the information in Figure 4.5, calculate (a) the number of milligrams of metoclopramide HCl in each milliliter of the prescription and (b) the number of milliliters of nasal spray that would provide a patient with an 80-mg dose of metoclopramide HCl.
18. If, in the above problem, each nasal spray actuation delivered 0.4 mL, how many full days would the prescription last if the patient administered the stated dose three times daily?

CALCQUIZ

4.A. Interpret the underlined portions taken directly from current product references[15]:
  (a) Dose of ritonavir when coadministered with fluconazole: <u>200 mg q6h × 4d</u>
  (b) Dose of epoetin alpha: <u>150 units/kg SC TIW</u>
  (c) Dose of acetylcysteine: for patients <u>>20 to <40 kg, 150 mg/kg</u>
  (d) Pediatric dose of cefuroxime axetil: <u>30 mg/kg/day, divided dose (b.i.d.)</u>
  (e) Dose of ciprofloxacin hydrochloride: <u>750 mg tablet q12h or 400 mg IV q8h</u>
  (f) Dose of interferon alpha-2b: <u>30 MIU/m2 TIW</u>
  (g) Infusion rate, rocuronium bromide: <u>4 mg/kg/min</u>
  (h) Dose of enoxaparin sodium injection: <u>1.5 mg/kg q.d. SC</u>
  (i) Dose of voriconazole: <u>200 mg po q12h × 8 d</u>
  (j) Dose of certolizumab pegol: <u>200 mg + MTX q2 wk</u>

4.B. The following are hospital medication orders and, in parenthesis, the product available in the pharmacy:
  (a) Furosemide 40 mg IV qd (10 mg/mL in 2-mL syringes)
  (b) Erythromycin 750 mg IV q6h (500 mg/vial)
  (c) Acyclovir 350 mg IV q8h (500 mg/vial)
  (d) MEGACE 40 mg PO tid (40 mg/mL oral suspension)
  (e) FORTAZ 2 g IV q8h (500 mg/vial)

For each, indicate the quantity to be provided daily by the pharmacy.

ANSWERS TO "CASE IN POINT" AND PRACTICE PROBLEMS

Case in Point 4.1

(a) Since aa. means "of each," 10 mg lisinopril and 10 mg hydrochlorothiazide are needed for each capsule. And since D.T.D. means "give of such doses," 30 capsules are to be prepared. Thus,
10 mg lisinopril × 30 (capsules) = 300 mg lisinopril and
10 mg hydrochlorothiazide × 30 (capsules) = 300 mg hydrochlorothiazide are needed to fill the prescription.

(b) Since q.s. ad means "a sufficient quantity to make," the total in each capsule is 300 mg. The amount of lactose per capsule would equal 300 mg *less* the quantity of the other ingredients (10 mg + 10 mg + 40 mg), or 240 mg. Thus,
240 mg lactose/capsule × 30 (capsules) = 7200 mg = 7.2 g lactose.

(c) Take one (1) capsule in the morning before breakfast.

Case in Point 4.2

(a) 12 total tablets and capsules.

(b) $$? \text{ mL} = \frac{1 \text{ mL}}{100 \text{ units}} \times \frac{35 \text{ units}}{\text{AM}}$$
$$= 0.35 \text{ mL in the AM}$$
$$? \text{ mL} = \frac{1 \text{ mL}}{100 \text{ units}} \times \frac{45 \text{ Units}}{\text{PM}}$$
$$= 0.45 \text{ mL in the PM}$$

(c) First 7 days: 2 tablets × 2 (twice daily) × 7 days = 28 tablets
Next 7 days: 1 tablet × 2 (twice daily) × 7 days = 14 tablets
Next 16 days: 1 tablet (daily) = 16 tablets
28 + 14 + 16 = 58 tablets.

(d) 1 capsule daily × 7 days = 7 capsules
1 capsule × 2 (twice daily) × (next) 10 days = 20 capsules
7 + 20 = 27 capsules taken with 33 capsules remaining.
Thus, nonadherence *would be* a concern.

Practice Problems

1. (a) Dispense 12 rectal suppositories.
   (b) Mix and make an isotonic solution. Dispense 120 mL.
   (c) Mix and divide into 40 powders.
   (d) Dispense six such doses. Do not repeat.
   (e) Mix and make ointment. Dispense 10 g.
   (f) Mix and make capsules. Dispense 48 such doses.
   (g) Mix and make a suspension containing 1 g per tablespoon. Dispense 60 mL.
   (h) Make one capsule. Dispense 36 such doses. Do not repeat.
   (i) Mix and make powder. Divide into 100 such doses.
   (j) Mix and make an intravenous injection.
   (k) Label: hydrocortisone, 20 mg tabs.
2. (a) Instill 2 drops in each eye every four (4) hours as needed for pain.
   (b) Take 1 tablespoonful in one-third glass of water every 6 hours.

(c) Apply morning and night as needed for pain.
(d) Instill 4 drops into the right ear morning and night.
(e) Take 1 teaspoonful in water every 4 or 5 hours as needed for pain.
(f) Apply ointment to the left eye as needed.
(g) Take 1 capsule with water at bedtime. Do not repeat.
(h) Instill 5 drops into each ear three times a day as needed.
(i) Place 1 tablet under the tongue, repeat if needed.
(j) Instill 2 drops into each eye of the newborn.
(k) Dilute with an equal volume of water and use as gargle every 5 hours.
(l) Take 2 capsules 1 hour prior to departure, then 1 capsule after 12 hours.
(m) Take 1 tablet as needed for shortness of breath.
(n) Take 1 tablet every morning for high blood pressure.
(o) Take 2 tablets every 6 hours around the clock for urinary tract infection.
(p) Take 2 teaspoonfuls four times a day after meals and at bedtime.
(q) Take 1 tablespoonful before meals three times a day.
(r) Add crushed tablet to pet's food once a day.

3. (a) AMBIEN 10 mg by mouth at every bedtime for 5 days
(b) 1000 mL of 5% dextrose in water every 8 hours intravenously with 20 milliequivalents of potassium chloride added to every third bottle
(c) Administer 10 mg of prochlorperazine intramuscularly every 3 hours, if there is need, for nausea and vomiting.
(d) One teaspoonful of minocycline hydrochloride suspension by mouth four times a day. Discontinue after 5 days.
(e) 10 mg of propranolol hydrochloride by mouth three times a day before meals and at bedtime
(f) 40 units of NPH 100-unit insulin subcutaneously every day in the morning
(g) 250 mg of cefamandole nafate intramuscularly every 12 hours
(h) 15 milliequivalents of potassium chloride by mouth twice a day after meals
(i) 1 mg of vincristine sulfate per square meter of patient's body surface area
(j) Administer 30 mg of flurazepam at bedtime as needed for sleep.
(k) Administer 20 milliequivalents of potassium chloride per liter in D5W (5% dextrose in water) at the rate of 84 milliliters per hour.
(l) Administer 2.5 grams per kilogram of body weight per day of amino acids in total parenteral nutrition.
(m) Start epoetin alfa (PROCRIT) immediately at 150 units per kilogram of body weight subcutaneously and then three times a week for 3 to 4 weeks.
(n) Methotrexate tablets, 2.5 mg each, to be taken three times a day 1 day a week
(o) Hydrochlorothiazide tablets, 12.5 mg, to be taken once each day in the morning

4. (a) 50 days
(b) yes

5. (a) 40 tablets.

6. (a) correct.

7. ℞ calls for *tablets* but label indicates *capsules*.
Sig: "in the morning" has been added, which may be correct if that is the prescriber's usual directive.
Refill "5" times is incorrect; the original filling of a prescription does not count as a refill.

℞ calls for drug name/strength on label; an omission.
It should be noted that after filling the prescription, the pharmacist would have added a prescription number, which would also appear on the label.

8. The words "all of the medicine" have been added and the numbers enhanced; this clarifies the directions and thus is positive. 250 *mL* should be 250 *mg*.
The prescription number should appear on the label.
9. Patient's name is incorrect. The active drug name *only* on the label is proper for a compounded prescription. The other ingredients are "pharmaceutic."
It should be noted that after filling the prescription, the pharmacist would have added a prescription number, which would also appear on the label.
10. (1) "QID" means four times a day
(2) Drug name is incorrect.
(3) Correct
11. Correct label.
12. Ritonavir: 600 mg twice a day orally for 7 days.
Theophylline: 3 mg per kilogram of body weight every 8 hours for 7 days.
13. 10 milli-international units per milliliter.
14. 6 million international units per square meter of body surface area three times a week.
15. (Take) 20 mg of simvastatin every evening.
16. (The drug combination of) lopinavir, 400 mg, and ritonavir, 100 mg, taken twice a day, plus efavirenz, 600 mg, taken once every day.
17. (a) 100 mg metoclopramide HCl/mL
(b) 0.8 mL nasal spray
18. 41 days

AUTHORS' EXTRA POINT A

DRUG NAMES

As stated in this chapter, drug substances may be prescribed by their nonproprietary (generic) name or by their brand (trademark) name. The designation of nonproprietary names is based on nomenclature reflecting a drug's chemical structure and/or pharmacologic activity. In the United States, each nonproprietary name is assigned by the *United States Adopted Names (USAN) Council*, which is cosponsored by the American Medical Association, the United States Pharmacopeial Convention, and the American Pharmacists Association.

To harmonize the program, the USAN Council works in conjunction with the federal Food and Drug Administration (FDA) as well as the World Health Organization (WHO) and the International Nonproprietary Name (INN) Expert Committee. Together with the British Approved Names (BANs) and the Japanese Approved Names (JANs), the *USP Dictionary of USAN and International Drug Names* database contains more than 8,400 nonproprietary drug name entries.[a]

Many of the same drug substances are approved for marketing and available internationally. In the United States, this approval is within the authority of the federal Food and Drug Administration.[b] There are many multinational pharmaceutical companies who engage in the worldwide development and marketing of pharmaceutical products. The brand names assigned to the same nonproprietary-named drug often differ country to country. The referenced International Drug Name Database contains more than 40,000 medication names from 185 countries and is presented in multiple languages.[c]

The nonproprietary names used in the calculation problems in this text are universal; however, the brand names by their very nature are not.

[a]http://library.dialog.com/bluesheets/html/bl0464.html

[b]Regulatory approval is within the purview of each country. In Canada, regulatory authority resides with Health Canada's Therapeutic Products Directorate (TPD). Within the European Union (EU), the 28 member countries depend collectively upon the European Medicines Evaluation Agency (EMEA) for drug approvals and regulation. A list of drug regulatory agencies worldwide may be found at http://www.regulatoryone.com/p/websites-of-regulatory-agencies.html

[c]http://www.drugs.com/international/

AUTHORS' EXTRA POINT B

ELECTRONIC PRESCRIPTIONS[a]

The overall integrated system of electronic health information includes *electronic health records* (EHRs), *computerized physician order entry* (CPOE), and *electronic prescriptions* (*e-prescriptions*). The system allows health care providers to electronically insert and access patients' vital medical information.

In the processing of electronic prescriptions, a complex network of pharmacies, payers, pharmacy benefit managers (PBMs), physicians, hospitals, health information exchanges (HIEs), and electronic health record systems (EHRs) must be connected in real time to assure patient eligibility, formulary data, and clinical requirements. As is shown in Figures 4.10 and 4.11, this information connectivity is facilitated by health information networks (Surescripts in the example), which notify providers of authorization status and requirements.

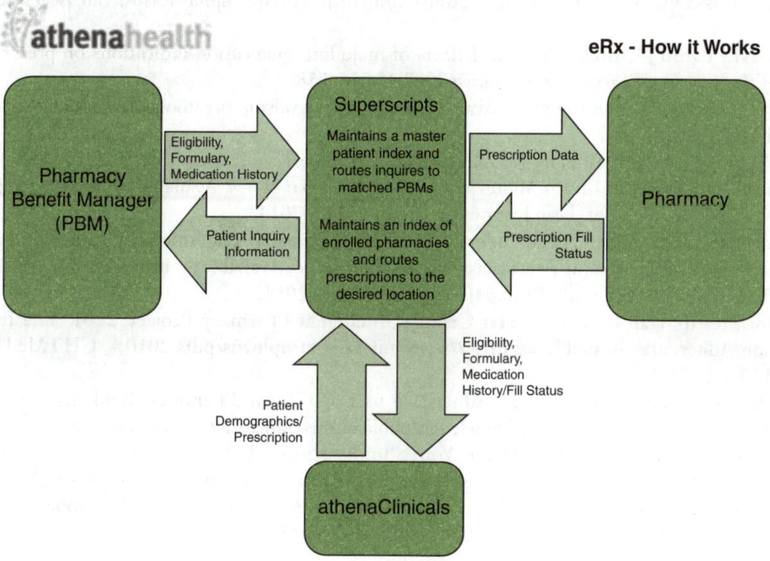

FIGURE 4.10 • Information connectivity in the processing and authorization of an e-prescription. *(Image provided through the courtesy of athenahealth, Inc. [Images © athenahealth, Inc., used with permission.] Additional information from http://surescripts.com/.)*

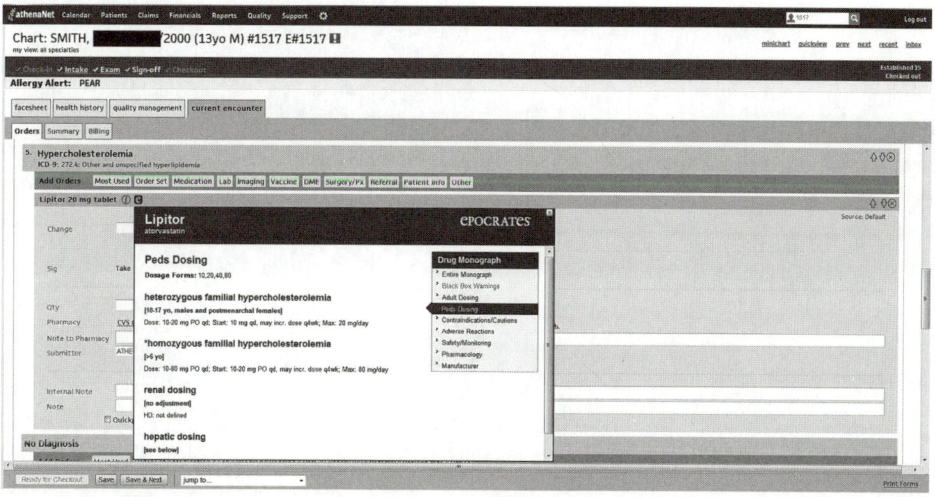

FIGURE 4.11 • An example of an e-prescription being ordered during a patient's visit with medical reference information embedded (Epocrates) to provide real-time decision clinical support. *(Image provided through the courtesy of athenahealth, Inc. [Images © athenahealth, Inc., used with permission.] Additional information from http://surescripts.com/.)*

References

1. Drug Quality and Security Act. Available at: https://www.govtrack.us/congress/bills/113/hr3204/text. Accessed April 27, 2014.
2. Draft Guidance. Pharmacy Compounding of Human Drug Products Under Section 503A of the Federal Food, Drug, and Cosmetic Act. U.S. Department of Health and Human Services, Food and Drug Administration, Center for Drug Evaluation and Research, 2013.
3. NCPDP Electronic Prescribing Standards. *National Council for Prescription Programs*. Available at: http://www.ncpdp.org/NCPDP/media/pdf/NCPDP-eprescribing-101-201308.pdf. Accessed May 1, 2014.
4. Kilbridge P. *E-Prescribing*. California HealthCare Foundation; 2001. Available at: http://www.chcf.org/~/media/MEDIA%20LIBRARY%20Files/PDF/E/PDF%20EPrescribing.pdf. Accessed May 1, 2014.
5. American College of Physicians. *Clinician's Guide to E-Prescribing*. Available at: http://www.acponline.org/running_practice/technology/eprescribing/clinicians_guide_eprescribing.pdf. Accessed May 1, 2014.
6. Hospital-Forms.com. Engineered Data, llc. Available at: http://www.hospital-forms.com. Accessed October 17, 2015.
7. Burnside NL, Bardo JA, Bretz CJ, et al. Effects of including medication indications on prescription labels. *Journal of the American Pharmacists Association* 2007;47:756–758.
8. Institute for Safe Medication Practices. Available at: http://www.ismp.org/tools/errorprone abbreviations.pdf. Accessed May 1, 2014.
9. Davis NM. A controlled vocabulary for reducing medication errors. *Hospital Pharmacy* 2000;35:227–228.
10. The Official "Do Not Use" List of Abbreviations. *The Joint Commission*. Available at: http://www.jointcommission.org/assets/1/18/Do_Not_Use_List.pdf. Accessed May 1, 2014.
11. Improving Medication Adherence in Older Adults. *Adult Medication*. The American Society on Aging and The American Society of Consultant Pharmacists Foundation; 2006. Available at: http://learning.rxassist.org/sites/default/files/Adult_Meducation%20All.pdf. Accessed May 1, 2014.
12. Center for Health Transformation. 21st Century Intelligent Pharmacy Project. 2101. The Importance of Medication Adherence. Available at: http://www.mirixa.com/uploads/pdfs/2010_-_CHTMedAdhrWp.pdf. Accessed May 1, 2014.
13. World Health Organization (WHO). Adherence to Long-Term Therapies: Evidence for Action, 2013. Available at: http://www.who.int/chp/knowledge/publications/adherence_report/en/. Accessed May 1, 2014.
14. Disposal of Unused Medicines: What You Should Know. U.S. Food and Drug Administration. Available at: http://www.fda.gov/Drugs/ResourcesForYou/Consumers/BuyingUsingMedicineSafely/EnsuringSafeUseofMedicine/SafeDisposalofMedicines/ucm186187.htm. Accessed October 17, 2015.
15. *Physicians' Desk Reference*. Montvale, NJ: PDR Network; 2011:65.

5

Density and Specific Gravity

OBJECTIVES

Upon successful completion of this chapter, the student will be able to:

- Define *density* and *specific gravity*, and determine each through appropriate calculations.
- Calculate specific gravity from data derived from the use of a pycnometer.
- Apply specific gravity in converting weight to volume and volume to weight.

Density

Density (*d*) is mass per unit volume of a substance. It is *usually* expressed as *grams per cubic centimeter* (*g/cc*). Because the *gram* is defined as the mass of 1 cc of water at 4°C, the density of water is *1 g/cc*. For our purposes, because the *United States Pharmacopeia*[1] states that 1 mL may be used as the equivalent of 1 cc, the density of water may be expressed as *1 g/mL*.

Density may be calculated by dividing mass by volume, that is:

$$\text{Density} = \frac{\text{Mass}}{\text{Volume}}$$

Thus, if 10 mL of sulfuric acid weighs 18 g, its density is:

$$\text{Density} = \frac{18\ (\text{g})}{10\ (\text{mL})} = \mathbf{1.8\ g/mL}$$

Specific Gravity

Specific gravity (*sp gr*) is a ratio, *expressed decimally*, of the weight of a substance to the weight of an equal volume of a substance chosen as a standard, both substances at the same temperature. It is useful to understand specific gravity as being a *relative value*, that is, the weight of a substance *relative* to the weight of a standard.

Water is used as the standard for the specific gravities of liquids and solids; the most useful standard for gases is hydrogen.

Specific gravity may be calculated by dividing the weight of a given substance by the weight of an equal volume of water, that is:

$$\text{Specific gravity} = \frac{\text{Weight of substance}}{\text{Weight of equal volume of water}}$$

Table 5.1 • SOME REPRESENTATIVE SPECIFIC GRAVITIES AT 25°C

Agent	SP GR
Ether (at 20°C)	0.71
Isopropyl alcohol	0.78
Acetone	0.79
Alcohol	0.81
Liquid petrolatum	0.87
Peppermint oil	0.90
Olive oil	0.91
Peanut oil	0.92
Cod liver oil	0.92
Castor oil	0.96
Water	**1.00**
Propylene glycol	1.03
Clove oil	1.04
Liquefied phenol	1.07
Polysorbate 80	1.08
Polyethylene glycol 400	1.13
Glycerin	1.25
Syrup	1.31
Hydrochloric acid	1.37
Nitric acid	1.42
Chloroform	1.47
Nitroglycerin	1.59
Phosphoric acid	1.70
Mercury	13.6

Thus, if 10 mL of sulfuric acid weigh 18 g and 10 mL of water, under similar conditions, weigh 10 g, the specific gravity of the acid is:

$$\text{Specific gravity} = \frac{18\ (\text{g})}{10\ (\text{g})} = \mathbf{1.8}$$

- *Substances that have a specific gravity less than 1 are lighter than water.*
- *Substances that have a specific gravity greater than 1 are heavier than water.*

Table 5.1 presents some representative specific gravities. Figure 5.1 depicts the layering of immiscible liquids due to their relative weights.

Although specific gravities may be expressed to as many decimal places as the accuracy of their determination warrants, in pharmacy practice, expressions to two decimal places generally suffice. In the *United States Pharmacopeia*, specific gravities are based on data from temperatures of 25°C, with the exception of that for alcohol that is based on 15.56°C by government regulation.[1]

Density versus Specific Gravity

The density of a substance is a concrete number (*1.8 g/mL* in the example), whereas specific gravity, being a ratio of like quantities, is an abstract number (*1.8* in the example). Whereas density varies with the units of measure used, specific gravity has no dimension and is therefore a constant value for each substance. Thus, whereas the density of water may be variously expressed as *1 g/mL*, *1000 g/L*, or *62½ lb/cu ft*, the specific gravity of water is always 1.

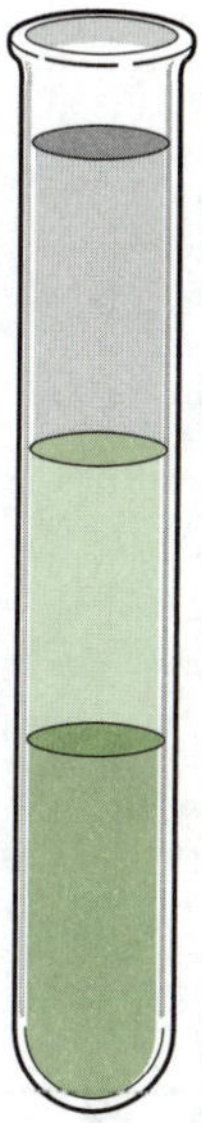

FIGURE 5.1 • Depiction of layering of immiscible liquids in a test tube, mineral oil being lighter than water and chloroform being heavier.

Calculating the Specific Gravity of Liquids

Known Weight and Volume

Apply the equation:

$$\text{Specific gravity} = \frac{\text{Weight of substance}}{\text{Weight of equal volume of water}}$$

(1) *If 54.96 mL of an oil weighs 52.78 g, what is the specific gravity of the oil?*

54.96 mL of water weighs 54.96 g

$$\text{Specific gravity of oil} = \frac{52.78\,(\text{g})}{54.96\,(\text{g})} = \mathbf{0.9603}$$

(2) *If a pint of a certain liquid weighs 601 g, what is the specific gravity of the liquid?*

1 pint = 16 fl. oz.
16 fl. oz. of water weighs 473 g

$$\text{Specific gravity of liquid} = \frac{601\,(\text{g})}{473\,(\text{g})} = \mathbf{1.27}$$

Pycnometer or Specific Gravity Bottle

A ***pycnometer*** is a special glass bottle used to determine specific gravity (Fig. 5.2). Pycnometers are generally available for laboratory use in volumes ranging from 1 to 50 mL. Pycnometers have fitted glass stoppers with a capillary opening to allow trapped air and excess fluid to escape. Some pycnometers have thermometers affixed in order to relate the specific gravity, as determined, with temperature.

In using a pycnometer, it is first weighed empty and then weighed again when filled to capacity with water. The weight of the water is calculated by difference. Since 1 g of water equals 1 mL, the exact volume of the pycnometer becomes known. Then, when any other

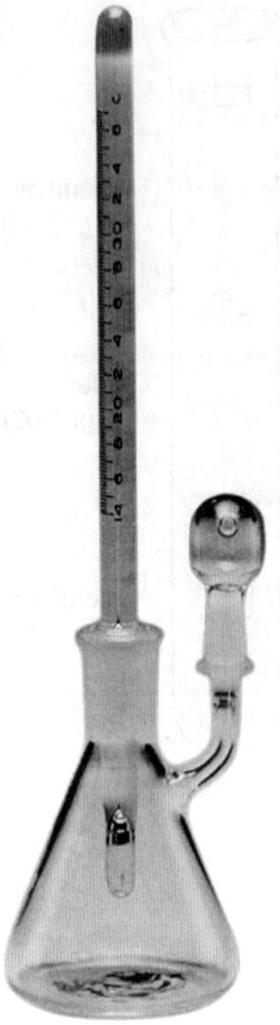

FIGURE 5.2 • Example of a *pycnometer* affixed with a thermometer. Pycnometers are used to determine the specific gravities of liquids at specific temperatures. See text for additional discussion. *(Courtesy of Kimble/Kontes Glass.)*

liquid subsequently is placed in the pycnometer, it is of *equal volume* to the water, and its specific gravity may be determined.

(1) *A 50-mL pycnometer is found to weigh 120 g when empty, 171 g when filled with water, and 160 g when filled with an unknown liquid. Calculate the specific gravity of the unknown liquid.*

$$\text{Weight of water}: 171\text{ g} - 120\text{ g} = 51\text{ g}$$

$$\text{Weight of unknown liquid}: 160\text{ g} - 120\text{ g} = 40\text{ g}$$

$$\text{Specific gravity} = \frac{\text{Weight of substance}}{\text{Weight of equal volume of water}}$$

$$\text{Specific gravity of unknown liquid} = \frac{40\text{ (g)}}{51\text{ (g)}} = \mathbf{0.78}$$

(2) *A specific gravity bottle weighs 23.66 g. When filled with water, it weighs 72.95 g; when filled with another liquid, it weighs 73.56 g. What is the specific gravity of the liquid?*

$$73.56\text{ g} - 23.66\text{ g} = 49.90\text{ g of liquid}$$

$$72.95\text{ g} - 23.66\text{ g} = 49.29\text{ g of water}$$

$$\text{Specific gravity of liquid} = \frac{49.90\text{ (g)}}{49.29\text{ (g)}} = \mathbf{1.012}$$

Use of Specific Gravity in Calculations of Weight and Volume

It is important to remember that specific gravity is a *factor* that expresses how much heavier or lighter a substance is than water, the standard with a specific gravity of 1.0. For example, a liquid with a specific gravity of 1.25 is 1.25 times as heavy as water, and a liquid with a specific gravity of 0.85 is 0.85 times as heavy as water.

Thus, if we had 50 mL of a liquid with a specific gravity of 1.2, it would weigh 1.2 times as much as an equivalent volume of water. An equivalent volume of water, 50 mL, would weigh 50 g, and therefore, the liquid would weigh 1.2 times that, or 60 g.

Calculating Weight, Knowing the Volume and Specific Gravity

Based on the explanation in the previous paragraphs, we can derive the following equation:

$$\text{Grams} = \text{Milliliters} \times \text{Specific gravity}$$

Although it is both obvious and true that one cannot multiply milliliters by specific gravity and have a product in grams, the equation "works" because the volume of the liquid in question is assumed to be the same volume as water for which milliliters equal grams. So, in essence, the true equation would be:

$$\text{Grams (other liquid)} = \text{Grams (of equal volume of water)} \times \text{Specific (gravity other liquid)}$$

(1) *What is the weight, in grams, of 3620 mL of alcohol with a specific gravity of 0.82?*

3620 mL of water weighs 3620 g

$3620 \text{ g} \times 0.82 = \mathbf{2968 \text{ g}}$

(2) *Sevoflurane (ULTANE) is a volatile liquid for inhalation with a specific gravity of 1.52. Calculate the weight of the contents of a bottle of 250 mL of the product.*

250 mL of water weighs 250 g

$250 \text{ g} \times 1.52 = \mathbf{380 \text{ g}}$

(3) *What is the weight, in grams, of 2 fl. oz. of a liquid having a specific gravity of 1.118?*

In this type of problem, it is best to convert the given volume to its metric equivalent first and then solve the problem in the metric system.

$2 \times 29.57 \text{ mL} = 59.14 \text{ mL}$

59.14 mL of water weighs 59.14 g

$59.14 \text{ g} \times 1.118 = \mathbf{66.12 \text{ g}}$

Calculating Volume, Knowing the Weight and Specific Gravity

By rearranging the previous equation, we can calculate the volume of a liquid using the equation:

$$\text{Milliliters} = \frac{\text{Grams}}{\text{Specific gravity}}$$

(1) *What is the volume, in milliliters, of 492 g of a liquid with a specific gravity of 1.40?*

492 g of water measure 492 mL

$$\frac{492 \text{ mL}}{1.40} = \mathbf{351 \text{ mL}}$$

(2) *What is the volume, in milliliters, of 1 lb of a liquid with a specific gravity of 1.185?*

1 lb = 454 g
454 g of water measure 454 mL

$$\frac{454 \text{ mL}}{1.185} = \mathbf{383.1\ mL}$$

(3) *What is the volume, in pints, of 50 lb of glycerin having a specific gravity of 1.25?*

50 lb = 454 g × 50 = 22,700 g
22,700 g of water measure 22,700 mL and 1 pint = 473 mL

$$\frac{22{,}700 \text{ mL}}{1.25} = 18{,}160 \text{ mL} \div 473 \text{ mL} = \mathbf{38.4\ pints}$$

Using Specific Gravity to Determine Weight/Volume Costs

(1) *What is the cost of 1000 mL of glycerin, specific gravity 1.25, bought at $5.43 per pound?*

1000 mL of water weighs 1000 g
Weight of 1000 mL of glycerin = 1000 g × 1.25 = 1250 g
1 lb = 454 g

$$\$5.43 \times \frac{1250 \text{ g}}{454 \text{ g}} = \mathbf{\$14.95}$$

(2) *What is the cost of 1 pint of chloroform, specific gravity 1.475, bought at $25.25 per pound?*

1 pint = 473 mL
473 mL of water weighs 473 g
Weight of 473 mL of chloroform = 473 g × 1.475 = 697.7 g
1 lb = 454 g

$$\$25.25 \times \frac{697.7 \text{ g}}{454 \text{ g}} = \mathbf{\$38.80}$$

Special Considerations of Specific Gravity

Pharmaceutical Applications

An interesting special application of specific gravity is in the use of automated, computer-controlled pharmaceutical equipment, termed *automated compounders*, in the preparation of multicomponent mixtures for parenteral nutrition (as describe in Chapter 14). In such systems, the measurement of the final volume of a mixture is determined by its weight divided by the solution's known specific gravity.[2] A complete explanation may be found in the indicated reference.

Clinical Application

Specific gravity is an important factor in urinalysis. In normal adults, the specific gravity of urine is usually within the range of 1.020 and 1.028 with a normal fluid intake (this range may vary with the reference source).[3]

Specific gravity is an indicator of both the concentration of particles in the urine and a patient's degree of hydration. A higher-than-normal specific gravity indicates that the urine is concentrated. This may be due to the presence of excess waste products or electrolytes in the urine, the presence of glucose (glucosuria) or protein (proteinuria), excessive water loss, decreased fluid intake, or other factors. A low specific gravity indicates that the urine is dilute, which may be a result of diabetes insipidus, renal disease (by virtue of the kidney's reduced ability to concentrate urine), increased fluid intake, intravenous hydration, or other factors.[4]

CASE IN POINT 5.1[5]

℞ Lactic acid
Salicylic acid aa. 1.5 g
Flexible collodion qs ad 15 mL
Sig: Apply one drop to wart twice a day
Label: Wart remover. For external use only

Lactic acid is available as a liquid containing 85 g of the acid in 100 g of solution (sp gr 1.21). Calculate the quantity of this solution, in milliliters, needed to fill the prescription.

CALCULATIONS CAPSULE

Specific Gravity

The specific gravity (sp gr) of a substance or a pharmaceutical preparation may be determined by the following equation:

$$\text{Specific gravity} = \frac{\text{Weight of substance (g)}}{\text{Weight of equal volume of water (g)}}$$

The following equation may be used to convert the volume of a substance or pharmaceutical preparation to its weight*:

$$\text{Weight of substance} = \text{Volume of substance} \times \text{Specific gravity}$$

Or simply,

$$\mathbf{g = mL \times sp\,gr}$$

The following equation may be used to convert the weight of a substance or pharmaceutical preparation to its volume[a]:

$$\text{Volume of substance} = \frac{\text{Weight of substance}}{\text{Specific gravity}}$$

Or simply,

$$\mathbf{mL = \frac{g}{sp\,gr}}$$

[a]The full explanation on why these equations work may be found in the section "Use of Specific Gravity in Calculations of Weight and Volume."

PRACTICE PROBLEMS

Calculations of Density

1. If 250 mL of alcohol weighs 203 g, what is its density?
2. A substance metal weighs 53.6 g and has a volume of 6 mL. Calculate its density.

Calculations of Specific Gravity

3. If 150 mL of a sorbitol solution weigh 170 g, what is its specific gravity?
4. If a liter of a cough syrup weighs 1285 g, what is its specific gravity?
5. If 500 mL of a solution weigh 650 g, what is its specific gravity?
6. If 2 fl. oz. of glycerol weigh 74.1 g, what is its specific gravity?
7. Five pints of a liquid weigh 2.79 kg. Calculate its specific gravity.
8. A pycnometer weighs 21.62 g. Filled with water, it weighs 46.71 g; filled with another liquid, it weighs 43.28 g. Calculate the specific gravity of the liquid.
9. A modified Ringer's Irrigation has the following formula:

Sodium chloride	8.6 g
Potassium chloride	0.3 g
Calcium chloride	0.33 g
PEG 3350	60 g
Water for injection to	1000 mL

   Assuming that 980 mL of water is used, calculate the specific gravity of the irrigation.

Calculations of Weight or Volume Using Specific Gravity

NOTE: Use the information in Table 5.1 as necessary.

10. α-Tocopherol is a form of vitamin E that is a yellow-brown viscous liquid with a density of 0.950 g/cm^3. Calculate its specific gravity.
11. A patient added a 17-g measured dose of polyethylene glycol 3350 (MIRALAX) to 180 mL of water to use as a laxative. If the volume of the resultant mixture was 195.6 mL, calculate the apparent density of polyethylene glycol 3350 and the specific gravity of the mixture.
12. If a pharmacist dissolves 1.2 g of a medicinal agent in 60 mL of a cough syrup having a specific gravity of 1.20. What is the specific gravity (to 3 decimal places) of the product if the addition of the medicinal agent increases the syrup's volume by 0.2 mL?
13. If a pharmacist adds 10 mL of purified water to 30 mL of a solution having a specific gravity of 1.30, calculate the specific gravity of the product (to three decimal places).
14. If a pharmacist combined 50-mL portions of three syrups having specific gravities of 1.10, 1.25, and 1.32, what would be the specific gravity (to two decimal places) of the combined product?
15. A laboratory utilizes a mixture of 10% dimethyl sulfoxide (DMSO) in the freezing and long-term storage of embryonic stem cells. If DMSO has a specific gravity of 1.1004, calculate the specific gravity, to four decimal places, of the mixture (assume water to be the 90% portion).

16. Calculate the weight, in grams, of 100 mL of each of the following:
    (a) Acetone
    (b) Liquid petrolatum
    (c) Syrup
    (d) Nitroglycerin
    (e) Mercury
17. What is the weight, in kilograms, of 5 liters of a liquid with a specific gravity of 1.84?
18. What is the weight, in kilograms, of 1 gallon of sorbitol solution having a specific gravity of 1.285?
19. If 500 mL of mineral oil are used to prepare a liter of mineral oil emulsion, how many grams of the oil, having a specific gravity of 0.87, would be used in the preparation of 1 gallon of the emulsion?
20. Calculate the volume, in milliliters, of 100 g of each of the following:
    (a) Peanut oil
    (b) Castor oil
    (c) Polysorbate 80
    (d) Phosphoric acid
    (e) Mercury
21. What is the volume, in milliliters, of 1 lb of benzyl benzoate having a specific gravity of 1.12?
22. Calculate the corresponding weights of liquefied phenol and propylene glycol needed to prepare 24 15-mL bottles of the following formula:

Liquefied phenol	0.4 mL
Camphor	0.5 g
Benzocaine	2.2 g
Ethanol	65 mL
Propylene glycol	17 mL
Purified water to	100 mL

23. Calculate the total weight of the following formula for a pediatric chewable gummy gel base for medication.

Gelatin	43.4 g
Glycerin	155 mL
Purified water	21.6 mL

24. Calculate the number of milliliters of polysorbate 80 required to prepare 48 100-g tubes of the following formula for a progesterone vaginal cream.

Progesterone, micronized	3 g
Polysorbate 80	1 g
Methylcellulose 2% gel	96 g

25. If fifty glycerin suppositories are made from the following formula, how many milliliters of glycerin, having a specific gravity of 1.25, would be used in the preparation of 96 suppositories?

Glycerin	91 g
Sodium stearate	9 g
Purified water	5 g

26. ℞ Testosterone propionate 2 g
Mineral oil, light 10 g
Polysorbate 80 1 g
Methylcellulose 2% gel 87 g

The specific gravity of light mineral oil is 0.85 and that of polysorbate 80 is 1.08. Calculate the milliliters of each needed to fill the prescription.

27. A formula for an anesthetic ointment is:

Benzocaine	200 g
Polyethylene glycol 400	600 g
Polyethylene glycol 3350 ad	1000 g

Polyethylene glycol 400 is a liquid, sp gr 1.13, benzocaine and polyethylene glycol 3350 are powders. How many milliliters of polyethylene glycol 400 would be used in the formula?

28. Prior to a computerized tomographic scan (CT scan) of the abdomen, a patient is instructed to drink 450 mL of a barium suspension. If the suspension has a specific gravity of 1.05, calculate the weight of the suspension.

Using Specific Gravity to Determine Weight/Volume Costs

29. An international supplier sells Indian castor oil at $1200 a metric ton (1000 kg). Using the information in Table 5.1 and the previously learned conversion factors, calculate the corresponding price of a pint of the oil.
30. The formula for 1000 g of polyethylene glycol ointment calls for 600 g polyethylene glycol 400. At $19.15 per pint, what is the cost of the polyethylene glycol 400, specific gravity 1.140, needed to prepare 4000 g of the ointment?

CALCQUIZ

5.A. Syrup, USP is prepared by dissolving 850 g of sucrose in sufficient purified water to make 1000 mL of syrup. Syrup has a specific gravity of 1.31. How many milliliters of water are used to prepare a liter of syrup?

5.B. A saturated solution of potassium iodide contains, in each 100 mL, 100 g of potassium iodide. The solubility of potassium iodide is 1 g in 0.7 mL of water. Calculate the specific gravity of the saturated solution.

5.C. Cocoa butter (theobroma oil) is used as a suppository base. It is a solid at room temperature, melts at 34°C, and has a specific gravity of 0.86. If a formula for medicated suppositories calls for 48 mL of theobroma oil, how many grams are equivalent?

ANSWERS TO "CASE IN POINT" AND PRACTICE PROBLEMS

Case in Point 5.1

Quantity of lactic acid needed to fill ℞ :1.5 g
Source of lactic acid: liquid containing 85 g/100 g; or, by using specific gravity:
100 g ÷ 1.21 = 82.64 mL
Thus, 85 g of lactic acid is in 82.64 mL of the source liquid.
By proportion:

$$\frac{85\text{ g}}{82.64\text{ mL}} = \frac{1.5\text{ g}}{\text{x mL}};\ \text{x} = 1.46\text{ mL}$$

Practice Problems

1. 0.812 g/mL
2. 8.933 g/mL
3. 1.133
4. 1.285
5. 1.30
6. 1.25
7. 1.18
8. 0.86
9. 1.05
10. 0.950
11. 1.09, density, and 1.01, specific gravity
12. 1.216
13. 1.225
14. 1.22
15. 1.0100
16. (a) 79 g acetone
    (b) 87 g liquid petrolatum
    (c) 131 g syrup
    (d) 159 g nitroglycerin
    (e) 1360 g mercury
17. 9.2 kg
18. 4.86 kg sorbitol solution
19. 1646.5 g mineral oil
20. (a) 108.7 mL peanut oil
    (b) 104.17 mL castor oil
    (c) 92.59 mL polysorbate 80
    (d) 58.82 mL phosphoric acid
    (e) 7.35 mL mercury
21. 405.36 mL benzyl benzoate
22. 1.54 g liquefied phenol
    63.04 g propylene glycol
23. 258.75 g
24. 44.44 mL polysorbate 80
25. 139.78 mL glycerin
26. 11.76 mL light mineral oil
    0.93 mL polysorbate 80
27. 530.97 mL polyethylene glycol 400
28. 472.5 g barium suspension
29. $ 0.54
30. $85.23

References

1. United States Pharmacopeial Convention. *United States Pharmacopeia 32 National Formulary* 27. Vol. 1. Rockville, MD: United States Pharmacopeial Convention; 2009:9.
2. American Society of Health-System Pharmacists. ASHP guidelines on the safe use of automated compounding devices for the preparation of parenteral nutrition admixtures. *American Journal of Health-System Pharmacy* 2000;57:1343–1348. Available at: http://www.ashp.org/s_ashp/docs/files/BP07/AutoIT_Gdl_Compounders.pdf. Accessed April 17, 2014.
3. Urine specific gravity. MedlinePlus. Available at: http://www.nlm.nih.gov/medlineplus/ency/article/003587.htm. Accessed March 6, 2011.
4. The Internet Pathology Laboratory for Medical Education. Urinalysis tutorial. Available at: http://library.med.utah.edu/WebPath/TUTORIAL/URINE/URINE.html. Accessed January 18, 2011.
5. Allen LV Jr, ed. *International Journal of Pharmaceutical Compounding* 1998;2:58.

6

Percent Strength, Ratio Strength, and Other Expressions of Concentration

OBJECTIVES

Upon successful completion of this chapter, the student will be able to:

- Perform calculations based on *percent weight in volume, percent volume in volume,* and *percent weight in weight.*
- Perform calculations based on *ratio strength.*
- Convert percent strength to ratio strength and ratio strength to percent strength.
- Utilize other expressions of concentration in calculations, as *parts per million* and *mg/mL.*

Percent

The term ***percent*** and the corresponding "%" sign indicate the number of *parts in a hundred.* The quantity also may be expressed as a common or decimal fraction. Thus, 50%, 50/100, and 0.5 are equivalent.

For the purposes of computation, percents are usually changed to equivalent decimal fractions. This change is made by dropping the percent sign (%) and dividing the expressed numerator by 100. Thus, 12.5% = 12.5/100, or 0.125, and 0.05% = 0.05/100, or 0.0005. We must not forget that in the reverse process (changing a decimal to a percent), the decimal is multiplied by 100 and the percent sign (%) is affixed.

Percent is an essential component of pharmaceutical calculations. It is used to (a) *express the strength* of a component in a pharmaceutical preparation as well as to (b) *determine the quantity* of a component to use when a certain percent strength is desired.

Percent Preparations

The percent concentrations of active and inactive constituents in various types of pharmaceutical preparations are defined as follows by the *United States Pharmacopeia*[1]:

Percent weight in volume (w/v) expresses the number of *grams* of a constituent in *100 mL* of solution or liquid preparation and is used regardless of whether water or another liquid is the solvent or vehicle. Expressed as: ____% *w/v.*

Percent volume in volume (v/v) expresses the number of *milliliters* of a constituent in *100 mL* of solution or liquid preparation. Expressed as: ____% *v/v.*

Percent weight in weight (w/w) expresses the number of *grams* of a constituent in *100 g* of solution or preparation. Expressed as: ____% *w/w.*

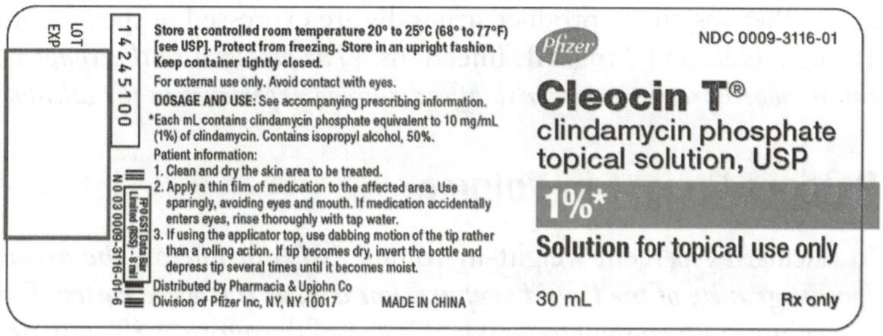

FIGURE 6.1 • A product label depicting the strength of the active ingredient on a w/v basis, 10 mg/mL. (From http://dailymed.nlm.nih.gov/dailymed/about.cfm)

The term *percent*, or the symbol %, when used *without qualification* means:

- For solutions or suspensions of solids in liquids, *percent weight in volume*
- For solutions of liquids in liquids, *percent volume in volume*
- For mixtures of solids or semisolids, *percent weight in weight*
- For solutions of gases in liquids, *percent weight in volume*

Figures 6.1 and 6.2 show product labels for different forms of clindamycin phosphate (CLEOCIN T), both 1% in strength. Figure 6.1 is the label of a topical solution containing active ingredient, 10 mg/mL (1% w/v), whereas Figure 6.2 is the label of a topical gel containing active ingredient, 10 mg/g (1% w/w).

Special Considerations in Percent Calculations

In general, the physical nature of the ingredients in a pharmaceutical preparation determines the basis of the calculation. That is, a powdered substance dissolved or suspended in a liquid vehicle would generally be calculated on a *weight-in-volume* basis; a powdered substance mixed with a solid or semisolid, such as an ointment base, would generally be calculated on a *weight-in-weight* basis; and a liquid component in a liquid preparation would be calculated on a *volume-in-volume* basis. *If the designation of the term of a calculation (e.g., w/v, w/w, or v/v) is not included in a problem, the appropriate assumption must be made.*

The use of *percent* to indicate the strength of a product generally is limited nowadays to certain topical products, such as ointments, creams, and eyedrops. However, there are some notable exceptions, such as 5% dextrose injection, used in intravenous infusions. In

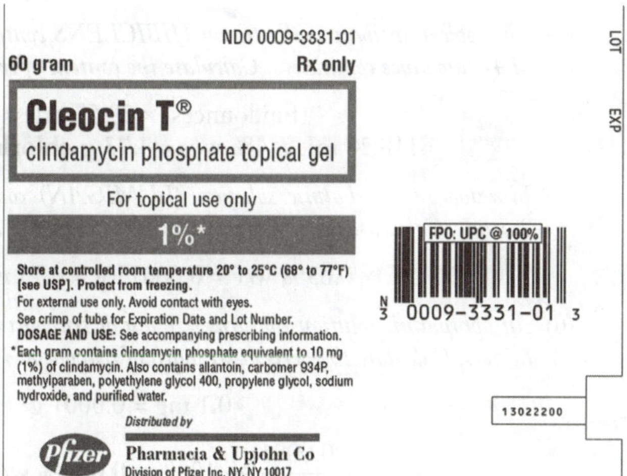

FIGURE 6.2 • A product label depicting the strength of the active ingredient on a w/w basis, 10 mg/g. (From http://dailymed.nlm.nih.gov/dailymed/about.cfm)

most other instances, product strengths are expressed in specific quantitative terms, such as 10-mg tablets and 2 mg/mL injections. [*The problems in this chapter take certain liberties from this standard practice in order to afford a broad experience in the calculations process.*]

Percent Weight in Volume

In calculating percent weight-in-volume (w/v) problems, ***the assumption is made that the specific gravity of the liquid preparation is 1, as if it were water.*** Thus, for example, 100 mL of a solution is assumed to weigh 100 g, and therefore, a 5% w/v preparation would contain 5 g of that ingredient [5% of (100 mL taken to be) 100 g].

Examples of Weight-in-Volume Calculations

(1) *How many grams of dextrose are required to prepare 4000 mL of a 5% solution?*

4000 mL represents 4000 g of solution
5% = 0.05
4000 g × 0.05 = **200 g**

Or, solving by dimensional analysis:

$$\frac{5\text{ g}}{100\text{ mL}} \times 4000\text{ mL} = \mathbf{200\text{ g dextrose}}$$

(2) *How many grams of potassium permanganate should be used in compounding the following prescription?*

℞	Potassium permanganate	0.02%
	Purified water ad	250 mL
	Sig. as directed	

250 mL represents 250 g of solution
0.02% = 0.0002
250 g × 0.0002 = **0.05 g potassium permanganate**

(3) *A cyclosporine ophthalmic emulsion (RESTASIS) contains 0.05% w/v cyclosporine in 0.4-mL vials. Calculate the content of cyclosporine, in milligrams, per vial.*

0.4 mL × 0.05% w/v = 0.0002 mL (equivalent in a w/v problem to 0.0002 g)
0.0002 = **0.2 mg cyclosporine**

(4) *The topical antibacterial solution HIBICLENS contains 4% w/v chlorhexidine gluconate in 4-fluidounce containers. Calculate the content of chlorhexidine gluconate, in grams.*

4 (fluidounces) × 29.57 mL = 118.28 mL
118.28 mL × 4% w/v = **4.73 g chlorhexidine gluconate**

(5) *Bimatoprost ophthalmic solution (LUMIGAN) contains 0.03% w/v of drug in each 2.5 mL. Calculate the micrograms of bimatoprost in a container of solution.*

2.5 mL × 0.03% w/v = 0.00075 g = 0.75 mg = **750 μg bimatoprost**

(6) *An ophthalmic solution contains 0.1 mg of travoprost* (TRAVATAN Z) *in 2.5 mL containers. Calculate the percent strength of travoprost in the solution.*

0.1 mg = 0.0001 g

$$\frac{0.0001\text{ g}}{2.5\text{ g}} \times 100\% = \mathbf{0.004\%\text{ w/v, travoprost}}$$

Percent Volume in Volume

Liquids are usually measured by volume, and the percent strength indicates the number of parts by volume of an ingredient contained in the total volume of the liquid preparation.

Examples of Volume-in-Volume Calculations

(1) *How many milliliters of liquefied phenol should be used in compounding the following prescription?*

℞ Liquefied phenol 2.5%
Calamine lotion ad 240 mL
Sig. for external use

240 mL × 0.025 = **6 mL**

Or, solving by dimensional analysis:

$$\frac{2.5\text{ mL}}{100\text{ mL}} \times 240\text{ mL} = \mathbf{6\text{ mL, liquefied phenol}}$$

(2) *In preparing 250 mL of a certain lotion, a pharmacist used 4 mL of liquefied phenol. What was the percent (v/v) of liquefied phenol in the lotion?*

$$\frac{250\text{ (mL)}}{4\text{ (mL)}} = \frac{100\ (\%)}{x\ (\%)}$$

$$x = \mathbf{1.6\%}$$

(3) *What is the percent strength v/v of a solution of 800 g of a liquid with a specific gravity of 0.8 in enough water to make 4000 mL?*

800 g of water measure 800 mL
800 mL ÷ 0.8 = 1000 mL of active ingredient

$$\frac{4000\text{ (mL)}}{1000\text{ (mL)}} = \frac{100\ (\%)}{x\ (\%)}$$

$$x = \mathbf{25\%}$$

Or, solving by dimensional analysis:

$$\frac{800\text{ mL}}{0.8} \times \frac{1}{4000\text{ mL}} \times 100\% = \mathbf{25\%}$$

(4) *If a veterinary liniment contains 30% v/v of dimethyl sulfoxide, how many milliliters of the liniment can be prepared from 1 lb of dimethyl sulfoxide (sp gr 1.10)?*

1 lb = 454 g
454 g of water measures 454 mL
454 mL ÷ 1.10 = **412.7 mL of dimethyl sulfoxide**

$$\frac{30\ (\%)}{100\ (\%)} = \frac{412.7\text{ (mL)}}{x\text{ (mL)}}$$

$$x = 1375.7 \text{ or } \mathbf{1376\text{ mL}}$$

Or, solving by dimensional analysis:

$$\frac{1\ \text{lb}}{30\%} \times \frac{454\ \text{g}}{1\ \text{lb}} \times \frac{1\ \text{mL}}{1\ \text{g}} \times \frac{1}{1.10} \times 100\% = 1375.7 \text{ or } \mathbf{1376\ mL}$$

Percent Weight in Weight

Percent weight in weight indicates the number of parts by weight of active ingredient contained in the total weight of the preparation.

Examples of Weight-in-Weight Calculations

(1) *A hydrocortisone cream contains 1% hydrocortisone. Calculate the grams of hydrocortisone used to prepare each 15-g tube of product.*

$1\% = 0.01$
$15\ \text{g} \times 0.01 = \mathbf{0.15\ g}$

(2) *FINACEA gel contains 15% azelaic acid in 50-g tubes. Calculate the grams of azelaic acid in each tube of product.*

$15\% = 0.15$
$50\ \text{g} \times 0.15 = \mathbf{7.5\ g}$

(3) *ANDROGEL 1.62% is a testosterone gel for topical use. Calculate the grams of gel required to provide a 40.5 mg dose of testosterone.*

1.62% = 1.62 g (testosterone)/100 g (gel) or 1620 mg (testosterone)/100 g (gel)

Thus,

$$\frac{1620\ \text{mg}}{100\ \text{g}} = \frac{40.5\ \text{mg}}{\text{x}} = \mathbf{2.5\ g\ gel}$$

Or,

$$40.5\ \text{mg} \times \frac{100\ \text{g}}{1.62\ \text{g}} \times \frac{1\ \text{g}}{1000\ \text{mg}} = \mathbf{2.5\ g\ gel}$$

Proof: 2.5 g (gel) × 1.62% (testosterone) = 0.0405 g or 40.5 mg testosterone

(4) *How many grams of a drug substance are required to make 120 mL of a 20% (w/w) solution having a specific gravity of 1.15?*

120 mL of water weigh 120 g
120 g × 1.15 = 138 g, weight of 120 mL of solution
138 g × 0.20 = **27.6 g** plus enough water to make 120 mL

Or, solving by dimensional analysis:

$$120\ \text{mL} \times \frac{1.15\ \text{g}}{1\ \text{mL}} \times \frac{20\%}{100\%} = \mathbf{27.6\ g}$$

Sometimes in a weight-in-weight calculation, the weight of one component is known but *not* the total weight of the intended preparation. This type of calculation is performed as demonstrated by the following example.

(5) *How many grams of a drug substance should be added to 240 mL of water to make a 4% (w/w) solution?*

100% – 4% = 96% (by weight) of water
240 mL of water weigh 240 g

$$\frac{96\,(\%)}{4\,(\%)} = \frac{240\,(\text{g})}{\text{x}\,(\text{g})}$$
$$\text{x} = \mathbf{10\ g}$$

It is usually impossible to prepare a specified *volume* of a solution or liquid preparation of given weight-in-weight percent strength because the volume displaced by the active ingredient cannot be known in advance. If an excess is acceptable, we may make a volume somewhat more than that specified by taking the given volume to refer to the solvent or vehicle and from this quantity calculating the weight of the solvent or vehicle (the specific gravity of the solvent or vehicle must be known). Using this weight, we may follow the method just described to calculate the corresponding weight of the active ingredient needed.

(6) *How should you prepare 100 mL of a 2% (w/w) solution of a drug substance in a solvent having a specific gravity of 1.25?*

100 mL of water weigh 100 g
100 g × 1.25 = 125 g, weight of 100 mL of solvent
100% – 2% = 98% (by weight) of solvent

$$\frac{98\,(\%)}{2\,(\%)} = \frac{125\,(\text{g})}{\text{x}\,(\text{g})}$$
$$\text{x} = \mathbf{2.55\ g}$$

Therefore, dissolve 2.55 g of drug substance in 125 g (or 100 mL) of solvent.

(7) *If 1500 g of a solution contains 75 g of a drug substance, what is the percent strength (w/w) of the solution?*

$$\frac{1500\,(\text{g})}{75\,(\text{g})} = \frac{100\,(\%)}{\text{x}\,(\%)}$$
$$\text{x} = \mathbf{5\%}$$

Or, solving by dimensional analysis:

$$\frac{75\ \text{g}}{1500\ \text{g}} \times 100\% = \mathbf{5\%}$$

(8) *If 5 g of boric acid are added to 100 mL of water, what is the percent strength (w/w) of the solution?*

100 mL of water weigh 100 g
100 g + 5 g = 105 g, weight of solution

$$\frac{105\,(\text{g})}{5\,(\text{g})} = \frac{100\,(\%)}{\text{x}\,(\%)}$$
$$\text{x} = \mathbf{4.76\%}$$

(9) *If 1000 mL of syrup with a specific gravity of 1.313 contain 850 g of sucrose, what is its percent strength (w/w)?*

1000 mL of water weigh 1000 g
1000 g × 1.313 = 1313 g, weight of 1000 mL of syrup

$$\frac{1313\text{ (g)}}{850\text{ (g)}} = \frac{100\text{ (\%)}}{x\text{ (\%)}}$$

$$x = \mathbf{64.7\%}$$

(10) *A 60-g tube of DESONATE gel contains 0.05% w/w desonide. Calculate the concentration of desonide on an mg/g basis.*

1 g × 0.05% w/w = 0.0005 g = **0.5 mg/g desonide**

(11) *DIPROLENE lotion contains 0.05% w/w betamethasone dipropionate. If the specific gravity of the lotion is 0.96, how many milligrams of betamethasone dipropionate would be present in a 60-mL container of the lotion?*

60 mL × 0.96 = 57.6 g
57.6 g × 0.05% = 0.0288 or 0.029 g = **29 mg betamethasone dipropionate**

(12) *What weight of a 5% (w/w) solution can be prepared from 2 g of active ingredient?*

$$\frac{5\text{ (\%)}}{100\text{ (\%)}} = \frac{2\text{ (g)}}{x\text{ (g)}}$$

$$x = \mathbf{40\ g}$$

(13) *How many milligrams of hydrocortisone should be used in compounding the following prescription?*

℞	Hydrocortisone	⅛%
	Hydrophilic ointment ad	10 g
	Sig. apply	

⅛% = 0.125%
10 g × 0.00125 = 0.0125 g or **12.5 mg hydrocortisone**

(14) *How many grams of benzocaine should be used in compounding the following prescription?*

℞	Benzocaine	2%
	Polyethylene glycol base ad	2 g
	Make 24 such suppositories	
	Sig. insert one as directed	

2 g × 24 = 48 g, total weight of mixture
48 g × 0.02 = **0.96 g benzocaine**

Or, solving by dimensional analysis:

$$24\text{ supp.} \times \frac{2\text{ g}}{1\text{ supp.}} \times \frac{2\%}{100\%} = \mathbf{0.96\ g\ benzocaine}$$

CALCULATIONS CAPSULE

Percent Concentration

The amounts of therapeutically active and/or inactive ingredients in certain types of pharmaceutical preparations are expressed in terms of their percent concentrations.

Unless otherwise indicated:

a. Liquid components in liquid preparations have *volume-in-volume* relationships with calculations following the equation:

mL of preparation × % concentration[a] = mL of component

b. Solid components in liquid preparations have *weight-in-volume* relationships with calculations following the equation:

mL of preparation × % concentration[a] = g of component

The terms of this equation are accepted due to the assumption that the specific gravity of the preparation is 1, as if it were water, and thus each milliliter represents the weight of 1 g.

c. Solid or semisolid components in solid or semisolid preparations have *weight-in-weight* relationships with calculations following the equation:

g of preparation × % concentration[a] = g of component

[a]In these equations, "% concentration" is expressed decimally (e.g., 0.05, *not* 5%).

Use of Percent in Compendial Standards

Percent is used in the *United States Pharmacopeia* to express the degree of tolerance permitted in the purity of single-chemical entities and in the labeled quantities of ingredients in dosage forms. For instance, according to the *United States Pharmacopeia*,[2] "Aspirin contains not less than 99.5% and not more than 100.5% of $C_9H_8O_4$ (pure chemical aspirin) calculated on the dried basis." Further, "Aspirin Tablets contain not less than 90.0% and not more than 110.5% of the labeled amount of $C_9H_8O_4$." Although dosage forms are formulated with the intent to provide 100% of the quantity of each ingredient declared on the label, some tolerance is permitted to allow for analytic error, unavoidable variations in manufacturing and compounding, and for deterioration to an extent considered insignificant under practical conditions.

The following problem demonstrates calculations involving percent in compendial standards.

If ibuprofen tablets are permitted to contain not less than 90% and not more than 110% of the labeled amount of ibuprofen, what would be the permissible range in content of the drug, expressed in milligrams, for ibuprofen tablets labeled 200 mg each?

90% of 200 mg = 180 mg
110% of 200 mg = 220 mg
Range = **180 mg to 220 mg ibuprofen**

CASE IN POINT 6.1[3] A patient with myasthenia gravis has undergone treatment to separate and remove certain abnormal antibodies and other unwanted elements from the blood (plasmapheresis). The desired red blood cell component is then returned back to the blood, but the patient has lost protein and blood volume.

The patient's physician orders 2000 mL of a 5% w/v solution of albumin in 0.9% w/v sodium chloride injection to replace lost protein and fluid.

In filling the order, the pharmacist decides to use a piece of automated equipment to compound the mixture. The equipment must be programmed with the specific gravities of the solutions being mixed. The pharmacist selects to use a 25% w/v albumin solution as the source of the albumin plus a 0.9% w/v sodium chloride injection.

From the literature, the pharmacist finds that 0.9% w/v sodium chloride has a specific gravity of 1.05. Using a precise 25-mL pycnometer with a tare weight of 28 g, the pharmacist fills it with the 25% w/v albumin solution and determines the weight of the flask and its content to be 58 g.

(a) What is the specific gravity of the albumin solution?
(b) How many milliliters of the 25% w/v albumin solution are needed to make 2000 mL containing 5% w/v albumin?
(c) What is the weight of the 25% w/v albumin solution needed to fill the order?
(d) If the pharmacist mixed the required number of milliliters of the 25% w/v albumin solution with a sufficient 0.9% w/v sodium chloride injection to make the required 2000 mL mixture, what would be the specific gravity of the resultant solution?

CASE IN POINT 6.2[3] A pharmacist receives the following prescription but does not have hydrocortisone powder on hand. However, the pharmacist does have an injection containing 100 mg of hydrocortisone per milliliter of injection. A search of the literature indicates that the injection has a specific gravity of 1.5.

℞	Hydrocortisone	1.5%
	Cold cream qs ad	30 g

(a) How many grams of hydrocortisone are needed to fill the prescription?
(b) How many milliliters of the hydrocortisone injection would provide the correct amount of hydrocortisone?
(c) How many grams of cold cream are required?

Ratio Strength

Percent strength itself indicates a ratio; that is, a solution which is 5% in strength represents the ratio of 5 parts in 100 parts, or the ratio 5:100. In expressing ratio strength, it is customary to have the first figure a *1*; thus, 5:100 would be reduced to 1:20.

When a ratio strength, for example, *1:1000*, is used to designate a concentration, it is to be interpreted as follows:

- *For solids in liquids = 1 g* of solute or constituent in *1000 mL* of solution or liquid preparation.

- *For liquids in liquids* = *1 mL* of constituent in *1000 mL* of solution or liquid preparation.
- *For solids in solids* = *1 g* of constituent in *1000 g* of mixture.

The ratio and percent strengths of any solution or mixture of solids are proportional, and either is easily converted to the other by the use of proportion.

Example Calculations Using Ratio Strength

(1) *Express 0.02% as a ratio strength.*

$$\frac{0.02\,(\%)}{100\,(\%)} = \frac{1\,(\text{part})}{x\,(\text{parts})}$$

$$x = 5000$$

Ratio strength = 1 : 5000

(2) *Express 1:4000 as a percent strength.*

$$\frac{4000\,(\text{parts})}{1\,(\text{part})} = \frac{100\,(\%)}{x\,(\%)}$$

$$x = \mathbf{0.025\%}$$

NOTE: To change ratio strength to percent strength, it is sometimes convenient to "convert" the last two zeros in a ratio strength to a percent sign (%) and change the remaining ratio first to a common fraction and then to a decimal fraction in expressing percent:

$$1{:}100 = \tfrac{1}{1}\% = 1\%$$
$$1{:}200 = \tfrac{1}{2}\% = 0.5\%$$
$$3{:}500 = \tfrac{3}{5}\% = 0.6\%$$
$$1{:}2500 = \tfrac{1}{25}\% = 0.04\%$$
$$1{:}10{,}000 = \tfrac{1}{100}\% = 0.01\%$$

(3) *A certain injectable contains 2 mg of a drug per milliliter of solution. What is the ratio strength (w/v) of the solution?*

$$2\text{ mg} = 0.002\text{ g}$$

$$\frac{0.002\,(\text{g})}{1\,(\text{g})} = \frac{1\,(\text{mL})}{x\,(\text{mL})}$$

$$x = 500\text{ mL.}$$

Ratio strength = 1 : 500

(4) *What is the ratio strength (w/v) of a solution made by dissolving five tablets, each containing 2.25 g of sodium chloride, in enough water to make 1800 mL?*

$$2.25\text{ g} \times 5 = 11.25\text{ g of sodium chloride}$$

$$\frac{11.25\,(\text{g})}{1\,(\text{g})} = \frac{1800\,(\text{mL})}{x\,(\text{mL})}$$

$$x = 160\text{ mL.}$$

Ratio strength = 1 : 160

In solving problems in which the calculations are based on ratio strength, it is sometimes convenient to translate the problem into one based on percent strength and to solve it accordingly.

(5) *How many grams of potassium permanganate should be used in preparing 500 mL of a 1:2500 solution?*

$$1{:}2500 = 0.04\%$$
$$500\ (g) \times 0.0004 = \mathbf{0.2\ g\ potassium\ permanganate}$$

Or,

1:2500 means 1 g in 2500 mL of solution

$$\frac{2500\ (mL)}{500\ (mL)} = \frac{1\ (g)}{x\ (g)}$$
$$x = \mathbf{0.2\ g\ potassium\ permanganate}$$

(6) *How many milligrams of gentian violet should be used in preparing the following solution?*

℞ Gentian violet solution 500 mL
1:10,000
Sig. instill as directed

$$1{:}10{,}000 = 0.01\%$$
$$500\ (g) \times 0.001 = 0.050 \text{ or } \mathbf{50\ mg\ gentian\ violet}$$

Or,

1:10,000 means 1 g of 10,000 mL of solution

$$\frac{10{,}000\ (mL)}{500\ (mL)} = \frac{1\ (g)}{x\ (g)}$$
$$x = 0.050\ g, \text{ or } \mathbf{50\ mg\ gentian\ violet}$$

(7) *How many milligrams of hexachlorophene should be used in compounding the following prescription?*

℞ Hexachlorophene 1:400
Hydrophilic ointment ad 10 g
Sig. apply

$$1{:}400 = 0.25$$
$$10\ (g) \times 0.0025 = 0.025\ g \text{ or } \mathbf{25\ mg\ hexachlorophene}$$

Or,

1:400 means 1 g in 400 g of ointment

$$\frac{400\ (g)}{10\ (g)} = \frac{1\ (g)}{x\ (g)}$$
$$x = 0.025\ g, \text{ or } \mathbf{25\ mg\ hexachlorophene}$$

Simple Conversions of Concentration to "mg/mL"

Occasionally, pharmacists, particularly those practicing in patient care settings, need to *convert rapidly* product concentrations expressed as percent strength, as ratio strength, or as grams per liter (as in IV infusions) *to milligrams per milliliter* (mg/mL). These conversions may be made quickly by using simple techniques. Some suggestions follow.

To convert *product percent strength to mg/mL*, multiply the percent strength, expressed as a whole number by 10.

(1) *Convert 4% (w/v) to mg/mL*

4×10	= **40 mg/mL**
Proof or alternate method: 4% (w/v)	= 4 g/100 mL
	= 4000 mg/100 mL
	= **40 mg/mL**

To convert *product ratio strengths to mg/mL*, divide the ratio strength by 1000.

(2) *Convert 1: 10,000 (w/v) to mg/mL*

$10{,}000 \div 1000$	= **1 mg/10 mL**
Proof or alternate method: 1:10,000 (w/v)	= 1 g/10,000 mL
	= 1000 mg/10,000 mL
	= **1 mg/10 mL**

To convert *product strengths expressed as grams per liter (g/L) to mg/mL*, convert the numerator of milligrams and divide by the number of milliliters in the denominator.

(3) *Convert a product concentration of 1 g per 250 mL to mg/mL*

$1000 \div 250$	= **4 mg/mL**
Proof or alternate method: 1 g/250 mL	= 1000 mg/250 mL = **4 mg/mL**

CALCULATIONS CAPSULE

Ratio Strength

The concentrations of very weak pharmaceutical preparations (usually weight-in-volume solutions) often are expressed in terms of their ratio strengths.

Ratio strength is another way of expressing percent strength. For example, a 1% w/v solution and a ratio strength of 1:100 w/v are equivalent.

The preferable style of a ratio strength is to have the numeric value of the solute as 1. This is accomplished when calculating a ratio strength, by setting up a proportion from the data as:

$$\frac{\text{g (given solute)}}{\text{mL (given solution)}} = \frac{1}{x}; \quad \text{then, 1 : value of x}$$

In using a ratio strength in a calculations problem, there are two options: (a) convert it to a percent strength and perform calculations in the usual manner, or (2) use the ratio strength directly in a problem-solving proportion.

(a) To convert a ratio strength to a percent strength; for example, 1:10,000 w/v:

$$\frac{1\text{ g}}{10{,}000\text{ mL}} = \frac{x\text{ (g)}}{100\text{ mL}}$$

Solving for x yields percent, by definition (parts per hundred).

(b) Problem-solving proportion, for example:

$$\frac{1\text{ g}}{10{,}000\text{ mL}} = \frac{x\text{ g}}{\text{(given quality, mL)}}; \quad x = \text{g in given mL}$$

Milligrams Percent

The term *milligrams percent* (mg%) expresses the number of milligrams of substance in 100 mL of liquid. It is used occasionally to denote the concentration of a drug or natural substance in a biologic fluid, as in the blood. Thus, the statement that the concentration of nonprotein nitrogen in the blood is 30 mg% means that each 100 mL of blood contains 30 mg of nonprotein nitrogen. However, the concentrations of substances in biologic fluids are more often expressed in milligrams per deciliter (mg/dL), which is a more accurate within the context of the *International System of Units.*

Parts per Million (PPM) and Parts per Billion (PPB)

The strengths of very dilute solutions are commonly expressed in terms of *parts per million (ppm)* or *parts per billion (ppb)*, that is, the number of parts of the agent per 1 million or 1 billion parts of the whole. For example, we are all familiar with fluoridated drinking water in which fluoride has been added at levels of between 1 to 4 parts per million (1:1,000,000 to 4:1,000,000) for the purpose of reducing dental caries.

We also are aware of and concerned with the presence of trace amounts of *contaminants* in our drinking water and food which can pose a risk to our health and safety. Many pharmacists serve on community committees and boards that address environmental issues. Although they may not refer to themselves as ***environmental pharmacists***, their backgrounds and interest in public health make them invaluable members of such bodies. Pharmacists have a special leadership role in providing guidance in the safe disposal of unused and/or expired medications.[4,5] Federal regulations and guidelines have been established to address this issue.[6,7]

Example Calculations of Parts per Million and Parts per Billion

(1) *Express 5 ppm of iron in water in percent strength and ratio strength.*

5 ppm = 5 parts in 1,000,000 parts = **1:200,000, ratio strength,** *and*
= **0.0005, percentage strength**

(2) *The concentration of a drug additive in an animal feed is 12.5 ppm. How many milligrams of the drug should be used in preparing 5.2 kg of feed?*

12.5 ppm = 12.5 g (drug) in 1,000,000 g (feed)

Thus,

$$\frac{1{,}000{,}000\text{ g}}{12.5\text{ g}} = \frac{5{,}200\text{ g}}{x\text{ g}}$$

$$x = 0.065\text{ g} = \mathbf{65\text{ mg}}$$

(3) *The drinking water in a community has detected lead in its drinking water at a level of 2.5 ppb. The EPA's MCL is set at 15 ppb. Express the difference between these two values as a ratio strength.*

15 ppb − 2.5 ppb = 12.5 ppb = 12.5:1,000,000,000 = **1:80,000,000**

PRACTICE PROBLEMS

Weight-in-Volume Calculations

1. CLOBEX lotion contains 0.05% w/v clobetasol propionate in 118 mL containers. Calculate the content of drug, in milligrams.
2. ℞ Ofloxacin ophthalmic solution 0.3%
   Disp. 10 mL
   How many milligrams of ofloxacin are contained in each milliliter of the dispensed prescription?
3.[8] ℞ Dexamethasone sodium phosphate 100 mg
   Sterile water for injection ad 100 mL
   Calculate the percent strength of dexamethasone sodium phosphate in the prescription.
4. If 100 mL of a pharmaceutical preparation contains 20 μL of a 50% w/v solution of benzalkonium chloride, what is the percent strength of that agent in the solution?
5. A tissue plasminogen activator (TPA) ophthalmic solution is prepared to contain 25 μg/100 μL.
   (a) Calculate the percent concentration of TPA in the solution.
   (b) What volume of a solution containing TPA, 50 mg/50 mL, should be used to prepare each 100 μL of the ophthalmic solution?
6. How many milligrams of methylparaben are needed to prepare 8 fluidounces of a solution containing 0.12% w/v of methylparaben?
7. A pharmacist emptied the contents of eight capsules, each containing 300 mg of clindamycin phosphate, into a liquid vehicle to prepare 60 mL of a suspension. Calculate the percent strength of clindamycin phosphate in the preparation.
8. ℞ Ketorolac ophthalmic solution 0.5%
   Disp. 5 mL
   Sig: One drop q.i.d. prn allergic conjunctivitis
   How many milligrams of the active constituent would be present in each drop of the ophthalmic solution if the dropper service delivers 20 drops per milliliter?
   (a) 0.25 mg
   (b) 25 mg
   (c) 0.025 mg
   (d) 1.25 mg
9. A formula for an antifungal shampoo contains 2% w/v ketoconazole. How many grams of ketoconazole would be needed to prepare 240 mL of the shampoo?
10. The biotechnology drug interferon gamma-1b (ACTIMMUNE) contains 100 mcg/0.5 mL. Calculate the percent strength of the solution.
11. Filgrastim (NEUPOGEN) prefilled syringes contain 480 mcg of active constituent in each 0.8 mL. The equivalent concentration is:
    (a) 0.6%
    (b) 0.384 mg/mL
    (c) 0.06%
    (d) 0.6 g/mL

12. Levofloxacin (LEVAQUIN) injection contains 5 mg/mL of levofloxacin and 5% of dextrose. How much of each would be delivered to a patient upon the administration of a 100-mL injection?
    (a) 5 g levofloxacin and 5 g dextrose
    (b) 50 mg levofloxacin and 5 g dextrose
    (c) 500 mg levofloxacin and 500 mg dextrose
    (d) 0.5 g levofloxacin and 5 g dextrose
13. An injection contains, in each milliliter, 60 μg of darbepoetin alfa (ARANESP), 0.05 mg of polysorbate 80, and 8.18 mg of sodium chloride. Calculate the percent of each in the injection.
14. An injection of adalimumab (HUMIRA) contains 40 mg/0.8 mL. Calculate the percent concentration of the injection.
15.[9] ℞

Erythromycin lactobionate	500 mg
Dexamethasone sodium phosphate	100 mg
Glycerin	2.5 mL
Sterile water for injection ad	100 mL
M. ft. ophthalmic solution	

    (a) What is the percent strength of erythromycin lactobionate in the prescription?
    (b) If glycerin has a specific gravity of 1.25, what is its percent concentration in the prescription?
16. CIPRODEX, an otic suspension, contains 0.3% w/v ciprofloxacin and 0.1% w/v dexamethasone in 7.5-mL drop containers. Calculate the quantities of each agent based on mg/mL.
17. A 180-mL bottle of an oral solution contains sodium oxybate, 0.5 g/mL. Calculate (a) the quantity of sodium oxybate, in grams, in the bottle and (b) the percent strength of sodium oxybate in the solution.
18. In the preparation of an intravenous infusion, a vial containing 115 mg of drug is diluted to 5 mL with sodium chloride for injection. Then, the contents of the vial are added to 110 mL of an infusion solution. Calculate the drug strength of the final infusion in (a) mg/mL, (b) percent strength, and (c) ratio strength.
19. An ophthalmic solution contains tafluprost, 0.0015% w/v, available in 0.3 mL pouches for single use. Calculate (a) the quantity of tafluprost, in micrograms, in each pouch and (b) the number of single-dose pouches that the manufacturer may prepare from each 1 g of drug.
20. A pharmacist adds 10 mL of a 20% w/v solution of a drug to 500 mL of D5W for parenteral infusion. What is the percentage strength of the drug in the infusion solution?
    (a) 2% v/v
    (b) 2% w/v
    (c) 1.96% w/v
    (d) 0.39% w/v
21. Calculate the percentage strength of an injection that contains 2 mg of hydromorphone hydrochloride in each milliliter of injection.
22. VIRAMUNE oral suspension contains 1% w/v of nevirapine. Calculate the milligrams of nevirapine present in a 240-mL bottle of the suspension.
23.[10] ℞

Misoprostol 200-μg tablets	12 tablets
Lidocaine hydrochloride	1 g
Glycerin qs ad	100 mL

Calculate the strength of misoprostol in the prescription.

(a) 2.4% w/v misoprostol
(b) 0.0002% w/v misoprostol
(c) 0.024 mg/mL misoprostol
(d) 2.4 mcg/mL misoprostol

24.[11] ℞

Fentanyl citrate	20 μg/mL
Bupivacaine hydrochloride	0.125%
Sodium chloride (0.9%) injection ad	100 mL

Calculate the percentage concentration of fentanyl citrate in the prescription.

25. Bepotastine besilate (BEPREVE) ophthalmic solution contains 1.5% w/v of the therapeutic agent. Express this concentration in mg/mL.
26. If 100 mL of a solution for patient-controlled anesthesia contains 200 mg of morphine sulfate and 8 mg of droperidol, calculate the percentage strength of each of these ingredients in the solution.
27. Oxycodone hydrochloride oral concentrate solution (OXYFAST) contains 20 mg/mL. If a dose of 0.75 mL is added to 30 mL of juice prior to administration, calculate (a) the milligrams of oxycodone hydrochloride administered and (b) the percent concentration of oxycodone hydrochloride in the drink.
28. A morphine sulfate extended-release liposome injection (DEPODUR) contains morphine sulfate 10 mg/mL of injection. Calculate the percent strength of morphine sulfate in the injection.
29. A topical solution contains 3% w/v hydroquinone. How many liters of the solution can be prepared from 30 g of hydroquinone?

Volume-in-Volume Calculations

30. What is the percent strength (v/v) if 225 g of a liquid having a specific gravity of 0.8 are added to enough water to make 1.5 L of the solution?
31. Cyclosporine (GENGRAF) capsules contain a dispersion of 25 mg of cyclosporine in a hydroalcoholic vehicle. The labeled content of absolute alcohol content is "12.8% v/v equivalent to 10.1% w/v." From these data, calculate the specific gravity of absolute alcohol.
32. A lotion vehicle contains 15% v/v of glycerin. How much glycerin should be used in preparing 5 gallons of the lotion?

    (a) 2271 g glycerin
    (b) 3339.7 mL glycerin
    (c) 2671.8 g glycerin
    (d) 3548.4 g glycerin

33. The formula for 1 L of an elixir contains 0.25 mL of a flavoring oil. What is the percent strength of the flavoring oil in the elixir?
34. A dermatologic lotion contains 1.25 mL of liquefied phenol in 500 mL. Calculate the percent strength of liquefied phenol in the lotion.

Weight-in-Weight Calculations

35. Each gram of LOTRISONE lotion contains 10 mg of clotrimazole and 0.643 mg of betamethasone dipropionate. Calculate the percent concentration of each of these two agents in the lotion.
36. A hemorrhoidal ointment contains, on a weight-in-weight basis, 46.6% mineral oil, 1% pramoxine HCl, and 12.5% zinc oxide in an ointment base. Calculate the grams of each ingredient, including the ointment base, in each 30-g tube.

37. What is the percentage strength (w/w) of a solution made by dissolving 62.5 g of potassium chloride in 187.5 mL of water?
38. If 500 g of dextrose are dissolved in 600 mL of water with a resultant final volume of 1 L, what is the percentage strength of dextrose in the solution on a w/w basis?
39. Hydromorphone hydrochloride suppositories contain 3 mg of active ingredient and weigh approximately 2 g each. What is the equivalent percentage strength?
    (a) 1.5%
    (b) 0.15%
    (c) 0.015%
    (d) None of the above
40. A metronidazole vaginal gel contains 0.75% of drug in 70-g tubes. An applicator will hold 5 g of gel for each administration. How much drug will be contained in each application?
    (a) 0.0375 mg metronidazole
    (b) 3.75 mg metronidazole
    (c) 37.5 mg metronidazole
    (d) 375 mg metronidazole
41. The percent of acyclovir and quantity of lidocaine in the filled prescription are:

℞	Acyclovir (ZOVIRAX)	5% cream
	Lidocaine 4% cream aa.	15 g

    (a) 3.75% acyclovir, 0.3 g lidocaine
    (b) 5% acyclovir, 1.2 g lidocaine
    (c) 2. 5% acyclovir, 0.6 g lidocaine
    (d) 2. 5% acyclovir, 1.2 g lidocaine
42. ANDROGEL 1.62% w/w is a testosterone gel applied topically in males for endogenous testosterone deficiency. For a starting dose of 40.5 mg testosterone, calculate the quantity, in grams, of gel administered.
43. DESONATE gel contains 0.05% w/w desonide. Calculate (a) the quantity of this agent, in grams, in each 60-g tube of product and (b) the concentration of desonide, in mg/g of gel.
44. Each gram of an ointment contains 2.5 mg of miconazole nitrate. The ointment is available in 50-g tubes. Calculate (a) the percent concentration of miconazole nitrate in the ointment and (b) the quantity of miconazole nitrate, in grams, in each tube of ointment.
45. A triamcinolone acetonide topical aerosol spray contains 0.147 mg of triamcinolone acetonide in each gram of product. Calculate the percent strength of triamcinolone acetonide in the product.
46. Calcipotriene (SORILUX) foam, 0.005% w/w, is supplied in containers holding 60 g of product. Calculate the number of milligrams of calcipotriene per container.
47. A topical gel contains 1.2% w/w clindamycin phosphate and 0.025% w/w tretinoin. Calculate the quantity of each of these ingredients on an mg/g basis.

Mixed Percent Calculations

48.[12]

℞	Progesterone, micronized	4 g
	Glycerin	5 mL
	Methylcellulose (1%) solution	50 mL
	Cherry syrup ad	100 mL

    (a) What is the percent concentration (w/v) of progesterone in the prescription?
    (b) What is the percent concentration (w/v) of methylcellulose in the prescription?

(c) What is the percent concentration (v/v and w/v) of glycerin (sp gr 1.25) in the prescription?

49.[13] ℞

Lactic acid	4 g
Salicylic acid	5 g
Trichloroacetic acid	2 g
Flexible collodion qs ad	100 g

Sig: wart remover. Use as directed.

(a) Flexible collodion contains 20% w/w camphor and 30% w/w castor oil. How many grams of each would be contained in 30 g of the mixture?
(b) The specific gravity of castor oil is 0.955. How many milliliters of the oil is contained in 30 g of the mixture?
(c) If the specific gravity of the mixture is 0.781, what are the percent w/v concentrations of lactic acid, salicylic acid, and trichloroacetic acid in the mixture?

Ratio Strength Calculations

50. Express each of the following as a percent strength:

(a) 1:1500
(b) 1:10,000
(c) 1:250
(d) 1:400
(e) 1:3300
(f) 1:4000

51. Express each of the following as a ratio strength:

(a) 0.125%
(b) 2.5%
(c) 0.80%
(d) 0.6%
(e) ⅓%
(f) ½%

52. Express each of the following concentrations as a ratio strength:
(a) 2 mg of active ingredient in 2 mL of solution
(b) 0.275 mg of active ingredient in 5 mL of solution
(c) 2 g of active ingredient in 250 mL of solution
(d) 1 mg of active ingredient in 0.5 mL of solution

53. A doxycycline calcium syrup is preserved with 0.08% w/v of methylparaben, 0.02% w/v of propylparaben, and 0.1% w/v of sodium metabisulfite. Express these concentrations as ratio strengths.

54. An injection contains 0.5% w/v of lidocaine hydrochloride and 1:200,000 w/v of epinephrine. Express the concentration of lidocaine hydrochloride as a ratio strength and that of epinephrine as a percent strength.

55. A sample of white petrolatum contains 10 mg of tocopherol per kilogram as a preservative. Express the amount of tocopherol as a ratio strength.

56. ℞

Potassium permanganate tablets	0.2 g
Disp.	#100

Sig: two tablets in 4 pt of water and use as directed.
Express the concentration, as a ratio strength, of the solution prepared according to the directions given in the prescription.

57. A skin test for fire ant allergy involves the intradermal skin prick of 0.05 mL of a 1:1,000,000 w/v dilution of fire ant extract. How many micrograms of extract would be administered in this manner?

58. An eyedrop has the following formula:

Fluorometholone	0.1% w/v
Neomycin sulfate	0.35% w/v
Benzalkonium chloride	0.004% w/v
Isotonic vehicle ad	5 mL

(a) Calculate the ratio strength of benzalkonium chloride in the formula.
(b) Calculate the quantity of fluorometholone, in milligrams, in the formula.

59. A lubricating eyedrop has the following formula:

Polyvinyl alcohol	1.4% w/v
Benzalkonium chloride	0.005% w/v
Sterile vehicle ad	10 mL

Calculate the equivalent ratio strength of the benzalkonium chloride

Parts per Million Calculations

60. Purified water contains not more than 10 ppm of total solids. Express this concentration as a percentage.
61. How many grams of sodium fluoride should be added to 100,000 L of drinking water containing 0.6 ppm of sodium fluoride to provide a recommended concentration of 1.75 ppm?
62. If a commercially available insulin preparation contains 1 ppm of proinsulin, how many micrograms of proinsulin would be contained in a 10-mL vial of insulin?

CALCQUIZ

6.A. AURALGAN Otic Drops contain:

Antipyrine	5.4%
Benzocaine	1.4%
Acetic acid	0.01%
u-Polycosanol 410	0.01%
Glycerin, ad	10 mL

(a) What would be the content of antipyrine, in mg/mL?
(b) If a patient used 5 drops of the otic solution, equivalent to 0.25 mL, how many milligrams of benzocaine would have been administered?
(c) How many microliters of acetic acid would be used to prepare the 10 mL of drops?
(d) What would be the equivalent ratio strength (v/v) of u-polycosanol 410?

6.B. Among its other ingredients, VISINE-A eyedrops contain the active ingredients: 0.025% w/v naphazoline hydrochloride and 0.3% w/v pheniramine maleate and 1:10,000 w/v benzalkonium chloride as a preservative. Calculate (a) the corresponding percent strength of benzalkonium chloride and (b) the quantities of each of the three ingredients in a 15-mL container.

6.C. An intravenous solution of AVELOX contains 400 mg of moxifloxacin hydrochloride (1.6 mg/mL). Calculate (a) the percent concentration of moxifloxacin hydrochloride and (b) the volume of solution in the product.

6.D. ATROVENT Nasal Spray contains 0.03% w/v of ipratropium bromide in a 30-mL metered dose container. If the container is calibrated to deliver 345 sprays, calculate (a) the volume of each spray, in microliters, and (b) the number of milligrams of ipratropium bromide in each spray.

6.E. A homeopathic teething gel states on its product label that it contains 0.0000003% alkaloid. Express the alkaloid content in ppm.

ANSWERS TO "CASE IN POINT" AND PRACTICE PROBLEMS

Case in Point 6.1

(a) 58 g (weight of filled pycnometer) – 28 g (weight of pycnometer) = 30 g (weight of 25 mL of albumin solution)

30 g ÷ 25 mL = 1.2, specific gravity of albumin solution

(b) 2000 mL × 0.05 (5%) = 100 g of albumin needed

$$\frac{25\text{ g}}{100\text{ mL}} = \frac{100\text{ g}}{\text{x mL}}; \quad \text{x} = 400\text{ mL, albumin solution needed}$$

(c) 400 mL × 1.2 (specific gravity) = 480 g, albumin solution needed

(d) 2000 mL (total solution) – 400 mL (albumin solution) = 1600 mL (0.9% sodium chloride solution)

1600 mL × 1.05 (specific gravity) = 1680 g (weight of 0.9% sodium chloride solution)

1680 g + 480 g = 2160 g (total weight of the 2000 mL)

2160 g ÷ 2000 mL = 1.08, specific gravity of the mixture

Case in Point 6.2

(a) 30 g × 0.015 (1.5% w/w) = 0.45 g hydrocortisone needed

(b) $\frac{0.1\text{ g}}{1\text{ mL}} = \frac{0.45\text{ g}}{\text{x mL}}$; x = 4.5 mL, hydrocortisone injection

(c) 4.5 mL × 1.5 (specific gravity) = 6.75 g (weight of hydrocortisone injection)

30 g – 6.75 g = 23.25 g cold cream needed

Practice Problems

1. 59 mg clobetasol propionate
2. 3 mg ofloxacin
3. 0.1% w/v dexamethasone sodium phosphate
4. 0.01% w/v benzalkonium chloride
5. (a) 0.025% w/v TPA
   (b) 0.025 mL
6. 283.9 mg methylparaben
7. 4% w/v clindamycin phosphate
8. (a) 0.25 mg ketorolac
9. 4.8 g ketoconazole
10. 0.02% w/v interferon gamma-1b
11. (c) 0.06%
12. (d) 0.5 g levofloxacin and 5 g dextrose
13. 0.006% w/v darbepoetin alpha, 0.005% w/v polysorbate 80, and 0.818% w/v sodium chloride
14. 5% w/v adalimumab
15. (a) 0.5% w/v erythromycin lactobionate
    (b) 3.125% w/v glycerin
16. 3 mg/mL ciprofloxacin and 1 mg/mL dexamethasone
17. (a) 90 g sodium oxybate
    (b) 50% w/v sodium oxybate
18. (a) 1 mg/mL
    (b) 0.1% w/v
    (c) 1:1000 w/v
19. (a) 4.5 mcg tafluprost
    (b) 222,222 pouches
20. (d) 0.39% w/v
21. 0.2% w/v hydromorphone
22. 2400 mg nevirapine
23. (c) 0.024 mg/mL misoprostol
24. 0.002% w/v fentanyl citrate
25. 15 mg bepotastine besilate/mL

26. 0.2% w/v morphine sulfate and 0.008% w/v droperidol
27. (a) 15 mg oxycodone hydrochloride
    (b) 0.049% w/v oxycodone hydrochloride
28. 1% w/v morphine sulfate
29. 1 L
30. 18.75% v/v
31. 0.79
32. (d) 3548.4 g glycerin
33. 0.025 v/v flavoring oil
34. 0.25% v/v liquefied phenol
35. 1% w/w clotrimazole and 0.0643% w/w betamethasone dipropionate
36. 13.98 g mineral oil
    0.3 g pramoxine HCl
    3.75 g zinc oxide
    11.97 g ointment base
37. 25% w/w potassium chloride
38. 45.45% w/w dextrose
39. (b) 0.15%
40. (c) 37.5 mg metronidazole
41. (c) 2.5% acyclovir, 0.6 g lidocaine
42. 2.5 g of testosterone gel
43. (a) 0.03 g desonide
    (b) 0.5 mg desonide/g gel
44. (a) 0.25% w/w miconazole nitrate
    (b) 0.125 g miconazole nitrate
45. 0.0147 % w/w triamcinolone acetonide
46. 3 mg calcipotriene
47. 12 mg/g clindamycin phosphate and
    0.25 mg/g tretinoin
48. (a) 4% w/v progesterone
    (b) 0.5% w/v methylcellulose
    (c) 5% v/v and 6.25% w/v glycerin
49. (a) 5.34 g camphor and 8.01 g castor oil
    (b) 8.39 mL castor oil
    (c) 3.12% w/v lactic acid, 3.91% w/v salicylic acid, and 1.56% w/v trichloroacetic acid
50. (a) 0.067%
    (b) 0.01%
    (c) 0.4%
    (d) 0.25%
    (e) 0.03%
    (f) 0.025%
51. (a) 1:800
    (b) 1:40
    (c) 1:125
    (d) 1:166.67 or 1:167
    (e) 1:300
    (f) 1:2000
52. (a) 1:1000
    (b) 1:18,182
    (c) 1:125
    (d) 1:500
53. 1:1250 w/v methylparaben
    1:5000 w/v propylparaben
    1:1000 w/v sodium metabisulfite
54. 1:200 w/v lidocaine hydrochloride
    0.0005% w/v epinephrine
55. 1:100,000 w/w tocopherol
56. 1:4730 w/v potassium permanganate
57. 0.05 μg fire ant extract
58. (a) 1:25,000 w/v benzalkonium chloride
    (b) 5 mg fluorometholone
59. 1:20,000 w/v benzalkonium chloride
60. 0.001% w/v
61. 115 g sodium fluoride
62. 10 μg proinsulin

References

1. United States Pharmacopeial Convention. *United States Pharmacopeia 32 National Formulary* 27. Vol. 1. Rockville, MD: United States Pharmacopeial Convention, 2009:8.
2. United States Pharmacopeial Convention. *United States Pharmacopeia 32 National Formulary* 27. Vol. 2. Rockville, MD: United States Pharmacopeial Convention, 2009:1582.
3. Flynn Warren, Clinical Pharmacist, Bishop, GA.

4. Johnson MG. Tools based on experiences of a community pharmacy providing destruction services for unwanted medications. *Journal of the American Pharmacists Association* 2010;50(3):388–392.
5. Gray-Winnett MD, Davis CS, Yokley SG, et al. From dispensing to disposal: the role of student pharmacists in medication disposal and implementation of a take-back program. *Journal of the American Pharmacists Association* 2010;50(5):613–618.
6. Office of National Drug Control Policy. *Proper Disposal of Prescription Drugs*. Washington, DC: Office of National Drug Control Policy; 2009. http://www.whitehousedrugpolicy.gov/publications. Accessed July 17, 2014.
7. Federal Register. *Secure and Responsible Drug Disposal Act of 2010*. Vol. 75. Federal Register; 2010:245.
8. Allen LV Jr, ed. Veterinary dexamethasone 0.1% ophthalmic ointment. *International Journal of Pharmaceutical Compounding* 1998;2:147.
9. Allen LV Jr, ed. Erythromycin and dexamethasone ophthalmic solution. *International Journal of Pharmaceutical Compounding* 2002;6:452.
10. Ford P. Misoprostol 0.0024% and lidocaine 1% in glycerin mouth paint. *International Journal of Pharmaceutical Compounding* 1999;3:48.
11. Allen LV Jr, ed. Fentanyl and bupivacaine injection for ambulatory pump reservoir. *International Journal of Pharmaceutical Compounding* 1997;1:178.
12. Allen LV Jr, ed. Progesterone Oral Suspension (40-mg/mL). *International Journal of Pharmaceutical Compounding* 1998;2:57.
13. Prince SJ. Calculations. *International Journal of Pharmaceutical Compounding* 2003;7:46.

7

Calculation of Doses: General Considerations

OBJECTIVES

Upon successful completion of this chapter, the student will be able to:

- Perform general dose calculations.
- Perform calculations relevant to specific dosing regimens.
- Apply dosing terminology correctly in performing pharmaceutical calculations.

Dose Definitions

The ***dose*** of a drug is the quantitative *amount* administered or taken by a patient for the intended medicinal effect. The dose may be expressed as a ***single dose***, the amount taken at one time; a ***daily dose***; or a ***total dose***, the amount taken during the course of therapy. A daily dose may be subdivided and taken in ***divided doses***, two or more times per day depending on the characteristics of the drug and the illness. The schedule of dosing (e.g., *four times per day for 10 days*) is referred to as the ***dosage regimen***.

Quantitatively, drug doses vary greatly among drug substances; some drugs have small doses, while other drugs have relatively large doses. The dose of a drug is based on its biochemical and pharmacologic activity, its physical and chemical properties, the dosage form used, the route of administration, and various patient factors. The dose of a drug for a particular patient may be determined in part on the basis of the patient's age, weight, body surface area, general physical health, liver and kidney function (for drug metabolism and elimination), and the severity of the illness being treated. Considerations of some specific patient parameters in dosing are presented in Chapter 8, and an introduction to ***pharmacokinetic*** dosing is presented in Chapter 22. Pharmacokinetic dosing takes into account a patient's ability to metabolize and eliminate drugs from the body due to impaired liver or renal function, which often necessitates a reduction in dosage.

The ***usual adult dose*** of a drug is the amount that ordinarily produces the medicinal effect intended in the adult patient. The ***usual pediatric dose*** is similarly defined for the infant or child patient. The "usual" adult and pediatric doses of a drug serve as a guide to physicians who may select to prescribe that dose initially or vary it depending on the assessed requirements of the particular patient. The ***usual dosage range*** for a drug indicates the quantitative range or amounts of the drug that may be prescribed within the guidelines of usual medical practice. Drug use and dose information is provided in the package inserts that accompany manufacturers' pharmaceutical products, from online resources, and through a variety of references such as *Drug Facts and Comparisons*[1]; *Physicians' Desk Reference*[2]; *Pediatric Dosage Handbook: Including Neonatal Dosing, Drug Administration, & Extemporaneous Preparations*[3]; *Geriatric Dosage Handbook*[4]; and *Drug Information Handbook*.[5]

The dose response of individuals varies as depicted in Figure 7.1 and may require dosage adjustment in a given patient. For certain conditions, as in the treatment of cancer patients, drug dosing is highly specialized and individualized. Frequently, combinations of drugs are

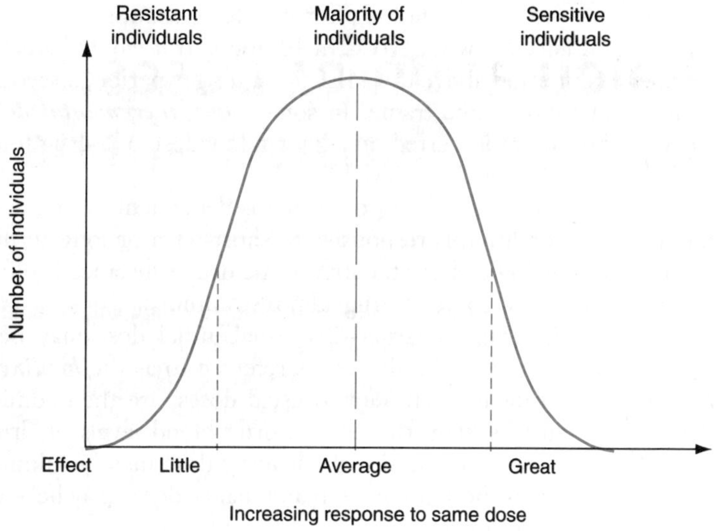

FIGURE 7.1 • Drug effect in a population sample.

used, with the doses of each adjusted according to the patient's response. Many anticancer drugs are administered *cyclically*, usually for 21 to 28 days, with a rest period between dosing cycles to allow recovery from the toxic effects of the drugs. As presented in Chapter 8, anticancer drugs are most commonly dosed on the basis of the patient's body surface area.

The ***median effective dose*** of a drug is the amount that produces the desired intensity of effect in 50% of the individuals tested. The ***median toxic dose*** of a drug is the amount that produces toxic effects in 50% of the individuals tested. Drugs intended to produce systemic effects must be absorbed or placed directly into the circulation and distributed in adequate concentrations to the body's cellular sites of action. For certain drugs, a correlation exists between drug dosage, the drug's blood serum concentration after administration, and the presentation and degree of drug effects. An average blood serum concentration of a drug can be measured, and the minimum concentration determined that can be expected to produce the drug's desired effects in a patient. This concentration is referred to as the ***minimum effective concentration*** (MEC). The base level of blood serum concentration that produces dose-related toxic effects is referred to as the ***minimum toxic concentration*** (MTC) of the drug.

Optimally, appropriate drug dosage should result in blood serum drug concentrations that are above the MEC and below the MTC for the period of time that drug effects are desired. As shown in Figure 7.2 for a hypothetical drug, the serum concentration of the

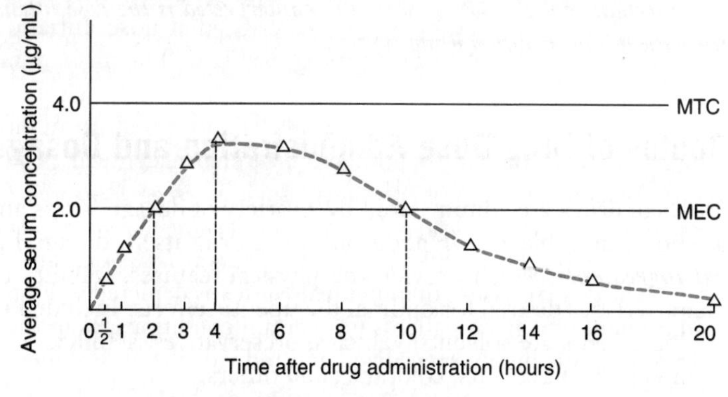

FIGURE 7.2 • Example of a blood level curve for a hypothetical drug as a function of the time after oral administration. (MEC, minimum effective concentration; MTC, minimum toxic concentration.)

drug reaches the MEC 2 hours after its administration, achieves a peak concentration in 4 hours, and falls below the MEC in 10 hours. If it would be desired to maintain the drug serum concentration above the MEC for a longer period, a second dose would be required at about an 8-hour time frame. In some cases, ***incremental dose escalation*** is employed whereby the patient is started on a known low dose of a drug followed by additional doses until the desired effect is achieved.

The *frequency or scheduling* of dosing is dependent on many factors including whether the illness or condition is responsive to short-term or long-term treatment; the physical–chemical and biologic characteristics of the drug substance itself; and features of the product formulation and route of drug administration.

For certain drugs, a larger-than-usual initial dose may be required to achieve the desired blood drug level. This dose is referred to as the ***loading dose***. Subsequent ***maintenance*** doses, similar in amount to usual doses, are then administered according to the dosage regimen to sustain the desired drug blood levels or drug effects. To achieve the desired drug blood level rapidly, the loading dose may be administered as an injection or oral liquid, whereas the subsequent maintenance doses may be administered in other forms, such as tablets or capsules.

As discussed later in this chapter, there are certain instances in which ***low-dose therapy*** or ***high-dose therapy*** is prescribed for a particular patient. And, for certain drugs, there may be different doses required depending on whether the use is for ***monotherapy***, that is, as the primary drug treatment, or ***adjunctive therapy***, that is, additional to or supportive of a different primary treatment.

Certain biologic or immunologic products, such as vaccines, may be administered in ***prophylactic doses*** to protect the patient from contracting a specific disease. Other products, such as antitoxins, may be administered in ***therapeutic doses*** to counter a disease after exposure or contraction. The doses of some biologic products, such as insulin, are expressed in ***units of activity***, derived from biologic assay methods. Calculations pertaining to these types of products are presented in Chapter 9.

Prefabricated products prepared on a large scale within the pharmaceutical industry and dispensed in community and institutional pharmacies generally contain the dosage strengths and dosage forms most often used. However, in instances in which the desired strength or dosage form is not available, pharmacists may be called upon to ***compound*** the preparation. Pharmaceutical products may be prepared to contain one or more therapeutic agents. Products containing more than one therapeutic agent are termed ***combination products***.

One of the primary responsibilities of the pharmacist is to check doses specified in prescriptions based on knowledge of the usual doses, usual dose ranges, and dosage regimens of the medicines prescribed. If an unusual dose is noted, the pharmacist is ethically bound to consult the physician to make certain that the dose as written or interpreted is the dose intended and that it is suitable for the patient and condition being treated.

Routes of Drug/Dose Administration and Dosage Forms

Doses of drugs are administered by a variety of dosage forms and routes of administration, as shown in Table 7.1. In addition to the drug itself, dosage forms contain ***pharmaceutical ingredients***, which provide the physical features, stability requirements, and aesthetic characteristics desired for optimal therapeutic effects. Included in the array of pharmaceutical ingredients are solvents, vehicles, preservatives, stabilizers, solubilizers, binders, fillers, disintegrants, flavorants, colorants, and others.

Table 7.1 • SELECTED ROUTES OF ADMINISTRATION AND REPRESENTATIVE DOSAGE FORMS

Route of Administration	Representative Dosage Forms
Oral (mouth, GI tract)	Tablets, capsules, lozenges, solutions, drops, syrups, and suspensions
Sublingual (under the tongue)	Tablets
Parenteral (injection)	Solutions and suspensions
Epicutaneous/transdermal (skin)	Ointments, creams, powders, lotions, aerosols, and patches
Conjunctival (eye)	Solutions, suspensions, and ointments
Intranasal (nose)	Solutions, sprays, and ointments
Intrarespiratory (lungs)	Aerosols and inhalant solutions
Rectal (rectum)	Ointments, creams, suppositories, solutions, and suspensions
Vagina (vagina)	Ointments, creams, tablets, suppositories, gels, solutions, and emulsion foams
Urethral (urethra)	Solutions and suppositories

With added pharmaceutical ingredients, the quantity of an active ingredient in a dosage form represents only a portion (often a small portion) of the total weight or volume of a product. For example, a tablet with 10 mg of drug actually could weigh many times that amount because of the added pharmaceutical ingredients.

Definitions of the various dosage forms and drug delivery systems are found in Appendix B.

Dose Measurement

In the institutional setting, doses are measured and administered by professional and paraprofessional personnel. A variety of measuring devices may be used, including calibrated cups and oral syringes for liquid oral medications (Figs. 7.3 and 7.4). For pediatric patients, use of oral syringes is recommended as a means of reducing medication dosing errors.[6] In hospitals, many medications are administered by injection and by intravenous infusion.

In the home setting, the patient, the caregiver, or, in the case of a child, the parent generally measures and administers oral medication. Liquids are measured using household measures such as teaspoons and tablespoons (Table 7.2), calibrated spoons or cups, oral

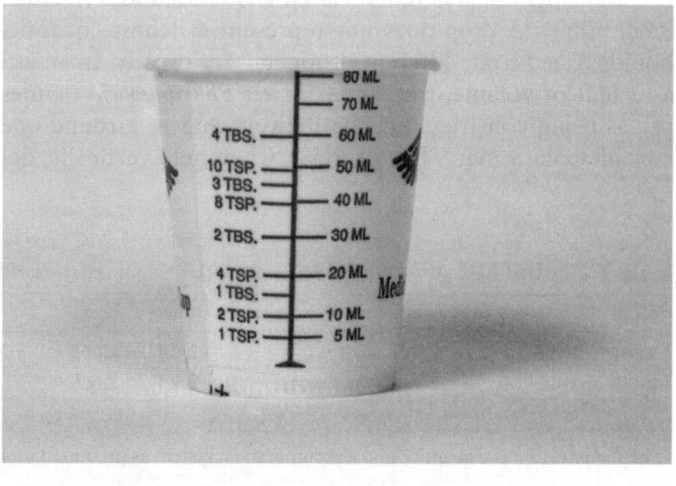

FIGURE 7.3 • An example of a calibrated medication cup for administering oral liquid medication.

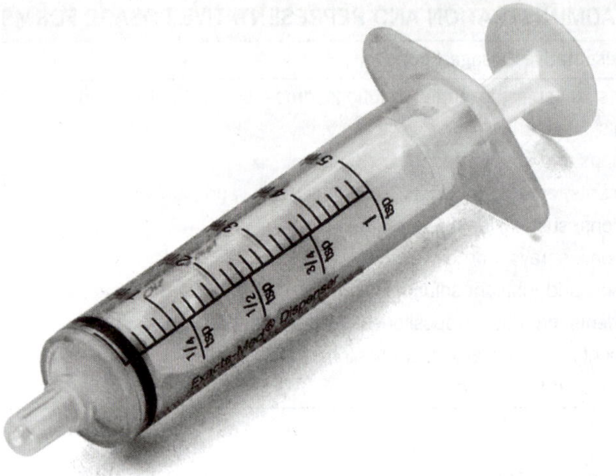

FIGURE 7.4 • An example of calibrated Exacta-Med Oral Dispenser for administering liquid medication to pediatric patients. *(Courtesy of Baxter Healthcare Corporation.)*

syringes, or drops. Patients being treated by home health care personnel may receive medications by all routes of administration including parenteral.

Teaspoon and Tablespoon

Household spoons vary greatly in capacities. Due to the variability in capacity, the Food and Drug Administration has issued the following statement: "*Do not use common household spoons to measure medicines for children since household spoons come in different sizes and are not meant for measuring medicines.*"[7] Instead, the FDA urges the use of the measuring device that accompanies a specific product or another device that is calibrated to deliver the recommended dose. A calibrated oral syringe often is a good option.

In approximate terms, and in dosage calculations, the teaspoon is considered to hold 5 mL of volume and the tablespoon 15 mL (Table 7.2).[8] Occasionally, a prescriber will indicate a teaspoonful dose by using the fluidram symbol (*fl℥*) in the *Signa* portion of a prescription, and the pharmacist interprets it accordingly.[a]

The Drop as a Unit of Measure

Occasionally, the *drop* (abbreviated *gtt*) is used as a measure for small volumes of liquid medications. A drop does not represent a definite quantity, because drops of different liquids issued from different droppers vary greatly. In an attempt to standardize the drop as a unit of volume, the *United States Pharmacopeia* defines the official medicine dropper as being constricted at the delivery end to a round opening with an external diameter of about 3 mm.[9] The dropper, when held vertically, delivers water in drops, each of

Table 7.2 • **USEFUL APPROXIMATE EQUIVALENT OF HOUSEHOLD MEASURE**

Household Measure (Abbreviation)	Ounce	Metric Measure
1 teaspoonful (tsp.)	≈1/6 fluidounce ≈	5 mL
1 tablespoonful (tbsp.)	≈1/2 fluidounce ≈	15 mL

[a]The *fluidram* (fl℥) is a quantity in the Apothecaries' system as presented in Appendix A.

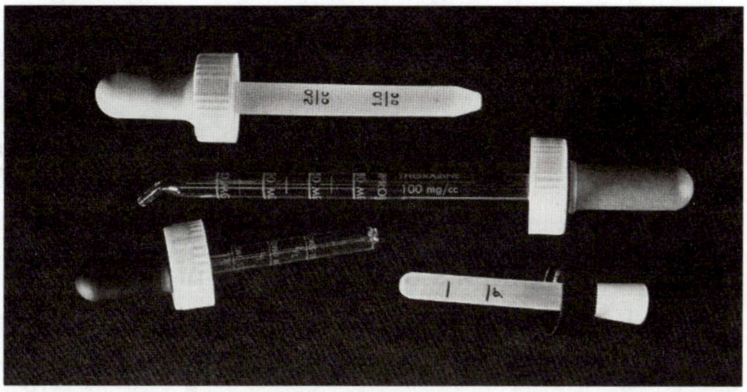

FIGURE 7.5 • Examples of calibrated droppers used in the administration of pediatric medications.

which weighs between 45 and 55 mg. Accordingly, the official dropper is calibrated to deliver approximately 20 drops of water per milliliter (i.e., 1 mL of water = 1 gram or 1000 mg ÷ 50 mg [ave.]/drop ≅ 20 drops).

It should be kept in mind that few medicinal liquids have the same surface and flow characteristics as does water, and therefore, the size of drops varies materially from one liquid to another. The drop should not be used as a measure for a specific liquid medication until the volume that the drop represents has been determined for that liquid. This determination is made by *calibrating* the dispensing dropper. Most manufacturers include a specially calibrated dropper along with their prepackaged medications for use by patients in measuring dosage. Examples of calibrated droppers are shown in Figure 7.5.

A dropper may be calibrated by counting the drops of a liquid as they fall into a graduate until a measurable volume is obtained. The number of drops per unit volume is then established (e.g., 20 drops/mL).

(1) *If a pharmacist counted 40 drops of a medication in filling a graduate cylinder to the 2.5-mL mark, how many drops per milliliter did the dropper deliver?*

$$\frac{40 \text{ (drops)}}{\text{x (drops)}} = \frac{2.5 \text{ (mL)}}{1 \text{ (mL)}}$$

$$\text{x} = \mathbf{16 \text{ drops mL}}$$

CASE IN POINT 7.1 A physician asks a pharmacist to calculate the dose of a cough syrup so that it may be safely administered dropwise to a child. The cough syrup contains the active ingredient dextromethorphan HBr, 30 mg/15 mL, in a 120-mL bottle.

Based on the child's weight and literature references, the pharmacist determines the dose of dextromethorphan HBr to be 1.5 mg for the child.

The medicine dropper to be dispensed with the medication is calibrated by the pharmacist and shown to deliver 20 drops of the cough syrup per 1 mL.

Calculate the dose, in drops, for the child.

General Dose Calculations

A pharmacist often needs to calculate the size of a dose, the number of doses, or the total quantity of medication to dispense. For these calculations, the following equation is useful *with the terms rearranged depending on the answer required.* In using the equation, the units of weight or volume must be the same for the total quantity and size of the dose.

$$\textbf{Number of doses} = \frac{\textbf{Total quantity}}{\textbf{Size of dose}}$$

Example Calculations of the Number of Doses

(1) *If the dose of a drug is 200 mg, how many doses are contained in 10 g?*

$$10 \text{ g} = 10{,}000 \text{ mg}$$

$$\text{Number of doses} = \frac{10{,}000 \text{ (mg)}}{200 \text{ (mg)}} = \textbf{50 doses}$$

Or, solving by dimensional analysis:

$$\frac{1 \text{ dose}}{200 \text{ mg}} \times \frac{1000 \text{ mg}}{1 \text{ g}} \times 10 \text{ g} = \textbf{50 doses}$$

(2) *If 1 tablespoonful is prescribed as the dose, approximately how many doses will be contained in 1 pint of the medicine?*

$$1 \text{ tablespoonful} = 15 \text{ mL}$$

$$1 \text{ pint} = 473 \text{ mL}$$

$$\text{Number of doses} = \frac{473 \text{ mL}}{15 \text{ mL}} = 31.5 \text{ or } \textbf{31 doses}$$

(3) *If the dose of a drug is 50 μg, how many doses are contained in 0.02 g?*

$$0.02 \text{ g} = 20 \text{ mg}$$

$$50 \text{ μg} = 0.05 \text{ mg}$$

$$\text{Number of doses} = \frac{20 \text{ (mg)}}{0.05 \text{ (mg)}} = \textbf{400 doses}$$

Example Calculations of the Size of a Dose

$$\textbf{Size of dose} = \frac{\textbf{Total quantity}}{\textbf{Number of doses}}$$

The *size of the dose* is expressed in whatever denomination is chosen for measuring the given total quantity.

(1) *How many teaspoonfuls would be prescribed in each dose of an elixir if 180 mL contained 18 doses?*

$$\text{Size of dose} = \frac{180 \text{ mL}}{18} = 10 \text{ mL} = \textbf{2 teaspoonfuls}$$

(2) *How many drops would be prescribed in each dose of a liquid medicine if 15 mL contained 60 doses? The dispensing dropper calibrates 32 drops/mL.*

$$15 \text{ mL} = 15 \times 32 \text{ drops} = 480 \text{ drops}$$

$$\text{Size of dose} = \frac{480 \text{ (drops)}}{60} = \textbf{8 drops}$$

Or, solving by dimensional analysis:

$$\frac{32 \text{ drops}}{1 \text{ mL}} \times \frac{1}{60 \text{ doses}} \times 15 \text{ mL} = \mathbf{8 \text{ drops/dose}}$$

Example Calculations of the Total Quantity of Product

Total quantity = numbers of doses × size of dose

It is convenient first to convert the given dose to the denomination in which the total quantity is to be expressed.

(1) *How many milliliters of a liquid medicine would provide a patient with 2 tablespoonfuls twice a day for 8 days?*

Number of doses = 16
Size of dose = 2 tablespoonfuls or 30 mL
Total quantity = 16 × 30 mL = **480 mL**

(2) *How many milliliters of a mixture would provide a patient with a teaspoonful dose to be taken three times a day for 16 days?*

Number of tsp doses = 16 × 3 = 48 tsp
Total quantity = 48 × 5 mL = **240 mL**

(3) *How many grams of a drug will be needed to prepare 72 dosage forms if each is to contain 30 mg?*

Number of doses = 72
Size of dose = 30 mg
Total quantity = 72 × 30 mg = 2160 mg = **2.16 g**

(4) *It takes approximately 4 g of ointment to cover an adult patient's leg. If a physician prescribes an ointment for a patient with total leg eczema to be applied twice a day for 1 week, which of the following product sizes should be dispensed: 15 g, 30 g, or 60 g?*

Number of doses = 2 per day × 7 days = 14
Size of dose = 4 g
Total quantity = 14 × 4 g = 56 g; thus 60 g product size

Additional Examples of Calculations of Dose

(1) *If 0.05 g of a substance is used in preparing 125 tablets, how many micrograms are represented in each tablet?*

$$0.05 \text{ g} = 50 \text{ mg} = 50{,}000 \ \mu\text{g}$$

$$\frac{50{,}000 \ (\mu\text{g})}{125} = \mathbf{400 \ \mu g}$$

Or, solving by dimensional analysis:

$$\frac{1{,}000{,}000 \ \mu\text{g}}{1 \text{ g}} \times \frac{1}{125 \text{ tablets}} \times 0.05 \text{ g} = \mathbf{400 \ \mu g/tablet}$$

(2) *If a preparation contains 5 g of a drug in 500 mL, how many grams are contained in each tablespoonful dose?*

1 tablespoonful = 15 mL

$$\frac{500\ (\text{mL})}{15\ (\text{mL})} = \frac{5\ (\text{g})}{\text{x}}$$

$$\text{x} = \mathbf{0.15\ g}$$

(3) *A cough mixture contains 48 mg of hydromorphone hydrochloride in 8 fl. oz. How many milligrams of hydromorphone hydrochloride are in each 2-teaspoonful dose?*

1 fl. oz. = 6 tsp
8 fl. oz. = 48 tsp
48 tsp ÷ 2 = 24 doses
48 tsp ÷ 24 = **2 mg**

Or,

$$\frac{48\ (\text{tsp})}{2\ (\text{tsp})} = \frac{48\ (\text{mg})}{\text{x}\ (\text{mg})}$$

$$\text{x} = \mathbf{2\ mg}$$

(4) *How many milligrams each of hydrocodone bitartrate and guaifenesin will be contained in each dose of the following prescription?*

℞ Hydrocodone bitartrate	0.12 g
Guaifenesin	2.4 g
Cherry syrup ad	120 mL

Sig. teaspoonful for cough
1 teaspoonful = 5 mL
120 ÷ 5 = 24 doses
0.12 g ÷ 24 = 0.005 g = **5 mg hydrocodone bitartrate** ***and***
2.4 g ÷ 24 = 0.1 g = **100 mg guaifenesin**

(5) *How many grams of a drug substance are required to make 120 mL of a solution each teaspoonful of which contains 3 mg of the drug substance?*

1 teaspoonful = 5 mL

$$\frac{5\ (\text{mL})}{120\ (\text{mL})} = \frac{3\ (\text{mg})}{\text{x}\ (\text{mg})}$$

$$\text{x} = 72\ \text{mg or } \mathbf{0.072\ g}$$

Or, solving by dimensional analysis:

$$\frac{1\ \text{g}}{1000\ \text{mg}} \times \frac{3\ \text{mg}}{5\ \text{mL}} \times 120\ \text{mL} = \mathbf{0.072\ g}$$

(6) *A physician ordered 500-mg capsules of tetracycline to be taken twice a day for 10 days. How many total grams of tetracycline would be prescribed?*

Size of dose = 500 mg
Total number of doses = 2 (a day) × 10 (days) = 20 doses
Total quantity = 500 mg × 20 (doses) = 10,000 mg = **10 g**

Dosing Options

Low-Dose and High-Dose Therapies

The administration of doses that are much smaller or much larger than the *usual dose* of a drug is referred to as *low-dose* or *high-dose* therapy, respectively. This terminology is different in intent from the normal variation in a standard dose based on a patient's age, weight, renal function, or other specific parameter.

The most common example of low-dose therapy is the use of aspirin in 81-mg amounts (rather than the usual dose of 325 mg) to lower the risk of heart attack and clot-related stroke. Other examples are low-dose oral contraceptive use[10] and low-dose postmenopausal hormone therapy.[11]

High-dose therapy is commonly associated with the chemotherapeutic treatment of cancer, in which there is an attempt, through increased dose intensity, to kill tumor cells. Other examples are the high-dose use of progestin in the treatment of endometriosis[12] and the high-dose influenza vaccination of the elderly.[13]

Pharmacists must be aware of the use of high-dose therapies while remaining vigilant in protecting patients against unintended high doses and consequent drug overdose.

Example Calculations of Low-Dose and High-Dose Therapies

(1) *If a patient is changed from a daily standard-dose postmenopausal product containing 0.625 mg of conjugated estrogens (CE) to a low-dose formulation containing 0.35 mg CE, how many milligrams less of CE would the patient take per week?*

0.625 mg − 0.35 mg = 0.275 mg × 7(days) = **1.925 mg conjugated estrogens**

(2) *To reduce the inflammation of an optic nerve, a patient is administered high-dose prednisone, 900 mg/day for 5 days by intravenous infusion. The usual daily dose of prednisone is 5 to 60 mg/day, depending on the condition being treated. Calculate the dose that the patient received, as a multiple of the highest usual daily dose.*

$$\frac{900\text{ mg}}{60\text{ mg}} = \textbf{15, multiple of the highest usual dose}$$

Fixed-Dose Combination Products

A variety of prescription and nonprescription products are available containing two or more therapeutic agents in fixed-dose combinations. An advantage of combination products is that two or more needed drugs may be taken in a single dose, which may be more convenient, enhance compliance, and be less expensive for the patient than taking the same drugs individually. A disadvantage is the relative inflexibility in dosing compared with individual drug dosing.

Whether the fixed-dose combination is a liquid (e.g., a syrup) or a solid (e.g., a tablet) dosage form, when a dose is taken, the component drugs are taken in a fixed-dose ratio. To provide some options in dosing, many combinations of prescription drugs are formulated into different strengths. For example, capsules containing amlodipine and benazepril HCl (LOTREL), two drugs used in the treatment of hypertension, are available in strengths of 2.5 mg/10 mg, 5 mg/10 mg, 5 mg/20 mg, 5 mg/40 mg, 10 mg/20 mg, and 10 mg/40 mg. The prescriber can select the desired combination.

Example Calculation Based on Fixed-Dose Combination Products

Valsartan and hydrochlorothiazide tablets are available separately or in combination in strengths of 80 mg/12.5 mg, 160 mg/12.5 mg, 160 mg/25 mg, and 320 mg/12.5 mg. If a patient was receiving the lowest-dose combination product and the physician wished to double the dose of hydrochlorothiazide, what is the option?

An additional prescription for 12.5 mg of hydrochlorothiazide or individual prescriptions for 80 mg of valsartan and 25 mg of hydrochlorothiazide may be written.

Tablet Splitting and Crushing

A number of tablets are ***scored***, or grooved, to allow breaking into approximately equal pieces (usually halves). This allows dosage flexibility, particularly when a patient is started at a half dose and then is titrated up to a full dosage level. It also enables a patient to take a product at a strength that is not otherwise available.

Some patients use tablet-splitting devices to cut scored or unscored tablets for economic reasons. For some medications, the price of tablets of twice the strength required is similar to the lower-strength tablets, and the patient can double his or her supply by tablet splitting. Unfortunately, this practice often results in unequal portions of tablets and thus in uneven doses.[14–17]

The federal Food and Drug Administration (FDA) has recommended that consumers consult with their health care professional before splitting a tablet to discuss the "splitability" of the product.[18] (Some products should not be split or crushed, but must remain intact for proper effects.) As a part of its drug approval process, the FDA verifies drug products that have been shown by testing procedures to be capable of being effectively split.[19,20]

Pharmacists can provide guidance to their patients by (a) verifying tablets that may be safely split, (b) suggesting that the entire dispensed supply of tablets *not* be split at one time but only as needed since split tablets may be more affected than whole tablets by factors such as heat and humidity, and (c) suggesting the best device for tablet splitting, especially for tablets of unique shape and size.

For tablets that *can* be crushed without destroying desired absorption characteristics, *tablet crushing* is a commonly employed practice for home or institutional patients who are unable to swallow intact solid dosage forms. In these instances, mortars and pestles or specially designed tablet crushers may be used (Fig. 7.6). After crushing, the resulting particles may be suspended in a beverage or mixed with a foodstuff such as applesauce or yogurt prior to administration.

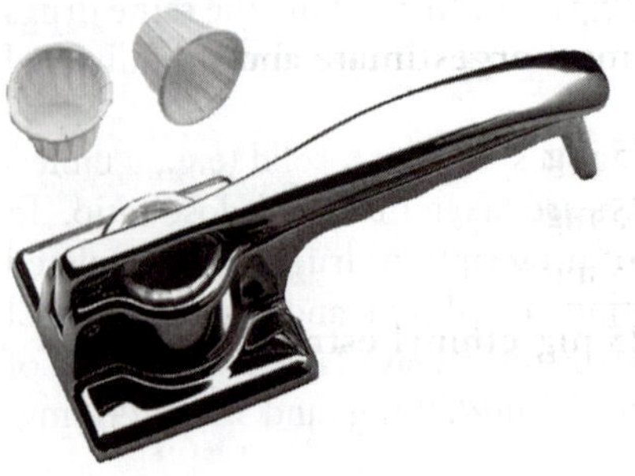

FIGURE 7.6 • An example of a tablet crusher. A tablet is placed in a paper cup, covered with a second cup, and then placed in the crusher. When the handles are gently squeezed, the pressure reduces the tablet to particles that may then be mixed with food or drink for administration. The device is used in patient care facilities and wherever a patient may have difficulty swallowing whole dosage units. *(Courtesy of Creative Living Medical, Brainerd, MN.)*

Example Calculation Based on Tablet Splitting

A patient attempted to split in half 20-mg unscored tablets of a drug, resulting in "half tablets" differing by 1.5 mg in drug content. Assuming a whole tablet was uniform in drug content, calculate the amount of drug in each "half tablet."

If L = larger "half" and S = smaller "half,"

then L + S = 20 mg

$$\frac{L - S = 1.5 \text{ mg}}{2\text{ L} = 21.5 \text{ mg}}$$

L = **10.75 mg**

S = 20 mg − 10.75 mg = **9.25 mg**

Proof: 10.75 mg − 9.25 mg = 1.5 mg difference in drug content and
10.75 mg + 9.25 mg = 20 mg total drug content

Special Dosing Regimens

Certain drugs have unique dosing regimens. Among them are chemotherapeutic agents (discussed in Chapter 8) and oral contraceptives. In the case of the latter, the prescribed regimen is based on a 28-day dosing cycle of 21 consecutive days of tablets containing a combination of estrogenic and progestational drugs followed by 7 consecutive days of tablets containing nondrug material. One tablet is taken daily, preferably at approximately the same time. The tablets generally are color-coded and packaged in special dispensers to facilitate compliance.

Another example of a drug having a special dosing regimen is methylprednisolone, as prescribed in dose packs containing 21 tablets of 4 mg each. The tablets are taken in *descending dosage* over a 6-day period in the treatment of responsive allergic and inflammatory conditions as contact dermatitis. In this regimen, 6 tablets are taken during the first day with 1 fewer tablet being taken each day thereafter.

Example Calculation Based on Special Dosing Regimen

The ORTHO TRI-CYCLEN LO 28-day regimen consists of norgestimate (N), ethinyl estradiol (EE), and nonmedicated tablets as follows:

7 white tablets containing 0.18 mg (N) + 0.025 mg (EE)
7 light blue tablets containing 0.215 mg (N) + 0.025 mg (EE)
7 dark blue tablets containing 0.25 mg (N) + 0.025 mg (EE)
7 green tablets containing 0 mg (N) + 0 mg (EE)

How many milligrams each of norgestimate and ethinyl estradiol are taken during each 28-day cycle?

Norgestimate:
0.18 mg × 7 = 1.26 mg
0.215 mg × 7 = 1.505 mg
0.25 mg × 7 = 1.75 mg

4.515 mg norgestimate and

Ethinyl estradiol:
0.025 mg × 7 = 0.175 mg
0.025 mg × 7 = 0.175 mg
0.025 mg × 7 = 0.175 mg

0.525 mg ethinyl estradiol

PRACTICE PROBLEMS

Doses: Solid Dosage Forms

1. The *ascending dose schedule* of ropinirole (REQUIP) in the treatment of Parkinson's disease is:

   Week 1: 0.25 mg three times a day
   Week 2: 0.5 mg three times a day
   Week 3: 0.75 mg three times a day
   Week 4: 1 mg three times a day

   How many 0.25-mg tablets would provide the 4 weeks of treatment?
2. The following regimen for oral prednisone is prescribed for a patient: 50 mg/day × 10 days; 25 mg/day × 10 days; 12.5 mg/day × 10 days; and 5 mg/day × 10 weeks. How many scored 25-mg tablets and how many 5-mg tablets should be dispensed to meet the dosing requirements?
3. A physician reduces a patient's once-daily dose of conjugated estrogen (PREMARIN) from tablets containing 0.625 mg to tablets containing 0.45 mg. What is the total reduction in conjugated estrogens taken, in milligrams, during a 30-day month?
4. A fixed-dose combination product contains amlodipine besylate and atorvastatin calcium (CADUET) for the treatment of both hypertension and hypercholesterolemia. If a physician starts a patient on a 5-mg/10-mg dose for 14 days and then raises the dose to 10 mg/20 mg, how many milligrams of each drug will the patient take during the first 30 days?
5. A patient cuts 100-mg scored tablets to take his 50-mg prescribed daily dose. A prescription for thirty 100-mg tablets costs $45, and a prescription for thirty 50-mg tablets costs $40. The patient asked the pharmacist to weigh an uncut tablet on an electronic balance into two "halves." The uncut tablet was found to weigh 240 mg, and the cut "halves" weighed 125 mg and 115 mg, respectively. (a) How much money did the patient save on a monthly basis by dosing with half tablets? (b) What was the percentage error in the weight of the cut tablets compared with "exact halves"?
6. The recommended dose of memantine HCl (NAMENDA) is:

   Week 1, 5 mg/day
   Week 2, 10 mg/day (5 mg b.i.d.)
   Week 3, 15 mg/day (10 mg a.m., 5 mg p.m.)
   Week 4, 20 mg/day (10 mg b.i.d.)

   How many 5-mg tablets must be dispensed for a 4-week supply of the medication?
7. Prior to a colonoscopy, a patient is instructed to take OSMOPREP tablets each of which contains 1.102 g sodium phosphate monobasic monohydrate and 0.398 g sodium phosphate dibasic anhydrous. The dose is:

   The evening before the procedure: 4 tablets with 8 ounces of clear liquids every 15 minutes for 5 cycles
   Starting 3 hours before the procedure: 4 tablets with 8 ounces of clear liquids every 15 minutes for 3 cycle

   How many tablets, how much liquid, and how much total sodium phosphates are taken?
   (a) 8 tablets, 16 ounces liquid, 2 g sodium phosphates
   (b) 16 tablets, 1000 mL liquid, 32 g sodium phosphates
   (c) 32 tablets, 1 quart liquid, 40 g sodium phosphates
   (d) 32 tablets, 0.5 gallon liquid, 48 g sodium phosphates

8. Varenicline tartrate (CHANTIX), for smoking cessation, is available in two strengths, 0.5-mg and 1-mg tablets. The dose is:
   Days 1 to 3: 0.5 mg once daily
   Days 4 to 7: 0.5 mg twice daily (AM and PM)
   Days 8 to end of treatment: 1 mg twice daily (AM and PM)
   The treatment period is 12 weeks. How many 0.5-mg tablets and 1-mg tablets should be dispensed?
   (a) 7 0.5-mg tablets and 11 1-mg tablets
   (b) 8 0.5-mg tablets and 84 1-mg tablets
   (c) 10 0.5-mg tablets and 84 1-mg tablets
   (d) 11 0.5-mg tablets and 154 1-mg tablets

Doses: Drops

9. A ciprofloxacin otic solution contains 0.5 mg of ciprofloxacin in a 0.25-mL single-dose package. Based on 20 drops/mL, (a) how many drops would be administered and (b) how many micrograms of ciprofloxacin would be in each drop?
10. ℞ Acetaminophen oral drops
    Disp. 15 mL
    Sig. 0.5 mL t.i.d.
    (a) If acetaminophen oral drops contain 1.5 g of acetaminophen per 15-mL container, how many milligrams are there in each prescribed dose?
    (b) If the dropper is calibrated to deliver 22 drops/mL, how many drops should be administered per dose?
11. RESTASIS ophthalmic emulsion contains 0.05% w/v cyclosporin. If a dose of one drop measures 28 μL, how many micrograms of cyclosporin are present?
12.[21] The oral dose of a drug is 2.5 mg. If a solution contains 0.5% w/v of the drug in a dropper bottle that delivers 12 drops/mL, how many drops would supply the dose?
13. Infants' MYLICON antigas drops contain 2 g of simethicone in a 30-mL container. (a) How many milligrams of simethicone are contained in each 0.3-mL dose? And if 12 doses per day are not to be exceeded, calculate the corresponding 12-dose (b) volume and (c) simethicone content.

Doses: Oral Liquids

14. Rimantadine HCl syrup contains 2.4 g of rimantadine HCl in each 240 mL of syrup. How many milligrams of rimantadine HCl would there be in 2.5 mL delivered by oral dispenser?
15. If a liquid medicine is to be taken three times daily, and if 180 mL are to be taken in 4 days, how many tablespoonfuls should be prescribed for each dose?
16. The usual starting dose of sodium oxybate is 4.5 g per night in two equally divided doses, taken 2.4 to 4 hours apart. A sodium oxybate oral solution is available in 180-mL bottles, containing sodium oxybate, 50% w/v. How many divided doses are available in each container?
17. The dose of posaconazole in the treatment of oropharyngeal candidiasis is 100 mg twice a day on the first day and then 100 mg once a day for the next 13 days. Posaconazole oral suspension (posaconazole, 40 mg/mL) is available in 4-fluidounce bottles. How many bottles should be dispensed to meet the dosing requirements?

18. A physician prescribes tetracycline HCl syrup for a patient who is to take 2 teaspoonfuls four times per day for 4 days, and then 1 teaspoonful four times per day for 2 days. How many milliliters of the syrup should be dispensed to provide the quantity for the prescribed dosage regimen?
19. Ipecac oral solution has the following formula:

Powdered ipecac	70 g
Glycerin	100 mL
Syrup ad	1000 mL

    Powdered ipecac contains 2 grams of the combined alkaloids emetine and cephaeline in each 100 grams of powder. Calculate the quantity of these alkaloids, in milligrams, in each 5-mL dose of ipecac oral solution.
20. A dose of digoxin for rapid digitalization is a total of 1 mg, divided into two or more portions at intervals of 6 to 8 hours. How many milliliters of digoxin elixir containing 50 μg/mL would provide the 1 mg dose?
21. Ciprofloxacin (CIPRO) oral suspension contains 250 mg of ciprofloxacin per 5 mL. A physician prescribed 125 mg of ciprofloxacin q.i.d. × 10 days. (a) How many doses are needed? (b) How many milliliters should be given per dose? (c) How many milliliters of ciprofloxacin oral suspension containing 250 mg per 5 mL should be dispensed?
22. A patient has been instructed to take 15 mL of alumina and magnesium oral suspension every other hour for four doses daily. How many days will two 12-fl. oz. bottles of the suspension last?
23. ℞ Dextromethorphan HBr 50 mg/tsp
    Guaifenesin syrup ad 120 mL
    Sig. ʒi q.i.d. a.c. & h.s.

    How many grams of dextromethorphan HBr would be needed to fill the prescription?
24. The dose of AUGMENTIN oral suspension for a patient is 5 mL b.i.d. Each 5 mL of suspension contains 400 mg of amoxicillin and 57 mg of clavulanic acid. If the suspension is to be taken for 10 days and is available in 50-mL, 75-mL, and 100-mL containers, calculate (a) the least wasteful package size to dispense and (b) total quantity of amoxicillin taken during the treatment period.

Doses: Injections

25. A physician ordered 20 mg of MEPERGAN and 0.3 mg of atropine sulfate to be administered preoperatively to a patient. MEPERGAN is available in a syringe containing 25 mg/mL, and atropine sulfate is in an ampul containing 0.4 mg per 0.5 mL. How many milliliters of each should be used in filling the medication order?
26. How many milliliters of an injection containing 250 mg of aminophylline in each 10 mL should be used in filling a medication order calling for 15 mg of aminophylline?
27.[22] Pediatric LANOXIN injection contains digoxin, 100 mcg/mL. What volume must be administered to provide a dose of 0.04 mg?
28. In treating Crohn's disease, the recommended dose of the monoclonal antibody adalimumab (HUMIRA) is 160 mg as the first dose, a second dose of 80 mg 2 weeks later, then a third dose of 40 mg 2 weeks after the second dose, and followed by a maintenance dose of 40 mg every 2 weeks. How many prefilled syringes, each containing adalimumab, 40 mg/0.8 mL, would be required for the initial 2 months of treatment?

29. BYETTA injection, as an adjunct for glycemic control in type 2 diabetes mellitus, contains 250 mcg of exenatide in each milliliter of solution. The injection is available in 1.2-mL prefilled pens. At a starting dose of 5 mcg b.i.d, (a) how many milliliters are injected per dose, (b) how many doses are contained in each pen, and (c) how many days will the dosing pen last the patient?
30. The biotechnology drug peginterferon alpha-2b is administered at a starting dose of 6 mcg for each kilogram of a patient's body weight (6 mcg/kg). The drug is available in single-use 0.74-mL injections containing 40 mcg/0.1 mL, 60 mcg/0.1 mL, or 120 mcg/0.1 mL. Which product size would be most efficacious for administration to a 156-lb patient?

Doses: Other Dosage Forms

31. The recommended maintenance dose of beclomethasone dipropionate (BECLOVENT), an aerosolized inhalant, is 100 mcg administered twice daily. The commercial inhaler delivers 50 mcg per metered inhalation and contains 200 inhalations. How many inhalers should be dispensed to a patient if a 60-day supply is prescribed?
32. A 16-week regimen for a brand of a nicotine patch calls for a patient to wear a 21-mg patch each day for the first 6 weeks, followed by a 14-mg patch each day for the next 2 weeks, and then a 7-mg patch for the next 2 weeks to conclude the treatment regimen. In all, how many milligrams of nicotine are administered?
33. A transdermal patch contains 5 mg of fentanyl and has a drug-release rate of 50 mcg/hour. The patch is worn for 72 hours. Calculate (a) the milligrams of fentanyl delivered daily, (b) the milligrams of fentanyl remaining in the patch when it is removed, and (c) the percentage of drug remaining in the patch when it is removed.
34. If a VENTOLIN inhaler contains 20 mg of albuterol, how many inhalation doses can be delivered if each inhalation dose contains 90 mcg?
35. FLONASE nasal spray contains 50 mcg of fluticasone propionate per actuation spray in each 100 mg of formulation. Each container provides 120 metered sprays. How many milligrams of fluticasone propionate are contained in each container?
36. The dose of diclofenac sodium (VOLTAREN GEL), when applied to the hands in the treatment of arthritic pain, is 2 g four times a day. The gel contains diclofenac sodium 1% and is available in 100-g tubes. How many grams of the drug diclofenac sodium would be administered per day, and how many days of treatment would be available per tube of gel?
    (a) 8 g diclofenac sodium per day for 8 days
    (b) 8 g diclofenac sodium per day for 12.5 days
    (c) 80 mg diclofenac sodium per day for 8 days
    (d) 0.08 g diclofenac sodium per day for 12.5 days
37. SYMBICORT 80/4.5 is an oral inhalation product containing 80 mcg of budesonide and 4.5 mcg of formoterol fumarate per inhalation. The dose is stated as "two inhalations twice daily." How much of *each drug* would be administered daily?
    (a) 160 mcg budesonide and 9 mcg formoterol fumarate
    (b) 0.32 mg budesonide and 0.18 mg formoterol fumarate
    (c) 320 mcg budesonide and 0.18 mg formoterol fumarate
    (d) 0.32 mg budesonide and 0.018 mg formoterol fumarate
38. An aerosol oral inhaler delivers, per actuation, 40 mcg of beclomethasone dipropionate. The recommended starting dose is 40 to 80 mcg twice daily. The highest recommended dose is 320 mcg twice daily. Compare the number of daily inhaler actuations to deliver the lowest starting dose and the highest recommended dose.

CALCQUIZ

7.A. The ophthalmic solution ALPHAGAN P contains 0.15% brimonidine tartrate in 10-mL containers. The recommended dose is one drop in the affected eye(s) three times daily. If a glaucoma patient doses each eye, and the dropper used delivers 20 drops/mL, calculate the quantity, in milligrams, of brimonidine tartrate administered each day.

7.B. The starting dose of sodium oxybate oral solution (XYREM) is 4.5 g/night divided into two equal doses and administered 2.5 to 4 hours apart. How many milliliters of the oral solution containing sodium oxybate, 500 mg/mL, should be administered in each divided dose?

7.C. A pediatric stool softener contains 393.3 mg of docusate sodium in each four fluid ounce (118 mL) container. If the labeled dose is 2 tablespoonful for a 5-year-old child, how many milligrams of docusate sodium would be contained per dose?

7.D. An oral inhalation (DULERA) to treat asthma provides in each inhalation 100 μg of mometasone furoate and 5 μg of formoterol fumarate. The recommended dose is "two inhalations twice daily (morning and evening)." Calculate the quantity, in milligrams, of each drug inhaled daily.

7.E. In an experiment of tablet-splitting effectiveness, a pharmacist had a pharmacy student split a previously weighed lisinopril tablet containing 20 mg of drug. On an electronic balance, the whole tablet weighed 111.62 mg. After splitting, one "half tablet" weighed 51.21 mg and the other "half," 58.49 mg. There was residue powder remaining. Calculate (a) the percent of lost tablet (residue), (b) the percent accuracy in actual weight (to ideal weight) for each "half tablet," and (c) the *supposed* quantity of drug, in milligrams (not assayed, of course) in each "half tablet."

ANSWERS TO "CASE IN POINT" AND PRACTICE PROBLEMS

Case in Point 7.1

First, calculate the volume of cough syrup containing the child's dose of 1.5 mg of dextromethorphan HBr:

$$\frac{30 \text{ mg}}{15 \text{ mL}} = \frac{1.5 \text{ mg}}{\text{x mL}}; \text{ x} = 0.75 \text{ mL}$$

Then determine the number of drops of cough syrup that will provide the 0.75-mL dose:

$$\frac{1 \text{ mL}}{20 \text{ drops}} = \frac{0.75 \text{ mL}}{\text{x drops}};$$

$$\text{x} = 15 \text{ drops of cough syrup}$$

Practice Problems

1. Two hundred ten 0.25-mg ropinirole tablets
2. Thirty-five 25-mg tablets and seventy 5-mg tablets
3. 5.25 mg conjugated estrogen
4. 230 mg amlodipine besylate and 460 mg atorvastatin calcium
5. (a) $17.50
   (b) 4.2%
6. 70 tablets
7. (d) 32 tablets, 0.5 gallon liquid, 48 g sodium phosphates
8. (d) 11 0.5-mg tablets and 154 1-mg tablets
9. (a) 5 drops ciprofloxacin otic solution
   (b) 100-μg ciprofloxacin/drop
10. (a) 50 mg acetaminophen
    (b) 11 drops
11. 14 mcg cyclosporine
12. 6 drops
13. (a) 20 mg simethicone
    (b) 3.6 mL of infants' MYLICON drops
    (c) 240 mg simethicone
14. 25 mg rimantadine HCl
15. 1 tablespoonful
16. 40 divided doses sodium oxybate oral solution
17. 1 bottle of posaconazole oral suspension
18. 200 mL tetracycline HCl syrup
19. 7 mg alkaloids
20. 20 mL digoxin elixir
21. (a) 40 doses
    (b) 2.5 mL/dose
    (c) 100 mL ciprofloxacin oral suspension
22. 11 + days
23. 1.2 g dextromethorphan HBr
24. (a) 100-mL package
    (b) 8000 mg or 8 g of amoxicillin
25. 0.8 mL MEPERGAN and 0.375 mL atropine sulfate injections
26. 0.6 mL aminophylline injection
27. 0.4 mL LANOXIN injection
28. 9 prefilled syringes, 40 mg/0.8 mL
29. (a) 0.02 mL per dose
    (b) 60 doses per pen
    (c) 30 days
30. 60 mcg/0.1 mL
31. 2 inhalers
32. 1176 mg nicotine
33. (a) 1.2 mg fentanyl
    (b) 1.4 mg fentanyl
    (c) 28%
34. 222 doses
35. 6 mg fluticasone propionate
36. (d) 0.08 g diclofenac sodium per day for 12.5 days
37. (d) 0.32 mg budesonide and 0.018 mg formoterol fumarate
38. 2 actuations (lowest daily starting dose) and 16 actuations (highest daily recommended dose)

References

1. *Drug Facts and Comparisons*. St. Louis, MO: Wolters Kluwer Health; 2014.
2. *Physicians' Desk Reference*. Montvale, NJ: Medical Economics; 2014:68.
3. Taketomo CK. *Pediatric & Neonatal Dosage Handbook*. 20th Ed. Hudson, OH: Lexicomp/Wolters Kluwer Health Clinical Solutions; 2013–2014.
4. Semla TP. *Geriatric Dosage Handbook*. 19th Ed. Hudson, OH: Lexicomp/Wolters Kluwer Health Clinical Solutions; 2013–2014.
5. *Drug Information Handbook*. 23rd Ed. Hudson, OH: Lexicomp/Wolters Kluwer Health Clinical Solutions; 2014–2015.
6. The Joint Commission. Available at: http://www.jointcommission.org/assets/1/18/SEA_39.PDF. Accessed May 1, 2014.

7. U.S. Food and Drug Administration. Use of over-the-counter cough and cold products in infants and children. Available at: http://www.fda.gov/Drugs/DrugSafety/DrugSafetyPodcasts/ucm077935.htm. Accessed July 24, 2014.
8. United States Pharmacopeial Convention. *United States Pharmacopeia 32 National Formulary* 27. Vol. 1. Rockville, MD: United States Pharmacopeial Convention; 2009:728.
9. United States Pharmacopeial Convention. *United States Pharmacopeia 32 National Formulary* 27. Vol. 1. Rockville, MD: United States Pharmacopeial Convention; 2009:604.
10. Actavis Pharma, Inc. LO LOESTRIN FE, product information. Available at: http://www.loloestrin.com/ Accessed July 24, 2014.
11. Santen RJ, Allred DC, Ardoin SP, et al. Postmenopausal hormone therapy: an endocrine society scientific statement. *J Clin Endocrinol Metab* 2010;95:S1–S66.
12. Available at: http://www.women.webmd.com/endometriosis/high-dose-progestin-for-endometriosis. Accessed July 25, 2014.
13. Foster SL, Moore WP. High-dose influenza vaccination in the elderly. *J Am Pharm Assoc* 2010;50:546–547.
14. Rashed SM, Nolly RJ, Robinson L, et al. Weight variability of scored and unscored split psychotropic drug tablets. *Hosp Pharm* 2003;38:930–934.
15. Hill SW, Varker AS, Karlage K, et al. Analysis of drug content and weight uniformity for half-tablets of 6 commonly split medications. *J Manag Care Pharm* 2009;15:253–261.
16. Verrue C, Mehuys E, Boussery K, et al. Tablet-splitting: a common yet not so innocent practice. *J Adv Nurs* 2010;67:26–32.
17. Green G, Berg C, Polli JE, et al. Pharmacopeial standards for the subdivision characteristics of scored tablets. *Pharmacopeial Forum* 2009;35:1598.
18. Food and Drug Administration, Department of Health and Human Services. Tablet splitting. Available at: http://www.fda.gov/Drugs/ResourcesForYou/Consumers/BuyingUsingMedicineSafely/EnsuringSafeUseofMedicine/ucm265754.htm. Accessed May 1, 2014.
19. Food and Drug Administration, Department of Health and Human Services. Best Practices for Tablet Splitting. Available at: http://www.fda.gov/Drugs/ResourcesForYou/Consumers/BuyingUsingMedicineSafely/EnsuringSafeUseofMedicine/ucm184666.htm. Accessed May 1, 2014.
20. Food and Drug Administration, Center for Drug Evaluation and Research, Department of Health and Human Services. Guidance for Industry: Tablet Scoring: Nomenclature, Labeling, and Data for Evaluation. Available at: http://www.fda.gov/downloads/Drugs/GuidanceComplianceRegulatoryInformation/Guidances/UCM269921.pdf. Accessed May 1, 2014.
21. Prince S. Calculations. *International Journal of Pharmaceutical Compounding* 2003;7:212.
22. Beach W. *College of Pharmacy*. Athens, GA: The University of Georgia; 2004.

8

Calculation of Doses: Patient Parameters

OBJECTIVES

Upon successful completion of this chapter, the student will be able to:

- Calculate doses based on factors of age, body weight, and body surface area.
- Utilize dosing tables and nomograms in calculations.
- Calculate doses for single and combination chemotherapy regimens.

As noted in the previous chapter, the ***usual dose*** of a drug is the amount that ordinarily produces the desired therapeutic response in the majority of patients in a general, or otherwise defined, population group. The drug's ***usual dosage range*** is the range of dosage determined to be safe and effective in that same population group. This provides the prescriber with dosing guidelines in initially selecting a drug dose for a particular patient and the flexibility to change that dose as the patient's clinical response warrants. Usual doses and dosage regimens are based on the results of clinical studies conducted during the drug development process as well as on clinical information gathered following the initial approval and marketing of the drug (*postmarketing surveillance/postmarketing studies*).

For certain drugs and for certain patients, drug dosage is determined on the basis of specific patient parameters. These parameters include the patient's age, weight, body surface area, and nutritional and functional status. Drug selection and drug dosage in patients who are pregnant and in nursing mothers are especially important considerations due to potential harm to the fetus or child.

Among patients requiring individualized dosage are neonates and other pediatric patients, elderly patients with diminished biologic functions, individuals of all age groups with compromised liver and/or kidney function (and thus reduced ability to metabolize and eliminate drug substances), critically ill patients, and patients being treated with highly toxic chemotherapeutic agents. Certain drugs with a narrow therapeutic window often require individualized dosing based on blood level determinations and therapeutic monitoring. Digoxin, for example, at a blood level of 0.9 to 2 ng/mL is considered therapeutic, but above 2 ng/mL, it is toxic.[1]

Since age, body weight, and body surface area are often-used factors in determining the doses of drugs for pediatric and elderly patients, these parameters represent the majority of the calculations presented in this chapter. The dosing of chemotherapeutic agents also is included because it represents a unique dosing regimen compared with most other categories of drugs.

Pediatric Patients

Pediatrics is the branch of medicine that deals with disease in children from birth through adolescence. Because of the range in age and bodily development in this patient population, the inclusive groups are defined further as follows: ***neonate*** (newborn), from birth to

1 month; ***infant***, 1 month to 1 year; ***early childhood***, 1 year through 5 years; ***late childhood***, 6 years through 12 years; and ***adolescence***, 13 years through 17 years of age.[2] A neonate is considered ***premature*** if born at less than 37 weeks' gestation.

Proper drug dosing of the pediatric patient depends on a number of factors, including the patient's age and weight, overall health status, the condition of such biologic functions as respiration and circulation, and the stage of development of body systems for drug metabolism (e.g., liver enzymes) and drug elimination (e.g., renal system). In the neonate, these biologic functions and systems are underdeveloped. Renal function, for example, develops over the span of the first 2 years of life. This fact is particularly important because the most commonly used drugs in neonates, infants, and young children are antimicrobial agents, which are eliminated primarily through the kidneys. If the rate of drug elimination is not properly considered, drug accumulation in the body could occur, leading to drug overdosage and toxicity. Thus, the use of ***pharmacokinetic*** data (i.e., the rates and extent of drug absorption, distribution, metabolism, and elimination; see Chapters 10 and 22), together with individual patient factors and therapeutic response, provides a rational approach to pediatric drug dosage calculations.[2]

Special Considerations in Dose Determinations for Pediatric Patients

The majority of medications commercially available are formulated and labeled for adult use. When used for the pediatric patient, appropriate dosage calculations must be made, and often, so must adjustments to the concentration of the medication. In the absence of a suitable commercial preparation, pharmacists may be called upon to compound a medication for a pediatric patient.

Among the special considerations in pediatric dosing are the following[3]:

- Doses should be based on accepted clinical studies as reported in the literature.
- Doses should be age appropriate and generally based on body weight or body surface area.
- Pediatric patients should be weighed as closely as possible to the time of admittance to a health care facility and that weight recorded in kilograms.
- As available, pediatric formulations rather than those intended for adults should be administered.
- All calculations of dose should be double-checked by a second health professional.
- All caregivers should be properly advised with regard to dosage, dose administration, and important clinical signs to observe.
- Calibrated oral syringes should be used to measure and administer oral liquids.

Doses of drugs used in pediatrics, including neonatology, may be found in individual drug product literature as well as in references, such as those listed at the conclusion of this chapter.[4,5]

CASE IN POINT 8.1 A hospital pharmacist is asked to determine the dose of clindamycin for a 3-day-old neonate weighing 3 lb 7 oz. In checking the literature, the pharmacist determines that the dose is listed as follows[4]:

<1200 g: 10 mg/kg/day divided q12h
<2000 g and 0 to 7 days old: 10 mg/kg/day divided q12h
<2000 g and >7 days old: 15 mg/kg/day divided q8h
>2000 g and 0 to 7 days old: 15 mg/kg/day divided q8h
>2000 g and >7 days old: 20 to 30 mg/kg/day divided q12h

Each divided dose is to be added to an intravenous infusion at the scheduled hour and infused over a period of 20 minutes.

The product shown in Figure 8.1 was used to prepare an IV bag containing 600 mg/50 mL of injectable solution. How many milliliters of this solution should be given for each divided dose?

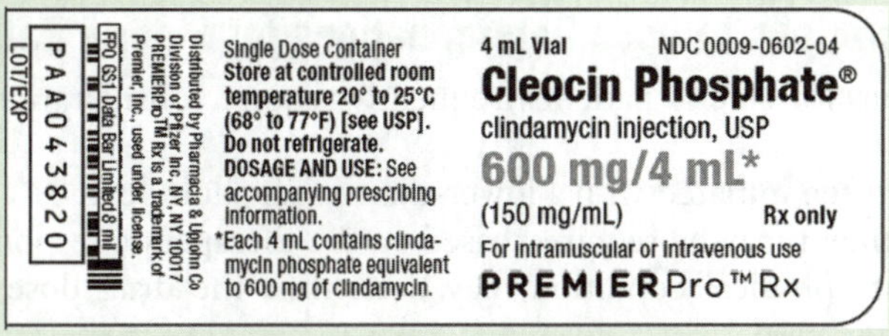

FIGURE 8.1 • Product label showing the drug concentration in mg/mL for an injectable product. *(Source: http://dailymed.nlm.nih.gov/dailymed/about.cfm. Courtesy of Pfizer, Inc.)*

CASE IN POINT 8.2 A pediatric patient is being administered enalaprilat (VASOTEC IV) every 12 hours by intravenous injection to manage hypertension and possible heart failure.[4] Based on a dose of 5 mcg/kg, the patient is receiving 55 mcg of enalaprilat per dose. The physician wishes to convert the patient to oral enalapril at a dosage of 100 mcg/kg as a single daily dose. The standard procedure is to crush a 2.5-mg tablet of enalapril, mix with sterile water to make 12.5 mL, and administer the appropriate dose using a calibrated oral dispenser. Calculate the dose, in milliliters, to be administered to this patient.

Geriatric Patients

Although the term *elderly* is subject to varying definitions with regard to chronologic age, it is clear that the functional capacities of most organ systems decline throughout adulthood, and important changes in drug response occur with advancing age. *Geriatric medicine* or *geriatrics* is the field that encompasses the management of illness in the elderly.

In addition to medical conditions affecting all age groups, some conditions are particularly common in the elderly, including degenerative osteoarthritis, congestive heart failure, venous and arterial insufficiency, stroke, urinary incontinence, prostatic carcinoma, parkinsonism, and Alzheimer's disease. Many elderly patients have coexisting pathologies that require multiple-drug therapies.

Most age-related physiologic functions peak before age 30, with subsequent gradual linear decline.[2] Reductions in physiologic capacity and function are cumulative, becoming more profound with age. Kidney function is a major consideration in drug dosing in the elderly because reduced function results in reduced drug elimination.

Because reduced kidney function increases the possibility of toxic drug levels in the body and adverse drug effects, initial drug dosing in the elderly patient often reflects a downward variance from the usual adult dose. There is also a frequent need for dosage adjustment or medication change due to adverse effects or otherwise unsatisfactory therapeutic outcomes.

There are a number of other common features of medication use in the elderly, including the long-term use of maintenance drugs; the need for multidrug therapy, with the attendant increased possibility of drug interactions and adverse drug effects; and difficulties in patient adherence. The latter is often due to impaired cognition, confusion over the various dosing schedules of multiple medications, and economic reasons in not being able to afford the prescribed medication.

Special Considerations in Dose Determinations for Elderly Patients

Dose determinations for elderly patients frequently require consideration of some or all of the following:

- Therapy is often initiated with a lower-than-usual adult dose.
- Dose adjustment may be required based on the therapeutic response.
- The patient's physical condition may determine the drug dose and the route of administration used.
- The dose may be determined, in part, on the patient's weight, body surface area, health and disease status, and pharmacokinetic factors.
- Concomitant drug therapy may affect drug/dose effectiveness.
- A drug's dose may produce undesired adverse effects and may affect patient adherence.
- Complex dosage regimens of multiple drug therapy may affect patient adherence.

The adult dose of a drug is 500 mg every 8 hours. For an elderly patient with impaired renal function, the dose is reduced to 250 mg every 6 hours. Calculate the reduction in the daily dose, in milligrams.

$$\text{Daily doses}: 500\text{ mg} \times 3 \text{ (every 8 hours)} = 1500\text{ mg}$$
$$250\text{ mg} \times 4 \text{ (every 6 hours)} = 1000\text{ mg}$$
$$1500\text{ mg} - 100\text{ mg} = \mathbf{500\text{ mg}}$$

Dosage Forms Applicable to Pediatric and Geriatric Patients

In the general population, solid dosage forms, such as tablets and capsules, are preferred for the oral administration of drugs because of their convenience, precise dose, ease of administration, ready identification, transportation, and lower cost per dose relative to other dosage forms. However, solid dosage forms are often difficult or impossible for the pediatric, geriatric, or infirm patient to swallow. In these instances, liquid forms are preferred, such as oral solutions, syrups, suspensions, and drops. With liquid forms, the dose can be adjusted by changing the volume administered. When necessary, liquid forms of medication may be administered by oral feeding tube. Pharmacists are sometimes asked to compound an oral liquid from a counterpart solid dosage form when a liquid product is not available. Chewable tablets and solid gel forms (medicated "gummy bears") that disintegrate or dissolve in the mouth are often used for pediatric and geriatric patients. In addition, and as noted in the previous chapter, *tablet splitting* and *tablet crushing* are options for individuals unable to swallow whole tablets.

For systemic effects, injections may be used rather than the oral route of administration when needed for pediatric and elderly patients, with the dose or strength of the preparation adjusted to meet the requirements of the individual patient.

Drug Dosage Based on Age

For reasons stated earlier, the young and the elderly require special dosing considerations based on factors characteristic of these groups.

Table 8.1 • ILLUSTRATIVE PEDIATRIC DOSAGES OF DIGOXIN BASED ON AGE AND WEIGHT[a]

Age	Digoxin Dose (μg/kg/day)
Premature	4–8
Full term	7–11
1–24 mo	11–18
2–5 y	9–13
5–10 y	6–11
Over 10 y	3–5

[a]These are illustrative doses. Specific pediatric doses for various age groups, clinical conditions, and by various routes of administration may be found at https://online.epocrates.com/u/102198/digoxin/Pediatric+Dosing.

Before the physiologic differences between adult and pediatric patients were clarified, the latter were treated with drugs as if they were merely miniature adults. Various rules of dosage in which the pediatric dose was a fraction of the adult dose, based on relative age, were created for youngsters (e.g., *Young's rule*). *Today these rules are not in general use because age alone is no longer considered a singularly valid criterion in the determination of accurate dosage for a child, especially when calculated from the usual adult dose, which itself provides wide clinical variations in response. Some of these rules are presented in the footnote for perspective and historical purposes.*[a]

Currently, when age *is* considered in determining dosage of a *potent* therapeutic agent, it is used generally in conjunction with another factor, such as weight. This is exemplified in Table 8.1, in which the dose of the drug digoxin is determined by a combination of the patient's age and weight.

---

[a]*Young's rule*, based on age:

$$\frac{\text{Age}}{\text{Age} + 12} \times \text{Adult dose} = \text{Dose for child}$$

Cowling's rule:

$$\frac{\text{Age at next birthday (in years)} \times \text{Adult dose}}{24} = \text{Dose for child}$$

Fried's rule for infants:

$$\frac{\text{Age (in months)} \times \text{Adult dose}}{150} = \text{Dose for infant}$$

Clark's rule, based on weight:

$$\frac{\text{Weight (in lb)} \times \text{Adult dose}}{\text{150 (average weight of adult in lb)}} = \text{Dose for child}$$

NOTE: The value of 150 in Fried's rule was an estimate of the age (12.5 years or 150 months) of an individual who would normally receive an adult dose, and the number 150 in Clark's rule was an estimate of the weight of an individual who likewise would receive an adult dose.

Example Calculations of Dose Based on Age

(1) *An over-the-counter cough remedy contains 120 mg of dextromethorphan in a 60-mL bottle of product. The label states the dose as 1½ teaspoonfuls for a child 6 years of age. How many milligrams of dextromethorphan are contained in the child's dose?*

$$1\tfrac{1}{2} \text{ teaspoonfuls} = 7.5 \text{ mL}$$

$$\frac{60 \text{ mL}}{120 \text{ mg}} = \frac{7.5 \text{ mL}}{x \text{ mg}}$$

$$x = \textbf{15 mg dextromethorphan}$$

(2) *The dose of a drug for an adolescent is acceptable as either 10 mg/kg or 300 mg. Calculate the difference in these alternative doses for a 9-year-old child weighing 70 lb.*

Dose at 10 mg/kg: 70 lb ÷ 2.2 lb/kg = 31.8 kg; 31.8 kg × 10 mg/kg = 318.2 mg
Difference in dose = 318.2 mg – 300 mg = **18.2 mg**

(3) *From the data in Table 8.1, calculate the dosage range for digoxin for a 20-month-old infant weighing 6.8 kg.*

$$\frac{11 \text{ mcg}}{x \text{ mcg}} = \frac{1 \text{ kg}}{6.8 \text{ kg}} \quad \text{and} \quad \frac{18 \text{ mcg}}{x \text{ mcg}} = \frac{1 \text{ kg}}{6.8 \text{ kg}}$$

$$x = 74.8 \text{ mcg} \quad \text{and} \quad x = 122.4 \text{ mcg}$$

Dosage range between 74.8 and 122.4 mcg digoxin

Drug Dosage Based on Body Weight

Drug doses based on weight are expressed as a specific quantity of drug per unit of patient weight, such as *milligrams of drug per kilogram of body weight* (abbreviated [*mg/kg*]). Dosing in this manner makes the quantity of drug administered specific to the weight of the patient being treated.

Example Calculations of Dose Based on Body Weight

A useful equation for the calculation of dose based on body weight is

$$\text{Patient's dose (mg)} = \text{Patient's weight (kg)} \times \frac{\text{Drug dose (mg)}}{1 \text{ (kg)}}$$

This equation is based on a drug dose in mg/kg and the patient's weight in kilograms. When different units are given or desired, other units may be substituted in the equation as long as the terms used are consistently applied.

(1) *The usual initial dose of chlorambucil is 150 mcg/kg of body weight. How many milligrams should be administered to a person weighing 154 lb?*
Solving by the equation:
150 mcg = 0.15 mg

$$\text{Patient's dose (mg)} = 154 \text{ lb} \times \frac{0.15 \text{ mg}}{2.2 \text{ lb}} = \textbf{10.5 mg chlorambucil}$$

Or, solving by ratio and proportion:
150 mcg = 0.15 mg 1 kg = 2.2 lb

$$\frac{2.2 \text{ lb}}{154 \text{ lb}} = \frac{0.15 \text{ mg}}{\text{x mg}}; \text{ x} = \mathbf{10.5 \text{ mg chlorambucil}}$$

Or, solving by dimensional analysis:

$$\frac{1 \text{ mg}}{1000 \text{ mcg}} \times \frac{150 \text{ mcg}}{1 \text{ kg}} \times \frac{1 \text{ kg}}{2.2 \text{ lb}} \times \frac{154 \text{ lb}}{1} = \mathbf{10.5 \text{ mg chlorambucil}}$$

(2) *The usual dose of sulfisoxazole for infants over 2 months of age and children is 60 to 75 mg/kg of body weight. What would be the usual range for a child weighing 44 lb?*

$$1 \text{ kg} = 2.2 \text{ lb}$$
$$20 \text{ kg} = 44 \text{ lb}$$
$$60 \text{ mg/kg} \times 20 \text{ kg} = 1200 \text{ mg}$$
$$75 \text{ mg/kg} \times 20 \text{ kg} = 1500 \text{ mg}$$

Thus, the **dosage range would be 1200 to 1500 mg**

(3) *The dose of minocycline to treat acne vulgaris is given as 1 mg/kg/day × 12 weeks. Tablet strengths available include 45 mg, 55 mg, 65 mg, 80 mg, 90 mg, 105 mg, and 115 mg of minocycline. What strength tablet and how many tablets should be prescribed for the entire course of treatment for a 100-lb patient?*

100 lb ÷ 2.2 lb/kg = 45.5 kg

1 mg/kg/day × 45.5 kg = 45.5 mg/day ≈ **45-mg minocycline tablets**, and

12 week × 7 day/week = 84 days; thus, **84 tablets required**

(4) *A dose of enoxaparin sodium injection (LOVENOX) is "1 mg/kg q12h SC." If a graduated prefilled syringe containing 80 mg/0.8 mL is used, how many milliliters should be administered per dose to a 154-lb patient?*

$$154 \text{ lb} \div 2.2 \text{ lb/kg} = 70 \text{ kg}$$
$$1 \text{ mg/kg} \times 70 \text{ kg} = 70 \text{ mg}$$
$$0.8 \text{ mL} \times \frac{70 \text{ mg}}{80 \text{ mg}} = \mathbf{0.7 \text{ mL enoxaparin sodium injection}}$$

CASE IN POINT 8.3 A hospital pharmacist is called to a pediatric nursing station to calculate the quantity of an injection to administer to a pediatric patient. The daily dose of the injection for the child's weight is stated as 15 mg/kg/day, divided into three equal portions. The child weighs 10 kg. The injection contains 5 mg/mL of the prescribed drug.

How many milliliters of injection should be administered?

Dosing Tables Based on Body Weight

For some drugs dosed according to body weight or body surface area, dosing tables appear in product literature to assist the physician and pharmacist. An example is presented in Table 8.2.

Table 8.2 • DOSING BY BODY WEIGHT FOR A HYPOTHETICAL DRUG

Body Weight		Total mg/day		
Kilograms	Pounds	0.5 mg/kg	1 mg/kg	2 mg/kg
40	88	20	40	80
50	110	25	50	100
60	132	30	60	120
70	154	35	70	140
80	176	40	80	160
90	198	45	90	180
100	220	50	100	200

(1) *Using Table 8.2 and a daily dose of 0.5 mg/kg, how many 20-mg capsules of the drug product should be dispensed to a patient weighing 176 lb if the dosage regimen calls for 15 weeks of therapy?*

$$2 \text{ capsules/day} \times 7 \text{ days/week} \times 15 \text{ weeks} = \mathbf{210\ capsules}$$

(2) *A pharmacist compounds a suspension from oseltamivir phosphate capsules to contain 15 mg of drug per milliliter. Using Table 8.3, calculate the single dose in milliliters for a pediatric patient weighing 40 lb.*

From Table 8.3, the dose for the pediatric patient is 45 mg.

$$45 \text{ mg} \times \frac{1 \text{ mL}}{15 \text{ mL}} = \mathbf{3\ mL,\ dose\ of\ oseltamivir\ phosphate\ suspension}$$

Drug Dosage Based on Body Surface Area

The *body surface area (BSA)* method of calculating drug doses is widely used for two types of patient groups: cancer patients receiving chemotherapy and pediatric patients.

Table 8.4 shows the *approximate* relation between body weight and body surface area, in square meters (m^2), based on average body dimensions. The average adult is considered to have a BSA of 1.73 m^2. Thus, in reading Table 8.4, a person with a BSA of 1.30 (or about 75% of that of the average adult) would receive about 75% of the adult dose.

Example Calculations of Dose Based on Body Surface Area

A useful equation for the calculation of dose based on BSA is:

Table 8.3 • DOSING OF OSELTAMIVIR PHOSPHATE IN THE TREATMENT OF INFLUENZA IN PEDIATRIC PATIENTS[a]

Body Weight	Recommended Dose × 5 Days
15 kg or less	30 mg twice daily
15.1 to 23 kg	45 mg twice daily
23.1 to 40 kg	60 mg twice daily
40.1 kg or more	75 mg twice daily

[a]Adapted from product literature for oseltamivir phosphate (TAMIFLU); Genentech, 2014 @ http://www.drugs.com/pro/tamiflu.html

Table 8.4 • APPROXIMATE RELATION OF SURFACE AREA AND WEIGHTS OF INDIVIDUALS OF AVERAGE BODY DIMENSION

Kilograms	Pounds	Surface Area in Square Meters	Percentage of Adult Dose[a]
2	4.4	0.15	9
3	6.6	0.20	11.5
4	8.8	0.25	14
5	11.0	0.29	16.5
6	13.2	0.33	19
7	15.4	0.37	21
8	17.6	0.40	23
9	19.8	0.43	25
10	22.0	0.46	27
15	33.0	0.63	36
20	44.0	0.83	48
25	55.0	0.95	55
30	66.0	1.08	62
35	77.0	1.20	69
40	88.0	1.30	75
45	99.0	1.40	81
50	110.0	1.51	87
55	121.0	1.58	91

[a]Based on average adult surface area of 1.73 m^2.

Adapted from Martin EW, et al. *Techniques of Medication.* J.B. Lippincott; 1969:31, who adapted it from *Modell's Drugs of Choice* (Mosby).

$$\text{Patient's dose} = \frac{\text{Patient's BSA (m}^2)}{1.73 \text{ m}^2} \times \text{Drug dose (mg)}$$

If the adult dose of a drug is 100 mg, calculate the approximate dose for a child with a BSA of 0.83 m², using (a) the equation and (b) Table 8.4.

(a) $\text{Child's dose} = \frac{0.83 \text{ m}^2}{1.73 \text{ m}^2} \times 100 \text{ mg} = 47.97$ or **48 mg**

(b) According to Table 8.4, a BSA of 0.83 m^2 represents 48% of the average adult BSA of 1.73 m^2; thus, the child dose would be 48% of the average adult dose:

$$100 \text{ mg} \times 0.48 = \mathbf{48 \text{ mg dose for child}}$$

Dosing Tables Based on Body Surface Area

For certain drugs, dosing tables may be provided to determine the approximate dose based on a patient's body surface area. Table 8.5 presents an example for a hypothetical drug.

Using Table 8.5, find the dose of the hypothetical drug at a dose level of 300 mg/m² for a child determined to have a BSA of 1.25 m². Calculate to verify.

From Table 8.5, the dose = 375 mg

From calculations, 300 mg/m^2 × 1.25 m^2 = 375 mg dose

Nomograms for Determining Body Surface Area

Most BSA calculations use a standard *nomogram,* which includes both weight and height. Nomograms for children and adults are shown in Figures 8.2 and 8.3. The BSA of an

Table 8.5 • PEDIATRIC DOSING GUIDELINE FOR A HYPOTHETICAL DRUG BASED ON BSA

	Dose Level			
Patient's BSA (m^2)	250 mg/m^2 Dose	300 mg/m^2 Dose	350 mg/m^2 Dose	400 mg/m^2 Dose
0.25	62.5 mg	75 mg	87.5 mg	100 mg
0.50	125 mg	150 mg	175 mg	200 mg
1.00	250 mg	300 mg	350 mg	400 mg
1.25	312.5 mg	375 mg	437.5 mg	500 mg
1.50	375 mg	450 mg	525 mg	600 mg

individual is determined by drawing a straight line connecting the person's height and weight. The point at which the line intersects the center column indicates the person's BSA in square meters. In the example shown in Figure 8.2, a child weighing 15 kg and measuring 100 cm in height has a BSA of 0.64 m^2.

(1) *If the adult dose of a drug is 75 mg, what would be the dose for a child weighing 40 lb and measuring 32 inches in height using the BSA nomogram?*

From the nomogram, the BSA = 0.60 m^2

$$\frac{0.60\ \text{m}^2}{1.73\ \text{m}^2} \times 75\ \text{mg} = \mathbf{26\ mg}$$

(2) *The usual pediatric dose of a drug is stated as 25 mg/m^2. Using the nomogram, calculate the dose for a child weighing 18 kg and measuring 82 cm in height.*

From the nomogram, the BSA = 0.60 m^2

$$25\ \text{mg} \times 0.60 = \mathbf{15\ mg}$$

The nomogram in Figure 8.3 designed specifically for determining the BSA of *adults* may be used in the same manner as the one previously described. The adult dose is then calculated as follows:

$$\frac{\text{BSA of adult (m}^2\text{)}}{1.73\ \text{m}^2} \times \text{Usual adult dose} = \text{Dose for adult}$$

CALCULATIONS CAPSULE

Dose Based on Body Surface Area

A useful equation for the calculation of dose based on body surface area is:

$$\text{Patient's dose} = \frac{\text{Patient's BSA (m}^2\text{)}}{1.73\ \text{m}^2} \times \text{Drug dose (mg)}$$

If there is need to determine a patient's BSA, a nomogram or the following equation may be used:

$$\text{Patient's BSA (m}^2\text{)} = \sqrt{\frac{\text{Patient's height (cm)} \times \text{Patient's weight (kg)}}{3600}}$$

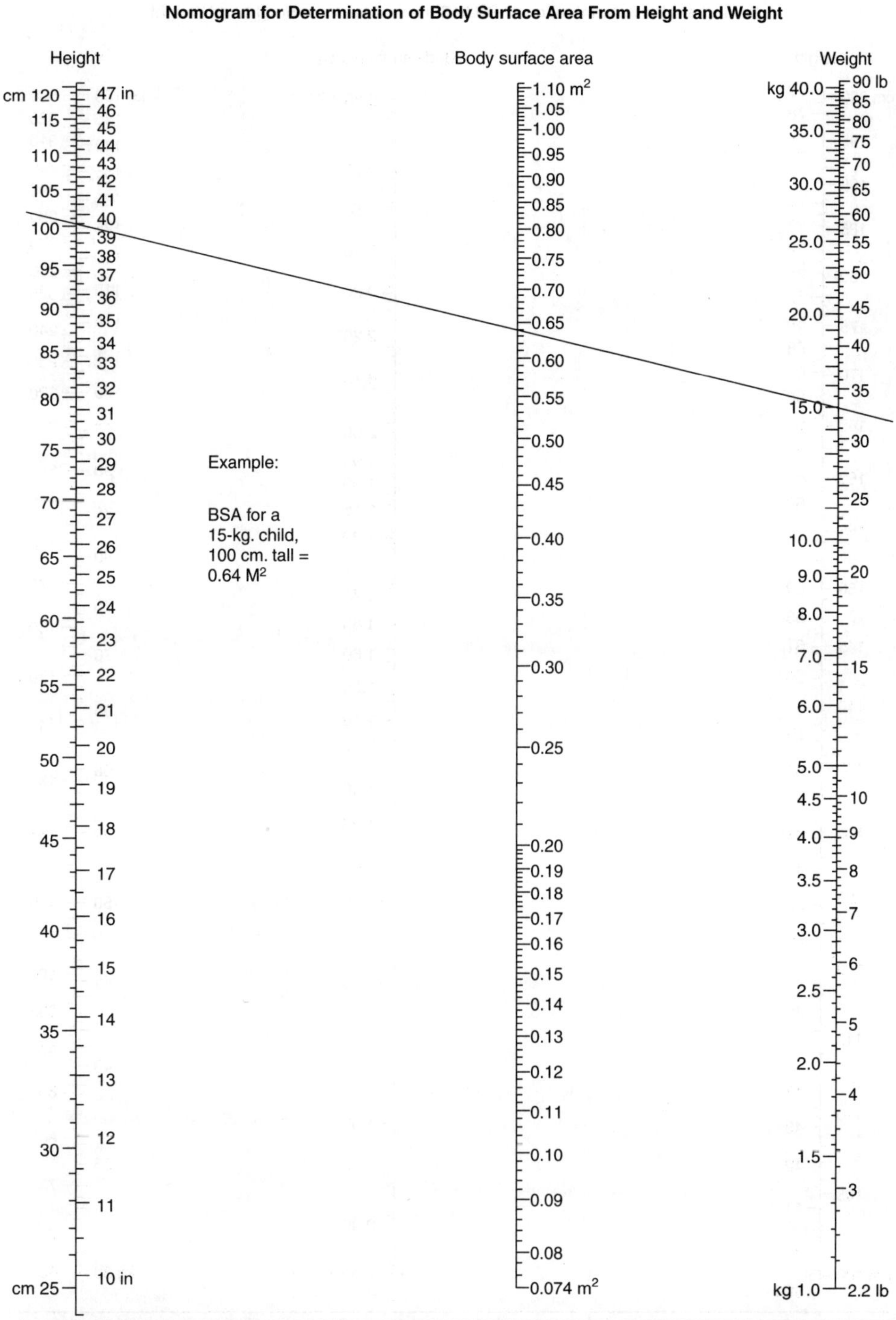

From the formula of Du Bois and Du Bois, *Arch Intern Med* 17, 863 (1916): $S = W^{0.425} \times H^{0.725} \times 71.84$, or $\log S = \log W \times 0.425 + \log H \times 0.725 + 1.8564$ (S = body surface in cm², W = weight in kg, H = height in cm).

FIGURE 8.2 • Body surface area of children. *(From Diem K, Lentner C, Geigy JR. Scientific Tables. 7th Ed. Basel, Switzerland: JR Geigy; 1970:538.)*

Nomogram for Determination of Body Surface Area from Height and Weight

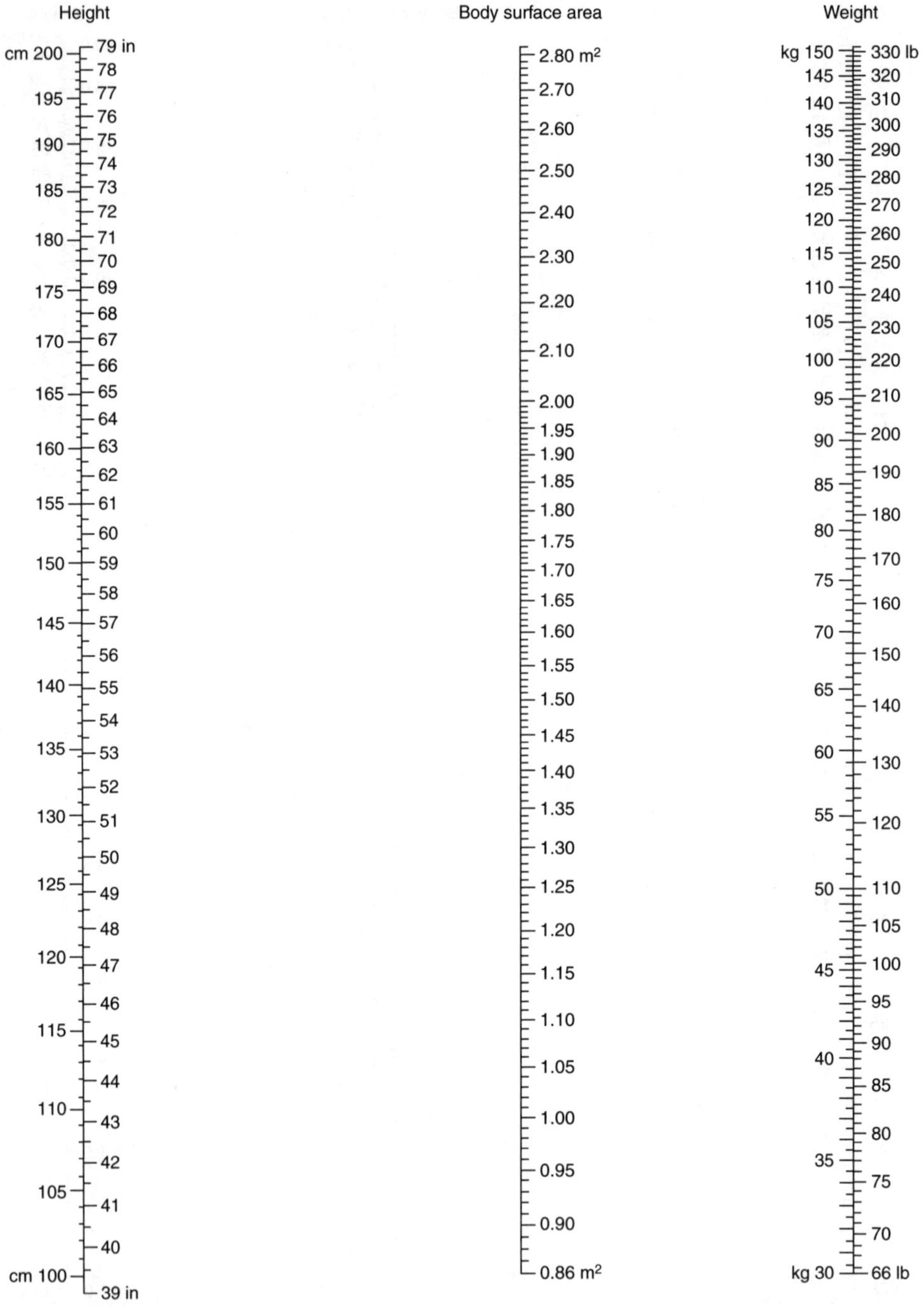

From the formula of Du Bois and Du Bois, *Arch Intern Med* 17, 863 (1916): $S = W^{0.425} \times H^{0.725} \times 71.84$, or $\log S = \log W \times 0.425 + \log H \times 0.725 + 1.8564$ (S = body surface in cm^2, W = weight in kg, H = height in cm).

FIGURE 8.3 • Body surface area of adults. *(From Diem K, Lentner C, Geigy JR. Scientific Tables. 7th Ed. Basel, Switzerland: JR Geigy; 1970:538.)*

(1) *If the usual adult dose of a drug is 120 mg, what would be the dose based on BSA for a person measuring 6 feet tall and weight 200 lb?*

$$\text{BSA (from the nomogram)} = 2.13 \text{ m}^2$$

$$\frac{2.13 \text{ m}^2}{1.73 \text{ m}^2} \times 120 \text{ mg} = 147.75 \text{ mg or } \mathbf{148 \text{ mg}}$$

(2) *If the dose of a drug is 5 mg/m², what would be the dose for a patient with a BSA of 1.9 m²?*

$$5 \text{ mg} \times 1.9 = \mathbf{9.5 \text{ mg}}$$

BSA Equation

In addition to the use of the nomogram, BSA may be determined through use of the following Mosteller formula[6]:

$$\text{BSA, m}^2 = \sqrt{\frac{\text{Ht (cm)} \times \text{Wt (kg)}}{3600}}$$

Calculate the BSA for a patient measuring 165 cm in height and weighing 65 kg.

$$\text{BSA, m}^2 = \sqrt{\frac{165 \text{ (cm)} \times 65 \text{ (kg)}}{3600}}$$

$$\text{BSA} = \mathbf{1.73 \text{ m}^2}$$

NOTE: For the sake of comparison, check Figure 8.3 to derive the BSA for the same patient using the nomogram.

Dosage Based on the Medical Condition to Be Treated

In addition to the factors previously discussed that might be used to determine a drug's dose, the medical condition to be treated and the severity of that condition must also be considered.

Table 8.6 presents an example of a dosage schedule for a drug based both on a patient's age and the medical condition to be treated.

Table 8.6 • PARENTERAL DOSAGE SCHEDULE FOR A HYPOTHETICAL ANTI-INFECTIVE DRUG BASED ON PATIENT AGE AND CONDITION BEING TREATED

	Dose	Route	Frequency
Adults			
Urinary tract infection	250 mg	IV or IM	q12h
Bone and joint infections	2 g	IV	q12h
Pneumonia	500 mg–1g	IV or IM	q8h
Mild skin infections	500 mg–1g	IV or IM	q8h
Life-threatening infections	2 g	IV	q8h
Lung infections (normal kidney function)	10 mg/kg (NMT 6 g/day)	IV	q8h
Neonates (up to 1 month)	30 mg/kg	IV	q12h
Infants and Children (1 mo to 12 y)	30–50 mg/kg (NMT 6 g/day)	IV	q8h

(1) *By using Table 8.6, calculate the IV drug dose for a 3-lb 3-oz neonate.*

$$3 \text{ lb} = 3 \times 454 \text{ g} = 1362 \text{ g}$$
$$3 \text{ oz} = 3 \times 28.35 \text{ g} = 85 \text{ g}$$
$$\text{Weight of neonate} = 1362 \text{ g} + 85 \text{ g} = 1447 \text{ g}$$
$$1447 \text{ g}/1000 = 1.447 \text{ kg}$$
$$30 \text{ mg/kg} \times 1.447 \text{ kg} = \mathbf{43.4 \text{ mg every 12 hours}}$$

(2) *By using Table 8.6, calculate the daily IV dose of the drug in the treatment of a lung infection for a patient weighing 160 lb.*

$$160 \text{ lb} \div 2.2 \text{ lb/kg} = 72.72 \text{ kg}$$
$$72.72 \text{ kg} \times 40 \text{ mg/kg/dose} = 2909 \text{ mg/dose (every 8 hours)}$$
$$2909 \text{ mg} \times 3 \text{ doses per day} = 8727 \text{ mg or } \mathbf{8.73 \text{ g daily dose}}$$

Dosage Adjustment Based on Coadministered Drugs

The usual dose of a drug may require adjusting based on the coadministration of another drug when there is a known or suspected risk for a drug interaction. Drug interactions may result in diminished drug efficacy and/or in increased toxicity due to a number of factors including those affecting a drug's pharmacokinetics (i.e., absorption, distribution, metabolism, and elimination).

The usual adult dose of colchicine in the prevention of gout flares is 6 mg once or twice a day. However, when coadministered with protease inhibitors (e.g., ritonavir), the dose is reduced to 0.3 mg once daily or once every other day. For "once every other day" treatment, how many whole or split 0.6-mg tablets are required for a 30-day supply?

15 days (of treatment) × 0.3 mg/day = 4.5 mg, colchicine
4.5 mg/0.6 mg (tablet) = **7.5 whole tablets or 15 split tablets**

Dosage Based on Reduced Kidney and/or Liver Function

The status of a patient's hepatic (liver) and renal (kidney) function plays a major role in determining drug dosage due to their roles in drug metabolism and elimination. Specific calculations of dosage based on reduced kidney function are presented in Chapter 10.

Other Patient Factors Affecting Drug Dosage and Utilization

In addition to factors of renal and/or hepatic impairment and age (pediatric, geriatric), other patient factors play a role in drug selection and dosage including gender, genetics (e.g., pharmacogenetics), metabolic disorders, pregnancy, breastfeeding, current health status, medical and medication history, and others.

Special Dosing Considerations in Cancer Chemotherapy

The term ***chemotherapy*** applies to the treatment of disease with chemical drugs or ***chemotherapeutic agents***. Chemotherapy is primarily associated with the treatment of cancer patients and is considered the mainstay of such treatment in that it is effective in widespread or metastatic cancer, whereas treatments such as surgery and radiation therapy are limited to specific body sites. Chemotherapeutic agents most often are administered orally, by intravenous injection, or by continuous intravenous infusion.

CASE IN POINT 8.4 A hospital pharmacist is consulted on the appropriate dose of lopinavir/ritonavir (KALETRA) oral solution in the treatment of an HIV-1 infection in a 12-month-old pediatric patient. The oral solution contains, in each milliliter, 80 mg of lopinavir and 20 mg of ritonavir, expressed as "KALETRA 80/20." According to the pharmacy's protocol, the pediatric dose for patients greater than 6 months of age, not receiving other concomitant therapy, may be calculated based on either BSA or body weight as follows:

- 230/57.5 mg/m², administered twice daily
- 12/3 mg/kg for patients <15 kg, administered twice daily
- 10/2.5 mg/kg for patients >15 kg administered twice daily

The patient measures 28 inches in length and weighs 22 lb.
(a) Calculate the single dose, in mg, using the BSA equation.
(b) Translate the calculated single dose from (a) into corresponding milliliters of the oral solution.
(c) Calculate the daily dose, in mg, based on the patient's weight.
(d) Translate the daily dose from (c) into corresponding milliliters of oral solution.

Although a single anticancer drug may be used in a patient's treatment plan, *combination chemotherapy* perhaps is more usual. By using combinations of drugs having different mechanisms of action against the target cancer cells, the effectiveness of treatment may be enhanced, lower doses used, and side effects reduced. The combination chemotherapy plans often include *two-agent regimens, three-agent regimens,* and *four-agent regimens.*[7–11]

Cancer chemotherapy is unique in the following ways:

- It may involve single or multiple drugs of well-established drug therapy regimens or protocols, or it may involve the use of investigational drugs as a part of a clinical trial.
- Combinations of drugs may be given by the same or different routes of administration, most often oral and/or intravenous.
- The drugs may be administered concomitantly or alternately on the same or different days during a prescribed treatment cycle (e.g., 28 days). The days of treatment generally follow a prescribed format of written instructions, with *D* for "day," followed by the day(s) of treatment during a cycle, with a dash (–) meaning "to" and a comma (,) meaning "and." Thus, *D 1–4* means "days 1 to 4," and *D1,4* means "days 1 and 4."[9]
- The drugs used in combination chemotherapy often fit into a standard drug/dosage regimen identified by abbreviations or *acronyms*. For example, a treatment for bladder cancer referred to as MVAC consists of methotrexate + vinblastine + doxorubicin (or actinomycin) + cisplatin; a treatment for colorectal cancer called FU/LU consists of fluorouracil + leucovorin; a treatment for lung cancer called PC consists of paclitaxel + carboplatin; and one for ovarian cancer called CHAD consists of cyclophosphamide + hexamethylmelamine + Adriamycin + diamminedichloroplatinum (cisplatin).

- In addition to the use of abbreviations for the drug therapy regimens, the drugs themselves are commonly abbreviated in medication orders, such as MTX for "methotrexate," DOX for "doxorubicin," VLB for "vinblastine," and CDDP for "cisplatin." Tables of standard chemotherapy treatments, dosing regimens, and abbreviations of the drugs and treatment regimens may be found in the indicated references.[7–11]
- For systemic action, chemotherapeutic agents are usually dosed based either on body weight or on body surface area. Often, the drug doses stated in standard regimens must be reduced, based on a particular patient's diminished kidney or liver function and, thus, his or her ability to metabolize and eliminate the drug(s) from the body.
- For certain patients, high-dose chemotherapy is undertaken in an effort to kill tumor cells.

To help prevent errors in chemotherapy, pharmacists must correctly interpret medication orders for the chemotherapeutic agents prescribed, follow the individualized dosing regimens, calculate the doses of each medication prescribed, and dispense the appropriate dosage forms and quantities/strengths required.[12]

Example Calculations of Chemotherapy Dosage Regimens

(1) *Regimen: VC*[11]
Cycle: 28 days; repeat for 2–8 cycles
Vinorelbine, 25 mg/m², IV, D 1,8,15,22
Cisplatin, 100 mg/m², IV, D 1

For each of vinorelbine and cisplatin, calculate the total intravenous dose per cycle for a patient measuring 5 feet 11 inches in height and weighing 175 lb.

From the nomogram for determining BSA, (a) find the patient's BSA and (b) calculate the quantity of each drug in the regimen.

(a) BSA ≐ **2.00 m²**

(b) Vinorelbine: 25 mg × 2.00 (BSA) × 4 (days of treatment) = **200 mg**

Cisplatin: 100 mg × 2.00 (BSA) × 1 = **200 mg**

(2) *Regimen: CMF*[11]
Cycle: 28 days
Cyclophosphamide, 100 mg/m²/day PO, D 1–14
Methotrexate, 40 mg/m², IV, D 2,8
Fluorouracil, 600 mg/m², IV, D 1,8

Calculate the total cycle dose for cyclophosphamide, methotrexate, and fluorouracil for a patient having a BSA of 1.5 m².

Cyclophosphamide:	100 mg × 1.5 (BSA) × 14 (days)	= 2100 mg = **2.1 g**
Methotrexate:	40 mg × 1.5 × 2	= **120 mg**
Fluorouracil:	600 mg × 1.5 × 2	= 1800 mg = **1.8 g**

(3) *Using Table* 8.7 *as a reference, calculate the quantities of doxorubicin and cyclophosphamide administered per treatment cycle to a woman measuring 5 feet 4 inches in height and weighing 142 lb during the "AC" protocol for breast cancer.*

BSA (from Table 8.2) = **1.70 m²**

1.70 m² × 60 mg/m² doxorubicin = **102 mg doxorubicin**

1.70 m² × 600 mg/m² cyclophosphamide = **1020 mg cyclophosphamide**

(4) *A variation of the "AC" protocol, referred to as "AC → T," follows 4 cycles of the AC protocol with paclitaxel (TAXOL), 175 mg/m² by intravenous infusion every 14 to 21 days*

Table 8.7 • EXAMPLES OF DOSAGE REGIMENS IN CANCER CHEMOTHERAPY[a]

Type of Cancer[b]	Abbreviation	Drug/Dose	Route	Day(s) of Administration per Treatment Cycle[c]
Bladder	MVAC	methotrexate, 30 mg/m^2	IV	days 1, 15, and 22
		vinblastine, 3 mg/m^2	IV	days 2, 15, and 22
		doxorubicin (Adriamycin),30 mg/m^2	IV	day 2
		cisplatin, 70 mg/m^2	IV	day 2
Breast	AC	doxorubicin (Adriamycin), 60 mg/m^2	IV	day 1
		cyclophosphamide, 600 mg/m^2	IV	day 1
Esophagus	DCF	docetaxel, 75 mg/m^2	IV	day 1
		cisplatin, 75 mg/m^2	IV	day 1
		5-fluorouracil, 750 mg/m^2/day	IV	days 1–5
Lung	CAE	cyclophosphamide, 1000 mg/m^2	IV	day 1
		doxorubicin, 45 mg/m^2	IV	day 1
		etoposide, 100 mg/m^2	IV	days 1–3
Stomach	ELF	etoposide, 120 mg/m^2	IV	days 1–3
		leucovorin, 150 mg/m^2	IV	days 1–3
		5-fluorouracil, 500 mg/m^2	IV	days 1–3

[a]Table from references.[8–11]

[b]Types of cancer are stated broadly and not differentiated by subclassifications.

[c]The frequency and number of treatment cycles vary according to the specific protocols employed.

for 4 cycles.[11] *Calculate the total quantity of paclitaxel, in milligrams, that the patient in the previous problem would receive during this treatment plan.*

$$\text{BSA} = 1.70\ \text{m}^2$$

$$1.70\ \text{m}^2 \times 175\ \text{mg/m}^2\ \text{paclitaxel} = 297.5\ \text{mg (per cycle)} \times 4\ \text{(cycles)}$$

$$= \mathbf{1190\ mg\ paclitaxel}$$

(5) *If an injection is available containing paclitaxel, 6 mg/mL, calculate the volume required per cycle to treat the patient in the previous problem.*

$$297.5\ \text{mg} \div 6\ \text{mg/mL} = \mathbf{49.6\ mL\ paclitaxel\ injection}$$

CASE IN POINT 8.5[13] In treating a 54-year-old female patient, an oncologist selects the drug temozolomide, an antitumor agent used in the treatment of refractory astrocytoma (brain tumor). The drug is used as part of a 28-day regimen, during which the first 5 days of treatment include temozolomide at a once-daily dose of 150 mg/m^2/day. The patient's medical chart indicates that she measures 5 feet in height and weighs 117 lb. The physician asks the pharmacist to determine the proper combination of available capsules to use in dosing the patient. The drug is available in capsules containing 5, 20, 100, and 250 mg of temozolomide. What combination of capsules would provide the daily dose of this drug?

PRACTICE PROBLEMS

Calculations Based on Body Weight

1. The dose of a drug is 500 mcg/kg of body weight. How many milligrams should be given to a child weighing 55 lb?
2. The dose of gentamicin for premature and full-term neonates is 2.5 mg/kg administered every 12 hours. What would be the daily dose for a newborn weighing 5.6 lb?
3. The dose of gentamicin for patients with impaired renal function is adjusted to ensure therapeutically optimal dosage. If the normal daily dose of the drug for adults is 3 mg/kg/day, administered in three divided doses, what would be the single (8-hour) dose for a patient weighing 165 lb and scheduled to receive only 40% of the usual dose, based on renal impairment?
4. A patient weighing 120 lb was administered 2.1 g of a drug supposed to be dosed at 30 mg/kg. Was the dose administered *correct*, or was it an *overdose*, or was it an *underdose*?
5. In a clinical trial of ciprofloxacin (CIPRO), pediatric patients were initiated on 6 to 10 mg/kg intravenously every 8 hours and converted to oral therapy, 10 to 20 mg/kg, every 12 hours. Calculate the ranges of the total daily amounts of ciprofloxacin that would have been administered intravenously and orally to a 40-lb child.
6. ℞ Erythromycin ethylsuccinate 400 mg/5 mL
   Disp. 100 mL
   Sig. _____ tsp. q.i.d. until all medication is taken.

   If the dose of erythromycin ethylsuccinate is given as 40 mg/kg/day
   (a) What would be the proper dose of the medication in the signa, if the prescription is for a 44-lb child?
   (b) How many days will the prescribed medication last?
7. If the pediatric dosage of chlorothiazide (DIURIL) is 10 to 20 mg/kg of body weight per day in a single dose or two divided doses, not to exceed 375 mg/day, calculate the *daily dosage range* of an oral suspension containing 250 mg chlorothiazide per 5 mL that should be administered to a 48-lb child.
8. Cyclosporine is an immunosuppressive agent administered before and after organ transplantation at a single dose of 15 mg/kg. How many milliliters of a 50-mL bottle containing 100 mg of cyclosporine per milliliter would be administered to a 140-lb kidney transplant patient?
9. The adult dose of a liquid medication is 0.1 mL/kg of body weight. How many teaspoonfuls should be administered to a person weighing 220 lb?
10. A hospitalist prescribed dimenhydrinate to treat a 48-lb child. The labeled dose of the drug is 1.125 mg/kg. The available oral solution contains dimenhydrinate, 12.5 mg/5 mL. Prior to administering the solution, the floor nurse decides to check her calculated dose of 9.8 mL with the hospital pharmacist. Were her calculations correct?
11. ℞ Fluconazole tabs 100 mg
    Disp. _____ tabs
    Sig: tab ii stat, then 3 mg/kg b.i.d. × 7 days thereafter.
    Calculate the number of tablets to dispense to a patient weighing 147 lb.
12. A physician desires a dose of 10 mcg/kg of digoxin for an 8-lb newborn child. How many milliliters of an injection containing 0.25 mg of digoxin per milliliter should be given?

13. Intravenous digitalizing doses of digoxin in children are 80% of oral digitalizing doses. Calculate the intravenous dose for a 5-year-old child weighing 40 lb if the oral dose is determined to be 10 mcg/kg.
14. An intratracheal suspension for breathing enhancement in premature infants is dosed at 2.5 mL/kg of birth weight. How many milliliters of the suspension should be administered to a neonate weighing 3 lb?
15. A 142-lb patient was receiving filgrastim (NEUPOGEN) in doses of 10 mcg/kg/day when, as a result of successful blood tests, the dose was lowered to 6 mcg/kg/day. Using an injection containing 0.3 mg filgrastim per 0.5 mL, calculate the previous and new dose to be administered.
    (a) 17.7 mL and 64.6 mL
    (b) 5.23 mL and 3.14 mL
    (c) 1.08 mL and 0.65 mL
    (d) 3.87 mL and 2.3 mL
16. A 25-lb child is to receive 4 mg of phenytoin per kilogram of body weight daily as an anticonvulsant. How many milliliters of pediatric phenytoin suspension containing 30 mg per 5 mL should the child receive?
17. The loading dose of digoxin in premature infants with a birth weight of less than 1.5 kg is 8 mcg/kg administered in three *un*equally divided doses (½, ¼, ¼) at 8-hour intervals. What would be the initial dose for an infant weighing 1.2 kg?
18. The pediatric dose of cefadroxil is 30 mg/kg/day. If a child was given a daily dose of 2 teaspoonfuls of a pediatric suspension containing 125 mg of cefadroxil per 5 mL, what was the weight, in pounds, of the child?
19. How many milliliters of an injection containing 1 mg of drug per milliliter of injection should be administered to a 6-month-old child weighing 16 lb to achieve a dose of 0.01 mg/kg?
20. Prior to hip replacement surgery, a patient receives an injection of an anticoagulant drug at a dose of 30 mg. Following the patient's surgery, the drug is injected at 1 mg/kg. For a 140-lb patient, calculate the total of the pre- and postsurgical doses.
21. Using Table 8.2 and a daily dose of 2 mg/kg, how many 20-mg capsules would a 176-lb patient be instructed to take per dose if the daily dose is to be taken in divided doses, q.i.d.?
22. For a 22-lb pediatric patient, the dose of cefdinir (OMNICEF) was determined to be 7 mg/kg. What quantity of an oral suspension containing 125 mg of cefdinir in each 5 mL should be administered?
    (a) 2.8 mL
    (b) 5.6 mL
    (c) 8.9 mL
    (d) 13.6 mL
23. How many capsules, each containing 250 mg of clarithromycin, are needed to provide 50 mg/kg/day for 10 days for a person weighing 176 lb?
24. If the pediatric dose of dactinomycin is 15 mcg/kg/day for 5 days, how many micrograms should be administered to a 40-lb child over the course of treatment?
25. If the administration of gentamicin at a dose of 1.75 mg/kg is determined to result in peak blood serum levels of 4 mcg/mL, calculate the dose, in milligrams, for a 120-lb patient that may be expected to result in a blood serum gentamicin level of 4.5 mcg/mL.

26. A medication order calls for tobramycin sulfate, 1 mg/kg of body weight, to be administered by IM injection to a patient weighing 220 lb. Tobramycin sulfate is available in a vial containing 80 mg per 2 mL. How many milliliters of the injection should the patient receive?
27. The usual pediatric dose of acyclovir is 20 mg/kg administered by infusion and repeated every 8 hours. What would be the single dose, in milligrams, for a child weighing 33 lb?
28. If the recommended dose of tobramycin for a premature infant is 4 mg/kg/day, divided into two equal doses administered every 12 hours, how many milligrams of the drug should be given every 12 hours to a 2.2-lb infant?
29. If a 3-year-old child weighing 35 lb accidentally ingested twenty 81-mg aspirin tablets, how much aspirin did the child ingest on a milligram per kilogram basis?
30. The recommended pediatric dose of epinephrine for allergic emergencies is 0.01 mg/kg. If a physician, utilizing this dose, administered 0.15 mg, what was the weight of the patient in pounds?
31. The initial maintenance dose of vancomycin for infants less than 1 week old is 15 mg/kg every 18 hours.
    (a) What would be the dose, in milligrams, for an infant weighing 2500 g?
    (b) How many milliliters of an injection containing 500 mg per 25 mL should be administered to obtain this dose?
32. The loading dose of indomethacin in neonates is 0.2 mg/kg of body weight by intravenous infusion.
    (a) What would be the dose for a neonate weighing 6 lb 4 oz?
    (b) How many milliliters of an injection containing 1 mg of indomethacin per 0.5 mL should be administered to obtain this dose?
33. ℞[13] Jimmy Jones Age: 8 years
    Wt: 88 lb
    Metronidazole suspension
    7.5 mg/kg/day
    M.ft. dose = 5 mL
    Sig: 5 mL b.i.d. × 10 days
    (a) How many milligrams of metronidazole will the patient receive per dose?
    (b) How many milliliters of the prescription should be prepared and dispensed?
    (c) If metronidazole is available in 250-mg tablets, how many tablets will be needed to fill the prescription?
34. ℞[13] Betty Smith Age: 4 years
    Weight: 52.8 lb
    Erythromycin ethylsuccinate (EES) 200 mg/5 mL
    Disp. 300 mL
    Sig: _____ mL q.i.d. until gone
    (a) If the dose of EES is 50 mg/kg/day, how many milliliters would provide each dose?
    (b) How many days would the prescription last the patient?

Calculations Based on Body Surface Area

NOTE: As needed, refer to the BSA nomograms, Mosteller Formula, and/or tables in this chapter.

35. If the daily dose of a drug is given in the literature as 8 mg/kg of body weight or 350 mg/m^2, calculate the dose on each basis for a patient weighing 150 lb and measuring 5 feet 8 inches in height.
36. If the dose of a drug is 10 mg/m^2/day, what would be the daily dose, in milligrams, for a child weighing 30 lb and measuring 26 inches in height?
37. The dose of mitomycin injection is 20 mg/m^2/day. Determine the daily dose for a patient who weighs 144 lb and measures 68 inches in height.
38. The pediatric starting dose of ritonavir (NORVIR) is 250 mg/m^2 by mouth twice daily. The available oral solution contains 600 mg of ritonavir in each 7.5 mL of solution. The correct volume and corresponding quantity of ritonavir to be administered to a child with a body surface area of 0.75 m^2 per dose is:
    (a) 5.6 mL (450.4 mg)
    (b) 2.8 mL (450.4 mg)
    (c) 2.8 mL (225.2 mg)
    (d) 2.3 mL (187.5 mg)
39. Calculate the dose for a child 4 years of age, 39 inches in height, and weighing 32 lb for a drug with an adult dose of 100 mg, using the following: (a) Young's rule, (b) Cowling's rule, (c) Clark's rule, and (d) BSA (use the BSA equation).
40. The daily dose of diphenhydramine HCl for a child may be determined on the basis of 5 mg/kg of body weight or on the basis of 150 mg/m^2. Calculate the dose on each basis for a child weighing 55 lb and measuring 40 inches in height.

Calculations of Chemotherapeutic Regimens

41. The drug cabazitaxel is used treating prostate cancer in doses of 25 mg/m^2. Calculate the dose for a patient measuring 73 inches in height and weighing 190 lb.
42. Calculate the quantities of each drug administered to a patient on day 2 of the ELF protocol if the patient's BSA is 1.64 m^2.
43. If the dose of etoposide for a patient on the CAE protocol is increased to 120 mg/m^2, calculate the increase in the dose, in milligrams, if the patient measures 150 cm and weighs 48 kg.
44. The drug carboplatin for ovarian carcinoma is administered intravenously at a dose of 360 mg/m^2 except in patients with impaired kidney function, in which case the dose is reduced by 30%. How many milligrams of the drug should be administered to a renally impaired patient measuring 5 feet 2 inches and weighing 110 lb?
45. A high-dose treatment of osteosarcoma includes the use of methotrexate at a starting dose of 12 g/m^2 as a 4-hour intravenous infusion. For a patient having a BSA of 1.7 m^2 and weighing 162 lb, calculate the dose on the basis of mg/kg/min.
46. A two-agent dosage regimen, termed MP, for the treatment of multiple myeloma is as follows[11]:

Melphalan	0.25 mg/kg, PO, D1–4/week × 6 weeks
Prednisone	2 mg/kg, PO, D1–4/week × 6 weeks

    (a) Calculate the total milligrams each of melphalan and prednisone taken per week by a patient who weighs 165 lb.
    (b) If melphalan is available in 2-mg tablets, how many tablets are required to dose this patient for the entire treatment cycle?
    (c) If the patient prefers prednisone oral solution to prednisone tablets, how many milliliters of the solution (5 mg/mL) should be dispensed weekly?

47. A three-agent dosage regimen, termed VAD, for the treatment of multiple myeloma includes the following drugs taken over a 28-day cycle[11]:

Vincristine	0.4 mg/day, CIVI, D 1–4
Doxorubicin	9 mg/m²/day, CIVI, D 1–4
Dexamethasone	40 mg/day, PO, D 1–4, 9–12, 17–20

Calculate the total quantity of each drug administered over the course of the treatment cycle for a patient with a BSA of 1.65 m².

48. A four-agent dosage regimen, termed MOPP, for the treatment of Hodgkin's lymphoma includes the following drugs taken over a 28-day cycle[11]:

Mechlorethamine	6 mg/m², IV, D 1,8
Vincristine	1.4 mg/m², IV, D 1,8
Procarbazine	100 mg/m²/day, PO, D 1–14
Prednisone	40 mg/m²/day, PO, D 1–14

Calculate the total number of 20-mg tablets of prednisone and 50-mg tablets of procarbazine to dispense to treat a patient with a BSA of 1.5 m² during the course of one treatment cycle.

49. The oncolytic agent lapatinib (TYKERB) is administered in the treatment of breast cancer in daily doses of 1250 mg for 21 consecutive days in combination with the drug capecitabine (XELODA), which is administered in doses of 1000 mg/m²/day during days 1 to 14 of the 21-day treatment cycle. Calculate the total quantity of *each drug* to be administered during the treatment cycle to a 5-feet 2-inch woman weighing 110 lb.
50. Among the single chemotherapeutic agents for breast cancer is docetaxel (TAXOTERE), which is administered @ 60 mg/m² IV every 3 weeks. Calculate the dose for a 5-feet-4-inch patient who weighs 160 lb.
51. Based on the dose calculated in the above problem, how many milliliters of an injection containing 80 mg/2 mL docetaxel would be administered per dose?
52. The chemotherapy regimen "CAF" during a 21-day cycle is[11]:

Cyclophosphamide	500 mg/m², D1
Doxorubicin	50 mg/m², D1
5-Fluorouracil	500 mg/m², D1,8

Calculate the dose of each drug/cycle for a patient with a BSA of 1.9 m².

Miscellaneous Practice Problems

53. The literature states the pediatric dose of the antibiotic clarithromycin as "7.5 mg/kg q12h." Calculate the daily dose in milligrams for a child weighing 55 lb.
54. If, in the previous problem, the medication is administered as a suspension containing 125 mg clarithromycin/5 mL, what volume should be administered for each single dose?
55. The recommended initial once-a-day dose of the neurologic drug divalproex sodium is 25 mg/kg/day, to be increased as indicated to an absolute maximum dose of 60 mg/kg/day. Calculate these quantities for a 182-lb patient.
56. Diproex sodium is available in 250 mg and 500 mg strength tablets. From the information in the previous problem, what strength tablet and quantity could a pharmacist recommend for an initial dose?

57. The recommended pediatric dose of leuprolide acetate suspension for intramuscular injection is 7.5 mg, once per month, for a child weighing 25 kg. What is the equivalent dose, based on mg/m^2, for this child measuring 36 inches in height? Use the BSA equation as needed.
58. The starting pediatric dose of ritonavir is 250 mg/m^2 twice daily. Calculate the single dose, in milliliters, of an oral solution containing 600 mg of ritonavir in 7.5 mL of solution, for a child with a body surface area of 0.64 m^2.
59. Beractant intratracheal sterile suspension may be administered to premature neonates within 15 minutes of birth, as indicated, for the prevention and treatment of respiratory distress syndrome. The suspension is available in 4-mL and 8-mL vials containing 25 mg of drug per milliliter. The dose is 100 mg/kg of birth weight. Calculate the dose of the suspension for a newborn weighing 1800 g.
60. The dose of the drug ixabepilone is 40 mg/m^2, but if a patient's BSA is above 2.2 m^2, the dose is calculated based on 2.2 m^2. Using Figure 8.3, determine which dose parameter should be used for a patient who is 6 feet tall and weighs 200 lb.
61. The pediatric dose of levothyroxine sodium is based on both age and body weight, according to the following:
    0 to 3 months, 10 to 15 mcg/kg/day
    3 to 6 months, 8 to 10 mcg/kg/day
    6 to 12 months, 6 to 8 mcg/kg/day
    1 to 5 years, 5 to 6 mcg/kg/day
    6 to 12 years, 4 to 5 mcg/kg/day

    Verify the correctness of a physician's order for the dispensing of 100-mcg tablets to be taken once a day by a 6-year-old child weighing 48 lb.
62. Levothyroxine sodium tablets may be crushed and suspended in water and administered by spoon or drop to infants and children who cannot swallow intact tablets. From the information in the previous problem, should a 25-mcg tablet, a 50-mcg tablet, or a 75-mcg tablet be crushed and suspended for administration to a 10-month-old infant weighing 17 lb?
63. The pediatric dose of nelarabine is 650 mg/m^2 administered intravenously over a period of 1 hour daily for 5 consecutive days. The drug is available in vials containing nelarabine, 250 mg/50 mL. Using Figure 8.2, calculate (a) the daily dose of drug, in milligrams, for a child weighing 15 kg and measuring 100 cm in height, and (b) the total volume of injection to infuse per treatment period.
64. The oral dose of topotecan in the treatment of small cell lung cancer is 2.3 $mg/m^2/day$ once daily for 5 consecutive days, repeated every 21 days. The medication is available in 0.25 mg and 1 mg capsules. Recommend the strength and number of capsules to dispense for the initial course of treatment of a patient who weighs 165 lb and measures 5 feet 11 inches in height. Use the BSA equation.
65. A patient who is 6 feet tall and weighs 187 lb has been given 170 mg of a medication based on a 2 mg/kg basis. Calculate the same dose, based on mg/m^2. Use the BSA equation as needed.
66. The recommended dosage of lapatinib for metastatic breast cancer is 1250 mg given orally once daily on days 1 to 21, in combination with capecitabine 2000 $mg/m^2/day$ given orally on days 1 to 14 of a 21-day cycle. How many 250-mg tablets of lapatinib and 150-mg *or* 500-mg tablets of capecitabine should be dispensed for each cycle of therapy for a patient with a calculated BSA of 1.75 m^2? (Also, refer to the package inserts *online* and think about the possible prescription-labeling instructions for the patient.).

67. Cefixime, an anti-infective agent, is available in oral suspensions of the following strengths: 100 mg/5 mL, 200 mg/5 mL, and 500 mg/5 mL. The pediatric dose is 8 mg/kg/day, administered in divided dosage. Calculate (a) the daily dose of cefixime for a 55-lb patient, (b) the most appropriate product strength to dispense, and (c) the quantity of oral suspension, in milliliters, required for a 10-day course of treatment.
68. Pertuzumab, for the treatment of late-stage breast cancer, is administered at an initial dose of 840 mg by intravenous infusion. It is coadministered every 3 weeks with trastuzumab 8 mg/kg and docetaxel 75 mg/m^2. Calculate the doses of trastuzumab and docetaxel, for a patient who is 60 inches in height and weighs 158 lb. Use the BSA equation as needed.

CALCQUIZ

8.A. The drug eribulin mesylate is used in late-stage metastatic breast cancer at an intravenous dose of 1.4 mg/m^2. It is administered on days 1 and 8 of a 21-day cycle. The dose is reduced by 20% for patients with moderate renal impairment. Calculate the reduced dose, in (a) mg/m^2, (b) mg/kg, and (c) the treatment-day dose, in milligrams, for a 110-lb patient measuring 5 feet 2 inches in height.

8.B. A parent takes her 5- and 7-year-old boys to the pediatrician, both with pharyngitis. The boys weigh 40 and 50 lb, respectively. The doctor prescribes an oral suspension of cefuroxime axetil (CEFTIN) at a dose of 20 mg/kg/day divided b.i.d. × 10 days. The suspension has a cefuroxime axetil concentration of 125 mg/mL. How many milliliters of suspension will be needed during the course of treatment?

8.C. The first-day loading dose of a drug is 70 mg/m^2 followed by a dose of 50 mg/m^2 daily thereafter. Irrespective of the patient's BSA, a dose is not to exceed 70 mg. For a 5-feet 8-inch 150-lb patient, calculate the (a) BSA using the Mosteller formula, (b) loading dose, and (c) maintenance dose, and indicate whether each dose is within the safe limit.

8.D. The pediatric oral dose of ciprofloxacin is given as 10 to 20 mg/kg every 8 hours, not to exceed a single dose of 400 mg irrespective of body weight. If a child weighing 55 lb is prescribed a one-teaspoonful dose of a 5% ciprofloxacin oral suspension every 8 hours, calculate whether or not the dose prescribed is within the therapeutic range.

8.E. The drug peginterferon alpha-2b is sometimes administered according to a "step-down" protocol from a starting dose of 1.5 mcg/kg/week to 1 mcg/kg/week to 0.5 mcg/kg/week. Calculate the three doses for a 5-feet 5-inch 132-lb patient (a) in micrograms and (b) on a mcg/m^2 basis.

ANSWERS TO "CASE IN POINT" AND PRACTICE PROBLEMS

Case in Point 8.1

The metric weight of a 3-lb 7-oz neonate is calculated:
1 lb = 454 g; 1 oz = 28.35 g
3 lb × 454 g/lb = 1362 g
7 oz × 28.35 g/oz = 198.45 g
1362 g + 198.45 g = 1560.45 g, weight of the neonate

According to the dosing table, the dose for a 3-day-old neonate weighing less than 2000 g is 10 mg/kg/day divided every 12 hours.

The dose, in mg, may be calculated by dimensional analysis:

$$\frac{1\text{ kg}}{1000\text{ g}} \times \frac{10\text{ mg}}{1\text{ kg/day}} \times 1560.45\text{ g}$$
$$= 15.6\text{ mg clindamycin/day}$$

Since the daily dose is administered in two divided doses, each divided dose is:

$$\frac{15.6\text{ mg}}{2}$$
$$= 7.8\text{ mg clindamycin every 12 hours}$$

The volume of injectable solution is then calculated:

$$\frac{50\text{ mL}}{600\text{ mg}} \times 7.8\text{ mg} = 0.65\text{ mL}$$

Case in Point 8.2

To calculate the oral dose of enalapril for the patient, it is necessary to know the patient's weight. This may be calculated from the intravenous dose:

$$\frac{1\text{ kg}}{5\text{ mcg}} \times 55\text{ mcg}$$
$$= 11\text{ kg, the weight of the patient}$$

Then, the oral dose may be calculated:

$$\frac{100\text{ mcg}}{1\text{ kg}} \times 11\text{ kg} = 1100\text{ mcg} = 1.1\text{ mg}$$

By crushing and mixing the 2.5-mg enalapril tablet with sterile water to make 12.5 mL, the oral dose may be calculated:

$$\frac{2.5\text{ mg}}{12.5\text{ mL}} = \frac{1.1\text{ mg}}{x\text{ mL}};\quad x = 5.5\text{ mL}$$

Case in Point 8.3

Daily dose: 15 mg/kg × 10 kg = 150 mg

Single dose: 150 mg ÷ 3 = 50 mg

$$\text{Quantity of injection: } 50\text{ mg} \times \frac{1\text{ mL}}{5\text{ mg}} = 10\text{ mL}$$

Case in Point 8.4

(a) 28 inches × 2.54 cm/1 inch = 71.12 cm
22 lb × 1 kg/2.2 lb = 10 kg

$$\text{BSA, m}^2 = \sqrt{\frac{\text{Ht (cm)} \times \text{Wt (kg)}}{3600}}$$

$$= \sqrt{\frac{71.12 \text{ (cm)} \times 10 \text{ (kg)}}{3600}}$$

$$= \sqrt{0.198}$$

$$\text{BSA, m}^2 = 0.44$$

230 mg (lopinavir) × 0.44 m^2 = 101.2 mg
57.5 mg (ritonavir) × 0.44 m^2 = 25.3 mg
Thus, 101.2 mg (lopinavir) and 25.3 mg (ritonavir)

(b) 101.2 mg × 1 mL/80 mg = 1.27 mL
25.3 mg × 1 mL/20 mg = 1.27 mL
Thus, 1.27 mL or 1.3 mL oral solution (administered by calibrated oral syringe).

(c) KALETRA, 12/3 mg/kg
12 mg (lopinavir)/kg × 10 kg = 120 mg (lopinavir, single dose)
3 mg (ritonavir)/kg × 10 kg = 30 mg (ritonavir, single dose)
Thus, 120 mg × 2 (doses/day) = 240 mg (lopinavir), and
30 mg × 2 (doses/day) = 60 mg (ritonavir)

(d) 240 mg (lopinavir) × 1 mL/80 mg = 3 mL
60 mg (ritonavir) × 1 mL/20 mg = 3 mL
Thus, 3 mL oral solution, daily dose (administered by calibrated oral syringe).

It should be noted that since the ratio of lopinavir to ritonavir in the oral solution is fixed, that is, 80 mg:20 mg (or 4 mg:1 mg), the calculation of one component will automatically yield the quantity of the second component.

Case in Point 8.5

To calculate the dose for the patient, the pharmacist must first determine the patient's body surface area. The pharmacist elects to use the following equation:

$$\text{BSA, m}^2 = \sqrt{\frac{\text{Ht (cm)} \times \text{Wt (kg)}}{3600}}$$

To use this equation, the patient's weight and height are converted to metric units:
Height = 5 feet = 60 inches × 2.54 cm/inch = 152.4 cm
Weight = 117 lb ÷ 2.2 lb/kg = 53.2 kg
Solving the equation:

$$\text{BSA, (m}^2\text{)} = \sqrt{\frac{152.4 \times 53.2}{3600}} = 1.50 \text{ m}^2$$

The daily dose is calculated as 150 mg/m^2 × 1.50 m^2 = 225 mg.

To obtain 225 mg, the patient may take two 100-mg capsules, one 20-mg capsule, and one 5-mg capsule daily.

Practice Problems

1. 12.5 mg
2. 12.73 mg gentamicin
3. 30 mg gentamicin
4. Overdose
5. IV: 327.3 to 545.5 mg ciprofloxacin
   Oral: 363.6 to 727.3 mg ciprofloxacin
6. (a) ½ tsp. (2.5 mL) erythromycin ethylsuccinate
   (b) 10 days
7. 4.4 to 7.5 mL chlorothiazide oral suspension
8. 9.55 mL cyclosporin
9. 2 tsp.
10. Yes, calculations were correct.
11. 30 tablets
12. 0.15 mL digoxin injection
13. 145.5 mcg digoxin
14. 3.41 mL
15. (c) 1.08 mL and 0.65 mL filgrastim injection
16. 7.58 mL phenytoin suspension
17. 4.8 mcg digoxin
18. 18.33 lb
19. 0.073 mL
20. 93.64 or 94 mg
21. 2 capsules
22. (a) 2.8 mL cefdinir oral suspension
23. 160 clarithromycin capsules
24. 1364 mcg dactinomycin
25. 107.39 mg gentamicin
26. 2.5 mL tobramycin injection
27. 300 mg acyclovir
28. 2 mg tobramycin
29. 101.83 mg/kg aspirin
30. 33 lb
31. (a) 37.5 g vancomycin
    (b) 1.875 mL vancomycin injection
32. (a) 0.57 mg indomethacin
    (b) 0.28 mL indomethacin injection
33. (a) 150 mg metronidazole
    (b) 100 mL
    (c) 12 metronidazole tablets
34. (a) 7.5 mL
    (b) 10 days
35. 545.5 mg and 630 mg
36. 4.5 mg
37. 35.4 mg mitomycin
38. 2.3 mL (187.5 mg) ritonavir
39. (a) 25 mg
    (b) 20.83 mg
    (c) 21.33 mg
    (d) 36.57 mg
40. (a) 125 mg diphenhydramine HCl
    (b) 120 mg diphenhydramine HCl
41. 52.7 mg cabazitaxel
42. 196.8 mg etoposide
    246 mg leucovorin
    820 mg 5-fluorouracil
43. 29.7 mg etoposide
44. 372.96 mg carboplatin
45. 1.15 mg/kg/min methotrexate
46. (a) 75 mg melphalan and 600 mg prednisone
    (b) 225 tablets
    (c) 120 mL prednisone oral solution
47. 1.6 mg vincristine
    59.4 mg doxorubicin
    480 mg dexamethasone
48. 42 procarbazine tablets
    42 prednisone tablets
49. 26.25 g lapatinib and 20.72 g capecitabine
50. 108.7 mg docetaxel
51. 2.7 mL docetaxel injection
52. 1900 mg 5-fluorouracil
    95 mg doxorubicin
    950 mg cyclophosphamide
53. 375 mg clarithromycin
54. 7.5 mL clarithromycin suspension
55. 2068.2 mg divalproex sodium, initial dose
    4963.6 mg divalproex sodium, maximum dose
56. Four 500-mg tablets, initial dose
57. 9.4 mg/m^2
58. 1 mL ritonavir oral solution
59. 7.2 mL beractant suspension
60. 40 mg/m^2
61. Correct

62. A 50-mcg levothyroxine sodium tablet
63. (a) 416 mg nelarabine
    (b) 416 mL nelarabine injection
64. Twenty 1-mg topotecan capsules (4/day) and ten 0.025 mg topotecan capsules (2/day)
65. 81.8 mg/m^2
66. One hundred five 250-mg lapatinib tablets and ninety-eight 500-mg capecitabine tablets
67. (a) 200 mg cefixime
    (b) 100 mg/5 mL
    (c) 100 mL cefixime suspension
68. 574.5 mg trastuzumab and 130.8 mg docetaxel

References

1. Ferri FF. *Practical Guide to the Care of the Medical Patient*. 8th Ed. Maryland Heights, MO: Elsevier; 2011.
2. Berkow R, ed. *The Merck Manual*. 16th Ed. Rahway, NJ: Merck Research Laboratories; 1992.
3. The Joint Commission. Available at: http://www.jointcommission.org/assets/1/18/SEA_39.PDF. Accessed May 5, 2014.
4. Gomella TL, ed. *Neonatology: Management, Procedures, On-Call Problems, Diseases, and Drugs*. 6th Ed. New York, NY: McGraw-Hill; 2009.
5. Taketomo CK. *Pediatric & Neonatal Dosage Handbook*. 20th Ed. Hudson, OH: Lexicomp/Wolters Kluwer Health Clinical Solutions; 2013–2014.
6. Mosteller RD. Simplified calculation of body surface area. *The New England Journal of Medicine* 1987;317:1098.
7. American Cancer Society. Available at: http://www.cancer.org/Treatment/TreatmentsandSideEffects/TreatmentTypes/index. Accessed February 10, 2011.
8. CancerTreatment.net. Available at: http://regimens.cancertreatment.net/. Accessed May 5, 2014.
9. Chemotherapy Advisor. Available at: http://www.chemotherapyadvisor.com/cancer-treatment-regimens/section/2412/. Accessed May 5, 2014.
10. National Cancer Institute. Available at: http://www.cancer.gov/cancertopics/druginfo/alphalist. Accessed May 5, 2014.
11. MediLexicon. Cancer drugs and oncology drugs. Available at: http://www.medilexicon.com/drugs-list/cancer.php. Accessed May 5, 2014.
12. Schwarz LR. Delivering cytotoxic chemotherapy safely in a community hospital. *Hospital Pharmacy* 1996;31:1108–1118.
13. Beach W. *College of Pharmacy*. Athens GA: The University of Georgia; 2004.

9

Calculations Involving Units of Activity and Other Measures of Potency

OBJECTIVES

Upon successful completion of this chapter, the student will be able to:

- Perform calculations involving units of activity and other measures of potency.

The potencies of some antibiotics, endocrine products, vitamins, products derived through biotechnology, and biologics (e.g., vaccines) are based on their *activity* and are expressed in terms of *units of activity*, in *micrograms per milligram*, or in other standardized terms of measurement. These measures of potency meet standards approved by the Food and Drug Administration as set forth in the *United States Pharmacopeia* (USP).[1] In addition, the World Health Organization (WHO) through the *International Pharmacopeia (IP)* provides internationally agreed upon standards for biological preparations, which define potency or activity, as expressed in *international units (I.U.* or *IU)*.[2]

The activity of a drug or biologic agent is determined by comparison against a corresponding *reference standard*—an authenticated specimen used in compendial tests and assays. The required potencies and respective weight equivalents for some drugs are given in Table 9.1. *A USP Unit for one drug has no relation to a USP Unit for another drug.*

Of the drugs for which potency is expressed in units, insulin is perhaps the most common. Commercially available types of insulin vary according to time for onset of action, peak action, and duration of action; however, all are standardized to contain either 100 or 500 insulin units per milliliter of solution or suspension. These products are labeled as "U-100" (Fig. 9.1) or "U-500." Insulin is dosed by the administration of a specific number of units. Specially calibrated insulin syringes (Fig. 9.2) or prefilled, dial-a-dose insulin pens (KwikPen [Lilly] and FlexPen [Novo Nordisk]) are employed.

CALCULATIONS CAPSULE

Units of Activity

The potency of many pharmaceutical products derived from biological sources is based on *units of activity.* Units of activity are determined against specific biologic standards and vary between products. Generally, there is an established relationship between a product's units of activity and a measurable quantity (e.g., units per milligram; units per milliliter). This relationship may be used in a ratio and proportion to determine either the number of units of activity or the weight or volume containing a specified number of units:

$$\frac{\text{Units of activity (given)}}{\text{Weight or volume (given)}} = \frac{\text{Units of activity (given or desired)}}{\text{Weight or volume (given or desired)}}$$

Table 9.1 • EXAMPLES OF DRUG POTENCY EQUIVALENTS

Drug	Units or μg of Potency Per Weight Equivalent[a]
Alteplase	580,000 USP Alteplase Units per mg of protein
Bacitracin zinc	NLT 65 Bacitracin Units per mg
Cefdinir	NLT 960 μg and NMT 1020 μg of cefdinir per mg
Clindamycin hydrochloride	NLT 800 μg of clindamycin per mg
Cod liver oil	In each gram: NLT 180 μg (600 USP Units) and NMT 750 μg (2500 USP Units) of Vitamin A and NLT 1.5 μg (60 USP Units) and NMT 6.25 μg (250 USP Units) of Vitamin D
Erythromycin estolate	NLT 600 μg of erythromycin per mg
Gentamicin sulfate	NLT 590 μg of gentamicin per mg
Heparin sodium	NLT 180 USP Heparin Units per mg
Insulin	NLT 26.5 USP Insulin Units per mg
Insulin glargine	27.5 units/mg
Insulin glulisine	28.7 units/mg
Insulin human	NLT 27.5 USP Insulin Human Units per mg
Insulin lispro	NLT 27 USP Insulin Lispro Units per mg
Interferon alpha-2b	2.6×10^8 international units per mg
Interferon alpha-n3	2×10^8 international units per mg
Interferon beta-1b	3.2×10^7 international units per mg
Neomycin sulfate	NLT 600 μg of neomycin per mg
Nystatin	NLT 4400 USP Nystatin Units per mg
Penicillin G benzathine	NLT 1090 and NMT 1272 Penicillin G Units per mg
Penicillin G potassium	NLT 1440 and NMT 1680 Penicillin G Units per mg
Penicillin V potassium	NLT 1380 and NMT 1610 Penicillin V Units per mg
Polymyxin B sulfate	NLT 6000 Polymyxin B Units per mg
Somatropin	3 international units per mg
Tobramycin	NLT 900 μg of tobramycin per mg
Vancomycin	NLT 900 μg vancomycin per mg
Vasopressin	NLT 300 Vasopressin Units per mg
Vitamin A	1 USP Vitamin A Unit equals the biologic activity of 0.3 μg of the all-*trans* isomer of retinol
Vitamin D	40 units per μg

[a]Data taken or derived from various literature sources including the *United States Pharmacopeia* and the *International Pharmacopeia.*

As noted previously in this text, medication errors can occur when the term *units* is abbreviated with a "*U*." For example, "100U" could be mistaken for "1000" units. Thus, it is recommended that the term *units* be spelled out as a matter of practice.

Another effort to reduce medication errors has been implemented by clarifying the contents of certain packages of multidose injections. Figure 9.3 shows the dual statement of strength in the labeling of a Heparin Sodium Injection in which the drug concentration for the entire contents (30,000 USP Units/30 mL) and the concentration per milliliter (1,000 USP Units/mL) are displayed.

Various Expressions of Potency

Biologics are preparations produced from a living source. They include vaccines, toxoids, and immune sera, used for the development of *immunity* or resistance to disease; certain antitoxins and antivenins, used as treatment against specific antigens; and toxins and skin

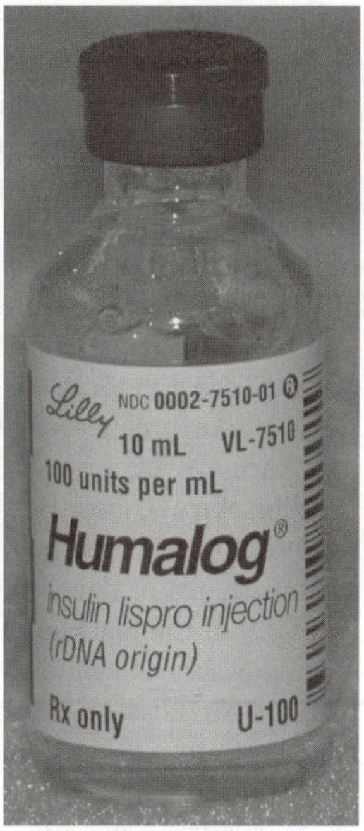

FIGURE 9.1 • Example of a pharmaceutical product standardized in units of activity.

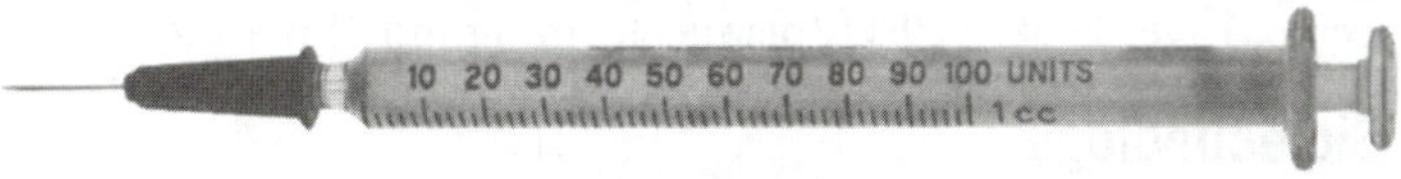

FIGURE 9.2 • Example of an insulin syringe calibrated in Units. *(Courtesy of Becton, Dickinson and Company.)*

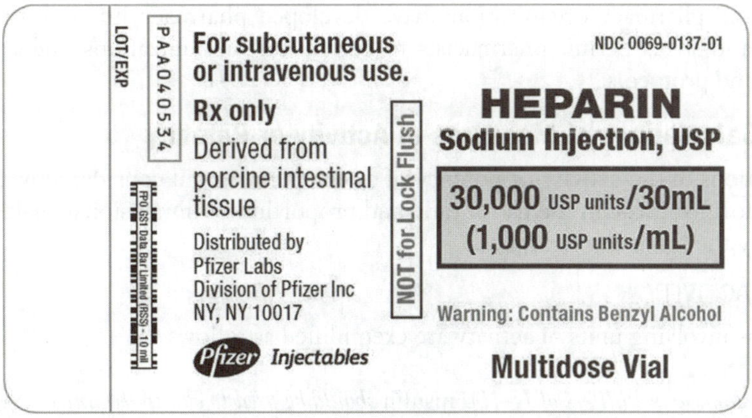

FIGURE 9.3 • Label for a multidose package of Heparin Sodium Injection, USP, displaying a dual statement of strength to clarify contents and reduce misinterpretation and medication errors. *(Source: http://dailymed.nlm.nih.gov/dailymed/about.cfm. Courtesy of Pfizer, Inc.)*

antigens, used as diagnostic aids. Biologics are prepared from human serum (e.g., immune globulin), horse serum (e.g., tetanus antitoxin), chick cell culture (e.g., measles virus vaccine), and other such animate media.

The strengths of the various biologic products are expressed in a number of ways. The strength of a bacterial vaccine commonly is expressed in terms of micrograms or units of antigen per milliliter. The strength of a viral vaccine is expressed most commonly in terms of the *tissue culture infectious dose* (*TCID*$_{50}$), which is the quantity of virus estimated to infect 50% of inoculated cultures. Viral vaccines may also be described in terms of units, micrograms of antigen, or number or organisms per milliliter. The strength of a toxoid is generally expressed in terms of *flocculating units (Lf Unit)*, with 1 Lf Unit having the capacity to flocculate or precipitate one unit of standard antitoxin.

Vaccines are available for a large number of diseases, including cervical cancer (human papillomavirus), hepatitis A and B, influenza, measles, mumps, pneumococcal, shingles (herpes zoster), smallpox, and tuberculosis. In addition, many additional vaccines are in various stages of development. The National Institute of Allergy and Infectious Diseases (NIAID) of the National Institutes of Health (NIH) lists all vaccines licensed for use in the United States as well as the status of vaccines in current research and development.[3] The Centers for Disease Control and Prevention (CDC) offers current guidelines for vaccine use in different population groups, as infants, children, adults, and pregnant women.[4]

Specific examples of the ***potency*** of vaccines expressed in terms other than weight are:

Hepatitis A vaccine, inactivated, 1440 EL.U (ELISA units) per 1-mL dose

Influenza virus vaccine, live (intranasal), $10^{6.5-7.5}$ FFU (fluorescent focus units) per 0.2-mL dose

Measles virus vaccine, live NLT 1000 TCID$_{50}$ (50% tissue culture infectious dose) in each 0.5-mL dose

Zoster Vaccine, Live, 19,400 PFU (plaque-forming units) per 0.65-mL dose

Products of Biotechnology

In addition to the biologic types of products described above, the activities of some products of *biotechnology* also are expressed in terms of units of activity (e.g., interferon alpha-2b contains 2.6×10^8 international units per milligram).

Pharmacy-Based Immunizations

Pharmacy-based immunization programs are commonplace nowadays. Many colleges of pharmacy and pharmacy organizations have developed pharmacy immunization training programs, and states permit pharmacists to administer immunizations under established guidelines and protocols.

Example Calculations of Measures of Activity or Potency

Determinations of the activity or potency of a biologic material considered in this chapter may be performed through the use of ratio and proportion or dimensional analysis, as demonstrated by the following examples.

UNITS OF ACTIVITY

Calculations involving units of activity are exemplified as follows.

(1) *How many milliliters of U-100* insulin *should be used to obtain 40 units of insulin?*

U-100 insulin contains 100 units/mL

$$\frac{100 \text{ (units)}}{40 \text{ (units)}} = \frac{1 \text{ (mL)}}{x \text{ (mL)}}$$

$$x = \mathbf{0.4\ mL\ U\text{-}100\ insulin}$$

Or, solving by dimensional analysis:

$$40 \text{ units} \times \frac{1 \text{ mL}}{100 \text{ units}} = \mathbf{0.4 \text{ mL U-100 insulin}}$$

(2) *A physician prescribed 100 units of insulin to be added to 500 mL of D5W in treating a patient with severe diabetic acidosis. How many milliliters of insulin injection concentrate, U-500, should be used?*

U-500 insulin contains 500 units/mL

$$\frac{500 \text{ (units)}}{100 \text{ (units)}} = \frac{1 \text{ (mL)}}{x \text{ (mL)}}$$

$$x = \mathbf{0.2 \text{ mL U-500 insulin}}$$

Or, solving by dimensional analysis:

$$100 \text{ units} \times \frac{1 \text{ mL}}{500 \text{ units}} = \mathbf{0.2 \text{ mL U-500 insulin}}$$

(3) *How many milliliters of a Heparin Sodium Injection containing 200,000 units in 10 mL should be used to obtain 5,000 heparin sodium units that are to be added to an intravenous dextrose solution?*

$$\frac{200{,}000 \text{ (units)}}{5000 \text{ (units)}} = \frac{10 \text{ (mL)}}{x \text{ (mL)}}$$

$$x = \mathbf{0.25 \text{ mL heparin sodium injection}}$$

(4) *If a 2.5-mL vial contains 100 units of onabotulinumtoxinA (BOTOX), and 0.1 mL is injected into each of five sites* during *a procedure, how many units of drug would remain in the vial?*

Used in procedure: $0.1 \text{ mL} \times 5 \text{ (sites)} = 0.5 \text{ mL}$

Remaining in vial: $2.5 \text{ mL} - 0.5 \text{ mL} = 2 \text{ mL}$

$$\frac{100 \text{ units} \times 2 \text{ mL}}{2.5 \text{ mL}} = \mathbf{80 \text{ units onabotulinumtoxinA}}$$

ACTIVITY BASED ON WEIGHT

Calculations involving the determination of activity per unit of weight are exemplified as follows.

If neomycin sulfate has a potency of 600 μg of neomycin per milligram, how many milligrams of neomycin sulfate would be equivalent in potency to 1 mg of neomycin?

$$\frac{600 \text{ (}\mu\text{g of neomycin)}}{1000 \text{ (}\mu\text{g of neomycin)}} = \frac{1 \text{ (mg of neomycin sulfate)}}{x \text{ (mg of neomycin sulfate)}}$$

$$x = \mathbf{1.67 \text{ mg neomycin sulfate}}$$

DOSE OR ANTIGEN CONTENT OF A BIOLOGIC BASED ON POTENCY

Calculations of the dose or the antigen content of a biologic product are exemplified as follows:

(1) *A biologic contains 50 Lf Units of diphtheria toxoid in each 2.5 mL of product. If a pediatric patient is to receive 10 Lf Units, how many milliliters of product should be administered?*

$$\frac{50 \text{ (Lf Units)}}{10 \text{ (Lf Units)}} = \frac{2.5 \text{ (mL)}}{x \text{ (mL)}}$$

$$x = \mathbf{0.5 \text{ mL}}$$

(2) *Measles virus vaccine live is prepared to contain 1000 $TCID_{50}$ per 0.5-mL dose. What is the $TCID_{50}$ content of a 50-mL multiple-dose vial of the vaccine?*

$$\frac{1000\ (TCID_{50})}{x\ (TCID_{50})} = \frac{0.5\ (mL)}{50\ (mL)}$$

$$x = \mathbf{100{,}000\ TCID_{50}}$$

CASE IN POINT 9.1[a] A pharmacist is asked to assist in determining the correct dose of epoetin alfa (PROCRIT) injection for a 76-year-old, 165-lb male patient suffering from anemia, in part due to chronic renal failure. The patient's initial hemoglobin is 9.2 g/dL.

The literature states the starting adult dose of epoetin alfa to be "50 to 100 units/kg SC TIW" to stimulate red blood cell production. Firstly, (a) what would be the correct interpretation of this dosage statement?[b]

The literature further states that the dose is to be *reduced* by 25% when the patient's hemoglobin reaches a level suitable to avoid transfusion or increases >1 g/dL in any 2-week period. The dose is to be *increased* to "300 units/kg TIW" after 2–4 weeks if the hemoglobin response is insufficient or if transfusions are still required.

Using epoetin alfa injection, 10,000 units/mL, and the minimal starting dose, calculate (b) the number of milliliters required for the initial dose and (c) the total number of milliliters to be administered during the first week of treatment. If the patient's hemoglobin increases to 10.5 g/dL after 2 weeks of treatment, what would be the new dose in (d) units of epoetin alfa and in (e) milliliters of injection?

[a]Case in Point courtesy of Flynn Warren, Bishop, GA.
[b]If unsure of the abbreviations, refer to Chapter 4 for guidance.

PRACTICE PROBLEMS

Authors' Note: some abbreviations in this section are as they appear in certain product literature, and their use here is strictly for instructional purposes and not an endorsement of style.

Units of Activity Calculations

1. How many milliliters of U-100 insulin zinc suspension should be used to obtain 18 units of insulin?
2. If a diabetic patient injects 20 units of insulin twice daily, how many days will a 10-mL vial of the U-100 product last the patient?
3. The biotechnology-derived product interferon beta-1b contains 32 million international units per milligram. Calculate the number of international units present in a vial containing 0.3 mg of interferon beta-1b.
4. ALFERON N injection contains 5 million international units of interferon alpha-n3 per milliliter. How many units will an injection of 0.05 mL deliver?
5. Insulin glargine (LANTUS) injection is available in 10-mL vials, containing 100 units/mL. How many milliliters would a patient administer for (a) a starting dose of 10 units and (b) a maintenance dose of 4 units?

6. The content of a vial of penicillin G potassium weighs 600 mg and represents 1 million units. How many milligrams are needed to prepare 15 g of an ointment that is to contain 15,000 units of penicillin G potassium per gram?
7. HUMALOG contains 100 units of insulin lispro (rDNA origin) per milliliter. How many complete days will a 3-mL HUMALOG PEN last a patient whose dose is 35 units bid?
8. A physician prescribes 2.5 million units of penicillin G potassium daily for 1 week. If 1 unit of penicillin G potassium equals 0.6 μg, how many tablets, each containing 250 mg, will provide the prescribed dosage regimen?
9. ℞

Penicillin G potassium	5000 units/mL
Isotonic sodium chloride solution ad	15 mL

Using soluble penicillin tablets, each containing 200,000 units of crystalline penicillin G potassium, explain how you would obtain the penicillin G potassium needed in compounding the prescription.

10. FOSAMAX PLUS D contains 70 mg alendronate and 140 mcg of vitamin D_3, the latter equivalent to 5600 international units of vitamin D. At a once-a-week dose, calculate the daily intake of vitamin D_3 in milligrams and units.
11. A vial for preparation of 100 mL of injection of the drug alteplase (ACTIVASE) contains 100 mg of drug equivalent to 58 million international units to be administered by intravenous infusion. Calculate (a) the units administered to a 176-lb patient at a dose of 0.9 mg/kg and (b) the milliliters of injection to use.
12. Calcitonin is available as an injection containing 200 international units per milliliter. Adult doses of up to 32 units per kilogram have produced no adverse effects. On this basis, if a 120-lb patient were administered 0.75 mL of injection, would adverse effects be anticipated?
13. A physician's hospital medication order calls for a patient to receive 1 unit of insulin injection subcutaneously for every 10 mg/dL of blood sugar over 175 mg/dL, with blood sugar levels and injections performed twice daily in the morning and evening. The patient's blood sugar was 200 mg/dL in the morning and 320 mg/dL in the evening. How many total units of insulin injection were administered?
14. A physician's hospital medication order calls for isophane insulin suspension to be administered to a 136-lb patient on the basis of 1 unit/kg per 24 hours. How many units of isophane insulin suspension should be administered daily?
15. Somatropin (NUTROPIN) contains 5 mg of drug equivalent to approximately 15 IU of drug in a vial to prepare 10 mL of injection. If the starting adult dose is 0.006 mg/kg, calculate the dose (a) in units and (b) in milliliters for a 132-lb patient.
16. Cod liver oil is available in capsules containing 0.6 mL per capsule. Using Table 9.1, calculate the amounts, in units, each of vitamins A and D in each capsule. The specific gravity of cod liver oil is 0.92.
17. A hepatitis B immune globulin contains 312 IU/mL. If the dose is 0.06 mL/kg for certain at-risk persons, calculate the dose (a) in units and (b) in milliliters for a 132-lb person.
18. If a 5-mL vial of HUMATROPE, a biosynthetic somatropin of rDNA origin, contains 5 mg of somatotropin equivalent to 13 IU, how many milligrams of somatotropin and how many IU would be administered in a 0.6-mL dose?

19. EPOGEN injection is available containing in each milliliter, 2000, 3000, 4000, or 10,000 units of epoetin alfa. If the staring dose for a 160-lb patient is prescribed at 50 units/kg, which of the following would provide that dose?
(a) 4 mL of 2000 units/mL
(b) 1 mL of 3000 units/mL
(c) 0.9 mL of 4000 units/mL
(d) 0.8 mL of 10,000 units/mL
20. The prophylactic dose of tetanus antitoxin is 1500 units for persons weighing less than 65 lb and 3000 to 5000 units for persons weighing more than 65 lb. The antitoxin is available in dose vials of 1500 units, 3000 units, 5000 units, and 20,000 units. Which vial should a pharmacist provide for administration to a patient weighing 25 kg?

Additional Calculations of Potency

21. The product CREON (pancrelipase) contains 3000 units of lipase, 9,500 units of protease, and 15,000 units of amylase in delayed-release capsules. The capsules are to be swallowed whole or the contents added uncrushed to food immediately prior to administration. The dose should not exceed 2500 lipase units/kg of body weight. If the contents of one capsule are added to 120 mL of the feeding formula for a 12-lb infant, is the dose within accepted limits?
22. Define "<1.75 mIU/mL" as stated in the package insert for the drug leuprolide acetate (LUPRON DEPOT-PED).
23. What is the numerical difference between "1 mIU" and "1 MIU?"
24. During cholecystography to determine gallbladder function, the contents of one bottle of cholecystokinin containing 75 units is dissolved in physiological saline solution to make 7.5 mL. Then, 1 unit per kilogram of body weight is administered by slow intravenous injection. Calculate the dose, in units, and the volume, in milliliters, to be administered to a patient weighing 154 pounds.
25. Using Table 9.1, calculate the clindamycin potency equivalence, in milligrams per milliliter, of a solution containing 1 g of clindamycin hydrochloride in 10 mL of solution.
26. Each 1-mL adult dose of hepatitis A vaccine contains 1440 EL.U. of viral antigen. What would be the pediatric dose of this vaccine if 360 EL.U. of viral antigen are to be administered?
(a) 0.8 mL
(b) 0.25 mL
(c) 4 mL
(d) 0.4 mL
27. Each 0.01 mL of a mumps vaccine contains 400 $TCID_{50}$ of the mumps virus. If the usual dose contains 20,000 $TCID_{50}$, how many milliliters of vaccine should be administered?
28. If a biologic product contains 7.5 Lf Units of diphtheria toxoid per 0.5 mL, how many flocculating units would be present in a 7.5-mL multiple-dose vial?
29. Zoster Vaccine Live (ZOSTAVAX) contains about 29,850 plaque-forming units (PFU) of attenuated virus per 0.1 cL. Approximately how many PFUs would be contained in each 0.65-mL dose?
(a) 45,900 PFU
(b) 4590 PFU
(c) 1940 PFU
(d) 19,400 PFU

CALCQUIZ

9.A. If a 5-mL quantity of a nystatin oral suspension is prepared to contain 500,000 USP Nystatin Units, using Table 9.1, calculate (a) the concentration of nystatin in the suspension in mg/mL. If a child's dose is 2 mL four times a day, how many (b) nystatin units and (c) milligrams of nystatin would be administered daily?

9.B. The drug dalteparin sodium (FRAGMIN) is administered by subcutaneous injection in patients with unstable angina or myocardial infarction at doses of 120 units/kg but not to exceed 10,000 units. Prefilled calibrated syringes are available with the following strengths (units/mL): 2500/0.2 mL, 5000/0.2 mL, 7500/0.3 mL, 10,000/0.4 mL, 12,500/0.5 mL, and 15,000/0.6 mL. Calculate (a) the most efficient product strength to use to dose a patient weighing 148 lb, (b) the volume of that injection to administer, and (c) the weight of a hypothetical patient, in pounds, to reach the maximum dose of 10,000 units.

9.C. An injection contains 5 million international units (MIU) of interferon alpha-n3 (ALFERON N) proteins per milliliter. The recommended dose is 0.05 mL. The literature states that the activity of interferon alpha-n3 is approximately equal to 2.6×10^8 international units/mg of protein. Calculate (a) the number of international units and (b) the micrograms of interferon alfa-n3 proteins administered per dose.

9.D. One general guideline for the maintenance dosing of heparin in pediatric patients is 100 units/kg every 4 hours, or 20,000 units/m^2/24 hour administered continuously. The available injection for use by intravenous infusion contains 1000 USP Heparin Units/mL. For a 44-lb child, measuring 42 inches in height, calculate the *difference* between the quantities of heparin administered over a 24-hour period in (a) heparin units, (b) in milligrams of heparin (sodium), and (c) in milliliters of heparin injection.

ANSWERS TO "CASE IN POINT" AND PRACTICE PROBLEMS

Case in Point 9.1

(a) TIW = three times a week (*It should be noted that although this abbreviation appears in the literature, it is considered error prone and thus its use is not approved by the Institute of Safe Medication Practices.*)
(b) 165 lb ÷ 2.2 lb/kg = 75 kg, weight of patient
Minimal starting dose = 50 units/kg; thus, 50 units × 75 (kg) = 3750 units
3750 units ÷ 10,000 units/mL = 0.375 mL of epoetin alfa injection
(c) 0.375 mL/dose × 3 (times per week) = 1.125 mL epoetin alfa injection
(d) Dose reduced by 25% or 937.5 units; thus, 3750 − 937.5 = 2812.5 units epoetin alfa
(e) 2812.5 units ÷ 10,000 units/mL = 0.28 mL epoetin alfa injection

Practice Problems

1. 0.18 mL U-100 insulin zinc suspension
2. 25 days
3. 9,600,000 units interferon beta 1-b
4. 250,000 international units
5. (a) 0.1 mL insulin glargine
(b) 0.04 mL insulin glargine

6. 135 mg penicillin G potassium
7. 4 days
8. 42 penicillin G potassium tablets
9. Dissolve 1 tablet in enough isotonic sodium chloride solution to make 8 mL, and take 3 mL of the dilution.
10. 800 units and 0.02 mg/day
11. (a) 41.76 million units alteplase
    (b) 72 mL alteplase injection
12. No
13. 17 units insulin
14. 61.82 units isophane insulin
15. (a) 1.08 units somatropin
    (b) 0.72 mL somatropin injection
16. 331.2 to 1380 units of vitamin A 33.12 to 138 units of vitamin D
17. (a) 1123.2 IU hepatitis B immune globulin
    (b) 3.6 mL hepatitis B immune globulin
18. 0.6 mg, and 1.56 or 1.6 IU somatropin
19. (c) 0.9 mL of 4000 units/mL
20. 1500-unit vial
21. Yes
22. Less than 1.75 milli-international units per milliliter
23. 1 billion international units
24. 70 Units/dose and 7 mL/dose
25. 80 mg/mL clindamycin
26. (b) 0.25 mL
27. 0.5 mL mumps vaccine
28. 112.5 Lf Units diphtheria toxoid
29. (d) 19,400 PFU

References

1. *United States Pharmacopeia 32 National Formulary 27*. Vol. 1. Rockville, MD: The United States Pharmacopeial Convention; 2009;419–420.
2. World Health Organization (WHO). Available at: http://www.who.int/biologicals/reference_preparations/en/. Accessed May 8, 2014.
3. National Institute of Allergy and Infectious Diseases. Vaccine Research Center. Available at: http://www.niaid.nih.gov/about/organization/vrc/Pages/default.aspx. Accessed May 8, 2014.
4. Centers for Disease Control and Prevention. Vaccines and Immunizations. Available at: http://www.cdc.gov/vaccines/. Accessed May 8, 2014.

10

Selected Clinical Calculations

OBJECTIVES

Upon successful completion of this chapter, the student will be able to:

- Calculate heparin doses from medication orders and standardized protocols.
- Utilize equianalgesic dose charts to determine appropriate doses of narcotic analgesics based on previous narcotic use.
- Calculate estimated creatinine clearance rates and apply in dose determinations.
- Calculate ideal body weight and adjusted body weight and apply in dose determinations.
- Calculate various cholesterol ratios and cholesterol reduction percent from clinical laboratory data.
- Convert blood serum chemistry values from *mg/dL* to *mmol/L* (international system).

Heparin-Dosing Calculations

Heparin, also known as unfractionated heparin or UFH, is a heterogenous group of mucopolysaccharides that have anticoagulant properties. Heparin slows clotting time. It is derived from the intestinal mucosa or other suitable tissues of domestic animals (often porcine) used for food by man. Salt forms of heparin, such as heparin sodium, are standardized to contain 180 USP Heparin Units in each milligram. Heparin salts are administered as sterile aqueous solutions by intravenous infusion, intermittent intravenous injection, or deep subcutaneous injection for the prophylaxis and treatment of venous thrombosis. The commercial preparations, available in single-use syringes and multiple-dose vials, indicate on their labeling the number of USP Heparin Units of activity contained per milliliter.

Although heparin is a treatment option for acute venous thromboembolism, its use carries with it the risk of hemorrhage. Patients especially at risk include elderly patients, postsurgical patients, patients with a history of peptic ulcers, severe renal, or hepatic failure, and patients who recently have taken other medications that affect blood clotting time.[1]

When heparin sodium is administered in therapeutic amounts, its dosage is adjusted according to the results of tests measuring the patient's level of blood coagulation, or activated partial thromboplastin time (aPTT). These tests are performed before each intravenous injection and approximately every 4 to 6 hours when administered by intravenous infusion or subcutaneously. In general, the aPTT value should be maintained at 1.5 to 2 times the patient's pretreatment aPTT value or, when the whole-blood clotting time is evaluated, approximately 2 to 3 times the control value.[1,2]

The dose varies depending on the circumstances. Bolus doses, given by direct intravenous injection, may be followed by intravenous infusion as a heparin drip. For prevention of thromboembolism following surgery (also known as low-dose heparin therapy), patients receive 5000 units given by deep subcutaneous injection 2 hours before surgery and an additional 5000 units every 8 to 12 hours thereafter as required. Heparin is also used in higher doses to treat patients with active phlebitis or with pulmonary emboli.[3]

In pediatric use, the initial dose may be 50 units/kg by intravenous infusion, followed by maintenance doses of 100 units/kg every 4 hours or 20,000 units/m^2/24 hours, infused continuously.[3]

Figure 10.1 presents a hospital form for an adult weight–based heparin protocol. The form allows physicians' orders for bolus doses, as well as protocols for intravenous heparin infusions. The values given in this figure may differ from heparin protocols at other institutions. Pharmacists must follow those used within their institutions of practice.

Low-molecular-weight heparins (LMWHs) are also used as antithrombotic agents and are the agents of choice in treating deep vein thrombosis and pulmonary embolus. The

CITY HOSPITAL

ADULT WEIGHT-BASED HEPARIN PROTOCOL

Standard Heparin IV Premixed Solution is 25,000 units in 250 mL (100 units per mL)
Initial laboratory tests (draw before starting heparin): aPTT, PT, CBC with platelet count
Day 2 and every 3 days thereafter: CBC with platelet count
aPTT six (6) hours after heparin infusion is started
aPTT six (6) hours after every change in heparin administration rate or bolus dose of heparin
Once a therapeutic aPTT level is reached, do an aPTT six (6) hours later
After two (2) consecutive therapeutic aPTT levels are obtained, do an aPTT daily at 0600
Discontinue all IM medications and other IM injections

Patient _______ MAY _______ MAY NOT receive drugs containing aspirin.

Patient _______ MAY _______ MAY NOT receive drugs containing non-steroidal antiinflammatory agents.

Bolus Dose	
__________ None	
__________ 80 units/kg (limit 8,000 units)	
__________ Other (specify: __________ units)	
Continuous infusion rate	
__________ 18 units/kg/h	
__________ Other (specify: __________ units/h)	
aPTT Value	**Heparin Dose Adjustments**
< 35 seconds	Bolus with 80 units/kg and increase infusion rate by 4 units/kg/h
35 to 45 seconds	Bolus with 80 units/kg and increase infusion rate by 2 units/kg/h
46 to 70 seconds	No change in infusion rate
71 to 90 seconds	Decrease infusion rate by 2 units/kg/h
> 90 seconds	Hold infusion for 1 hour; when restarted, decrease infusion rate by 3 units/kg/h
DATE	TIME
	M.D.

FIGURE 10.1 • Example of hospital form for adult weight–based heparin protocol. *(Courtesy of Nina Morris, Southwestern Oklahoma State University, Weatherford, OK.)*

products currently on the market in the United States are enoxaparin sodium (LOVENOX) and dalteparin sodium (FRAGMIN). Heparin has a molecular weight ranging from 3000 to 30,000 daltons, whereas LMWHs are fragments of heparin with mean molecular weights of 4000 to 6000 daltons.[4] These shorter compounds may be administered subcutaneously (rather than intravenously, as is heparin), they interfere less with platelet function, and they generally have a more predictable anticoagulant response that does not require monitoring of clotting times.

Special Considerations in Heparin Management

Heparin is a very useful but potentially dangerous agent. It is administered only when necessary and with extreme caution. Hemorrhage is a distinct risk with heparin use, requiring patients to be closely monitored. Pediatric patients and seniors are among those who require particular care in dosing. Heparin-dosing errors can result from miscommunication (as with the use of the abbreviation "u" for units), from miscalculation of the appropriate dose, or from the administration of a product of incorrect strength. To reduce the likelihood of the latter, products are available in which the strengths are made distinctive by use of stark color-coding and bold, tall-letter labeling.

Example Calculations of Heparin Dosing

(1) *An intravenous infusion contained 20,000 units of heparin sodium in 1000 mL of D5W. The rate of infusion was set at 1600 units/h for a 160-lb patient. Calculate (a) the concentration of heparin sodium in the infusion, in units/mL; (b) the length of time the infusion would run, in hours; and (c) the dose of heparin sodium administered to the patient, on a unit/kg/min basis.*

(a) $\frac{20{,}000 \text{ units}}{1000 \text{ mL}} = 20 \text{ units/mL}$

(b) $\frac{20{,}000 \text{ units}}{1600 \text{ units/h}} = 12.5 \text{ hours}$

(c) 160 pounds = 72.7 kg

12.5 hours = 750 minutes

$$\frac{20{,}000 \text{ units}}{750 \text{ minutes}} = 26.67 \text{ units/min}$$

(d) $\frac{26.67 \text{ units/min}}{72.7 \text{ kg}} = 0.37 \text{ units/kg/min}$

(2) *A patient weighing 80 kg was given an initial bolus dose of heparin and a heparin drip for the first 6 hours. Using Figure* 10.1, *what was the total amount of heparin administered in this period?*

Bolus dose [80 units/kg]:

$$\frac{80 \text{ units}}{\text{kg}} \times 80 \text{ kg} = 6400 \text{ units}$$

Heparin infusion [18 units/kg/h]:

$$\frac{18 \text{ units}}{\text{kg/h}} \times 80 \text{ kg} \times 6 \text{ hours} = 8640 \text{ units}$$

$$6400 \text{ units} + 8640 \text{ units} = \mathbf{15{,}040 \text{ units}}$$

(3) *After 6 hours, the aPTT for the patient in example problem 2 is 102 seconds. Use Figure* 10.1 *to determine any changes necessary in his heparin therapy, and calculate a new flow rate for the infusion in mL/h using the standard heparin IV solution.*

According to Figure 10.1, the infusion for a patient with an aPTT of greater than 90 seconds should be stopped for 1 hour and then decreased by 3 units/kg/h when resumed. The new infusion rate would then be calculated as follows:

$$\frac{18 \text{ units}}{\text{kg/h}} - \frac{3 \text{ units}}{\text{kg/h}} = \frac{15 \text{ units}}{\text{kg/h}}$$

$$\frac{15 \text{ units}}{\text{kg/h}} \times 80 \text{ kg} = \frac{1200 \text{ units}}{\text{h}} \times \frac{250 \text{ mL}}{25{,}000 \text{ units}} = \mathbf{12\ mL/h}$$

(4) *Heparin sodium may be administered to children by intermittent intravenous infusion every 4 hours at doses ranging from 50 to 100 units/kg of body weight. Using an injection containing heparin, 5000 units/mL, calculate the daily dosage range, in milliliters, for a 50-lb child.*

$$\frac{50 \text{ to } 100 \text{ units}}{\text{kg/dose}} \times \frac{1 \text{ kg}}{2.2 \text{ lb}} \times 50 \text{ lb} = 1136.36 \text{ to } 2272.73 \text{ units/dose}$$

$$\frac{1136.36 \text{ to } 2272.73 \text{ units}}{\text{dose}} \times \frac{6 \text{ doses}}{\text{day}} = 6818.18 \text{ to } 13{,}636.36 \text{ units/day}$$

$$\frac{6818.18 \text{ to } 13{,}636.36 \text{ units}}{\text{day}} \times \frac{1 \text{ mL}}{5000 \text{ units}} = \mathbf{1.36\ to\ 2.73\ mL/day}$$

(5) *The pediatric maintenance dose of heparin sodium is stated in the literature as 20,000 units/m²/24 hours. Using the BSA nomogram in Chapter 8, and a heparin sodium injection containing heparin sodium, 1000 units/mL, calculate the daily volume of injection to administer to a 25-lb child measuring 22 inches in height.*

$$\text{BSA} = 0.37 \text{ m}^2$$

$$\frac{20{,}000 \text{ units}}{\text{m}^2} \times 0.37 \text{ m}^2 = 7400 \text{ units}$$

$$7400 \text{ units} \times \frac{1 \text{ mL}}{1000 \text{ units}} = \mathbf{7.4\ mL\ injection}$$

Example Calculations of Low-Molecular-Weight Heparin Dosing

The recommended dose of dalteparin sodium (FRAGMIN) for patients undergoing hip replacement surgery is 2500 international units within 2 hours before surgery, 2500 units 4 to 8 hours after surgery, and 5000 units daily for 5 to 10 days, starting on the postoperative day. How many milliliters from a vial containing 10,000 units/mL should be administered (a) before surgery, (b) after surgery, and (c) the day following surgery?

(a) $\frac{1 \text{ mL}}{10{,}000 \text{ units}} \times 2500 \text{ units} = 0.25 \text{ mL}$

(b) Same as (a) = 0.25 mL

(c) $\frac{1 \text{ mL}}{10{,}000 \text{ units}} \times 5000 \text{ units} = 0.5 \text{ mL}$

CASE IN POINT 10.1[a] A 198-lb hospitalized patient is placed on heparin therapy to treat a pulmonary embolism. The patient requires a bolus injection followed by a heparin infusion. The hospital follows the protocol shown in Figure 10.1.

The hospital pharmacist has heparin available for bolus doses containing 5000 units/mL in 5-mL vials and heparin for intravenous infusion in 250-mL infusion bags each containing 25,000 units of heparin.

(a) How many milliliters of the 5000 units/mL injection should the pharmacist recommend as a bolus dose?

(b) How many milliliters per hour of the heparin infusion should the pharmacist instruct the nurse to deliver, based on the standard infusion protocol?

(c) If the intravenous set is programmed to deliver 60 drops per milliliter, what should be the flow rate, in drops per minute, to deliver the mL/h required in answer (b)?

(d) How long will the 250-mL infusion bag last, in hours?

[a]Case in Point courtesy of Flynn Warren, Bishop, GA.

Use of Equianalgesic Dosing Charts

Narcotic analgesics, also termed opioid analgesics, are widely prescribed to relieve moderate to severe pain. They are used in cases of acute pain, such as due to an injury or surgery, and in cases of chronic pain due to cancer, musculoskeletal conditions, and other illnesses. In cases of chronic pain, when the patient will most likely be on a narcotic analgesic for an extended period of time, the goal of therapy is usually to relieve the patient's pain enough that he or she can continue a normal lifestyle but without overmedicating the patient and causing unwanted side effects of constant drowsiness, lethargy, and constipation. Once a patient is established on a chronic narcotic analgesic therapy, changes often need to be made to manage the patient's pain without overly sedating the patient. Furthermore, the patient may be switched to a different narcotic analgesic medication if he or she has developed a tolerance to the current medication regimen, cannot tolerate the adverse effects of the current medication, or desires a more convenient formulation or dosing schedule. In these cases, an equianalgesic dosing chart, such as in Table 10.1, is used to determine the appropriate dose of the new medication to ensure that the patient receives adequate pain relief with minimal adverse effects. An equianalgesic dosing chart is used to estimate the dose of the new narcotic analgesic to be used, and the patient should still be monitored for pain relief and presence of side effects. Most of the published charts are limited to adult patients weighing greater than 50 kg, and recommend a reduced dosage for elderly patients and patients with renal or hepatic insufficiency. In addition, clinicians may reduce the stated equivalent dose due to the potential for incomplete cross-tolerance between opioid analgesics. To use the equianalgesic dosing chart, the daily dose of the current medication is determined from the dose and dosage regimen, compared to the daily dose in the chart, and then converted to the dose and dosage regimen for new medication.

Whereas Table 10.1 provides equianalgesic dosing for opioids acting as full agonists at the mu opioid receptor, a different chart is utilized for opioid analgesics with different pharmacological profiles (Table 10.2). These include buprenorphine (a partial agonist at mu opioid receptors), nalbuphine and butorphanol (opioid agonist–antagonists, which

Table 10.1 • OPIOID ANALGESICS: APPROXIMATE EQUIANALGESIC DOSES FOR ADULTS[a]

	Equianalgesic Dose	
Opioid	**Oral**	**Parenteral**
Codeine	200 mg	NA
Fentanyl	NA	0.1 mg
Hydrocodone	30–45 mg	NA
Hydromorphone	7.5 mg	1.5 mg
Levorphanol	4 mg (acute); 1 mg (chronic)	NA
Meperidine	300 mg	75 mg
Morphine	30 mg	10 mg
Oxycodone	20 mg	NA
Oxymorphone	10 mg	1 mg

[a]Adapted with permission from Drug Facts & Comparisons. *Facts & Comparisons eAnswers [database online]*. St. Louis, MO: Clinical Drug Information LLC; 2015.

block mu receptors and stimulate kappa opioid receptors), and pentazocine (an agonist at kappa receptors and weakly blocking at mu receptors). The dosing chart for these opioids determines a dose equivalent to 10 mg of parenteral morphine. The clinician may then use this morphine dose to convert to another opioid analgesic by consulting the equianalgesic dosing chart in Table 10.1.

Drug-specific conversion charts are available for certain opioid analgesics. For example, Table 10.3 provides equivalent dosing for conversion from an existing narcotic analgesic to the highly potent fentanyl transdermal system. Table 10.4 lists ratios to guide conversion from hydrocodone, oxycodone, methadone, or morphine to oxymorphone extended-release tablets. If a patient is changing to or from one of these narcotic analgesic medications, it is important for the clinician to consult these drug-specific charts to guide accurate and appropriate dosing.

Table 10.2 • OPIOID AGONIST–ANTAGONIST ANALGESICS: APPROXIMATE EQUIANALGESIC DOSES FOR ADULTS[a]

Agonist–Antagonist		**Dose Equivalent to 10 mg Parenteral Morphine**
Buprenorphine	IM IV Sublingual Transdermal	0.3 mg
Butorphanol	IM IV Nasal	2 mg
Nalbuphine	SC/IM IV	10 mg
Pentazocine	SC/IM IV	30 mg

[a]Adapted with permission from Drug Facts & Comparisons. *Facts & Comparisons eAnswers [database online]*. St. Louis, MO: Clinical Drug Information LLC; 2015.

Table 10.3 • FENTANYL TRANSDERMAL DOSAGE CONVERSION GUIDELINES[a,b]

Current Analgesic	Daily Dosage (mg/day)			
Oral morphine	60–134	135–224	225–314	315–404
IM/IV morphine	10–22	23–37	38–52	53–67
Oral oxycodone	30–67	67.5–112	112.5–157	157.5–202
Oral codeine	150–447			
Oral hydromorphone	8–17	17.1–28	28.1–39	39.1–51
IV hydromorphone	1.5–3.4	3.5–5.6	5.7–7.9	8–10
IM meperidine	75–165	166–278	279–390	391–503
Oral methadone	20–44	45–74	75–104	105–134
Recommended fentanyl transdermal system dose				
Fentanyl transdermal system	25 mcg/h	50 mcg/h	75 mcg/h	100 mcg/h

[a]Adapted with permission from Drug Facts & Comparisons. *Facts & Comparisons eAnswers [database online].* St. Louis, MO: Clinical Drug Information LLC; 2015.

[b]This table should not be used to convert fentanyl transdermal to other therapies because the conversion to fentanyl transdermal is conservative. Use of this table for conversion to other analgesic therapies can overestimate the dose of the new agent. Overdosage of the new analgesic agent is possible.

Example Calculations Using Equianalgesic Dosing Charts

(1) *A patient is taking LORTAB 7.5-mg tablets containing 7.5 mg of hydrocodone bitartrate and 325 mg of acetaminophen to manage his chronic back pain. His current dosage is two tablets every 6 hours, but his pain management doctor would like to switch him to hydromorphone hydrochloride tablets to better alleviate his pain. Hydromorphone hydrochloride tablets are available in strengths of 2, 4, and 8 mg and should be administered every 4 to 6 hours. Determine the dose of hydromorphone hydrochloride for this patient.*

$$\frac{7.5 \text{ mg hydrocodone}}{\text{tablet}} \times \frac{2 \text{ tablets}}{\text{dose}} \times \frac{4 \text{ doses}}{\text{day}} = 60 \text{ mg hydrocodone/day}$$

According to the chart in Table 10.1, 30 mg of hydrocodone is equivalent to 7.5 mg of hydromorphone taken orally.

$$\frac{60 \text{ mg hydrocodone}}{\text{day}} \times \frac{7.5 \text{ mg hydromorphone}}{30 \text{ mg hydrocodone}} = 15 \text{ mg hydromorphone/day}$$

Table 10.4 • CONVERSION FACTORS TO OXYMORPHONE ER TABLETS[a]

Prior Oral Opioid	Approximate Oral Conversion Factor
Oxymorphone	1
Hydrocodone	0.5
Oxycodone	0.5
Methadone	0.5
Morphine	0.333

[a]Adapted with permission from Drug Facts & Comparisons. *Facts & Comparisons eAnswers [database online].* St. Louis, MO: Clinical Drug Information LLC; 2015.

Since the patient is accustomed to taking the current medication every 6 hours, this dosage regimen would probably be most effective for him.

$$\frac{15 \text{ mg hydromorphone}}{\text{day}} \times \frac{1 \text{ day}}{4 \text{ doses}} = \mathbf{3.75\ mg/dose}$$

The patient should begin with hydromorphone hydrochloride 4-mg tablets every 6 hours and monitored for relief of pain symptoms as well as for adverse effects.

(2) *CR is a 57-year-old male patient who is 6 feet 1 inch tall and weighs 212 lb. He is receiving a 20-mg intravenous injection of pentazocine lactate every 4 hours to control his pain after an injury due to a motorcycle accident. His physician wishes to switch him to an oral dose of meperidine hydrochloride so that he can move into a rehabilitation facility. What would be the equivalent dose of meperidine hydrochloride for this patient?*

According to Table 10.2, a 30-mg injection of pentazocine is equivalent to a 10-mg injection of morphine; therefore, the amount of morphine represented by a 20-mg injection of pentazocine can be calculated as:

$$\frac{10 \text{ mg morphine}}{30 \text{ mg pentazocine}} \times 20 \text{ mg pentazocine} = 6.67 \text{ mg morphine}$$

According to Table 10.1, a 10-mg injection of morphine is equivalent to 300 mg of meperidine given orally. The oral dose of meperidine for this patient can be calculated as:

$$\frac{300 \text{ mg meperidine}}{10 \text{ mg morphine}} \times 6.67 \text{ mg morphine} = \mathbf{200\ mg\ meperidine}$$

The patient can take two 100-mg meperidine hydrochloride tablets every 4 hours to manage his pain.

(3) *A cancer patient is taking one 20-mg oxycodone tablet q.i.d. to manage her pain. (a) What is the total daily oxycodone dose for this patient? (b) The patient's pain management physician decides to switch her to fentanyl transdermal patches. What strength of fentanyl patch should he prescribe?*[5]

(a) $\frac{20 \text{ mg}}{\text{tablet}} \times \frac{4 \text{ tablets}}{\text{day}} = \mathbf{80\ mg/day}$

(b) According to Table 10.3, a patient receiving an oral oxycodone dose of 67.5 to 112 mg/day of oral oxycodone should begin with a 50 mcg/h fentanyl patch.

(4) *A patient with a spinal injury is taking one 15-mg tablet of immediate-release morphine sulfate every 4 hours for pain. His physician wants to switch him to oxymorphone hydrochloride extended-release tablets to better manage his pain, and reserve the immediate-release morphine tablets for breakthrough pain. The oxymorphone hydrochloride extended-release (ER) tablets should be given every 12 hours. Calculate the appropriate dose for this patient.*

First, the daily dose of morphine sulfate must be calculated:

$$\frac{15 \text{ mg}}{\text{dose}} \times \frac{6 \text{ doses}}{\text{day}} = 90 \text{ mg/day}$$

According to Table 10.4, a conversion factor of 0.333 should be used to convert an oral dose of morphine to oxymorphone ER tablets.

$$\frac{90 \text{ mg morphine}}{\text{day}} \times 0.333 = 29.97 \text{ mg} \approx 30 \text{ mg oxymorphone ER/day}$$

Since the oxymorphone ER tablets are to be given every 12 hours, the single dose can be calculated as:

$$\frac{30 \text{ mg oxymorphone ER}}{\text{day}} \times \frac{1 \text{ day}}{2 \text{ doses}} = \mathbf{15\ mg\ oxymorphone\ ER/day}$$

Therefore, one 15-mg oxymorphone ER tablet should be given to this patient every 12 hours.

CASE IN POINT 10.2[6] The usual recommended dose of butorphanol tartrate nasal spray is one spray containing 1 mg of drug, and the nasal spray solution contains the drug at a concentration of 10 mg/mL. Calculate (a) the volume of solution delivered with each dose; (b) the number of doses contained in the 2.5-mL manufacturer's container; and (c) the number of tablets, containing 5 mg of hydrocodone bitartrate and 300 mg of acetaminophen, needed to produce the 1-mg dose of butorphanol tartrate.

Dosage Calculations Based on Creatinine Clearance

The two major mechanisms by which drugs are eliminated from the body are through hepatic (liver) metabolism and renal (kidney) excretion. When renal excretion is the major route, a loss of kidney function will dramatically affect the rate at which the drug is cleared from the body.

With many drugs, it is important to reach and maintain a specific drug concentration in the blood to realize the proper therapeutic effect. The initial blood concentration attained from a specific dose depends, in part, on the weight of the patient and the volume of body fluids in which the drug is distributed.

The kidneys receive about 20% of the cardiac output (blood flow) and filter approximately 125 mL of plasma per minute. As kidney function is lost, the quantity of plasma filtered per minute decreases, with an accompanying decrease in drug clearance. The filtration rate of the kidney can be estimated by a number of methods. One of the most useful, however, is the estimation of the creatinine clearance rate (CrCl) through the use of the following empiric formulas based on the patient's age, weight, and serum creatinine (S_{cr}) value. Creatinine, which is a breakdown product from creatine produced in muscle metabolism, is generally produced at a constant rate and in quantities that depend on the muscle mass of the patient. Females usually have a lower serum creatinine than males due to less muscle mass. Because creatinine is eliminated from the body essentially through renal filtration, reduced kidney performance results in a reduced CrCl. The normal adult value of serum creatinine is 0.6 to 1.3 mg/dL (the range varies with the laboratory used as the reference source). The CrCl represents the volume of blood plasma that is cleared of creatinine by kidney filtration and usually expressed in milliliters per minute.

In addition to the Jelliffe and Cockcroft-Gault equations, other equations are used to estimate creatinine clearance for special patient populations such as pediatric patients and elderly patients.[10]

By the Jelliffe equation[7,8]:
For males:

$$\text{CrCl} = \frac{98 - 0.8 \times (\text{Patient's age in years} - 20)}{\text{Serum creatinine in mg/dL}}$$

For females:

$$\text{CrCl} = 0.9 \times \text{CrCl determined using formula for males}$$

By the Cockcroft-Gault equation[9]:
For males:

$$\text{CrCl} = \frac{(140 - \text{Patient's age in years}) \times \text{Body weight in kg}}{72 \times \text{Serum creatinine in mg/dL}}$$

For females:

$$\text{CrCl} = 0.85 \times \text{CrCl determined using formula for males}$$

Example Calculations of Creatinine Clearance

(1) *Determine the creatinine clearance rate for an 80-year-old male patient weighing 70 kg and having a serum creatinine of 2 mg/dL. Use both the Jelliffe and Cockcroft-Gault equations.*

By the Jelliffe equation:

$$\text{CrCl} = \frac{98 - 0.8 \times (80 - 20)}{2\ (\text{mg/dL})}$$

$$= \frac{98 - (0.8 \times 60)}{2\ (\text{mg/dL})} = \frac{98 - 48}{2\ (\text{mg/dL})} = \frac{50}{2\ (\text{mg/dL})}$$

$$= \mathbf{25\ mL/min}$$

By the Cockcroft-Gault equation:

$$\text{CrCl} = \frac{(140 - 80) \times 70}{72 \times 2\ (\text{mg/dL})}$$

$$= \frac{60 \times 70}{144}$$

$$= \frac{4200}{144}$$

$$= \mathbf{29.2\ mL/min}$$

(2) *A 70-year-old gentleman and his 68-year-old wife have their annual physical exams. He weighs 160 lb and she 126 lb. His blood work reveals a serum creatinine of 1.3 mg/dL and hers is 1.1 mg/dL. Using the Cockcroft-Gault equation, calculate their respective creatinine clearance rates.*

$$\text{His CrCl} = \frac{(140 - 70) \times 72.7}{72 \times 1.3} = \mathbf{54.4\ mL/min}$$

$$\text{Her CrCl} = 0.85 \times \frac{(140 - 68) \times 57.3}{72 \times 1.1} = \mathbf{44.3\ mL/min}$$

ADJUSTING CREATININE CLEARANCE FOR BODY SURFACE AREA

It is sometimes desirable to adjust the calculated creatinine clearance for body surface area to account for this possible variable in determining drug dosage. This adjustment is accomplished through the use of a nomogram or equation to determine body surface area (BSA), as described previously in Chapter 8, and the following formula:

$$\frac{\text{BSA}}{1.73} \times \text{CrCl} = \text{Adjusted CrCl}$$

If a patient weighing 120 lb and measuring 60 inches in height has a calculated creatinine clearance of 40 mL/min, adjust the CrCl based on body surface area.

Using the nomogram in Chapter 8, the patient's BSA is determined to be 1.50 m^2.

$$\frac{1.50\ \text{m}^2}{1.73\ \text{m}^2} \times 40\ \text{mL/min} = \mathbf{34.68\ mL/min,\ adjusted\ CrCl}$$

Normal CrCl may be considered 100 mL/min. Thus, in the preceding example, the patient would exhibit about 35% of normal creatinine clearance.

USE OF CREATININE CLEARANCE IN DETERMINING DOSES

The CrCl method for determining drug dose is used with various drugs in which renal function is a factor. Meperidine, for example, is dosed based on creatinine clearance as follows:

CrCl = 10 – 50 mL/min, give 75% of usual dose
CrCl < 10 mL/min, give 50% of usual dose

The patient in example problem 2 on page 174 has a serum creatinine of 2.4 mg/dL. Using the Cockcroft-Gault equation, determine if the meperidine dose should be adjusted for kidney function.

$$212\ \text{lb} \times \frac{1\ \text{kg}}{2.2\ \text{lb}} = 96.36\ \text{kg}$$

$$\text{CrCl} = \frac{(140 - 57) \times 96.36}{72 \times 2.4} = 46.29\ \text{mL/min}$$

According to the dosing information, 75% of the dose should be given. Since the dose calculated in example problem 2 on page 174 is 200 mg, the patient should receive 200 mg × 75% = **150 mg based on his renal function.**

For certain drugs, tables of dosage guidelines may be presented in the labeling/literature to adjust for impaired renal function. For example, the usual dose of the anti-infective drug ceftazidime is 1 g every 8 to 12 hours, with dosage adjusted based on the location and severity of the infection and the patient's renal function. For adult patients with impaired renal function, guidelines for dosage based on creatinine clearance are given in Table 10.5.

Using Table 10.5, *determine the dose and daily dose schedule for a 62-year-old female patient weighing 70 kg with a serum creatinine of 1.8 mg/dL.*

$$\text{CrCl} = 0.85 \times \frac{(140 - 62) \times 70}{72 \times 1.8} = 35.81\ \text{mL/min}$$

According to the table, a patient with a creatinine clearance of 31 to 50 mL/min should receive **a dose of 1 g every 12 hours.**

Table 10.5 • CREATININE CLEARANCE DOSING GUIDELINES FOR CEFTAZIDIME (IV OR IM)[a]

Renal Function	Creatinine Clearance (mL/min)	Dose	Frequency
Normal to mild impairment	100–51	1 g	q8–12 h
Moderate impairment	50–31	1 g	q12h
Severe impairment	30–16	1 g	q24h
Very severe impairment	15–6	500 mg	q24h
Essentially none	<5	500 mg	q48h

[a]Adapted from product literature for FORTAZ (ceftazidime). Available at http://www.accessdata.fda.gov/drugsatfda_docs/label/2014/050578s055,050634s023lbledt.pdf. Accessed February 23, 2015.

CALCULATIONS CAPSULE

Creatinine Clearance Equations[7–9]

Jelliffe equation

For males:

$$CrCl = \frac{98 - 0.8 \times (\text{Patient's age in years} - 20)}{\text{Serum creatinine in mg/dL}}$$

For females:

$$CrCl = 0.9 \times CrCl \text{ determined by equation for males}$$

Cockcroft-Gault equation

For males:

$$CrCl = \frac{(140 - \text{Patient's age in years}) \times \text{pt. wt., kg}}{72 \times \text{Serum creatinine in mg/dL}}$$

For females:

$$CrCl = 0.85 \times CrCl \text{ determined using for males}$$

Adjusting CrCl for body surface area

$$\frac{BSA}{1.73} \times CrCl = \text{Adjusted CrCl}$$

Dosage Calculations Based on Ideal Body Weight and Adjusted Body Weight

The ideal body weight (IBW) provides an excellent estimation of the distribution volume, particularly for some polar drugs that are not well distributed in adipose (fat) tissue. The IBW may be calculated through the use of the following formulas based on the patient's height and gender.

For males:

IBW = 50 kg + 2.3 kg for each inch of patient height over 5 feet

or in pounds

110 lb + 5 lb for each inch over 5 feet

For females:

IBW = 45.5 kg + 2.3 kg for each inch of patient height over 5 feet

or in pounds

100 lb + 5 lb for each inch over 5 feet

Adjusted body weight may be used in calculating dosages for obese patients using the following equation:[11]

$$\text{Adjusted body weight} = [(\text{ABW} - \text{IBW}) \times 0.25] + \text{IBW},$$

where ABW is the patient's actual body weight.

Clinical controversy exists over the use of actual body weight, IBW, or an adjusted body weight to determine dosages, and specific references should be consulted to determine the most appropriate dose for a patient.[12–14]

Example Calculations of Ideal Body Weight and Adjusted Body Weight

(1) *Calculate the ideal body weight in pounds and kilograms for a male patient weighing 164 lb and measuring 5 feet 8 inches in height.*

$$\text{IBW} = 110 \text{ lb} + (8 \times 5 \text{ lb}) = 110 \text{ lb} + 40 \text{ lb} = \mathbf{150\ lb}$$

$$\text{IBW} = 50 \text{ kg} + (8 \times 2.3 \text{ kg}) = 50 \text{ kg} + 18.4 \text{ kg} = \mathbf{68.4\ kg}$$

(2) *Calculate the ideal body weight, in kilograms, for a female patient weighing 60 kg and measuring 160 cm in height.*

$$160 \text{ cm} \times \frac{1 \text{ inch}}{2.54 \text{ cm}} = 62.99 \text{ inches} \approx 5 \text{ feet } 3 \text{ inches}$$

$$\text{IBW} = 45.5 \text{ kg} + (3 \times 2.3 \text{ kg}) = 45.5 \text{ kg} + 6.9 \text{ kg} = \mathbf{52.4\ kg}$$

(3) *Calculate the ideal body weight and adjusted body weight, in kilograms, for a male patient who is 6 feet 1 inch tall and weighs 255 lb.*

$$\text{IBW} = 50 \text{ kg} + (13 \times 2.3 \text{ kg}) = 50 \text{ kg} + 29.9 \text{ kg} = \mathbf{79.9\ kg}$$

$$\text{ABW} = 255 \text{ lb} \times \frac{1 \text{ kg}}{2.2 \text{ lb}} = 115.91 \text{ kg}$$

$$\text{Adjusted body weight} = [(115.91 \text{ kg} - 79.9 \text{ kg}) \times 0.25] + 79.9 \text{ kg} = 9 \text{ kg} + 79.9 \text{ kg} = \mathbf{88.9\ kg}$$

Drug-Specific Clinical Equations

For certain clinical conditions, there are equations that are useful for determining patient requirements. For example, the following is used in determining the amount of iron required to bring hemoglobin (Hb) values to normal levels:

$$\text{Iron required (mg)} = \text{Body weight (lb)} \times 0.3 \times \left[100 - \frac{\text{Hb (g/dL)} \times 100}{14.8 \text{ g/dL}}\right]$$

In the equation, 14.8 g/dL is the normal value of hemoglobin in adults and the factor 0.3 is its iron content (percent).[15]

Using the equation for determining iron deficiency, calculate the number of milliliters of an iron dextran solution containing 50 mg/mL of iron to be administered to a 150-lb patient with a hemoglobin value of 10 g/dL.

$$\text{Iron required (mg)} = 150 \times 0.3 \times \left[100 - \frac{10 \times 100}{14.8}\right]$$

$$= 150 \times 0.3 \times 32.4$$

$$= 1458 \text{ mg}$$

$$\text{by proportion, } \frac{50 \text{ mg}}{1458 \text{ mg}} = \frac{1 \text{ mL}}{x \text{ mL}}$$

x = **29 mL iron dextran solution**

Therapeutic Drug Monitoring

Also termed ***drug therapy monitoring***, this process often includes the analysis of blood serum samples to ensure optimum drug therapy. This is especially important for categories of drugs in which the margin between safe and toxic levels is narrow. Data are available indicating these levels.[16] The drugs presented in this chapter are but a few of those requiring specific types of dosing. Many other drugs, including aminoglycoside antibiotics (gentamicin, tobramycin, amikacin), theophylline, digoxin, and warfarin, require dosing based on plasma levels of the drug, specific laboratory values, creatinine clearance, and IBW. Clinical reference sources should be consulted when dosing drugs with specific and complex dosing parameters.

CASE IN POINT 10.3[a] A 35-year-old male patient weighing 180 lb and standing 5 feet 8 inches tall has been diagnosed with AIDS. His physician prescribes lamivudine (EPIVIR) as a component of his treatment program and knows that the dose of the drug must be adjusted based on the patient's renal function. Laboratory tests indicate that the patient's serum creatinine is 2.6 mg/dL and has held at the same level for 5 days.

(a) Calculate the patient's IBW and use in subsequent calculations if the IBW is lower than the patient's actual weight.
(b) Calculate the patient's CrCl by the Cockcroft-Gault equation.
(c) Select the appropriate dose of lamivudine from the dosing schedule:

Creatinine Clearance	Initial Dose	Maintenance Dose
<5 mL/min	50 mg	25 mg once daily
5–14 mL/min	150 mg	50 mg once daily
15–29 mL/min	150 mg	100 mg once daily
30–49 mL/min	150 mg	150 mg once daily

[a]Case in Point courtesy of Flynn Warren, Bishop, GA.

Clinical Laboratory Tests

It is common practice in assessing health status to analyze biologic fluids, especially blood and urine, for specific chemical content. The clinical laboratory tests used, known as *chemistries*, analyze samples for such chemicals as glucose, cholesterol, total lipids, creatinine, blood urea nitrogen (BUN), bilirubin, potassium, sodium, calcium, carbon dioxide, and other substances, including drugs following their administration. Blood chemistries are performed on plasma (the fluid part of the blood) or serum (the watery portion of clotted blood). Depending on the laboratory equipment used as well as patient factors (such as age and gender), the "usual" amount of each chemical substance varies, with no single "normal" value, but rather a common range. For example, the reference range of glucose in serum is, by some laboratories, 65 to 115 mg/dL and that for creatinine is 0.5 to 1.7 mg/dL.

Table 10.6 presents examples of the normal ranges of serum chemistry values for some commonly analyzed blood components. The "conversion factors" shown are used to convert the units most often used in the United States to those of the international system. For example, a cholesterol reading of 180 (mg/dL) may be recorded as 4.65 millimoles per liter (mmol/L or mM).

Low-density lipoprotein cholesterol (LDL-C), high-density lipoprotein (HDL-C), and total cholesterol (TC) are each measured in assessing a patient's risk for atherosclerosis.[17] The greatest risk comes from the non–high-density lipoprotein cholesterol (non–HDL-C), particularly in patients with high serum levels of triglycerides (TG or TGR). In addition, certain accompanying patient factors are considered added risk factors and affect the LDL-C goal for a particular patient. These include personal and/or familial history of coronary heart disease, atherosclerotic disease, diabetes, hypertension, and cigarette smoking. Table 10.7 presents categories of cholesterol and triglyceride blood levels. Furthermore, total cholesterol is calculated by adding triglyceride level divided by five, HDL, and LDL levels (i.e., $TC = TG/5 + HDL + LDL$).

There are two "cholesterol ratios" that are considered clinically relevant to risk assessment for cardiovascular disease. One is the ratio of total cholesterol to HDL cholesterol, the target being 5:1 or less. The other ratio used in assessing risk is LDL:HDL with the target being 3:1 or less.[18] Greater proportions of HDL are considered to lower risk of cardiovascular disease. In addition, the percent reduction required to achieve a goal level of LDL cholesterol may be calculated as the difference in values as a percent of the current level. The difference in values is calculated by subtracting the patient's desired LDL from the current measured LDL level, then dividing it by the current LDL level.

Table 10.6 • EXAMPLES OF NORMAL RANGES OF SERUM CHEMISTRY VALUES[a]

Laboratory Test	Normal Values (Range, in US Units)	Conversion Factor (Multiply)	International System[b]
Albumin	3.6–5 g/dL	10	36–50 g/L
Calcium	8.6–10.3 mg/dL	0.25	2.2–2.6 mmol/L
Cholesterol, total	<200 mg/dL	0.026	<5.2 mmol/L
HDL cholesterol	≥60 mg/dL	0.026	≥1.56 mmol/L
LDL cholesterol	<130 mg/dL	0.026	<3.38 mmol/L
Glucose	65–115 mg/dL	0.055	3.58–6.39 mmol/L
Triglycerides	<150 mg/dL	0.011	<1.65 mmol/L
Creatinine	0.5–1.7 mg/dL	88.4	44.2–150.28 μmol/L
Urea nitrogen (BUN)	8–25 mg/dL	0.357	2.86–8.93 mmol/L

[a] *Normal* values shown may vary between test laboratories and may be referred to as "reference," "healthy," or "goal" values.
[b] The international system is generally expressed in mmol (or other units) per liter.

Table 10.7 • CATEGORIES OF CHOLESTEROL AND TRIGLYCERIDE BLOOD LEVELS[a]

Blood Level (Fasting)	Clinical Category
Total cholesterol (TC) levels:	
<200 mg/dL	Desirable
200–239 mg/dL	Borderline high
240 mg/dL and above	High
Low-density cholesterol (LDL):	
<100 mg/dL	Optimal
100–129 mg/dL	Near optimal
130–159 mg/dL	Borderline high
160–189 mg/dL	High
190 mg/dL and above	Very high
High-density cholesterol (HDL):	
<40 mg/dL	Low level/increased risk
40–50 mg/dL (men); 50–59 mg/dL (women)	Average level/average risk
60 mg/dL and above	High level/less than average risk
Triglycerides (TRG):	
<150 mg/dL	Desirable
150–199 mg/dL	Borderline high
200–499 mg/dL	High
500 mg/dL and above	Very high

[a]National Heart, Lung, and Blood Institute; National Institutes of Health; Public Health Service; U.S. Department of Health and Human Services. NIH Publication No. 05–3290. Available at http://www.nhlbi.nih.gov/health/public/heart/chol/wyntk.htm. Accessed March 2, 2011.

Example Calculations Involving Clinical Laboratory Tests

(1) *If a patient is determined to have a serum cholesterol level of 200 mg/dL, what is the equivalent value expressed in terms of millimoles (mmol) per liter?*

Molecular Weight (m.w. of cholesterol) = 387

1 mmol cholesterol = 387 mg

200 mg/dL = 2000 mg/L

$$\frac{387\ (\text{mg})}{2000\ (\text{mg})} = \frac{1\ (\text{millimole})}{x\ (\text{millimoles})}$$

$$x = \mathbf{5.17\ mmol/L}$$

(2) *Calculate the TC:HDL ratio when the total cholesterol is 240 mg/dL and the HDL cholesterol is 60 mg/dL, and identify if the ratio is within the desirable range.*

240 mg/dL:60 mg/dL = **4:1**

The ratio is less than the maximum desired level of 5:1.

(3) *If 160 mg/dL is a patient's current LDL level and the desired level is 100 mg/dL, calculate the percent reduction required.*

Difference in values: 160 mg/dL – 100 mg/dL = 60 mg/dL

Difference as a percent of current level: $\frac{60\ \text{mg/dL}}{160\ \text{mg/dL}} \times 100\% = \mathbf{37.5\%}$

PRACTICE PROBLEMS

Heparin-Dosing Calculations

1. A hospital pharmacy order calls for 5000 units of heparin to be administered to a patient, twice daily, subcutaneously, for the prevention of thrombi. The pharmacist has on hand a vial containing 10,000 Heparin Units/mL. How many milliliters of the injection should be administered for each dose?
2. A physician orders 1500 units of heparin to be administered by intravenous infusion per hour. The pharmacy provides a heparin intravenous bag containing 25,000 units of heparin in 250 mL of D5W. How many milliliters should be administered per minute?
3.[19] A male patient weighing 76 kg is placed on heparin therapy for the prevention of deep vein thrombosis after surgery.
   (a) How many milliliters of a heparin injection containing 5000 units/mL should be administered for a loading dose of 80 units/kg?
   (b) What should be the infusion rate, in mL/h, using a solution that contains heparin 25,000 units/500 mL, to administer 18 units/kg/h?
   (c) Six hours after heparin therapy is initiated, the patient's aPTT is found to be 75 seconds. Adjust the infusion rate, in mL/h, according to the heparin protocol (Fig. 10.1).
4.[19] A blood sample taken from a 113-lb patient 6 hours after heparin therapy is initiated shows an aPTT of 24 seconds. Calculate (a) the bolus dose and (b) the infusion rate, in mL/h, according to the heparin protocol (Fig. 10.1).
5. Enoxaparin sodium (LOVENOX) injection, a low-molecular-weight heparin, contains 150 mg/mL in 0.8-mL prefilled syringes. The recommended dose for knee replacement surgery is 30 mg every 12 hours. How many milliliters of the injection should be administered per dose?

Equianalgesic Dosing Calculations

6. A patient has been taking acetaminophen 300 mg with codeine 30 mg (TYLENOL with CODEINE #3) tablets and wishes to switch to acetaminophen/hydrocodone tablets due to nausea and constipation caused by the codeine. The patient has been taking one tablet every 4 to 6 hours. What would be the most appropriate dose and dosage regimen for the acetaminophen/hydrocodone tablets?
   (a) One 2.5-mg hydrocodone/325-mg acetaminophen tablet every 4 to 6 hours
   (b) One 5-mg hydrocodone/300-mg acetaminophen tablet every 4 to 6 hours
   (c) One 7.5-mg hydrocodone/300-mg acetaminophen tablet every 6 hours
   (d) One 10-mg hydrocodone/325-mg acetaminophen tablet every 6 hours
7. TC is a 52-year-old female patient who is receiving 0.5 mL of a 50 mcg/mL injection of fentanyl citrate (SUBLIMAZE) every 2 hours following surgery to manage her pain. Her physician wants to change to oral oxycodone hydrochloride given every 4 hours so she can be discharged from the hospital. What strength of oxycodone hydrochloride tablets should be used for this patient?
   (a) 20-mg tablets
   (b) 15-mg tablets
   (c) 10-mg tablets
   (d) 5-mg tablets

8. IH is a 42-year-old male patient suffering from chronic back pain due to a workplace injury. He is currently taking one-half of a 2-mg levorphanol tartrate tablet every 6 hours to manage his pain but consults his doctor about switching to BUTRANS weekly buprenorphine transdermal patches for convenience. BUTRANS transdermal delivery systems are available in strengths of 5, 7.5, 10, 15, and 20 mcg/h. What strength of patch should be used for this patient?
9. NT is taking two PERCOCET tablets each containing 7.5 mg of oxycodone and 325 mg of acetaminophen every 4 hours to manage his pain. His physician wants to switch him to oxymorphone extended-release tablets (OPANA ER) for improved pain control. Oxymorphone extended-release tablets are available in strengths of 5, 7.5, 10, 15, 20, 30, and 40 mg to be given every 12 hours. What should be the dose and dosage regimen for this patient?
10. A patient is receiving morphine sulfate intravenously via a patient controlled analgesia (PCA) pump. The concentration of the solution is 15 mg/mL and is being infused at a rate of 0.1 mL/h. The patient may access a 2-mg bolus dose every hour for breakthrough pain and is currently using an average of 8 doses per day. The patient's caregiver requests that the patient be converted to a fentanyl transdermal patch (DURAGESIC) for a "more safe dosage form". What strength of fentanyl patch would be most effective for this patient?

Creatinine Clearance Calculations

11. Use both the Jelliffe equation and the Cockcroft-Gault equation to calculate the creatinine clearance rate for a 24-year-old male patient weighing 70 kg with a serum creatinine of 1 mg/dL.
12. If the patient in problem 11 is 5 feet 8 inches tall, adjust the creatinine clearance calculated by the Cockcroft-Gault equation based on body surface area.
13. The usual adult dose of levofloxacin is a 500-mg initial dose followed by subsequent doses of 250 mg every 24 hours for 10 days. For patients with a CrCl of less than 19 mL/min, doses following the initial dose are administered every 48 hours. How many 250-mg levofloxacin tablets should be dispensed to a 75-year-old, 160-lb female patient with a serum creatinine of 1.32 mg/dL? (Use the Cockcroft-Gault equation to determine creatinine clearance.)
14. Using Table 10.5, what would be the dose and dosage schedule of ceftazidime for an 84-year-old male patient weighing 60 kg, measuring 66 inches in height, and having a serum creatinine level of 4.22 mg/dL? (Use the Cockcroft-Gault equation to determine creatinine clearance.)

Ideal Body Weight and Adjusted Body Weight Calculations

15. Calculate the ideal body weight in pounds and kilograms for an 87-year-old female patient who is 5 feet 1 inch tall and weighs 111 lb.
16. Calculate the adjusted body weight in kilograms for a 50-year-old male patient who is 5 feet 11 inches tall and weighs 288 lb.
17. The initial dose for atracurium besylate is 0.4 mg/kg and should be dosed based on IBW for obese patients.[12] How much of a 10-mg/mL injection should be administered to a 42-year-old male patient who is 6 feet 2 inches tall and weighs 262 lb?
18. DT is a 61-year-old female patient with primary humoral immunodeficiency. She is 5 feet 6 inches tall and weighs 303 lb. The dosing range for human immune globulin (BIVIGAM) is 300 to 800 mg/kg given intravenously every 3 to 4 weeks, and the patient's adjusted body weight should be used for dosing this drug since she is obese.[12] What would be the dose range for this patient?

Clinical Laboratory Test Calculations

19. If a serum sample is determined to contain 270 mg/dL of cholesterol, what is the concentration of cholesterol (m.w. 386) in terms of millimoles per liter?
20. The normal blood level of theophylline is 0.055 to 0.11 mmol/L. Determine the amount range, in micrograms, of theophylline that would be contained in a 5-mL blood sample to fall within this range. (m.w. theophylline = 180.17)
21. Among clinical recommendations to prevent cardiovascular disease in women is the maintenance of lipid levels as follows: low-density lipoproteins (LDL) <100 mg/dL; high-density lipoproteins (HDL) >50 mg/dL; and triglycerides (TG) <150 mg/dL.[20] Which of the following meet these criteria?
    (a) LDL <2.6 mmol/L
    (b) HDL >1.3 mmol/L
    (c) TG <1.65 mmol/L
    (d) All of the above
22. If a patient is instructed by her physician to reduce her LDL cholesterol level from 130 mg/dL to 100 mg/dL, calculate the percent reduction required.
23. A patient has an HDL of 50 mg/dL, an LDL of 150 mg/dL, and a TG of 85 mg/dL. Calculate the (a) TC:HDL ratio and (b) LDL percent reduction required for a goal of 100 mg/dL.
24. On the basis of the information in Table 10.6, calculate the mmol/L of glucose equivalent to a value of 140 mg/dL.
    (a) 7.7 mmol/L
    (b) 2.5 mmol/L
    (c) 5.4 mmol/L
    (d) 6.2 mmol/L

CALCQUIZ

10.A. When a PTT was performed on the patient described in "Case in Point 10.1," the patient's value was 40 seconds. Based on the protocol in Figure 10.1, calculate (a) the needed bolus dose, in units, and (b) the new infusion rate, in mL/h, using heparin injection, 25,000 units/250 mL.

10.B. A patient has been receiving an intravenous infusion of fentanyl citrate (SUBLIMAZE) at a rate of 15 mcg/h for pain management during an extended 4-day hospital stay. His physician wishes to prescribe oxymorphone ER (OPANA ER) tablets to be administered every 12 hours to allow the patient to return home. Should 15-, 20-, 30-, or 40-mg oxymorphone ER tablets be prescribed for this patient to receive an equivalent dose for his pain?

10.C. Based on creatinine clearance, the dose of a drug is:
CrCl = 8–10 mL/min; dose = 2.43 mg/kg every 24 hours, divided into two doses
CrCl = 11–20 mL/min; dose = 3.58 mg/kg every 24 hours, divided into two doses
CrCl = 21–40 mL/min; dose = 5.87 mg/kg every 24 hours as a single dose.

For a 52-year-old male patient weighing 155 lb and measuring 69 inches with a serum creatinine of 2.6 mg/dL, calculate the per-dose volume to administer of an injection containing drug, 80 mg/mL.

10.D. A hospital order for midazolam for maintenance of sedation at a rate of 0.05 mg/kg/h is received for a patient. The patient is a 33-year-old female patient who is 5 feet 4 inches tall and weighs 164 lb. Because she is obese, the patient should receive a dose based on her ideal body weight.[12] Calculate the infusion rate for an IV solution with a midazolam concentration of 0.5 mg/mL.

10.E. Calculate the total cholesterol in a patient with a HDL of 87 mg/dL, LDL of 152 mg/dL, and a TRG of 50 mg/dL. Also, which of the following are correct?
(a) HDL:LDL ratio ≈ 1:1.7
(b) TC:HDL ratio ≈ 2.9:1
(c) HDL = high risk
(d) LDL = low risk
(e) TRG = low risk
(f) After being placed on a statin drug, the patient's LDL dropped to 106 mg/dL, equivalent to a 30% reduction.

ANSWERS TO "CASE IN POINT" AND PRACTICE PROBLEMS

Case in Point 10.1

(a) Patient's weight in kg:

$$198\ \text{lb} \times \frac{1\ \text{kg}}{2.2\ \text{lb}} = 90\ \text{kg}$$

Bolus dose: 80 units heparin/kg

$$\frac{80\ \text{units}}{\text{kg}} \times 90\ \text{kg} = 7200\ \text{units}$$

$$7200\ \text{units} \times \frac{1\ \text{mL}}{5000\ \text{units}} = 1.44\ \text{mL}$$

(b) Infusion rate: 18 units/kg/h

$$18\ \text{units/kg/h} \times 90\ \text{kg} = 1620\ \text{units/h}$$

$$\frac{250\ \text{mL}}{25{,}000\ \text{units}} \times \frac{1620\ \text{units}}{1\ \text{h}} = 16.2\ \text{mL/h}$$

(c) $\frac{16.2\ \text{mL}}{1\ \text{h}} \times \frac{60\ \text{drops}}{1\ \text{mL}} \times \frac{1\ \text{h}}{60\ \text{min}} = 16.2\ \text{or}\ 16\ \text{drops/min}$

(d) $250\ \text{mL} \times \frac{1\ \text{h}}{16.2\ \text{mL}} = 15.43\ \text{h}$

Case in Point 10.2

(a) $\frac{1\ \text{mg}}{\text{dose}} \times \frac{1\ \text{mL}}{10\ \text{mg}} = 0.1\ \text{mL/dose}$

(b) $2.5\ \text{mL} \times \frac{1\ \text{dose}}{0.1\ \text{mL}} = 25\ \text{doses}$

(c) According to Table 10.2, a 2-mg intranasal dose of butorphanol tartrate is equivalent to 10 mg of parenteral morphine.

$$1 \text{ mg butorphanol} \times \frac{10 \text{ mg morphine}}{2 \text{ mg butorphanol}} = 5 \text{ mg morphine}$$

According to Table 10.1, a 10-mg parenteral dose of morphine is equivalent to 30 mg of hydrocodone given orally.

$$5 \text{ mg morphine} \times \frac{30 \text{ mg hydrocodone}}{10 \text{ mg morphine}} = 15 \text{ mg hydrocodone}$$

$$15 \text{ mg hydrocodone} \times \frac{1 \text{ tablet}}{5 \text{ mg hydrocodone}} = 3 \text{ tablets}$$

Case in Point 10.3

(a)

$$\text{IBW} = 50 \text{ kg} + (2.3 \times 8 \text{ inches}) = 68.4 \text{ kg}$$

$$\text{Patient's actual weight} = 180 \text{ lb} \times 1 \text{ kg}/2.2 \text{ lb} = 81.8 \text{ kg}$$

(b) $$\text{CrCl} = \frac{[(140 - 35) \times 68.4 \text{ kg}]}{72 \times 2.6 \text{ mg/dL}} = \frac{7182}{187.2} = 38.37 \text{ mL/min}$$

(c) Dose = 150 mg initially and 150 mg maintenance dose once daily

Practice Problems

1. 0.5 mL heparin injection
2. 0.25 mL/min
3. (a) 1.22 mL heparin injection
   (b) 27.36 mL/h
   (c) 24.32 mL/h
4. (a) 4109.09 units
   (b) 11.3 mL/h
5. 0.2 mL enoxaparin sodium injection
6. (b) One 5-mg hydrocodone/300-mg acetaminophen tablet every 4 to 6 hours
7. (c) 10-mg tablets
8. 10-mcg/h transdermal patch
9. 20-mg tablet every 12 hours
10. 75-mcg/h transdermal patch
11. 94.8 mL/min (Jelliffe)
    112.78 mL/min (Cockcroft-Gault)
12. 118.64 mL/min
13. 12 levofloxacin tablets
14. 500 mg ceftazidime every 24 hours
15. 105 lb
    47.8 kg
16. 89.2 kg
17. 3.29 mL atracurium besylate injection
18. 23.67 to 63.13 g human immune globulin
19. 6.99 mmol/L
20. 49.55 to 99.09 mcg
21. (d) All of the above
22. 23.08%
23. (a) 4.34:1 = TC:HDL ratio
    (b) 33.33%
24. (a) 7.78 mmol/L

References

1. Heparin dosing. Available at: http://www.rxkinetics.com/heparin.html. Accessed June 25, 2014.
2. Heparin Sodium Injection, USP. Available at: http://www.hospira.com/Images/EN-3340_32-92402_1.pdf. Accessed July 16, 2014.
3. Heparin Sodium. Drug Facts & Comparisons. *Facts & Comparisons [database online]*. St. Louis, MO: Wolters Kluwer Health, Inc.; 2014.
4. Bontempo FA, Hassett AC. Low molecular weight heparin. Available at: http://www.itxm.org/tmu/tmu1996/tmu6-96.htm. Accessed July 16, 2014.
5. Stockton SJ. Calculations. *International Journal of Pharmaceutical Compounding* 2014;18:320.
6. Stockton SJ. Calculations. *International Journal of Pharmaceutical Compounding* 2009;13:239.
7. Jelliffe RW. Estimations of creatinine clearance when urine cannot be collected. *Lancet* 1971;1:975.
8. Jelliffe RW. Creatinine clearance bedside estimate. *Annals of Internal Medicine* 1973;79:604.
9. Cockcroft DW, Gault MH. Prediction of creatinine clearance from serum creatinine. *Nephron* 1976;16:31.
10. Dowling TC. Evaluation of kidney function. In: DiPiro JT, Talbert RL, Yee GC, et al., eds. *Pharmacotherapy: A Pathophysiologic Approach, 9th Ed. [book online]*. New York, NY: McGraw-Hill; 2014.
11. Chessman KH, Kumpf VJ. Assessment of nutrition status and nutrition requirements. In: DiPiro JT, Talbert RL, Yee GC, et al., eds. *Pharmacotherapy: A Pathophysiologic Approach, 9th Ed. [book online]*. New York, NY: McGraw-Hill; 2014.
12. Drug Dosing in Obesity Reference Table. Available at: http://clincalc.com/kinetics/obesitydosing.aspx. Accessed February 22, 2015.
13. Ng JK, Schulz LT, Rose WE, et al. Daptomycin dosing based on ideal body weight versus actual body weight: comparison of clinical outcomes. *Antimicrobial Agents in Chemotherapy* 2014;58(1):88–93. Available at: http://www.ncbi.nlm.nih.gov/pubmed/24145531. Accessed February 22, 2015.
14. ASCO Guideline Recommends the Use of Actual Body Weight to Calculate Appropriate Dose of Chemotherapy Drugs for Obese Patients. Available at: http://www.asco.org/press-center/asco-guideline-recommends-use-actual-body-weight-calculate-appropriate-dose. Accessed February 22, 2015.
15. Alldredge BK, Corelli RL, Ernst ME, et al., eds. *Koda-Kimble & Young's Applied Therapeutics: The Clinical Use of Drugs*. 10th Ed. Baltimore, MD: Wolters Kluwer Health/Lippincott Williams & Wilkins; 2013:238.
16. Drug levels. Drug Facts & Comparisons. *Facts & Comparisons [Database Online]*. St. Louis, MO: Wolters Kluwer Health, Inc.; 2015.
17. National Cholesterol Education Program Report. *Circulation* 2004;110:227–239. Available at: http://www.circulationaha.org. Accessed March 1, 2011.
18. Herrier RN, Apgar DA, Boyce RW, et al. Dyslipidemia. In: Herrier RN, Apgar DA, Boyce RW, et al., eds. *Patient Assessment in Pharmacy* [book online]. New York, NY: McGraw-Hill; 2015.
19. Ansel HC, Prince SJ. Pharmaceutical calculations. In: *The Pharmacist's Handbook*. Baltimore, MD: Lippincott Williams & Wilkins; 2004:236–240.
20. Women's health: What's hot. *Pharmacy Today* 2007;13(9):28.

11

Isotonic and Buffer Solutions

OBJECTIVES

Upon successful completion of this chapter, the student will be able to:

- Calculate the dissociation factor (*i*) of a chemical agent.
- Calculate the sodium chloride equivalent (*E*-value) of a chemical agent.
- Demonstrate by calculation whether a solution is hypotonic, isotonic, or hypertonic.
- Perform calculations required in the preparation of isotonic solutions.
- Calculate the pH of a buffer solution.
- Determine the amounts of components needed to prepare a buffer at a specific pH.

When a solvent passes through a semipermeable membrane from a dilute solution into a more concentrated one, the concentrations become equalized and the phenomenon is known as ***osmosis***. The pressure responsible for this phenomenon is termed ***osmotic pressure*** and varies with the nature of the solute.

If the solute is a nonelectrolyte, its solution contains only molecules and the osmotic pressure varies with the concentration of the solute. If the solute is an electrolyte, its solution contains ions and the osmotic pressure varies with both the concentration of the solute and its degree of dissociation. Thus, solutes that dissociate present a greater number of particles in solution and exert a greater osmotic pressure than do *un*dissociated molecules.

Two solutions that have the same osmotic pressure are termed ***isosmotic***. Many solutions intended to be mixed with body fluids are designed to have the same osmotic pressure for greater patient comfort, efficacy, and safety. A solution having the same osmotic pressure as a *specific* body fluid is termed ***isotonic*** (meaning of equal tone) with *that* specific body fluid.

Solutions of *lower* osmotic pressure than that of a body fluid are termed ***hypotonic***, whereas those having a *higher* osmotic pressure are termed ***hypertonic***. Pharmaceutical dosage forms intended to be added directly to the blood or mixed with biological fluids of the eye, nose, and bowel are of principal concern to the pharmacist in their preparation and clinical application.

Special Clinical Considerations of Tonicity

It is generally accepted that for ophthalmic and parenteral administration, isotonic solutions are better tolerated by the patient than those at the extremes of hypo- and hypertonicity. With the administration of an isotonic solution, there is a homeostasis with the body's intracellular fluids. Thus, *in most instances*, preparations that are isotonic, or nearly so, are preferred. However, there are exceptions, as in instances in which hypertonic solutions are used to "draw" fluids out of edematous tissues and into the administered solution.

Most ophthalmic preparations are formulated to be isotonic, or approximately isotonic, to duplicate ophthalmic tears for the comfort of the patient. These solutions are also prepared and buffered at an appropriate pH, both to reduce the likelihood of irritation to the eye's tissues and to maintain the stability of the preparations.

Injections that are not isotonic should be administered slowly and in small quantities to minimize tissue irritation, pain, and cell fluid imbalance. The tonicity of small-volume injections is generally inconsequential when added to large-volume parenteral infusions because of the presence of tonic substances, such as sodium chloride or dextrose in the large-volume infusion, which serve to adjust the tonicity of the smaller added volume.[1]

Intravenous infusions, which are hypotonic or hypertonic, can have profound adverse effects because they generally are administered in large volumes.[1] Large volumes of *hypertonic* infusions containing dextrose, for example, can result in hyperglycemia, osmotic diuresis, and excessive loss of electrolytes. Excess infusions of *hypotonic* fluids can result in the osmotic hemolysis of red blood cells and surpass the upper limits of the body's capacity to safely absorb excessive fluids. Even isotonic fluids, when infused intravenously in excessive volumes or at excessive rates, can be deleterious due to an overload of fluids placed into the body's circulatory system.

Physical/Chemical Considerations in the Preparation of Isotonic Solutions

The calculations involved in preparing isotonic solutions may be made in terms of data relating to the colligative properties of solutions. Theoretically, any one of these properties may be used as a basis for determining tonicity. Practically and most conveniently, a comparison of freezing points is used for this purpose. It is generally accepted that −0.52°C is the freezing point of both blood serum and lacrimal fluid.

When 1g molecular weight of any nonelectrolyte, that is, a substance with negligible dissociation, such as boric acid, is dissolved in 1000 g of water, the freezing point of the solution is about 1.86°C below the freezing point of pure water. By simple proportion, therefore, we can calculate the weight of any nonelectrolyte that should be dissolved in each 1000 g of water if the solution is to be isotonic with body fluids.

Boric acid, for example, has a molecular weight of 61.8; thus (in theory), 61.8 g in 1000 g of water should produce a freezing point of −1.86°C. Therefore:

$$\frac{1.86\ (°\text{C})}{0.52\ (°\text{C})} = \frac{61.8\ (\text{g})}{\text{x}\ (\text{g})}$$

$$\text{x} = 17.3\ \text{g}$$

In short, 17.3 g of boric acid in 1000 g of water, having a weight-in-volume strength of approximately 1.73%, should make a solution isotonic with lacrimal fluid.

With electrolytes, the problem is not so simple. Because osmotic pressure depends more on the number of particles, substances that dissociate have a tonic effect that increases with the degree of dissociation; the greater the dissociation, the smaller the quantity required to produce any given osmotic pressure. If we assume that sodium chloride in weak solutions is about 80% dissociated, then each 100 molecules yields 180 particles, or 1.8 times as many particles as are yielded by 100 molecules of a nonelectrolyte. This dissociation factor, commonly symbolized by the letter *i*, must be included in the proportion when we seek to determine the strength of an isotonic solution of sodium chloride (m.w. 58.5):

$$\frac{1.86\ (°C) \times 1.8}{0.52\ (°C)} = \frac{58.5\ (g)}{x\ (g)}$$

$$x = 9.09\ g$$

Hence, 9.09 g of sodium chloride in 1000 g of water should make a solution isotonic with blood or lacrimal fluid. In practice, a 0.9% w/v sodium chloride solution is considered isotonic with body fluids.

Simple isotonic solutions may then be calculated by using this formula:

$$\frac{0.52 \times \text{molecular weight}}{1.86 \times \text{dissociation } (i)} = \text{g of solute per 1000 g of water}$$

The value of i for many medicinal salts has not been experimentally determined. Some salts are exceptional (such as zinc sulfate, with only 40% dissociation and an i value therefore of 1.4), but most medicinal salts approximate the dissociation of sodium chloride in weak solutions. If the number of ions is known, we may use the following values, lacking better information:

Nonelectrolytes and substances of slight dissociation: 1.0
Substances that dissociate into 2 ions: 1.8
Substances that dissociate into 3 ions: 2.6
Substances that dissociate into 4 ions: 3.4
Substances that dissociate into 5 ions: 4.2

A special problem arises when a prescription directs us to make a solution isotonic by adding the proper amount of a tonicity agent (such as sodium chloride or boric acid) to the solution containing the active ingredient. Given a 0.5% w/v solution of sodium chloride, we may easily calculate that 0.9 g – 0.5 g = 0.4 g of additional sodium chloride that should be contained in each 100 mL if the solution is to be made isotonic with a body fluid. But how much sodium chloride should be used in preparing 100 mL of a 1% w/v solution of atropine sulfate, which is to be made isotonic with lacrimal fluid? The answer depends on *how much sodium chloride is in effect represented by the atropine sulfate.*

The relative tonic effect of two substances—that is, the quantity of one that is equivalent in tonic effects to a given quantity of the other—may be calculated if the quantity of one having a certain effect in a specified quantity of solvent is divided by the quantity of the other having the same effect in the same quantity of solvent. For example, we calculated that 17.3 g of boric acid per 1000 g of water and 9.09 g of sodium chloride per 1000 g of water are both instrumental in making an aqueous solution isotonic with lacrimal fluid. If, however, 17.3 g of boric acid are equivalent in tonicity to 9.09 g of sodium chloride, then 1 g of boric acid must be the equivalent of 9.09 g ÷ 17.3 g or 0.52 g of sodium chloride. Similarly, 1 g of sodium chloride must be the "tonicic equivalent" of 17.3 g ÷ 9.09 g or 1.9 g of boric acid.

We have seen that one quantity of any substance should in theory have a constant tonic effect if dissolved in 1000 g of water: 1 g molecular weight of the substance divided by its i or dissociation value. Hence, the relative quantity of sodium chloride that is the tonicic equivalent of a quantity of boric acid may be calculated by these ratios:

$$\frac{58.5 \div 1.8}{61.8 \div 1.0} \text{ or } \frac{58.5 \times 1.0}{61.8 \times 1.8}$$

and we can formulate a convenient rule: *quantities of two substances that are tonicic equivalents are proportional to the molecular weights of each multiplied by the* i *value of the other.*

To return to the problem involving 1 g of atropine sulfate in 100 mL of solution:

Molecular weight of sodium chloride = 58.5; $i = 1.8$
Molecular weight of atropine sulfate = 695; $i = 2.6$

$$\frac{695 \times 1.8}{58.5 \times 2.6} = \frac{1\ (g)}{x\ (g)}$$

x = 0.12 g of sodium chloride represented by 1 g of atropine sulfate

Therefore, the sodium chloride equivalent, or *E*-value, of atropine sulfate is 0.12. Because a solution isotonic with lacrimal fluid should contain the equivalent of 0.9 g of sodium chloride in each 100 mL of solution, the difference to be added must be 0.9 g − 0.12 g = 0.78 g of sodium chloride.

Rearranging the information for calculating the *E*-value of boric acid or atropine sulfate, the following equation can be used to calculate the sodium chloride equivalent of any substance:

$$\frac{\text{Molecular weight of sodium chloride}}{i \text{ Factor of sodium chloride}} \times \frac{i \text{ factor of the substance}}{\text{Molecular weight of the substance}} = \text{Sodium chloride equivalent}$$

Table 11.1 gives the *sodium chloride equivalents* (*E*-values) of each of the substances listed. These values were calculated according to the rule stated previously using the general dissociation factors listed on page 191 or adapted from tables listing experimental values. ***If the amount of a substance included in a prescription is multiplied by its sodium chloride equivalent, the amount of sodium chloride represented by that substance is determined.***

Table 11.1 • SODIUM CHLORIDE EQUIVALENTS (*E*-VALUES)

Substance	Molecular Weight	Ions	Sodium Chloride Equivalent (E-value)[a]
Antipyrine	188	1	0.17
Atropine sulfate·H_2O	695	3	0.12
Benoxinate hydrochloride	345	2	0.17
Benzalkonium chloride	360	2	0.16
Benzyl alcohol	108	1	0.17
Boric acid	61.8	1	0.52
Brimonidine tartrate	442	2	0.13
Chlorobutanol	177	1	0.24
Cocaine hydrochloride	340	2	0.17
Cromolyn sodium	512	2	0.14
Cyclopentolate hydrochloride	328	2	0.18
Demecarium bromide	717	3	0.12
Dextrose (anhydrous)	180	1	0.18
Dextrose·H_2O	198	1	0.16
Ephedrine hydrochloride	202	2	0.29
Ephedrine sulfate	429	3	0.2
Epinephrine bitartrate	333	2	0.18
Fluorescein sodium	376	3	0.31

Table 11.1 • SODIUM CHLORIDE EQUIVALENTS (*E*-VALUES) (*Continued*)

Substance	Molecular Weight	Ions	Sodium Chloride Equivalent (E-value)[a]
Glycerin	92	1	0.35
Homatropine hydrobromide	356	2	0.17
Hydroxyamphetamine hydrobromide	232	2	0.25
Idoxuridine	354	1	0.09
Lidocaine hydrochloride	289	2	0.2
Mannitol	182	1	0.18
Morphine sulfate·$5H_2O$	759	3	0.11
Moxifloxacin hydrochloride	438	2	0.13
Naphazoline hydrochloride	247	2	0.27
Oxymetazoline hydrochloride	297	2	0.22
Penicillin G potassium	372	2	0.18
Phenobarbital sodium	254	2	0.24
Phenylephrine hydrochloride	204	2	0.32
Physostigmine salicylate	413	2	0.16
Pilocarpine hydrochloride	245	2	0.24
Potassium chloride	74.5	2	0.76
Potassium iodide	166	2	0.34
Potassium nitrate	101	2	0.58
Potassium phosphate, monobasic	136	2	0.43
Procaine hydrochloride	273	2	0.21
Proparacaine hydrochloride	331	2	0.15
Scopolamine hydrobromide·$3H_2O$	438	2	0.12
Silver nitrate	170	2	0.33
Sodium bicarbonate	84	2	0.65
Sodium borate·$10H_2O$	381	5	0.42
Sodium carbonate·H_2O	124	3	0.6
Sodium chloride	58	2	1
Sodium citrate·$2H_2O$	294	4	0.31
Sodium iodide	150	2	0.39
Sodium lactate	112	2	0.52
Sodium phosphate, dibasic, anhydrous	142	3	0.53
Sodium phosphate, dibasic·$7H_2O$	268	3	0.29
Sodium phosphate, monobasic, anhydrous	120	2	0.49
Sodium phosphate, monobasic·H_2O	138	2	0.42
Tetracaine hydrochloride	301	2	0.18
Tetracycline hydrochloride	481	2	0.12
Tetrahydrozoline hydrochloride	237	2	0.25
Timolol maleate	432	2	0.14
Tobramycin	468	1	0.07
Tropicamide	284	1	0.09
Urea	60	1	0.53
Xylometazoline hydrochloride	281	2	0.21
Zinc chloride	136	3	0.62
Zinc sulfate·$7H_2O$	288	2	0.16

[a]Calculated based on general dissociation constant or adapted from Allen LV, ed. *Remington: The Science and Practice of Pharmacy.* London, UK: Pharmaceutical Press; 2013:652–662 and O'Neil MJ, ed. *The Merck Index.* Vol. 13. Whitehouse Station, NJ: Merck & Co., Inc.; 2001:MISC-32–MISC-42.

The procedure for the *calculation of isotonic solutions with sodium chloride equivalents* may be outlined as follows:

STEP 1. Calculate the amount of sodium chloride *represented* by each ingredient in a prescription by multiplying the amount of each ingredient by its sodium chloride equivalent.

STEP 2. Calculate the amount of sodium chloride, alone, that would be contained in an isotonic solution of the volume specified in the prescription, namely, *the amount of sodium chloride in a 0.9% solution of the specified volume.*

STEP 3. Subtract the amount of sodium chloride represented by the ingredients in the prescription (*Step 1*) from the amount of sodium chloride, alone, that would be represented in the specific volume of an isotonic solution (*Step 2*). The answer represents the amount of sodium chloride to be added to make the solution isotonic.

STEP 4. If an agent other than sodium chloride, such as boric acid, dextrose, or mannitol, is to be used to make a solution isotonic, divide the amount of sodium chloride (*Step 3*) by the sodium chloride equivalent of the other substance.

Example Calculations of the *i* Factor

(1) *Zinc sulfate is a 2-ion electrolyte, dissociating 40% in a certain concentration. Calculate its dissociation (i) factor.*

On the basis of 40% dissociation, 100 particles of zinc sulfate will yield:

40 zinc ions
40 sulfate ions
<u>60</u> undissociated particles
or 140 particles

Because 140 particles represent 1.4 times as many particles as were present before dissociation, the dissociation (*i*) factor is **1.4.**

(2) *Zinc chloride is a 3-ion electrolyte, dissociating 80% in a certain concentration. Calculate its dissociation (i) factor.*

On the basis of 80% dissociation, 100 particles of zinc chloride will yield:

80 zinc ions
80 chloride ions
80 chloride ions
<u>20</u> undissociated particles
or 260 particles

Because 260 particles represents 2.6 times as many particles as were present before dissociation, the dissociation (*i*) factor is **2.6.**

Example Calculations of the Sodium Chloride Equivalent (*E*-values)

(1) *Papaverine hydrochloride* (m.w. 376) *is a 2-ion electrolyte, dissociating 80% in a given concentration. Calculate its sodium chloride equivalent.*

Because papaverine hydrochloride is a 2-ion electrolyte, dissociating 80%, its *i* factor is 1.8.

$$\frac{58.5}{1.8} \times \frac{1.8}{376} = \mathbf{0.16}$$

(2) *Calculate the sodium chloride equivalent for glycerin, a nonelectrolyte with a molecular weight of 92.*[2]

Glycerin, *i* factor = 1.0

$$\frac{58.5}{1.8} \times \frac{1.0}{92} = \mathbf{0.35}$$

(3) *Calculate the sodium chloride equivalent for timolol maleate (TIMOPTIC), which dissociates into two ions and has a molecular weight of 432.*[2]

Timolol maleate, *i* factor = 1.8

$$\frac{58.5}{1.8} \times \frac{1.8}{432} = \mathbf{0.14}$$

(4) *Calculate the sodium chloride equivalent for fluorescein sodium, which dissociates into three ions and has a molecular weight of 376.*[2]

Fluorescein sodium, *i* factor = 2.6

$$\frac{58.5}{1.8} \times \frac{2.6}{376} = \mathbf{0.22}$$

Note that the calculated value differs from the value in Table 11.1 (0.31). This is most likely due to using the general dissociation factor of 2.6 rather than the specific dissociation factor for fluorescein sodium. The value reported in Table 11.1 is an experimentally determined value.

(5) *The agent brimonidine tartrate (ALPHAGAN P) has a molecular weight of 442 and dissociates into two ions when in solution. It is used as a 0.1% ophthalmic solution in the treatment of glaucoma. Calculate (a) the sodium chloride equivalent of brimonidine tartrate and (b) whether, without additional formulation agents, a 0.1% solution would be isotonic, hypotonic, or hypertonic with tears.*

(a) $\frac{58.5}{1.8} \times \frac{1.8}{442}$ = **0.13 sodium chloride equivalent**

(b) Arbitrarily select a volume of solution as a basis for the calculation. The commercial product is available in 10-mL containers, so that volume would be a good choice.

For isotonicity, a 10-mL volume would require the following amount of sodium chloride or its equivalent:

10 mL × 0.9% w/v = 0.09 g sodium chloride or its equivalent

A 10-mL volume of a 0.1% w/v solution of brimonidine tartrate would contain

10 mL × 0.1% w/v = 0.01 g brimonidine tartrate

Applying the sodium chloride equivalent (0.13):

0.01 g brimonidine tartrate × 0.13 = 0.0013 g of sodium chloride equivalence

Thus, this solution would be **hypotonic**.

(6) *If 1 g of epinephrine bitartrate, when dissolved in water, prepares 20 mL of an isotonic solution, calculate its sodium chloride equivalent.*

20 mL of an isotonic *sodium chloride* solution would be calculated by

20 mL × 0.9% w/v = 0.18 g sodium chloride (in 20 mL of solution)

Therefore, 1 g of epinephrine bitartrate is equal in tonic effect to 0.18 g sodium chloride, and thus, its sodium chloride equivalent is 0.18.

Example Calculations of Tonicic Agent Required

(1) *How many grams of sodium chloride should be used in compounding the following prescription?*

℞	Homatropine hydrobromide	0.6 g
	Sodium chloride	qs
	Purified water ad	30 mL
	Make isoton. sol.	
	Sig. for the eye	

STEP 1.

$$0.6\text{ g} \times \frac{1000\text{ mg}}{1\text{ g}} \times 0.17 \text{ (from Table 11.1)}$$

= 102 mg of sodium chloride represented by the homatromine HBr

STEP 2.

$$30\text{ mL} \times \frac{0.9\text{ g}}{100\text{ mL}} \times \frac{1000\text{ mg}}{1\text{ g}}$$

= 270 mg of sodium chloride in 30 mL of an isotonic sodium chloride solution

STEP 3. 270 mg (from *Step 2*) – 102 mg (from *Step 1*) = **168 mg of sodium chloride to be used**

(2) *How many grams of boric acid should be used in compounding the following prescription?*

℞	Proparacaine hydrochloride	0.5%
	Pilocarpine hydrochloride	2%
	Boric acid	qs
	Purified water ad	60 mL
	Make isoton. sol.	
	Sig. one drop in each eye	

STEP 1. Proparacaine HCl:

$$\frac{0.5\text{ g}}{100\text{ mL}} \times \frac{1000\text{ mg}}{1\text{ g}} \times 60\text{ mL} = 300\text{ mg} \times 0.15 = 45\text{ mg of sodium chloride represented}$$

Pilocarpine HCl:

$$\frac{2\text{ g}}{100\text{ mL}} \times \frac{1000\text{ mg}}{1\text{ g}} \times 60\text{ mL} = 1200\text{ mg} \times 0.24 = 288\text{ mg of sodium chloride represented}$$

Total: 45 mg + 288 mg = 333 mg of sodium chloride represented by both ingredients

STEP 2.

$$\frac{0.9\text{ g}}{100\text{ mL}} \times \frac{1000\text{ mg}}{1\text{ g}} \times 60\text{ mL}$$

= 540 mg of sodium chloride in 60 mL of an isotonic sodium chloride solution

STEP 3. 540 mg (from *Step 2*) – 333 mg (from *Step 1*) = 207 mg of sodium chloride required to make the solution isotonic

But because the prescription calls for boric acid:

STEP 4. 207 mg ÷ 0.52 = **398.08 mg of boric acid to be used**

(3) *How many grams of potassium nitrate should be used to make the following prescription isotonic?*

℞	Sol. silver nitrate	60 mL
	1:500 w/v	
	Make isoton. sol.	
	Sig. for eye use	

STEP 1.

$$\frac{1\text{ g}}{500\text{ mL}} \times \frac{1000\text{ mg}}{1\text{ g}} \times 60\text{ mL} = 120\text{ mg silver nitrate} \times 0.33$$
$$= 39.6\text{ mg of sodium chloride represented}$$

STEP 2.

$$\frac{0.9\text{ g}}{100\text{ mL}} \times \frac{1000\text{ mg}}{1\text{ g}} \times 60\text{ mL}$$

= 540 mg of sodium chloride in 60 mL of an isotonic sodium chloride solution

STEP 3. 540 mg (from *Step 2*) – 39.6 mg (from *Step 1*) = 500.4 mg of sodium chloride required to make solution isotonic

Because, in this solution, sodium chloride is incompatible with silver nitrate, the tonicity agent of choice is potassium nitrate. Therefore,

STEP 4. 500.4 mg ÷ 0.58 (sodium chloride equivalent of potassium nitrate) = **862.76 mg of potassium nitrate to be used**

(4) *How many grams of sodium chloride should be used in compounding the following prescription?*

℞	Ingredient X	0.5 g
	Sodium chloride	qs
	Purified water ad	50 mL
	Make isoton. sol.	
	Sig. eyedrops	

Let us assume that ingredient X is a new substance for which no sodium chloride equivalent is to be found in Table 11.1 and that its molecular weight is 295 and its *i* factor is 2.4. The sodium chloride equivalent of ingredient X may be calculated as follows:

$$\frac{58.5}{1.8} \times \frac{2.4}{295} = 0.26\text{, the sodium chloride equivalent for ingredient X}$$

Then,

STEP 1.

$$0.5\text{ g} \times \frac{1000\text{ mg}}{1\text{ g}} \times 0.26 = 130\text{ mg of sodium chloride represented by ingredient X}$$

STEP 2.

$$\frac{0.9\text{ g}}{100\text{ mL}} \times \frac{1000\text{ mg}}{1\text{ g}} \times 50\text{ mL}$$

= 450 mg of sodium chloride in 50 mL of an isotonic sodium chloride solution

STEP 3. 450 mg (from *Step 2*) – 130 mg (from *Step 1*) = **320 mg of sodium chloride to be used**

Preparing Isotonic Solutions by Volume Adjustment

As a convenience in compounding, a method of preparing isotonic solutions by volume adjustment may be employed. The method, once described in the *United States Pharmacopeia–National Formulary*,[3] is based on the following:

By adding purified water to a 1-g quantity of a drug with a known E-value, a calculated volume of an isotonic solution may be prepared. Then, by diluting this volume of solution with an isotonic vehicle, the drug strength may be reduced while maintaining the solution's isotonicity.

For example, 1 g of tetracaine hydrochloride ($E = 0.18$) can prepare 20 mL of an isotonic solution, calculated as follows:

$$\frac{0.18 \text{ g [sodium chloride (equiv.)]}}{\text{x mL (isotonic solution)}} = \frac{0.9 \text{ g (sodium chloride)}}{100 \text{ mL (isotonic solution)}}; \text{x} = 20 \text{ mL}$$

This isotonic solution would contain 5% w/v tetracaine hydrochloride (1 g/20 mL). If a solution of lesser strength is desired, a calculated quantity of an isotonic vehicle, such as 0.9% sodium chloride, may be added. For example, if a 1% w/v solution of tetracaine hydrochloride is desired, a total volume of 100 mL (1 g tetracaine hydrochloride/100 mL) may be prepared by adding 80 mL of isotonic vehicle to the 20 mL of the 5% w/v solution.

(1) *If pilocarpine hydrochloride has a sodium chloride equivalent of 0.24, (a) how many milliliters of isotonic solution may be prepared from 1 g of the drug, and (b) how many milliliters of 0.9% w/v sodium chloride solution may be added to the resultant solution to prepare an isotonic solution having a 1.5% w/v concentration of pilocarpine hydrochloride?*

(a) $$\frac{0.24 \text{ g [sodium chloride (equiv.)]}}{\text{x mL (isotonic solution)}} = \frac{0.9 \text{ g (sodium chloride)}}{100 \text{ mL (isotonic solution)}}; \text{x} = \mathbf{26.67 \text{ mL}}$$

(b) Although there are a number of ways to solve this problem, use of the equation in Chapter 15 is perhaps the most convenient method:

1st quantity (Q1) × 1st concentration (C1) = 2nd quantity (Q2) × 2nd concentration (C2)

First, one must calculate the concentration of pilocarpine hydrochloride in 26.67 mL of solution:

$$\frac{1 \text{ g}}{26.67 \text{ mL}} \times 100\% = 3.75\% \text{ w/v}$$

Then, applying the above equation:
26.67 mL (Q1) × 3.75% (C1) = x mL (Q2) × 1.5% (C2)

$$\text{x} = \frac{26.67 \text{ mL} \times 3.75\%}{1.5\%} = 66.68 \text{ mL}$$

Thus, 66.68 mL of solution may be prepared, and **40.01 mL** (66.68 mL – 26.67 mL) of 0.9% sodium chloride solution should be added.

Proof that the concentration of pilocarpine hydrochloride is 1.5%:

$$\frac{1 \text{ g pilocarpine HCl}}{66.68 \text{ mL}} \times 100\% = 1.4997 \text{ or } 1.5\% \text{ w/v pilocarpine HCl}$$

Other examples of calculated volumes of isotonic solutions that may be prepared from 1 g of drug are given in Table 11.2 and available from other references.[3,4]

(2) *Determine the volume of purified water and 0.9% w/v sodium chloride solution needed to prepare 20 mL of a 1% w/v solution of hydromorphone hydrochloride (E = 0.22).*

STEP 1. 20 mL × 1% w/v = 0.2 g hydromorphone hydrochloride needed

STEP 2. 0.2 g (hydromorphone hydrochloride) × 0.22 (*E*-value) = 0.044 g (sodium chloride equivalence)

Table 11.2 • EXAMPLES OF ISOTONIC SOLUTIONS THAT MAY BE PREPARED FROM 1 g QUANTITIES OF DRUGS[a]

Drug, 1 g	Volume of Isotonic Solution, mL
Boric acid	57.8
Ephedrine sulfate	22.2
Phenylephrine hydrochloride	35.6
Pilocarpine hydrochloride	26.7
Tetracaine hydrochloride	20.0
Zinc sulfate·$7H_2O$	17.8

[a]Calculated from the *E*-values in Table 11.1.

$$\frac{0.044\ \text{g}}{\text{x mL}} = \frac{0.9\ \text{g NaCl}}{100\ \text{mL}};$$ x = **4.89 mL of an isotonic solution of hydromorphone hydrochloride may be prepared by the addition of a sufficient quantity (qs) of purified water.**

STEP 3. 20 mL – 4.89 mL = **15.11 mL 0.9% w/v sodium chloride solution required**

Proof: 20 mL × 0.9% = 0.18 g sodium chloride or equivalent required
0.2 × 0.22 = 0.044 g (sodium chloride represented by 0.2 g hydromorphone hydrochloride)
15.11 mL × 0.9% = 0.136 g sodium chloride present
0.044 g + 0.136 g = 0.18 g sodium chloride required for isotonicity

Use of Freezing Point Data in Isotonicity Calculations

Freezing point data (ΔT_f) can be used in isotonicity calculations when the agent has a tonicic effect and does not penetrate the biologic membranes in question (e.g., red blood cells). As stated previously, the freezing point of both blood and lacrimal fluid is –0.52°C. Thus, a pharmaceutical solution that has a freezing point of –0.52°C is considered isotonic.

Representative data on freezing point depression by medicinal and pharmaceutical substances are presented in Table 11.3. Although these data are for solution strengths of 1% ($\Delta T_f^{1\%}$), data for other solution strengths and for many additional agents may be found in physical pharmacy textbooks and in the literature.

Freezing point depression data may be used in isotonicity calculations as shown by the following.

Example Calculations Using Freezing Point Data

How many milligrams each of sodium chloride and lidocaine hydrochloride are required to prepare 30 mL of a 1% solution of lidocaine hydrochloride isotonic with tears?

To make this solution isotonic, the freezing point must be lowered to –0.52°C. From Table 11.3, it is determined that a 1% solution of lidocaine hydrochloride has a freezing point lowering of 0.063°C. Thus, sufficient sodium chloride must be added to lower the freezing point an additional 0.457°C (0.52°C – 0.063°C).

Also from Table 11.3, it is determined that a 1% solution of sodium chloride lowers the freezing point by 0.58°C. By proportion:

$$\frac{1\%\ \text{NaCl}}{\text{x\% NaCl}} = \frac{0.58°\text{C}}{0.457°\text{C}}$$

x = 0.79% sodium chloride needed to lower the freezing point by 0.457°C and, therefore, required to make the solution isotonic

Table 11.3 • FREEZING POINT DATA FOR SELECT AGENTS

Agent	Freezing Point Depression, 1% Solutions ($\Delta T_f^{1\%}$)
Atropine sulfate	0.07
Boric acid	0.29
Chlorobutanol	0.14
Dextrose	0.09
Ephedrine sulfate	0.13
Epinephrine bitartrate	0.10
Glycerin	0.20
Homatropine hydrobromide	0.11
Lidocaine hydrochloride	0.063
Lincomycin	0.09
Morphine sulfate	0.08
Naphazoline hydrochloride	0.16
Physostigmine salicylate	0.09
Sodium bisulfite	0.36
Sodium chloride	0.58
Sulfacetamide sodium	0.14
Zinc sulfate	0.09

Thus, to make 30 mL of solution,

30 mL × 1% = 0.3 g = **300 mg lidocaine hydrochloride**, and

30 mL × 0.79% = 0.24 g = **236.68 mg sodium chloride**

NOTE: Should a prescription call for more than one medicinal and/or pharmaceutic ingredient, the sum of the freezing points is subtracted from the required value in determining the additional lowering required by the agent used to provide isotonicity.

CALCULATIONS CAPSULE

Isotonicity

To calculate the "equivalent tonic effect" to sodium chloride represented by an ingredient in a preparation, multiply its weight by its *E*-value:

$$g \times \text{E-value} = \text{g, equivalent tonic effect to sodium chloride}$$

To make a solution isotonic, calculate and ensure the quantity of sodium chloride and/or the equivalent tonic effect of all other ingredients to total 0.9% w/v in the preparation:

$$\frac{\text{g (NaCl)} + \text{g (NaCl tonic equivalents)}}{\text{mL (preparation)}} \times 100 = 0.9\%\ \text{w/v}$$

To make an isotonic solution from a drug substance, add sufficient water by the equation:

$$\frac{\text{g (drug substance)} \times \text{E-value (drug substance)}}{0.009} = \text{mL water}$$

This solution may then be made to any volume with isotonic sodium chloride solution to maintain its isotonicity.

The *E*-value can be derived from the same equation, given the grams of drug substance and the milliliters of water required to make an isotonic solution.

CASE IN POINT 11.1[a] A local ophthalmologist is treating one of his patients for a post-LASIK eye infection that is not responding to topical ciprofloxacin. These infections, although rare, can occur after laser in situ keratomileusis (LASIK) surgery for vision correction.

Topical amikacin sulfate has been shown to be effective for the treatment of eye infections due to ciprofloxacin-resistant *Pseudomonas*,[5,6] *Burkholderia ambifaria*,[7] *Mycobacterium chelonae*, and *Mycobacterium fortuitum*.[8–10]

The ophthalmologist prescribes 60 mL of a 2.5% amikacin sulfate isotonic solution, two drops in the affected eye every 2 hours.

Amikacin sulfate USP ($C_{22}H_{43}N_5O_{13} \cdot 2H_2SO_2$), m.w., 781.76, is an aminoglycoside-type antibiotic containing three ions.

(a) Determine the weight in grams of amikacin sulfate needed to prepare the solution.
(b) Calculate the sodium chloride equivalent (*E*-value) for amikacin sulfate.
(c) Calculate the amount of sodium chloride needed to make the prepared solution isotonic.
(d) How many milliliters of 23.5% sodium chloride injection should be used to obtain the needed sodium chloride?

[a]Case in Point courtesy of W. Beach, Athens, GA.

CASE IN POINT 11.2[11] A formula for a compounded ophthalmic solution is shown below:

℞	Tobramycin sulfate		300 mg
	Diclofenac sodium		100 mg
	Sodium chloride		806 mg
	Sterile water for injection	qs	100 mL

This formula combines the antibacterial action of tobramycin sulfate with the anti-inflammatory and analgesic properties of diclofenac sodium. It should be prepared in an aseptic environment such as a laminar flow hood and has a beyond-use date of up to 3 days if stored in the refrigerator.

(a) Tobramycin sulfate [$(C_{18}H_{37}N_5O_9)_2 \cdot 5H_2SO_4$] is a 7-ion electrolyte and has a molecular weight of 1425.45. Assuming that it dissociates 80% at a certain concentration, calculate the dissociation factor (*i*) and sodium chloride equivalent (*E*-value) for tobramycin sulfate.
(b) The potency of tobramycin sulfate is 634 to 739 mcg of tobramycin activity per milligram. What is the amount range of tobramycin activity in this formulation?
(c) Diclofenac sodium ($C_{14}H_{10}Cl_2NNaO_2$) is a 2-ion electrolyte with an average dissociation factor of 1.8 and a molecular weight of 318.13. Calculate the *E*-value for diclofenac sodium.
(d) Is the amount of sodium chloride listed in the formulation correct to make the solution isotonic?
(e) How much of each ingredient would be needed to prepare 20 mL of the compounded solution?
(f) How much of a tobramycin sulfate injectable solution with a concentration of 80 mg/2 mL would be needed to prepare 20 mL of the compounded solution?

Buffers and Buffer Solutions

When a minute amount of hydrochloric acid is added to pure water, a significant increase in *hydrogen-ion* concentration occurs immediately. In a similar manner, when a minute amount of sodium hydroxide is added to pure water, it causes a correspondingly large increase in the *hydroxide-ion* concentration. These changes take place because water alone cannot neutralize even traces of acid or base, that is, it has no ability to resist changes in hydrogen-ion concentration or pH. A solution of a neutral salt, such as sodium chloride, also lacks this ability. Therefore, it is said to be *unbuffered*.

The presence of certain substances or combinations of substances in aqueous solution imparts to the system the ability to maintain a desired pH at a relatively constant level, even with the addition of materials that may be expected to change the hydrogen-ion concentration. These substances or combinations of substances are called ***buffers***, and solutions of them are called ***buffer solutions***. By definition, then, a ***buffer solution*** is a system, usually an aqueous solution, that possesses the property of resisting changes in pH with the addition of small amounts of an acid or base.

Buffers are used to establish and maintain an ion activity within rather narrow limits. In pharmacy, the most common buffer systems are used in (i) the preparation of such dosage forms as injections and ophthalmic solutions, which are placed directly into pH-sensitive body fluids; (ii) the manufacture of formulations in which the pH must be maintained at a relatively constant level to ensure maximum product stability; and (iii) pharmaceutical tests and assays requiring adjustment to or maintenance of a specific pH for analytic purposes.

A buffer solution is usually composed of a weak acid and a salt of the acid, such as acetic acid and sodium acetate, or a weak base and a salt of the base, such as ammonium hydroxide and ammonium chloride. Typical buffer systems that may be used in pharmaceutical formulations include the following pairs: acetic acid and sodium acetate, boric acid and sodium borate, and sodium phosphate monobasic and sodium phosphate dibasic. Formulas for standard buffer solutions for pharmaceutical analysis are given in the *United States Pharmacopeia*.[12]

In the selection of a buffer system, due consideration must be given to the dissociation constant of the weak acid or base to ensure maximum buffer capacity. This dissociation constant, in the case of an acid, is a measure of the strength of the acid; the more readily the acid dissociates, the higher its dissociation constant and the stronger the acid. Selected dissociation constants, or K_a values, are given in Table 11.4.

Table 11.4 • DISSOCIATION CONSTANTS OF SOME WEAK ACIDS AT 25°C

Acid	K_a
Acetic	1.75×10^{-5}
Barbituric	1.05×10^{-4}
Benzoic	6.30×10^{-5}
Boric	6.4×10^{-10}
Formic	1.76×10^{-4}
Lactic	1.38×10^{-4}
Mandelic	4.29×10^{-4}
Salicylic	1.06×10^{-3}

The dissociation constant, or K_a value, of a weak acid is given by the equation:

$$K_a = \frac{(H^+)(A^-)}{(HA)} \quad \text{where } A^- = \text{salt}, \quad HA = \text{acid}$$

Because the numeric values of most dissociation constants are small numbers and may vary over many powers of 10, it is more convenient to express them as negative logarithms:

$$pK_a = -\log K_a$$

When equation $K_a = \frac{(H^+)(A^-)}{(HA)}$ is expressed in logarithmic form, it is written:

$$pK_a = -\log (H^+) - \log \frac{\text{salt}}{\text{acid}}$$

and because $pH = -\log (H^+)$:

$$\text{then} \quad pK_a = pH - \log \frac{\text{salt}}{\text{acid}}$$

$$\text{and} \quad pH = pK_a + \log \frac{\text{salt}}{\text{acid}}$$

Buffer Equation

The equation just derived is the Henderson-Hasselbalch equation for weak acids, commonly known as the ***buffer equation***.

Similarly, the dissociation constant, or K_b value, of a weak base is given by the equation:

$$K_b = \frac{(B^+)(OH^-)}{(BOH)} \quad \text{in which } B^+ = \text{salt} \quad \text{and } BOH = \text{base}$$

and the buffer equation for weak bases, which is derived from this relationship, may be expressed as:

$$pH = pK_w - pK_b + \log \frac{\text{base}}{\text{salt}}$$

The buffer equation is useful for calculating (1) the pH of a buffer system if its composition is known and (2) the molar ratio of the components of a buffer system required to give a solution of a desired pH. The equation can also be used to calculate the change in pH of a buffered solution with the addition of a given amount of acid or base.

pK$_A$ VALUE OF A WEAK ACID WITH KNOWN DISSOCIATION CONSTANT

Calculating the pK_a value of a weak acid, given its dissociation constant, K_a:

The dissociation constant of acetic acid is 1.75×10^{-5} at 25°C. Calculate its pK_a value.

$$pK_a = -\log K_a = -\log(1.75 \times 10^{-5}) = \mathbf{4.76}$$

PH VALUE OF A SALT/ACID BUFFER SYSTEM

Calculating the pH value:

What is the pH of a buffer solution prepared with 0.05 M sodium borate and 0.005 M boric acid? The pK_a value of boric acid is 9.24 at 25°C.

Note that the ratio of the components of the buffer solution is given in molar concentrations.

Using the buffer equation for weak acids:

$$\begin{aligned} pH &= pK_a + \log\frac{\text{salt}}{\text{acid}} \\ &= 9.24 + \log\frac{0.05}{0.005} \\ &= 9.24 + \log 10 \\ &= 9.24 + 1 \\ &= \mathbf{10.24} \end{aligned}$$

pH VALUE OF A BASE/SALT BUFFER SYSTEM

Calculating the pH value:

What is the pH of a buffer solution prepared with 0.05 M ammonia and 0.05 M ammonium chloride? The K_b value of ammonia is 1.80×10^{-5} at *25°C.*

Using the buffer equation for weak bases:

$$pH = pK_w - pK_b + \log\frac{\text{base}}{\text{salt}}$$

Because the K_w value for water is 10^{14} at 25°C, $pK_w = 14$.

$$pK_b = -\log K_b = -\log(1.80 \times 10^{-5}) = 4.74$$

$$pH = 14 - 4.74 + \log\frac{0.05}{0.05} = \mathbf{9.26}$$

MOLAR RATIO OF SALT/ACID FOR A BUFFER SYSTEM OF DESIRED pH

Calculating the molar ratio of salt/acid required to prepare a buffer system with a desired pH value:

What molar ratio of salt/acid is required to prepare a sodium acetate–acetic acid buffer solution with a pH of 5.76? The pK_a value of acetic acid is 4.76 at 25°C.

Using the buffer equation:

$$pH = pK_a + \log\frac{\text{salt}}{\text{acid}}$$

$$\begin{aligned} \log\frac{\text{salt}}{\text{acid}} &= pH - pK_a \\ &= 5.76 - 4.76 = 1 \end{aligned}$$

$$\text{antilog of } 1 = 10$$

$$\text{ratio} = 10/1 \text{ or } \mathbf{10{:}1}$$

QUANTITY OF COMPONENTS IN A BUFFER SOLUTION TO YIELD A SPECIFIC VOLUME

Calculating the amounts of the components of a buffer solution required to prepare a desired volume, given the molar ratio of the components and the total buffer concentration:

The molar ratio of sodium acetate to acetic acid in a buffer solution with a pH of 5.76 is 10:1. Assuming the total buffer concentration is 0.022 mol/L, how many grams of sodium acetate (m.w. 82) and how many grams of acetic acid (m.w. 60) should be used in preparing a liter of the solution?

Because the molar ratio of sodium acetate to acetic acid is 10:1,

$$\text{the mole fraction of sodium acetate} = \frac{10}{1+10} \text{ or } \frac{10}{11}$$

$$\text{and the mole fraction of acetic acid} = \frac{1}{1+10} \text{ or } \frac{1}{11}$$

If the total buffer concentration = 0.022 mol/L,

$$\text{Concentration of sodium acetate} = \frac{10}{11} \times 0.022\ \text{mol/L} = 0.02\ \text{mol/L}$$

$$\text{Concentration of acetic acid} = \frac{1}{11} \times 0.022\ \text{mol/L} = 0.002\ \text{mol/L}$$

$$\text{Amount of sodium acetate} = 0.02\ \text{mol/L} \times 82\ \text{g/mol} \times 1\ \text{L} = 1.64\ \text{g}$$

$$\text{Amount of acetic acid} = 0.002\ \text{mol/L} \times 60\ \text{g/mol} \times 1\ \text{L} = 0.12\ \text{g}$$

The efficiency of buffer solutions—that is, their specific ability to resist changes in pH—is measured in terms of *buffer capacity*; the *smaller* the pH change with the addition of a given amount of acid or base, the *greater* the buffer capacity of the system. Among other factors, the buffer capacity of a system depends on (1) the relative concentration of the buffer components and (2) the ratio of the components. For example, a 0.5-*M* acetate buffer at a pH of 4.76 would have a higher buffer capacity than a 0.05-*M* buffer.

If a strong base such as sodium hydroxide is added to a buffer system consisting of sodium acetate and acetic acid, the base is neutralized by the acetic acid forming more sodium acetate, and the resulting *increase* in pH is slight. Actually, the addition of the base increases the concentration of sodium acetate and decreases *by an equal amount* the concentration of acetic acid. In a similar manner, the addition of a strong acid to a buffer system consisting of a weak base and its salt would produce only a small *decrease* in pH.

CHANGE IN pH WITH ADDITION OF AN ACID OR BASE

Calculating the change in pH of a buffer solution with the addition of a given amount of acid or base:

Calculate the change in pH after adding 0.04 mol of sodium hydroxide to a liter of a buffer solution containing 0.2 M concentrations each of sodium acetate and acetic acid. The pK_a value of acetic acid is 4.76 at 25°C.

The pH of the buffer solution is calculated by using the buffer equation as follows:

$$\begin{aligned} pH &= pK_a + \log\frac{\text{salt}}{\text{acid}} \\ &= 4.76 + \log\frac{0.2}{0.2} \\ &= 4.76 + \log 1 \\ &= 4.76 \end{aligned}$$

The addition of 0.04 mol of sodium hydroxide converts 0.04 mol of acetic acid to 0.04 mol of sodium acetate. Consequently, the concentration of acetic acid is *decreased* and the concentration of sodium acetate is *increased* by equal amounts, according to the following equation:

$$pH = pK_a + \log\frac{\text{salt} + \text{base}}{\text{acid} - \text{base}}$$

$$pH = pK_a + \log\frac{0.2 + 0.04}{0.2 - 0.04}$$

$$= pK_a + \log\frac{0.24}{0.16}$$

$$= 4.76 + 0.1761 = 4.9361 \text{ or } 4.94$$

Because the pH before the addition of the sodium hydroxide was 4.76, the change in pH = 4.94 − 4.76 = 0.18 unit.

PRACTICE PROBLEMS

Calculations of Tonicity

1. Isotonic sodium chloride solution contains 0.9% w/v sodium chloride. If the *E*-value of boric acid is 0.52, calculate the percentage strength (w/v) of an isotonic solution of boric acid.
2. Sodium chloride is a 2-ion electrolyte, dissociating 90% in a certain concentration. Calculate (a) its dissociation factor and (b) the freezing point of a molal solution.
3. A solution of anhydrous dextrose (m.w. 180) contains 25 g in 500 mL of water. Calculate the freezing point of the solution.
4. Procaine hydrochloride (m.w. 273) is a 2-ion electrolyte, dissociating 80% in a certain concentration.
   (a) Calculate its dissociation factor.
   (b) Calculate its sodium chloride equivalent.
   (c) Calculate the freezing point of a molal solution of procaine hydrochloride.
5. The freezing point of a molal solution of a nonelectrolyte is −1.86°C. What is the freezing point of a 0.1% solution of zinc chloride (m.w. 136), dissociating 80%? (For lack of more definite information, assume that the volume of the molal solution is approximately 1 liter.)
6. ℞

Ephedrine sulfate	0.3 g
Sodium chloride	qs
Purified water ad	30 mL
Make isoton. sol.	
Sig. use as directed	

   How many milligrams of sodium chloride should be used in compounding the prescription?

7. ℞

Benoxinate hydrochloride	0.4% w/v
Fluorescein sodium	0.25% w/v
Sodium chloride	qs
Purified water qs	30 mL
Make isoton. sol.	
Sig. use in the eye	

   How much sodium chloride should be used in compounding the prescription?

8. ℞

Zinc sulfate	0.06 g
Boric acid	qs
Purified water ad	30 mL
Make isoton. sol.	
Sig. drop in eyes	

   How much boric acid should be used in compounding the prescription?

9. ℞

Cromolyn sodium	4% (w/v)
Benzalkonium chloride	1:10,000 (w/v)
Buffer solution (pH 5.6)	qs
Water for injection ad	10 mL
Sig. one (1) drop in each eye b.i.d.	

   How many milliliters of the buffer solution ($E = 0.30$) should be used to render the solution isotonic? (For lack of more definite information, assume that the specific gravity of the buffer solution is 1.)

10. Dextrose, anhydrous 2.5%
    Sodium chloride qs
    Sterile water for injection ad 1000 mL
    Label: Isotonic dextrose and saline solution
    How many grams of sodium chloride should be used in preparing the solution?
11. A sterile ophthalmic preparation contains 0.6% besifloxacin ($E = 0.08$) in a 5-mL container. Calculate the quantity of sodium chloride required for isotonicity.
12. Calculate the *effective quantity (g) of sodium chloride related to tonicity* in 100 mL of an intravenous fluid labeled "5% dextrose in 0.45% sodium chloride," and indicate whether the solution is isotonic, hypotonic, or hypertonic.
13. ℞ Brimonidine tartrate 30 mg
    Timolol maleate 75 mg
    Chlorobutanol 50 mg
    Sodium chloride qs
    Purified water qs 15 mL
    Make isoton. sol.
    Sig. for the eye
    How many milligrams of sodium chloride should be used in compounding the prescription?
14. ℞ Tetracaine hydrochloride 0.1 g
    Zinc sulfate 0.05 g
    Boric acid qs
    Purified water ad 30 mL
    Make isoton. sol.
    Sig. drop in eye
    How much boric acid should be used in compounding the prescription?
15. ℞ Sol. homatropine hydrobromide 1% 15 mL
    Make isoton. sol. with boric acid
    Sig. for the eye
    How many milligrams of boric acid should be used in compounding the prescription?
16. ℞ Procaine Hydrochloride 1%
    Sodium Chloride qs
    Sterile Water for Injection ad 100
    Make isoton. sol.
    Sig. For injection.
    How many grams of sodium chloride should be used in compounding the prescription?
17. ℞ Phenylephrine hydrochloride 1%
    Chlorobutanol 0.5%
    Sodium chloride qs
    Purified water ad 15 mL
    Make isoton. sol.
    Sig. use as directed
    How many milliliters of a 0.9% solution of sodium chloride should be used in compounding the prescription?

18. ℞ Oxymetazoline hydrochloride ½%
Boric acid solution qs
Purified water ad 15 mL
Make isoton. sol.
Sig. for the nose, as decongestant

How many milliliters of a 5% solution of boric acid should be used in compounding the prescription?

19. ℞ Ephedrine hydrochloride 0.5 g
Chlorobutanol 0.25 g
Dextrose, monohydrate qs
Rose water ad 50 mL
Make isoton. sol.
Sig. nose drops

How many grams of dextrose monohydrate should be used in compounding the prescription?

20. ℞ Naphazoline hydrochloride 1%
Sodium chloride qs
Purified water ad 30 mL
Make isoton. sol.
Sig. use as directed in the eye

How many milligrams of sodium chloride should be used in compounding the prescription? Use the freezing point depression method or the sodium chloride equivalent method.

21. ℞ Moxifloxacin hydrochloride 110 mg
Chlorobutanol 50 mg
Sodium chloride qs
Purified water ad 20 mL
Make isoton. sol.
Sig. eye drops

How many milligrams of sodium chloride should be used in compounding the prescription?

22. How many milligrams of sodium chloride may be used in the preparation of 15 mL of an eye drop containing 1% tropicamide and 0.5% chlorobutanol to render the solution isotonic with tears?
(a) 18 mg
(b) 31.5 mg
(c) 103.5 mg
(d) 135 mg

23. ℞ Monobasic sodium phosphate, anhydrous 5.6 g
Dibasic sodium phosphate, anhydrous 2.84 g
Sodium chloride qs
Purified water ad 1000 mL
Label: Isotonic buffer solution, pH 6.5

How many grams of sodium chloride should be used in preparing the solution?

24. How many grams of anhydrous dextrose should be used in preparing 1 liter of a ½% isotonic ephedrine sulfate nasal spray?

25. ℞ Xylometazoline hydrochloride 0.8% w/v
Chlorobutanol 0.5% w/v
Purified water qs 100 mL
Make isoton. sol. and buffer to pH 6.5
Sig. nose drops

You have on hand an isotonic buffered solution, pH 6.5. How many milliliters of purified water and how many milliliters of the buffered solution should be used in compounding the prescription?

26. ℞ Tobramycin 0.75%
Tetracaine hydrochloride Sol. 2% 15 mL
Sodium chloride qs
Purified water ad 30 mL
Make isoton. sol.
Sig. for the eye

The 2% solution of tetracaine hydrochloride is already isotonic. How many milliliters of a 0.9% solution of sodium chloride should be used in compounding the prescription?

27. Determine if the following commercial products are hypotonic, isotonic, or hypertonic:
   (a) An ophthalmic solution containing 40 mg/mL of cromolyn sodium and 0.01% of benzalkonium chloride in purified water.
   (b) A parenteral infusion containing 20% (w/v) of mannitol.
   (c) A 500-mL large volume parenteral containing D5W (5% w/v of anhydrous dextrose in sterile water for injection).
28. For agents having the following sodium chloride equivalents, calculate the percentage concentration of an isotonic solution:
   (a) 0.20
   (b) 0.32
   (c) 0.61
29. How many milliliters each of purified water and an isotonic sodium chloride solution should be used to prepare 30 mL of a 1% w/v isotonic solution of fentanyl citrate ($E = 0.11$)?
30. Using the E-values in Table 11.1, calculate the number of milliliters of water required to make an isotonic solution from 0.3 g of each of the following:
   (a) Antipyrine
   (b) Chlorobutanol
   (c) Ephedrine sulfate
   (d) Silver nitrate
   (e) Zinc sulfate
31. Calculate the E-values for each of the following, given that the number of milliliters of water shown will produce an isotonic solution from 0.3 g of drug substance.
   (a) Apomorphine hydrochloride, 4.7 mL water
   (b) Aminocaproic acid, 8.7 mL water
   (c) Prilocaine hydrochloride, 7.7 mL water
   (d) Procainamide hydrochloride, 7.3 mL water
   (e) Gentamicin sulfate, 1.7 mL water

32. COSOPT ophthalmic solution contains dorzolamide hydrochloride 22.26 mg/mL, timolol maleate 6.83 mg/mL, benzalkonium chloride 0.0075% w/v, and mannitol for tonicity.[13] Dorzolamide hydrochloride has a molecular weight of 360.91 and is a 2-ion electrolyte that dissociates 78% in a certain concentration. The *E*-values for the other ingredients can be found in Table 11.1. How much of each ingredient would be needed to prepare enough solution to fill five hundred 10-mL bottles?

Calculations of Buffer Solutions

33. The dissociation constant of ethanolamine is 2.77×10^{-5} at 25°C. Calculate its pK_b value.
34. What is the pH of a buffer solution prepared with 0.055 M sodium acetate and 0.01 M acetic acid? The pK_a value of acetic acid is 4.76 at 25°C.
35. What molar ratio of salt to acid would be required to prepare a buffer solution with a pH of 4.5? The pK_a value of the acid is 4.05 at 25°C.
36. What is the change in pH on adding 0.02 mol of sodium hydroxide to a liter of a buffer solution containing 0.5 M of sodium acetate and 0.5 M acetic acid? The pK_a value of acetic acid is 4.76 at 25°C.
37. The molar ratio of salt to acid needed to prepare a sodium acetate–acetic acid buffer solution is 1:1. Assuming that the total buffer concentration is 0.1 mol/L, how many grams of sodium acetate (m.w. 82) should be used in preparing 2 liters of the solution?
38. What is the change in pH with the addition of 0.01 mol hydrochloric acid to a liter of a buffer solution containing 0.05 M of ammonia and 0.05 M of ammonium chloride? The K_b value of ammonia is 1.80×10^{-5} at 25°C.
39. Calculate the pH of the following buffer:

Sodium phosphate, dibasic	6.2 g
Sodium phosphate, monobasic	4.5 g
Water qs	1000 mL

The pK_a value of sodium phosphate monobasic is 7.21 at 25°C and serves as an acid in this buffer because it is more acidic than sodium phosphate dibasic. The molecular weight of sodium phosphate monobasic is 120 and of sodium phosphate dibasic is 142.

40. What is the pH change in the buffer in problem 39 if 3 mL of a 5-M hydrochloric acid solution are added to the buffer? Assume negligible volume displacement by the hydrochloric acid solution.

CALCQUIZ

11.A. A 3-mL container of a 0.5% ophthalmic solution of moxifloxacin hydrochloride (m.w. 401; *i* = 1.8) is prepared in an aqueous solution of 0.45% sodium chloride. Calculate the quantity, in milligrams, of boric acid required to render the solution isotonic.

11.B. How many grams of boric acid should be used to render this prescription isotonic?

℞ Tetracaine hydrochloride	0.5%
0.1% Epinephrine bitartrate in NSS	10 mL
Boric acid, qs	
Purified water, ad	30 mL

11.C. A formulation pharmacist has developed an injection for dental local anesthesia that contains the following agents:

Lidocaine hydrochloride	1%
Epinephrine bitartrate	1:50,000
Sodium chloride	6.5 mg/mL
Potassium metabisulfite	1.2 mg/mL
Edetate disodium	0.25 mg/mL
Sterile purified water, ad	1.7 mL

Using the following data, determine the *total tonic effect,* expressed in terms of percent strength of "sodium chloride" or its equivalent.
Lidocaine hydrochloride ($E = 0.2$)
Epinephrine bitartrate ($E = 0.18$)
Potassium metabisulfite (m.w. 222; $i = 2.6$)
Edetate disodium (m.w. 372; $i = 2.6$)

11.D. A FLEET saline enema delivers in each 118 mL 19 g monobasic sodium phosphate (monohydrate) and 7 g dibasic sodium phosphate (heptahydrate). Calculate the product's percent strength in terms of "sodium chloride or its equivalent," and indicate whether the enema is hypotonic, isotonic, or hypertonic.

11.E. What would be the pH of a buffer solution prepared with 0.5 M dibasic sodium phosphate and 1 M monobasic sodium phosphate? The pK_a of monobasic sodium phosphate is 7.21 at 25°C.

ANSWERS TO "CASE IN POINT" AND PRACTICE PROBLEMS

Case in Point 11.1

(a) 60 mL × 2.5% w/v = 1.5 g amikacin sulfate

(b) Sodium chloride m.w. = 58.5
Amikacin m.w. = 781.76

$$i = 2.6$$

$$\frac{58.5}{1.8} \times \frac{2.6}{781.76} = E$$

$$E = 0.108$$

(c) 60 mL × 0.9% w/v = 0.54 g sodium chloride
1.5 g (amikacin sulfate) × 0.108 (NaCl equivalent) = 0.162 g
0.54 g − 0.162 g = 0.378 g sodium chloride required for isotonicity

(d) $\frac{23.5\text{ g}}{100\text{ mL}} = \frac{0.378\text{ g}}{\text{x mL}}$;

x = 1.61 mL sodium chloride injection

Case in Point 11.2

(a) On the basis of 80% dissociation, 100 particles of tobramycin sulfate will yield:
80 × 2 = 160 tobramycin ions
80 × 5 = 400 sulfate ions
20 undissociated particles
580 total particles

$$i = \frac{580 \text{ particles}}{100 \text{ particles}} = 5.8$$

$$\text{E-value} = \frac{58.5}{1.8} \times \frac{5.8}{1425.45} = 0.132$$

(b) $$300 \text{ mg tobramycin sulfate} \times \frac{634 \text{ mcg tobramycin}}{1 \text{ mg tobramycin sulface}} \times \frac{1 \text{ mg}}{1000 \text{ mcg}}$$
$$= 190.2 \text{ mg tobramycin}$$

$$300 \text{ mg tobramycin sulfate} \times \frac{739 \text{ mcg tobramycin}}{1 \text{ mg tobramycin sulfate}} \times \frac{1 \text{ mg}}{1000 \text{ mcg}}$$
$$= 221.7 \text{ mg tobramycin}$$

Amount range = 190.2 to 221.7 mg tobramycin activity

(c) $$\text{E-value} = \frac{58.5}{1.8} \times \frac{1.8}{318.13} = 0.184$$

(d) 300 mg tobramycin sulfate × 0.132 = 39.6 mg sodium chloride equivalent
100 mg diclofenac sodium × 0.184 = 18.4 mg sodium chloride equivalent
39.6 mg + 18.4 mg + 806 mg = 864 mg sodium chloride equivalent

Since 100 mL of an isotonic solution would contain 0.9 g or 900 mg of sodium chloride, the solution is slightly hypotonic. According to the calculations of *E*-values for the ingredients, an additional 900 mg – 864 mg = 36 mg of sodium chloride should be added.

(e) $$\text{Formula conversion factor} = \frac{20 \text{ mL}}{100 \text{ mL}} = 0.2$$

Tobramycin sulfate: 300 mg × 0.2 = 60 mg
Diclofenac sodium: 100 mg × 0.2 = 20 mg
Sodium chloride: 806 mg × 0.2 = 161.2 mg
Sterile water for injection: qs 20 mL

(f) $$60 \text{ mg} \times \frac{2 \text{ mL}}{80 \text{ mg}} = 1.5 \text{ mL of injectable solution}$$

Practice Problems

1. 1.73% w/v
2. (a) 1.9
   (b) –3.53°C
3. –0.52°C
4. (a) 1.8
   (b) 0.21
   (c) –3.35°C
5. –0.036°C
6. 210 mg sodium chloride
7. 226.35 mg sodium chloride
8. 500.77 mg boric acid
9. 0.113 mL buffer solution
10. 4.5 g sodium chloride
11. 42.6 mg sodium chloride
12. 1.35 g sodium chloride, hypertonic
13. 108.6 mg sodium chloride
14. 469.23 mg boric acid
15. 210.58 mg boric acid

16. 0.69 g sodium chloride
17. 7.67 mL sodium chloride solution
18. 4.56 mL boric acid solution
19. 1.53 g dextrose monohydrate
20. 186.21 mg sodium chloride (freezing point method) or 189 mg sodium chloride (sodium chloride equivalent method)
21. 153.7 mg sodium chloride
22. (c) 103.5 mg sodium chloride
23. 4.751 g sodium chloride
24. 44.44 g anhydrous dextrose
25. qs 32 mL purified water
    68 mL buffered solution
26. 13.25 mL sodium chloride solution
27. (a) Hypotonic
    (b) Hypertonic
    (c) Isotonic
28. (a) 4.5%
    (b) 2.81%
    (c) 1.48%
29. 3.67 mL purified water
    26.33 mL sodium chloride solution
30. (a) qs 5.67 mL water
    (b) qs 8 mL water
    (c) qs 6.67 mL water
    (d) qs 11 mL water
    (e) qs 5.33 mL water
31. (a) 0.14
    (b) 0.26
    (c) 0.23
    (d) 0.22
    (e) 0.051
32. 111.3 g dorzolamide ride, 34.15 g timolc 375 mg benzalkoniur 127.89 g mannitol
33. 4.56
34. 5.5
35. 2.82:1
36. 0.03 unit
37. 8.2 g
38. 0.18 unit
39. 7.28
40. 0.33 unit

References

1. Ingham A, Poon CY. Tonicity, osmoticity, osmolality, and osmolarity. In: Allen LV, ed. *Remington: The Science and Practice of Pharmacy*. Vol. 22. Philadelphia, PA: Pharmaceutical Press; 2013:641–646.
2. Ansel HC, Prince SJ. *Pharmaceutical Calculations: The Pharmacist's Handbook*. Baltimore, MD: Lippincott Williams & Wilkins; 2004:111.
3. Pharmaceutical Dosage Forms. US Pharmacopeial Convention, Inc. *United States Pharmacopeia 21–National Formulary 16*. Rockville, MD: US Pharmacopeial Convention, Inc.; 1985.
4. Allen LV, Ansel HC. *Ansel's Pharmaceutical Dosage Forms and Drug Delivery Systems*. Vol. 10. Baltimore, MD: Lippincott Williams & Wilkins; 2014:612.
5. Titcomb LC. Topical ocular antibiotics: part 2. *Pharmaceutical Journal* 2000;264:441–445.
6. Garg P, Sharma S, Rao GN. Ciprofloxacin-resistant *pseudomonas keratitis*. *Ophthalmology* 1999;106: 1319–1323.
7. Matoba AY. Polymicrobial keratitis secondary to *Burholderia ambifaria*, enterococcus, and *staphylococcus aureus* in a patient with herpetic stromal keratitis. *American Journal of Ophthalmology* 2003;136:748–749.
8. Chung MS, Goldstein MH, Driebe WT, et. al. *Mycobacterium chelonae* keratitis after laser in situ keratomileusis successfully treated with medical therapy and flap removal. *American Journal of Ophthalmology* 2000;129:382–384.
9. Chandra NS, Torres MF, Winthrop KL, et. al. Cluster of *Mycobacterium Chelonae* keratitis cases following laser in-situ keratomileusis. *American Journal of Ophthalmology* 2001;132:819–830.
10. Ford JG, Huang AJW, Pflugfelder SC, et. al. Nontuberculous mycobacterial keratitis in south Florida. *Ophthalmology* 1998;105:1652–1658.
11. Allen LV. Tobramycin sulfate 0.3% and diclofenac sodium 0.1% ophthalmic solution. *International Journal of Pharmaceutical Compounding* 2010;14:74.
12. Buffer Solutions. US Pharmacopeial Convention, Inc. *United States Pharmacopeia 37-National Formulary 32 [book online]*. Rockville, MD: US Pharmacopeial Convention, Inc.; 2014.
13. Cosopt (dorzolamide hydrochloride-timolol maleate ophthalmic solution) [product label information]. U.S. Food and Drug Administration. Department of Health and Human Services. [U.S. Food and Drug Administration Website.] Available at: http://www.accessdata.fda.gov/drugsatfda_docs/label/2010/020869s036lbl.pdf. Accessed January 9, 2015.

12

Electrolyte Solutions: Milliequivalents, Millimoles, and Milliosmoles

OBJECTIVES

Upon successful completion of this chapter, the student will be able to:

- Determine the molecular weight of an electrolyte from atomic or formula weights as well as the valence and the number of ions produced upon dissociation.
- Calculate problems involving milliequivalents and apply these principles to products used for electrolyte replacement.
- Calculate problems involving millimoles and micromoles and understand their use in pharmacy practice.
- Calculate problems involving milliosmoles and osmolarity and apply these principles to solutions primarily used for intravenous infusions.

As noted in Chapter 11, the molecules of chemical compounds in solution may remain intact, or they may dissociate into particles known as ***ions***, which carry an electric charge. Substances that are not dissociated in solution are called ***nonelectrolytes*** and those with varying degrees of dissociation are called ***electrolytes***. Urea and dextrose are examples of nonelectrolytes in body water; sodium chloride in body fluids is an example of an electrolyte.

Electrolyte ions in the blood plasma include the cations Na^+, K^+, Ca^{2+}, and Mg^{2+} and the anions Cl^-, HCO_3^-, HPO_4^{2-}, SO_4^{2-}, organic acids, and protein. Electrolytes in body fluids play an important role in maintaining the acid–base balance. They also play a part in controlling body water volumes and help regulate metabolism.

Applicable Dosage Forms

Electrolyte preparations are used in the treatment of disturbances of the electrolyte and fluid balance in the body. They are provided by the pharmacy as oral solutions, syrups, tablets, capsules, and, when necessary, intravenous infusions.

Milliequivalents

A *chemical unit*, the ***milliequivalent (mEq)***, is used almost exclusively in the United States by clinicians, physicians, pharmacists, and manufacturers to express the concentration of electrolytes in solution. This unit of measure is related to the total number of ionic charges in solution, and it takes note of the valence of the ions. In other words, it is a unit of measurement of the amount of *chemical activity* of an electrolyte.

Table 12.1 • BLOOD PLASMA ELECTROLYTES IN MILLIEQUIVALENTS PER LITER (mEq/L)

Cations	mEq/L	Anions	mEq/L
Na^+	142	HCO_3^-	24
K^+	5	Cl^-	105
Ca^{2+}	5	HPO_4^{2-}	2
Mg^{2+}	2	SO_4^{2-}	1
		Org. Ac.⁻	6
		Proteinate⁻	16
	154		154

Under normal conditions, blood plasma contains 154 mEq of cations and an equal number of anions (Table 12.1). However, it should be understood that normal laboratory values of electrolytes vary, albeit within a rather narrow range, as shown in Table 12.2. The total concentration of cations always equals the total concentration of anions. Any number of milliequivalents of Na^+, K^+, or any cation always reacts with precisely the same number of milliequivalents of Cl^-, HCO_3^-, or any anion. ***For a given chemical compound, the milliequivalents of cation equals the milliequivalents of anion equals the milliequivalents of the chemical compound.***

In preparing a solution of K^+ ions, a potassium salt is dissolved in water. In addition to the K^+ ions, the solution will also contain negatively charged ions. These two components will be chemically equal, in that the milliequivalents of one are equal to the milliequivalents of the other. Dissolving 40 mEq of potassium chloride in water results in a solution that contains 40 mEq of K^+ per liter *and* 40 mEq of Cl^-. Interestingly, the solution will *not* contain the *same weight* of each ion.

A milliequivalent represents the amount, in milligrams, of a solute equal to 1/1000 of its gram equivalent weight, taking into account the valence of the ions. The milliequivalent expresses the chemical activity or combining power of a substance relative to the activity of 1 mg of hydrogen. Thus, based on the atomic weight and valence of the species, 1 mEq is represented by 1 mg of hydrogen, 20 mg of calcium, 23 mg of sodium, 35.5 mg of chlorine, 39 mg of potassium, and so forth.

A key element in converting between the *weight* of an electrolyte (i.e., milligrams) and its *chemical activity* (i.e., milliequivalents) is the valence of the substance, and the total valence of the cation or anion in the compound must be taken into account. Sodium chloride, for example, has a total valence of one because there is one sodium cation with a +1 charge and

Table 12.2 • USUAL REFERENCE RANGE OF BLOOD SERUM VALUES FOR SOME ELECTROLYTES[a]

Cation/Anion	mEq/L	SI Units (mmol/L)
Sodium	135–145	135–145
Potassium	3.5–5.5	3.5–5.5
Calcium	4.6–5.5	2.3–2.75
Magnesium	1.5–2.5	0.75–1.25
Chloride	96–106	96–106
Carbon dioxide	24–30	24–30
Phosphorus	2.5–4.5	0.8–1.5

[a]Reference ranges may vary slightly between clinical laboratories based, in part, on the analytical methods and equipment used.

Table 12.3 • VALUES FOR SOME IMPORTANT IONS

Ion	Formula	Valence	Atomic or Formula Weight	Equivalent Weight[a]
Aluminum	Al^{3+}	3	27	9
Ammonium	NH_4^+	1	18	18
Calcium	Ca^{2+}	2	40	20
Ferric	Fe^{3+}	3	56	18.7
Ferrous	Fe^{2+}	2	56	28
Lithium	Li^+	1	7	7
Magnesium	Mg^{2+}	2	24	12
Potassium	K^+	1	39	39
Sodium	Na^+	1	23	23
Acetate	$C_2H_3O_2^-$	1	59	59
Bicarbonate	HCO_3^-	1	61	61
Carbonate	CO_3^{2-}	2	60	30
Chloride	Cl^-	1	35.5	35.5
Citrate	$C_6H_5O_7^{3-}$	3	189	63
Gluconate	$C_6H_{11}O_7^-$	1	195	195
Hydroxide	OH^-	1	17	17
Lactate	$C_6H_5O_3^-$	1	89	89
Phosphate, monobasic	$H_2PO_4^-$	1	97	97
Phosphate, dibasic	HPO_4^{2-}	2	96	48
Sulfate	SO_4^{2-}	2	96	48

[a] $\text{Equivalent weight} = \dfrac{\text{Atomic or formula weight}}{\text{Valence}}$

one chloride anion with a –1 charge in the compound. However, sodium citrate has a total valence of three because there are three sodium ions with a +1 charge (for a total of +3) and one citrate ion with a –3 charge. Knowing the valence of various compounds is essential in the calculation of milliequivalents. Important values for some ions are presented in Table 12.3, and a complete listing of atomic weights is provided on the back pages of this text.

Example Calculations of Milliequivalents

The following conversion can be used to convert milligrams to milliequivalents and vice versa:

$$\frac{\text{Molecular weight}}{\text{Valence}} = \frac{\text{mg}}{\text{mEq}}$$

(1) A physician prescribes 10 mEq of potassium chloride for a patient. How many milligrams of KCl would provide the prescribed quantity?

$$\text{Molecular weight of KCl} = 39\ (K^+) + 35.5\ (Cl^-) = 74.5$$

$$\text{Valence} = 1$$

$$\text{Conversion} = \frac{74.5\text{ mg}}{1\text{ mEq}}$$

$$10\text{ mEq} \times \frac{74.5\text{ mg}}{1\text{ mEq}} = \mathbf{745\ mg}$$

(2) *If a patient is prescribed 300 mg of potassium chloride, what is the corresponding mEq?*
See example problem 1 for molecular weight and conversion for KCl.

$$300\ \text{mg} \times \frac{1\ \text{mEq}}{74.5\ \text{mg}} = \mathbf{4.03\ mEq}$$

(3) *A physician prescribes 3 mEq/kg of NaCl to be administered to a 165-lb patient. How many milliliters of a half-normal saline solution (0.45% NaCl) should be administered?*

$$\text{Molecular weight of NaCl} = 23\ (Na^+) + 35.5\ (Cl^-) = 58.5$$

$$\text{Valence} = 1$$

$$\text{Conversion} = \frac{58.5\ \text{mg}}{1\ \text{mEq}}$$

$$\frac{3\ \text{mEq}}{\text{kg}} \times \frac{1\ \text{kg}}{2.2\ \text{lb}} \times 165\ \text{lb} = 225\ \text{mEq}$$

$$225\ \text{mEq} \times \frac{58.5\ \text{mg}}{1\ \text{mEq}} \times \frac{1\ \text{g}}{1000\ \text{mg}} = 13.16\ \text{g}$$

$$13.16\ \text{g} \times \frac{100\ \text{mL}}{0.45\ \text{g}} = \mathbf{2925\ mL}\ \text{of 0.45\% NaCl solution}$$

(4) *What is the concentration, in milligrams per milliliter, of a solution containing 2 mEq of potassium chloride (KCl) per milliliter?*
See example problem 1 for molecular weight and conversion for KCl.

$$\frac{2\ \text{mEq}}{\text{mL}} \times \frac{74.5\ \text{mg}}{1\ \text{mEq}} = \mathbf{149\ mg/mL}$$

(5) *What is the concentration, in grams per milliliter, of a solution containing 4 mEq of calcium chloride ($CaCl_2 \cdot 2H_2O$) per milliliter?*

$$\text{Molecular weight of } CaCl_2 \cdot 2H_2O = 40\ (Ca^{2+}) + [2 \times 35.5(Cl^-)] + [2 \times 18\ (H_2O)] = 147$$

$$\text{Valence} = 2$$

$$\text{Conversion} = \frac{147\ \text{mg}}{2\ \text{mEq}}$$

NOTE: The water of hydration molecules should be accounted for in the molecular weight but does not interfere in determination of valence.

$$\frac{4\ \text{mEq}}{\text{mL}} \times \frac{147\ \text{mg}}{2\ \text{mEq}} \times \frac{1\ \text{g}}{1000\ \text{mg}} = \mathbf{0.29\ g/mL}$$

(6) *What is the percent (w/v) concentration of a solution containing 100 mEq of ammonium chloride per liter?*

$$\text{Molecular weight of } NH_4Cl = 18\ (NH_4^+) + 35.5\ (Cl^-) = 53.5$$

$$\text{Valence} = 1$$

$$\text{Conversion} = \frac{53.5\ \text{mg}}{1\ \text{mEq}}$$

$$\frac{100\ \text{mEq}}{\text{L}} \times \frac{53.5\ \text{mg}}{1\ \text{mEq}} \times \frac{1\ \text{g}}{1000\ \text{mg}} \times \frac{1\ \text{L}}{1000\ \text{mL}} \times 100 = \mathbf{0.54\%\ w/v}$$

(7) *A solution contains 10 mg/100 mL of K^+ ions. Express this concentration in terms of milliequivalents per liter.*

$$\text{Molecular weight of } K^+ = 39$$

$$\text{Valence} = 1$$

$$\text{Conversion} = \frac{39 \text{ mg}}{1 \text{ mEq}}$$

$$\frac{10 \text{ mg}}{100 \text{ mL}} \times \frac{1 \text{ mEq}}{39 \text{ mg}} \times \frac{1000 \text{ mL}}{\text{L}} = \mathbf{2.56\ mEq/L}$$

(8) *A solution contains 10 mg/100 mL of Ca^{2+} ions. Express this concentration in terms of milliequivalents per liter.*

$$\text{Molecular weight of } Ca^{2+} = 40$$

$$\text{Valence} = 2$$

$$\text{Conversion} = \frac{40 \text{ mg}}{2 \text{ mEq}}$$

$$\frac{10 \text{ mg}}{100 \text{ mL}} \times \frac{2 \text{ mEq}}{40 \text{ mg}} \times \frac{1000 \text{ mL}}{\text{L}} = \mathbf{5\ mEq/L}$$

(9) *A magnesium (Mg^{2+}) level in blood plasma is determined to be 2.5 mEq/L. Express this concentration in terms of milligrams per liter.*

$$\text{Molecular weight of } Mg^{2+} = 24$$

$$\text{Valence} = 2$$

$$\text{Conversion} = \frac{24 \text{ mg}}{2 \text{ mEq}}$$

$$\frac{2.5 \text{ mEq}}{\text{L}} \times \frac{24 \text{ mg}}{2 \text{ mEq}} = \mathbf{30\ mg/L}$$

(10) *An aluminum hydroxide gel suspension contains 320 mg of aluminum hydroxide in each teaspoonful dose. How many milliequivalents of aluminum would a patient receive each day if he is ingesting two teaspoonfuls of the suspension four times daily?*

$$\text{Molecular weight of } Al(OH)_3 = 27\,(Al^{3+}) + [3 \times 17\,(OH^-)] = 78$$

$$\text{Valence} = 3$$

$$\text{Conversion} = \frac{78 \text{ mg}}{3 \text{ mEq}}$$

$$\frac{320 \text{ mg } Al(OH)_3}{\text{tsp}} \times \frac{2 \text{ tsp}}{\text{dose}} \times \frac{4 \text{ doses}}{\text{day}} = 2560 \text{ mg } Al(OH)_3/\text{day}$$

$$\frac{2560 \text{ mg } Al(OH)_3}{\text{day}} \times \frac{3 \text{ mEq}}{78 \text{ mg}} = 98.46 \text{ mEq } Al(OH)_3/\text{day}$$

$$= \mathbf{98.46\ mEq\ Al^{3+}/day}$$

(11) *How many milliequivalents of magnesium are represented in an 8-mL dose of an injectable solution containing 50% w/v magnesium sulfate heptahydrate?*

$$\text{Molecular weight of } MgSO_4 \cdot 7H_2O = 24\,(Mg^{2+}) + 96\,(SO_4^{\,2-}) + [7 \times 18\,(H_2O)] = 246$$

$$\text{Valence} = 2$$

$$\text{Conversion} = \frac{246 \text{ mg}}{2 \text{ mEq}}$$

$$8 \text{ mL} \times \frac{50 \text{ g } MgSO_4 \cdot 7H_2O}{100 \text{ mL}} \times \frac{1000 \text{ mg}}{1 \text{ g}} = 4000 \text{ mg } MgSO_4 \cdot 7H_2O$$

$$4000 \text{ mg } MgSO_4 \cdot 7H_2O \times \frac{2 \text{ mEq}}{246 \text{ mg}} = 32.52 \text{ mEq } MgSO_4 \cdot 7H_2O$$

$$= \mathbf{32.52 \text{ mEq } Mg^{2+}}$$

(12) *How many milliequivalents of Na^+ would be contained in a 30-mL dose of the following solution?*

Sodium phosphate, dibasic, heptahydrate	18 g
Sodium phosphate, monobasic, monohydrate	48 g
Purified water ad	100 mL

Each salt is considered separately in solving the problem.
Sodium phosphate, dibasic, heptahydrate:

$$\text{Molecular weight of } Na_2HPO_4 \cdot 7H_2O = [2 \times 23\,(Na^+)] + 96\,(HPO4^{2-}) + [7 \times 18\,(H_2O)] = 268$$

$$\text{Valence} = 2$$

$$\text{Conversion} = \frac{268 \text{ mg}}{2 \text{ mEq}}$$

$$\frac{18 \text{ g } Na_2HPO_4 \cdot 7H_2O}{100 \text{ mL}} \times \frac{30 \text{ mL}}{\text{dose}} = 5.4 \text{ g } Na_2HPO_4 \cdot 7H_2O/\text{dose}$$

$$\frac{5.4 \text{ g } Na_2HPO_4 \cdot 7H_2O}{\text{dose}} \times \frac{1000 \text{ mg}}{1 \text{ g}} \times \frac{2 \text{ mEq}}{268 \text{ mg}} = 40.3 \text{ mEq } Na_2HPO_4 \cdot 7H_2O/\text{dose}$$

$$= 40.3 \text{ mEq } Na^+/\text{dose}$$

Sodium phosphate, monobasic, monohydrate:

$$\text{Molecular weight of } NaH_2PO_4 \cdot H_2O = 23\,(Na^+) + 97\,(H_2PO_4^{\,-}) + 18\,(H_2O) = 138$$

$$\text{Valence} = 1$$

$$\text{Conversion} = \frac{138 \text{ mg}}{1 \text{ mEq}}$$

$$\frac{48 \text{ g } NaH_2PO_4 \cdot H_2O}{100 \text{ mL}} \times \frac{30 \text{ mL}}{\text{dose}} = 14.4 \text{ g } NaH_2PO_4 \cdot H_2O/\text{dose}$$

$$\frac{14.4\text{g } NaH_2PO_4 \cdot H_2O}{\text{dose}} \times \frac{1000 \text{ mg}}{1\text{g}} \times \frac{1 \text{ mEq}}{138\text{mg}} = 104.35 \text{ mEq } NaII_2PO_4 \cdot II_2O/\text{dose}$$

$$= 104.35 \text{ mEq } Na^+/\text{dose}$$

$$\text{Total} = 40.3 \text{ mEq } Na^+/\text{dose} + 104.35 \text{ mEq } Na^+/\text{dose} = \mathbf{144.65 \text{ mEq } Na^+/\text{dose}}$$

CASE IN POINT 12.1[a] A hospital pharmacist receives a medication order calling for 10 mEq of calcium to be added to a 500-mL bag of normal saline solution. The intravenous fluid is to be administered at a rate of 0.5 mEq of calcium per hour. The pharmacist has available 10-mL vials of a 10% injection of calcium chloride dihydrate. (a) How many milliliters of this injection should be added to the bag of IV fluid to make the desired product? (b) If the nurse administering the IV fluid uses an intravenous set that delivers 12 drops/mL, how many drops per minute should be delivered to provide the desired dose?

[a]Problem courtesy of Flynn Warren, Bishop, GA.

CASE IN POINT 12.2 A patient is to receive 0.12 mEq of ferrous gluconate per kilogram of body weight each day divided into three doses. (a) If the patient weighs 132 lb, how many milliliters of a compounded syrup containing 300 mg of ferrous gluconate per teaspoonful should be administered for each dose? (b) How much ferrous gluconate would be needed to prepare 6 fl. oz. of the compounded syrup?

Millimoles and Micromoles

Molar concentrations [as millimoles per liter (mmol/L) and micromoles per liter (μmol/L or mcmol/L)] are used in the International System (SI), which is employed in European countries and in many others throughout the world. Milliequivalents are used almost exclusively in the United States to express concentrations of electrolyte ions in a solution; however, millimoles and micromoles are sometimes used in expressions of clinical laboratory values. In some electrolyte solutions, determining the valence of the ions can be quite complicated, such as in the case of the phosphate ion, which can exist in a monovalent ($H_2PO_4^-$), divalent (HPO_4^{2-}), or trivalent (PO_4^{3-}) form. Millimoles are often used to express concentrations in these types of solutions as well.

A ***mole*** is the molecular weight of a substance in grams. A ***millimole*** is one-thousandth of a mole and is, therefore, the molecular weight of a substance in milligrams. Similarly, a ***micromole*** is one-millionth of a mole, which is the molecular weight of a substance in micrograms. For example, the molecular weight of sodium chloride is 58.5 g/mol but can be converted to milligrams and millimoles as follows:

$$\frac{58.5 \text{ g}}{\text{mol}} \times \frac{1000 \text{ mg}}{\text{g}} \times \frac{1 \text{ mol}}{1000 \text{ mmol}} = 58.5 \text{ mg/mmol}$$

Similarly, the molecular weight can also be converted to micrograms and micromoles. Notice that millimolar conversions do not take into account the valence of an electrolyte as do milliequivalent conversions. Therefore, for monovalent species, the numeric values of the milliequivalent and millimole are identical. Similar to milliequivalents, the millimoles of the compound are equal to the millimoles of the cation, which are equal to the millimoles of the anion, but this does not hold true for the actual weights of the ions.

Example Calculations of Millimoles and Micromoles

The following conversion can be used to convert milligrams to millimoles and vice versa:

$$\text{molecular weight} = \frac{\text{mg}}{\text{mmol}}$$

The following conversion can be used to convert micrograms to micromoles and vice versa:

$$\text{molecular weight} = \frac{\text{mcg}}{\text{mcmol}}$$

(1) *How many millimoles of monobasic sodium phosphate monohydrate (m.w. 138) are present in 100 g of the substance?*

$$100\text{ g} \times \frac{1000\text{ mg}}{\text{g}} \times \frac{1\text{ mmol}}{138\text{ mg}} = \mathbf{724.64\ mmol}$$

(2) *What is the weight, in milligrams, of 5 mmol of potassium phosphate dibasic?*

$$\text{Molecular weight of } K_2HPO_4 = [2 \times 39\,(K^+)] + 96\,(HPO_4^{2-}) = 174$$

$$5\text{ mmol} \times \frac{174\text{ mg}}{1\text{ mmol}} = \mathbf{870\ mg}$$

(3) *Convert the trough plasma range of 0.5 μg/mL to 2 μg/mL for tobramycin (m.w. = 467.52) to μmol/L.*[1]

$$\frac{0.5\ \mu\text{g}}{1\text{ mL}} \times \frac{1\ \mu\text{mol}}{467.52\ \mu\text{g}} \times \frac{1000\text{ mL}}{1\text{ L}} = 1.07\ \mu\text{mol/L}$$

$$\frac{2\ \mu\text{g}}{1\text{ mL}} \times \frac{1\ \mu\text{mol}}{467.52\ \mu\text{g}} \times \frac{1000\text{ mL}}{1\text{ L}} = 4.28\ \mu\text{mol/L}$$

$$\text{Range} = \mathbf{1.07\ to\ 4.28\ \mu mol/L}$$

(4) *If lactated Ringer's injection contains 20 mg of calcium chloride dihydrate ($CaCl_2 \cdot 2H_2O$) in each 100 mL, calculate the millimoles of calcium present in 1 L of lactated Ringer's injection.*

$$\text{Molecular weight of } CaCl_2 \cdot 2H_2O = 40\,(Ca^{2+}) + [2 \times 35.5\,(Cl^-)] + [2 \times 18\,(H_2O)] = 147$$

$$\frac{20\text{ mg } CaCl_2 \cdot 2H_2O}{100\text{ mL}} \times \frac{1000\text{ mL}}{\text{L}} \times 1\text{ L} = 200\text{ mg } CaCl_2 \cdot 2H_2O$$

$$200\text{ mg } CaCl_2 \cdot 2H_2O \times \frac{1\text{ mmol}}{147\text{ mg } CaCl_2 \cdot 2H_2O} = 1.36\text{ mmol } CaCl_2 \cdot 2H_2O$$

$$= \mathbf{1.36\ mmol\ Ca^{2+}}$$

(5) *How many micromoles of calcium are present in each milliliter of lactated Ringer's injection?*

$$\frac{1.36\text{ mmol}}{\text{L}} \times \frac{1\text{ L}}{1000\text{ mL}} \times \frac{1000\text{ mcmol}}{\text{mmol}} = \mathbf{1.36\ mcmol/mL}$$

(6) *A patient is receiving a slow intravenous infusion containing 40 mEq of potassium chloride in 1000 mL of fluid. If, after 12 hours, 720 mL of infusion had been infused, how many millimoles of potassium chloride were administered?*

Molecular weight of KCl = 39 (K^+) + 35.5 (Cl^-) = 74.5

$$720 \text{ mL} \times \frac{40 \text{ mEq}}{1000 \text{ mL}} = 28.8 \text{ mEq of KCl administered}$$

$$28.8 \text{ mEq} \times \frac{74.5 \text{ mg}}{1 \text{ mEq}} \times \frac{1 \text{ mmol}}{74.5 \text{ mg}} = \mathbf{28.8 \text{ mmol}}$$

NOTE: Since potassium chloride is monovalent, the amount in milliequivalents and the amount in millimoles are the same.

(7) *A medication order calls for 1.8 g of potassium chloride in 60 mL of solution. How many millimoles of KCl are contained in each milliliter?*

See example problem 6 for molecular weight of KCl.

$$\frac{1.8 \text{ g}}{60 \text{ mL}} \times \frac{1000 \text{ mg}}{\text{g}} \times \frac{1 \text{ mmol}}{74.5 \text{ mg}} = \mathbf{0.403 \text{ mmol/mL}}$$

(8) *Calculate the concentrations in mmol/L for each of the following infusion solutions: (a) 5% NaCl, (b) 3% NaCl, (c) 0.9% NaCl (NSS), (d) 0.45% NaCl (half-NSS), and (e) 0.2% NaCl.*

(a) Molecular weight of NaCl = 23 (Na^+) + 35.5 (Cl^-) = 58.5

$$\frac{5 \text{ g}}{100 \text{ mL}} \times \frac{1000 \text{ mg}}{\text{g}} \times \frac{1000 \text{ mL}}{\text{L}} \times \frac{1 \text{ mmol}}{58.5 \text{ mg}} = \mathbf{854.7 \text{ mmol/L}}$$

(b) $$\frac{3 \text{ g}}{100 \text{ mL}} \times \frac{1000 \text{ mg}}{\text{g}} \times \frac{1000 \text{ mL}}{\text{L}} \times \frac{1 \text{ mmol}}{58.5 \text{ mg}} = \mathbf{512.82 \text{ mmol/L}}$$

(c) $$\frac{0.9 \text{ g}}{100 \text{ mL}} \times \frac{1000 \text{ mg}}{\text{g}} \times \frac{1000 \text{ mL}}{\text{L}} \times \frac{1 \text{ mmol}}{58.5 \text{ mg}} = \mathbf{153.85 \text{ mmol/L}}$$

(d) $$\frac{0.45 \text{ g}}{100 \text{ mL}} \times \frac{1000 \text{ mg}}{\text{g}} \times \frac{1000 \text{ mL}}{\text{L}} \times \frac{1 \text{ mmol}}{58.5 \text{ mg}} = \mathbf{76.92 \text{ mmol/L}}$$

(e) $$\frac{0.2 \text{ g}}{100 \text{ mL}} \times \frac{1000 \text{ mg}}{\text{g}} \times \frac{1000 \text{ mL}}{\text{L}} \times \frac{1 \text{ mmol}}{58.5 \text{ mg}} = \mathbf{34.19 \text{ mmol/L}}$$

Osmolarity

As indicated in Chapter 11, osmotic pressure is important to biologic processes that involve the diffusion of solutes or the transfer of fluids through semipermeable membranes. The labels of solutions that provide intravenous replenishment of fluid, nutrients, or electrolytes, and the osmotic diuretic mannitol are required to state the osmolar concentration. This information indicates to the practitioner whether the solution is hypoosmotic, isoosmotic, or hyperosmotic with regard to biologic fluids and membranes.

Osmotic pressure is proportional to the ***total number*** of particles in solution. The unit used to measure osmotic concentration is the ***milliosmole*** (mOsmol). For dextrose, a nonelectrolyte, 1 mmol (1 formula weight in milligrams) represents 1 mOsmol. This relationship is not the same with electrolytes, however, because the total number of particles in solution depends on the degree of dissociation of the substance in question. Assuming complete dissociation, 1 mmol of NaCl represents 2 mOsmol ($Na^+ + Cl^-$) of total particles, 1 mmol of $CaCl_2$ represents 3 mOsmol ($Ca^{2+} + 2Cl^-$) of total particles, and 1 mmol of sodium citrate ($Na_3C_6H_5O_7$) represents 4 mOsmol ($3Na^+ + C_6H_5O_7^-$) of total particles.

The milliosmolar value of *separate* ions of an electrolyte may be obtained by dividing the concentration, in milligrams per liter, of the ion by its atomic weight. The milliosmolar value of the *whole* electrolyte in solution is equal to the sum of the milliosmolar values of the separate ions. According to the *United States Pharmacopeia*, the ideal osmolar concentration may be calculated according to the equation[2]:

$$\text{mOsmol/L} = \frac{\text{Concentration of substance (g/L)}}{\text{Molecular weight (g)}} \times \text{Number of species} \times 1000$$

Furthermore, the osmolar concentration is the total of the osmotic concentration of all solutes in a solution, so each solute must be included in the calculation of osmolarity of a particular solution as example problem 6 demonstrates.

In practice, as the concentration of the solute increases, physicochemical interaction among solute particles increases and actual osmolar values decrease when compared to ideal values. Deviation from ideal conditions is usually slight in solution within the physiologic range and for more dilute solutions, but for highly concentrated solutions, the actual osmolarities may be appreciably lower than ideal values. For example, the ideal osmolarity of 0.9% sodium chloride injection is:

$$\text{mOsmol/L} = \frac{9\text{ g/L}}{50.5\text{ g}} \times 2 \times 1000 \times 307.69\text{ mOsmol/L}$$

Because of bonding forces, however, the number of species is slightly less than 2 for solutions of sodium chloride at this concentration, and the actual measured osmolarity of the solution is about 286 mOsmol/L.

Some pharmaceutical manufacturers label electrolyte solutions with ideal or stoichiometric osmolarities calculated by the equation just provided, whereas others list experimental or actual osmolarities. The pharmacist should be aware of this distinction.

A distinction also should be made between the terms *osmolarity* and *osmolality*. Whereas ***osmolarity*** is the *milliosmoles of solute per liter of solution*, ***osmolality*** is the *milliosmoles of solute per kilogram of solvent*. For dilute aqueous solutions, osmolarity and osmolality are nearly identical. For more concentrated solutions, however, the two values may be quite dissimilar. The pharmacist should pay particular attention to a product's label statement regarding osmolarity versus osmolality.

Normal serum osmolality is considered to be within the range of 275 to 300 mOsmol/kg. The contribution of various constituents to the osmolality of normal serum is shown in Table 12.4. *Osmometers* are commercially available for use in the laboratory to measure osmolality.[3] Abnormal blood osmolality that deviates from the normal range can occur in association with shock, trauma, burns, water intoxication (overload), electrolyte imbalance, hyperglycemia, or renal failure.[3]

Example Calculations of Milliosmoles

The equation adapted from the USP used in the previous example can be used to determine osmolarity, or the following conversion can be used to convert milligrams to milliosmoles and vice versa:

$$\frac{\text{Molecular weight}}{\text{Number of species produced by dissociation}} = \frac{\text{mg}}{\text{mOsmol}}$$

Table 12.4 • THE CONTRIBUTION OF VARIOUS CONSTITUENTS OF NORMAL HUMAN SERUM TO THE TOTAL SERUM OSMOTIC PRESSURE[a]

Constituent	Mean Concentration (mEq/L)	Osmotic Pressure (mOsmol/kg of water)[b]	Percentage of Total Osmotic Pressure
Sodium	142.0	139.0	48.3
Potassium	5.0	4.9	1.7
Calcium	2.5	1.2	0.4
Magnesium	2.0	1.0	0.3
Chloride	102.0	99.8	34.7
Bicarbonate	27.0	26.4	9.2
Proteinate	16.0	1.0	0.3
Phosphate	2.0	1.1	0.4
Sulfate	1.0	0.5	0.2
Organic anions	3.5	3.4	1.2
Urea	30 (mg/100 mL)	5.3	1.8
Glucose	70 (mg/100 mL)	4.1	1.4
Totals		287.7 mOsmol/kg	99.9%
Observed normal mean		289.0 mOsmol/kg	

[a]From Chughtai MA, Hendry EB. Serum electrolytes, urea, and osmolality in cases of chloride depletion. *Clinical Biochemistry* 1967;1:91. Adapted from *Fluid and Electrolytes*. Chicago, IL: Abbott Laboratories, 1970.

[b]Water content of normal serum taken as 94 g/100 mL.

(1) *A solution contains 10% of anhydrous dextrose in water for injection. How many milliosmoles per liter are represented by this concentration?*

Molecular weight of anhydrous dextrose = 180

Dextrose does not dissociate, therefore the "number of species" = 1

$$\text{Conversion} = \frac{180\text{ mg}}{1\text{ mOsmol}}$$

$$\frac{10\text{ g}}{100\text{ mL}} \times \frac{1000\text{ mg}}{\text{g}} \times \frac{1000\text{ mL}}{\text{L}} \times \frac{1\text{ mOsmol}}{180\text{ mg}} = \mathbf{555.56\ mOsmol/L}$$

Or, utilizing the equation:

$$\frac{10\text{ g}}{100\text{ mL}} \times \frac{1000\text{ mL}}{\text{L}} = 100\text{ g/L}$$

$$\frac{100\text{ g/L}}{180} \times 1 \times 1000 = \mathbf{555.56\ mOsmol/L}$$

(2) *A solution contains 156 mg of K^+ ions per 100 mL. How many milliosmoles are represented in a liter of the solution?*

Molecular weight of K^+ = 39

Number of species = 1

$$\text{Conversion} = \frac{39\text{ mg}}{1\text{ mOsmol}}$$

$$\frac{156\text{ mg}}{100\text{ mL}} \times \frac{1000\text{ mL}}{\text{L}} \times 1\text{ L} \times \frac{1\text{ mOsmol}}{39\text{ mg}} = \mathbf{40\ mOsmol}$$

(3) *Calculate the osmolarity of a 3% hypertonic sodium chloride solution. Assume complete dissociation.*

$$\text{Molecular weight of NaCl} = 23\ (Na^+) + 35.5\ (Cl^-) = 58.5$$

$$\text{Number of species} = 2\ (Na^+ \text{ and } Cl^-)$$

$$\text{Conversion} = \frac{58.5 \text{ mg}}{2 \text{ mOsmol}}$$

$$\frac{3 \text{ g}}{100 \text{ mL}} \times \frac{1000 \text{ mg}}{\text{g}} \times \frac{1000 \text{ mL}}{\text{L}} \times \frac{2 \text{ mOsmol}}{58.5 \text{ mg}} = \mathbf{1025.64 \text{ mOsmol/L}}$$

(4) *Calcium chloride dihydrate injection is a 10% solution of* $CaCl_2 \cdot 2H_2O$. *How many milliosmoles are present in a 10-mL vial? Assume complete dissociation.*

$$\text{Molecular weight of } CaCl_2 \cdot 2H_2O = 40\ (Ca^{2+}) + [2 \times 35.5\ (Cl^-)] + [2 \times 18\ (H_2O)] = 147$$

$$\text{Number of species} = 3\ (Ca^{2+} \text{ and } 2Cl^-)$$

$$\text{Conversion} = \frac{147 \text{ mg}}{3 \text{ mOsmol}}$$

$$\frac{10 \text{ g}}{100 \text{ mL}} \times \frac{1000 \text{ mg}}{\text{g}} \times 10 \text{ mL} \times \frac{3 \text{ mOsmol}}{147 \text{ mg}} = \mathbf{20.41 \text{ mOsmol}}$$

(5) *If a pharmacist wished to prepare 100 mL of a solution containing 50 mOsmol of calcium chloride, how many grams of calcium chloride would be needed? Assume complete dissociation.*

$$\text{Molecular weight of } CaCl_2 = 40\ (Ca^{2+}) + [2 \times 35.5\ (Cl^-)] = 111$$

$$\text{Number of species} = 3\ (Ca^{2+} \text{ and } 2Cl^-)$$

$$\text{Conversion} = \frac{111 \text{ mg}}{3 \text{ mOsmol}}$$

$$50 \text{ mOsmol} \times \frac{111 \text{ mg}}{3 \text{ mOsmol}} \times \frac{1 \text{ g}}{1000 \text{ mg}} = \mathbf{1.85 \text{ g}}$$

(6) *What is the osmolarity of a solution containing 5% dextrose and 0.45% sodium chloride (D5½NS)? Assume complete dissociation.*

Because this solution contains two ingredients, the osmolarity of each must be calculated then added to determine the total osmolarity of the solution. Molecular weight, number of species, and conversion determinations for dextrose and sodium chloride are shown in example problems 1 and 3.

Dextrose:

$$\frac{5 \text{ g}}{100 \text{ mL}} \times \frac{1000 \text{ mg}}{\text{g}} \times \frac{1000 \text{ mL}}{\text{L}} \times \frac{1 \text{ mOsmol}}{180 \text{ mg}} = 277.78 \text{ mOsmol/L}$$

Sodium chloride:

$$\frac{0.45 \text{ g}}{100 \text{ mL}} \times \frac{1000 \text{ mg}}{\text{g}} \times \frac{1000 \text{ mL}}{\text{L}} \times \frac{2 \text{ mOsmol}}{58.5 \text{ mg}} = 153.85 \text{ mOsmol/L}$$

$$\text{Total} = 277.78 \text{ mOsmol/L} + 153.85 \text{ mOsmol/L} = \mathbf{431.62 \text{ mOsmol/L}}$$

(7) *PLASMA-LYTE 56 contains 32 mg of magnesium acetate tetrahydrate, 128 mg of potassium acetate, and 234 mg of sodium chloride in each 100 mL of solution.*[4] *What is the osmolarity of this solution? Assume complete dissociation.*

Magnesium acetate tetrahydrate ($Mg(C_2H_3O_2)_2 \cdot 4H_2O$):

$$\text{Molecular weight} = 24\ (Mg^{2+}) + [2 \times 59\ (C_2H_3O_2^-)] + [4 \times 18\ (H_2O)] = 214$$

$$\text{Number of species} = 3\ (Mg^{2+} \text{ and } 2C_2H_3O_2^-)$$

$$\text{Conversion} = \frac{214 \text{ mg}}{3 \text{ mOsmol}}$$

$$\frac{32 \text{ mg}}{100 \text{ mL}} \times \frac{1000 \text{ mL}}{\text{L}} \times \frac{3 \text{ mOsmol}}{214 \text{ mg}} = 4.49 \text{ mOsmol/L}$$

Potassium acetate ($KC_2H_3O_2$):

$$\text{Molecular weight} = 39\ (K^+) + 59\ (C_2H_3O_2^-) = 98$$

$$\text{Number of species} = 2\ (K^+ \text{ and } C_2H_3O_2^-)$$

$$\text{Conversion} = \frac{98 \text{ mg}}{2 \text{ mOsmol}}$$

$$\frac{128 \text{ mg}}{100 \text{ mL}} \times \frac{1000 \text{ mL}}{\text{L}} \times \frac{2 \text{ mOsmol}}{98 \text{ mg}} = 26.12 \text{ mOsmol/L}$$

Sodium chloride (NaCl):

$$\frac{234 \text{ mg}}{100 \text{ mL}} \times \frac{1000 \text{ mL}}{\text{L}} \times \frac{2 \text{ mOsmol}}{58.5 \text{ mg}} = 80 \text{ mOsmol/L}$$

Total = 4.49 mOsmol/L + 26.12 mOsmol/L + 80 mOsmol/L = **110.61 mOsmol/L**

(8) *Calculate the milliequivalents of sodium, potassium, and chloride, the millimoles of anhydrous dextrose, and the osmolarity of the following parenteral fluid. Assume complete dissociation.*

Dextrose, anhydrous	50 g
Sodium chloride	4.5 g
Potassium chloride	1.49 g
Water for injection, ad	1000 mL

Sodium chloride:

$$4.5 \text{ g} \times \frac{1000 \text{ mg}}{\text{g}} \times \frac{1 \text{ mEq}}{58.5 \text{ mg}} = 76.92 \text{ mEq NaCl} = \mathbf{76.92\ mEq\ Na^+}$$

and 76.92 mEq Cl^-

$$\frac{4.5 \text{ g}}{1000 \text{ mL}} \times \frac{1000 \text{ mg}}{\text{g}} \times \frac{1000 \text{ mL}}{\text{L}} \times \frac{2 \text{ mOsmol}}{58.5 \text{ mg}} = 153.85 \text{ mOsmol/L}$$

Potassium chloride:

$$1.49 \text{ g} \times \frac{1000 \text{ mg}}{\text{g}} \times \frac{1 \text{ mEq}}{74.5 \text{ mg}} = 20 \text{ mEq KCl} = \mathbf{20\ mEq\ K^+} \text{ and } 20 \text{ mEq } Cl^-$$

$$\frac{1.49 \text{ g}}{1000 \text{ mL}} \times \frac{1000 \text{ mg}}{\text{g}} \times \frac{1000 \text{ mL}}{\text{L}} \times \frac{2 \text{ mOsmol}}{74.5 \text{ mg}} = 40 \text{ mOsmol/L}$$

Dextrose:

$$50\text{ g} \times \frac{1000\text{ mg}}{\text{g}} \times \frac{1\text{ mmol}}{180\text{ mg}} = \mathbf{277.78\text{ mmol}}$$

$$\frac{50\text{ g}}{1000\text{ mL}} \times \frac{1000\text{ mg}}{\text{g}} \times \frac{1000\text{ mL}}{\text{L}} \times \frac{1\text{ mOsmol}}{180\text{ mg}} = 277.78\text{ mOsmol/L}$$

76.92 mEq Na^+, 20 mEq K^+, 76.92 mEq + 20 mEq = **96.92 mEq Cl^-**

277.78 mmol dextrose

Osmolarity = 153.85 mOsmol/L + 40 mOsmol/L + 277.78 mOsmol/L = **471.62 mOsmol/L**

Clinical Considerations of Water and Electrolyte Balance

Maintaining body water and electrolyte balance is an essential component of good health. Water provides the environment in which cells live and is the primary medium for the ingestion of nutrients and the excretion of metabolic waste products. Normally, the osmolality of body fluid is maintained within narrow limits through dietary input, the regulatory endocrine processes, and balanced output via the kidneys, lungs, skin, and the gastrointestinal system.

In clinical practice, fluid and electrolyte therapy are undertaken either to provide maintenance requirements or to replace serious losses or deficits. Body losses of water and/or electrolytes can result from a number of causes, including vomiting, diarrhea, profuse sweating, fever, chronic renal failure, diuretic therapy, surgery, and others. The type of therapy undertaken (i.e., oral or parenteral) and the content of the fluid administered depend on a patient's specific requirements.

For example, a patient taking diuretics may simply require a daily oral potassium supplement along with adequate intake of water. An athlete may require rehydration with or without added electrolytes. Hospitalized patients commonly receive parenteral maintenance therapy of fluids and electrolytes to support ordinary metabolic function. In severe cases of deficit, a patient may require the prompt and substantial intravenous replacement of fluids and electrolytes to restore acute volume losses resulting from surgery, trauma, burns, or shock.

The composition of body fluids generally is described with regard to body compartments: ***intracellular*** (within cells), ***intravascular*** (blood plasma), or ***interstitial*** (between cells in the tissue). Intravascular and interstitial fluids commonly are grouped together and termed ***extracellular*** fluid. The usual reference ranges of electrolytes in blood plasma are shown in Table 12.2. Although all electrolytes and nonelectrolytes in body fluids contribute to osmotic activity, sodium and chloride exert the principal effect in *extra*cellular fluid, and potassium and phosphate predominate in *intra*cellular fluid.

Since cell membranes generally are freely permeable to water, the osmolality of the extracellular fluid (about 290 mOsmol/kg water) is about equal to that of the intracellular fluid. Therefore, the plasma osmolality is a convenient and accurate guide to intracellular osmolality and may be approximated by the formula[5]:

$$\text{Plasma osmolality (mOsmol/kg)} = 2\,[\text{plasma Na}] + \frac{[\text{BUN}]}{2.8} + \frac{[\text{Glucose}]}{18}$$

where sodium (Na) concentration is in mEq/L, and blood urea nitrogen (BUN) and glucose concentrations are in mg/100 mL (mg/dL).

Example Calculation of Plasma Osmolality

Estimate the plasma osmolality from the following data: sodium, 135 mEq/L; blood urea nitrogen, 14 mg/dL; and glucose, 90 mg/dL.

$$\text{Plasma osmolality} = 2[135\ \text{mEq/L}] + \frac{[14\ \text{mg/dL}]}{2.8} + \frac{[90\ \text{mg/dL}]}{18} = 280\ \text{mOsmol/kg}$$

CALCULATIONS CAPSULE

Milliequivalents, Millimoles, and Milliosmoles

To calculate milliequivalents (mEq), use the following conversion:

$$\frac{\text{Molecular weight}}{\text{Valence}} = \frac{\text{mg}}{\text{mEq}}$$

where "valence" is the total valence of the cation or anion in the compound.

To calculate millimoles (mmol), use the following conversion:

$$\text{Molecular weight} = \frac{\text{mg}}{\text{mmol}}$$

To calculate milliosmoles (mOsmol), use the following conversion:

$$\frac{\text{Molecular weight}}{\text{Number of species produced by dissociation}} = \frac{\text{mg}}{\text{mOsmol}}$$

where "number of species produced by dissociation" is one for substances that do not dissociate, two for substances that dissociate into two ions, three for substances that dissociate into three ions, and so on.

Osmolarity (mOsmol/L) is the total number of milliosmoles of solute(s) per liter of solution.

CASE IN POINT 12.3[a] A hospital pharmacist fills a medication order calling for an intravenous fluid of dextrose 5% in a 0.9% sodium chloride injection and 40 mEq of potassium chloride in a total volume of 1000 mL. The intravenous infusion is administered through an IV set that delivers 15 drops per milliliter. The infusion has been running at a rate of 12 drops per minute for 15 hours.

During the 15-hour period:

(a) How many mEq of KCl have been administered?

(b) How many grams of KCl have been administered?

(c) How many millimoles of KCl have been administered?

(d) What is the total osmolarity of the intravenous fluid?

[a]Problem courtesy of Flynn Warren, Bishop, GA.

PRACTICE PROBLEMS

Calculations Based on Millimoles, Micromoles, and Milliequivalents

1. Convert blood plasma range of 11 to 25 mcmol/L of copper (m.w. = 63.55) to mcg/mL.
2. A preparation contains, in each milliliter, 236 mg of dibasic potassium phosphate (m.w. = 174.18) and 224 mg of monobasic potassium phosphate (m.w. = 136.09). Calculate the total concentration of phosphate, in mmol/mL, and potassium, in mEq/mL, in the preparation.[6]
3. A 10-mL ampul contains 2.98 g of potassium chloride. What is the concentration of the solution in milliequivalents per milliliter?
4. A 154-lb patient is to receive 36 mg/kg of ammonium chloride. How many milliliters of an ammonium chloride (NH_4Cl—m.w. 53.5) injection containing 5 mEq/mL should be added to the patient's intravenous infusion?
5. A sterile solution of potassium chloride contains 2 mEq/mL. If a 20-mL ampul of the solution is diluted to 1 liter, what is the percentage strength of the resulting solution?
6. A certain electrolyte solution contains, as one of the ingredients, the equivalent of 4.6 mEq of calcium per liter. How many grams of calcium chloride dihydrate ($CaCl_2 \cdot 2H_2O$—m.w. 147) should be used in preparing 20 liters of the solution?
7. Ammonium chloride injection contains 267.5 mg of NH_4Cl (m.w. 53.5) per milliliter. How many mEq of ammonium chloride are present in a 20-mL vial?
8. A solution contains, in each 5 mL, 0.5 g of potassium acetate ($C_2H_3KO_2$—m.w. 98), 0.5 g of potassium bicarbonate ($KHCO_3$—m.w. 100), and 0.5 g of potassium citrate monohydrate ($C_6H_5K_3O_7 \cdot H_2O$—m.w. 324). How many milliequivalents of potassium (K^+) are represented in each 5 mL of the solution?
9. How many grams of sodium chloride should be used in preparing 20 liters of a solution containing 154 mEq/L?
10. Sterile solutions of potassium chloride containing 5 mEq/mL are available in 20-mL containers. Calculate the amount, in grams, of potassium chloride in the container.
11. How many milliliters of a solution containing 2 mEq of potassium chloride per milliliter should be used to obtain 2.98 g of potassium chloride?
12. A patient is given 125 mg of phenytoin sodium ($C_{15}H_{11}N_2NaO_2$—m.w. 274) three times a day. How many milliequivalents of sodium are represented in the daily dose?
13. If a 40-mL vial of sodium chloride is added to a 1-L container of water for injection, calculate the concentration of sodium chloride, in mEq/mL in the original vial, if the resultant dilution is 0.56% in strength.
14. How many grams of sodium bicarbonate ($NaHCO_3$—m.w. 84) should be used in preparing a liter of a solution to contain 44.6 mEq per 50 mL?
15. A liter of an electrolyte solution contains the following: 131 mEq Na^+, 111 mEq Cl^-, 5 mEq K^+, 29 mEq $C_3H_5O_3^-$ (lactate), and 4 mEq Ca^{2+}. Convert each of these values to mmol/L.
16. Sterile sodium lactate solution is available commercially as a $^1/_6$-molar solution of sodium lactate in water for injection. How many milliequivalents of sodium lactate ($C_3H_5NaO_3$—m.w. 112) would be provided by a liter of the solution?
17. A certain electrolyte solution contains 0.9% of sodium chloride in 10% dextrose solution. Express the concentration of sodium chloride (NaCl) in terms of milliequivalents per liter.

18. ℞ Potassium chloride 10%
Cherry syrup q.s. ad 480 mL
Sig. tablespoonful b.i.d.
How many milliequivalents of potassium chloride are represented in each prescribed dose?
19. How many milliequivalents of potassium are in 5 million units of penicillin V potassium ($C_{16}H_{17}KN_2O_6S$—m.w. 388)? One milligram of penicillin V potassium represents 1380 penicillin V units.
20. The normal potassium level in the blood plasma is 17 mg% (17 mg/100 mL). Express this concentration in terms of milliequivalents per liter.
21. How many grams of potassium citrate ($C_6H_5K_3O_7 \cdot H_2O$—m.w. 324) should be used in preparing 500 mL of a potassium ion elixir so as to supply 15 mEq of K in each 5-mL dose?
22. A potassium supplement tablet contains 2.5 g of potassium bicarbonate ($KHCO_3$—m.w. 100). How many milliequivalents of potassium (K^+) are supplied by the tablet?
23. Ringer's injection contains 0.86% of sodium chloride, 0.03% of potassium chloride, and 0.033% of calcium chloride dihydrate. Calculate the sodium, potassium, calcium, and chloride content in mEq/L.
24. Calculate the mEq of Na^+ in each gram of ampicillin sodium ($C_{16}H_{18}N_3NaO_4S$—m.w. 371).
25. A 20-mL vial of concentrated ammonium chloride solution containing 5 mEq/mL is diluted to 1 liter with sterile distilled water. Calculate (a) the total milliequivalent value of the ammonium ion in the dilution and (b) the percentage strength of the dilution.
26. If a liter of an intravenous fluid contains 5% dextrose and 34 mEq sodium (as NaCl), calculate the percent strength of sodium chloride in the solution.
27. How many milliequivalents of potassium would be supplied daily by the usual dose (0.3 mL three times a day) of saturated potassium iodide solution? Saturated potassium iodide solution contains 100 g of potassium iodide per 100 mL.
28. An intravenous solution calls for the addition of 25 mEq of sodium bicarbonate. How many milliliters of 8.4% w/v sodium bicarbonate injection should be added to the formula?
29. Calcium gluconate ($C_{12}H_{22}CaO_{14}$—m.w. 430) injection 10% is available in a 10-mL ampul. How many milliequivalents of Ca^{2+} does the ampul contain?
30. A flavored potassium chloride packet contains 1.5 g of potassium chloride. How many milliequivalents of potassium chloride are represented in each packet?
31. How many milliequivalents of Li^+ are provided by a daily dose of four 300-mg tablets of lithium carbonate (LITHOBID) (Li_2CO_3—m.w. 74)?
32. Magnesium chloride is available as magnesium chloride hexahydrate in an injectable solution that supplies 1.97 mEq of magnesium per milliliter. What is the percent strength of magnesium chloride hexahydrate in this solution?
33. A patient is to receive 10 mEq of potassium gluconate ($C_6H_{11}KO_7$—m.w. 234) four times a day for 3 days. If the dose is to be one teaspoonful in a cherry syrup vehicle, (a) how many grams of potassium gluconate should be used and (b) what volume, in milliliters, should be dispensed to provide the prescribed dosage regimen?
34. A physician wishes to administer 1,200,000 units of penicillin G potassium every 4 hours. If 1 unit of penicillin G potassium ($C_{16}H_{17}KN_2O_4S$—m.w. 372) equals 0.6 mcg, how many milliequivalents of K^+ will the patient receive in a 24-hour period?

35. Five milliliters of lithium citrate syrup contain the equivalent of 8 mEq of Li^+. Calculate the equivalent, in milligrams, of lithium carbonate (Li_2CO_3—m.w. 74) in each 5-mL dose of the syrup.
36. How many milligrams of magnesium sulfate ($MgSO_4$—m.w. 120) should be added to an intravenous solution to provide 5 mEq of Mg^{2+} per liter?
37. K-TAB, a slow-release potassium chloride tablet, contains 750 mg of potassium chloride in a wax/polymer matrix. How many milliequivalents of potassium chloride are supplied by a dosage of one tablet three times a day?
38. An electrolyte solution contains 222 mg of sodium acetate ($C_2H_3NaO_2$—m.w. 82) and 15 mg of magnesium chloride ($MgCl_2$—m.w. 95) in each 100 mL. Express these concentrations in milliequivalents of Na^+ and Mg^{2+} per liter.
39. MARBLEN LIQUID contains 520 mg of calcium carbonate and 400 mg of magnesium carbonate in each teaspoonful dose. If a patient takes two teaspoonfuls after every meal, how many milliequivalents of calcium and magnesium is she receiving per day assuming that she eats three meals per day?
40. A patient has a sodium deficit of 168 mEq. How many milliliters of isotonic sodium chloride solution (0.9% w/v) should be administered to replace the deficit?
41. A normal 70 kg (154 lb) adult has 80 to 100 g of sodium. It is primarily distributed in the extracellular fluid. Body retention of 1 g additional of sodium results in excess body water accumulation of approximately 310 mL. If a person retains 100 mEq of extra sodium, how many milliliters of additional water could be expected to be retained?
42. A patient receives 3 liters of an electrolyte fluid containing 234 mg of sodium chloride (NaCl—m.w. 58.5), 125 mg of potassium acetate ($C_2H_3KO_2$—m.w. 98), and 21 mg of magnesium acetate ($Mg(C_2H_3O_2)_2$—m.w. 142) per 100 mL. How many milliequivalents each of Na^+, K^+, and Mg^{2+} does the patient receive?
43. Magnesium citrate laxative solution (CITROMA) contains 1.745 g of magnesium citrate per fluid ounce of solution. Express the concentration of magnesium in this solution as milliequivalents per milliliter.
44. The usual adult dose of calcium for elevating serum calcium is 7 to 14 mEq. How many milliliters of a calcium gluceptate injection, each milliliter of which provides 18 mg of elemental calcium, would provide the recommended dosage range?
45. The oral pediatric maintenance solution PEDIALYTE liquid has the following electrolyte content per liter: sodium, 45 mEq; potassium, 20 mEq; chloride, 35 mEq; and citrate, 30 mEq. Calculate the equivalent quantities of each in terms of milligrams.
46. Calculate the milliequivalents of chloride per liter of the following parenteral fluid:

Sodium chloride	516	mg
Potassium chloride	89.4	mg
Calcium chloride, anhyd.	27.8	mg
Magnesium chloride, anhyd.	14.2	mg
Sodium lactate, anhyd.	560	mg
Water for injection ad	100	mL

47. The pediatric infusion rate for potassium is 5 mEq/h. If 9 mL of a 39.2% solution of potassium acetate ($KC_2H_3O_2$) is diluted to 1 L of infusion solution, calculate the proper infusion rate in mL/h.

48. GOLYTELY, a colon lavage preparation, contains the following mixture of dry powder in each packet to prepare one gallon of solution:

Sodium sulfate	21.5 g
Sodium chloride	5.53 g
Potassium chloride	2.82 g
Sodium bicarbonate	6.36 g
Polyethylene glycol (3350)	227.1 g

Calculate the milliequivalents each of sodium and chloride present in the prepared solution.

49. PHOSPHA 250 NEUTRAL tablets contain 852 mg dibasic sodium phosphate anhydrous, 155 mg monobasic potassium phosphate, and 130 mg monobasic sodium phosphate monohydrate in each tablet. Determine the amount, in milliequivalents, of sodium and potassium in each tablet and the amount, in millimoles, of phosphate in each tablet.

50. TPN ELECTROLYTES solution contains the electrolytes shown below.

Calcium chloride	16.5 mg/mL
Magnesium chloride	25.4 mg/mL
Potassium chloride	74.6 mg/mL
Sodium acetate	121 mg/mL
Sodium chloride	16.1 mg/mL

(a) How many milliequivalents of sodium are contained in 5 mL of this solution?
(b) Express the concentration of magnesium chloride as mmol/mL.

Calculations Including Milliosmoles

51. At 3:00 P.M., a pharmacist received an order to add 30 mEq/L of potassium chloride to the already running intravenous fluid for a patient. After checking the medication order, the pharmacist found that the patient is receiving a 5% dextrose/0.9% sodium chloride infusion at a rate of 85 mL/h and that the patient's liter of fluid was started at 1:30 PM.[7]
(a) Assuming that it took 30 minutes to provide the needed potassium chloride to the floor nurse, how many milliequivalents of potassium chloride should have been added to the patient's running IV fluid to achieve the ordered concentration?
(b) How many milliliters of an injection containing 2 mEq of potassium chloride/mL should have been used to supply the amount of potassium chloride needed?
(c) What was the osmolarity of the infusion with the potassium chloride added? Assume complete dissociation of the sodium chloride and potassium chloride.

52. A solution contains 322 mg of Na^+ ions per liter. How many milliosmoles are represented in the solution?

53. A solution of sodium chloride contains 77 mEq/L. Calculate its osmolar strength in terms of milliosmoles per liter. Assume complete dissociation.

54. Calculate the osmolarity, in milliosmoles per liter, of a parenteral solution containing 2 mEq/mL of potassium acetate ($KC_2H_3O_2$—m.w. 98).

55. Calculate (a) the milliequivalents per milliliter, (b) the total milliequivalents, and (c) the osmolarity of a 500-mL parenteral fluid containing 5% w/v of sodium bicarbonate.
56. What is the osmolarity of an 8.4% w/v solution of sodium bicarbonate?
57. A hospital medication order calls for the administration of 100 g of mannitol to a patient as an osmotic diuretic over a 24-hour period. Calculate (a) how many milliliters of a 15% w/v mannitol injection should be administered per hour and (b) how many milliosmoles of mannitol (m.w. 182) would be represented in the prescribed dosage.
58. What would be the osmolarity of 500 mL of a solution containing 5% w/v dextrose, 0.3% w/v sodium chloride, and 30 mEq of potassium acetate?
59. Magnesium citrate laxative solution (CITROMA) contains 1.745 g of magnesium citrate per fluid ounce of solution. Calculate the osmolarity of this solution.
60. What would be the osmolarity of 1000 mL of a solution containing 10% w/v dextrose, 0.225% w/v sodium chloride, and 15 mEq of calcium gluconate?
61. How many (a) millimoles, (b) milliequivalents, and (c) milliosmoles of calcium gluconate ($Ca(C_6H_{11}O_7)_2$—m.w. 430) are represented in 15 mL of a 10% w/v calcium gluconate solution?
62. The information for a cardioplegic solution states that each 100 mL of solution contains calcium chloride dihydrate USP 17.6 mg, magnesium chloride hexahydrate USP 325.3 mg, potassium chloride USP 119.3 mg, and sodium chloride USP 643 mg, in water for injection USP. The information also gives electrolyte content per liter (not including ions for pH adjustment) as sodium (Na^+) 110 mEq, magnesium (Mg^{2+}) 32 mEq, potassium (K^+) 16 mEq, calcium (Ca^{2+}) 2.4 mEq, and chloride (Cl^-) 160 mEq. Osmolar concentration 304 mOsmol/liter (calc.).[8] Calculate the labeled concentrations to determine their accuracy.
63. NAUZENE contains in each tablespoonful dose 4.17 g of fructose (m.w. = 180), 921 mg of sodium citrate dihydrate, and 4.35 g of dextrose. (a) What would be the osmolarity of this solution? (b) If a patient ingests the maximum daily dose of 120 mL of NAUZENE, how many milliequivalents of sodium would he ingest?
64. Estimate the plasma osmolality, in milliosmoles per kilogram, from the following data: sodium, 139 mEq/L; blood urea nitrogen, 26 mg/100 mL; and glucose, 100 mg/dL.
65. A patient undergoes a CHEM-7 blood test with the following results:

Sodium	146 mEq/L
Potassium	4.8 mEq/L
Chloride	108 mEq/L
Bicarbonate	28 mEq/L
BUN	23 mg/dL
Creatinine	1.1 mg/dL
Glucose	134 mg/dL

Estimate the plasma osmolality for this patient.

CALCQUIZ

NOTE: *In solving the following problems, refer to Table 12.3 as needed.*

12.A. A veterinarian ordered a liter of *Hartmann's Irrigation* (lactated Ringer's irrigation) with the following formula:

Sodium chloride	600 mg
Sodium lactate	310 mg
Potassium chloride	30 mg
Calcium chloride, dihydrate	20 mg
Water for injection, ad	100 mL

Calculate the mEq/L of Na^+, K^+, Ca^{2+}, Cl^-, and $C_3H_5O_3^-$.

12.B. Calculate the content of *Hartmann's Irrigation* in mOsmol/L.

12.C. A multiple electrolytes injection (PLASMA-LYTE 148) contains the following electrolytes in each 100 mL:

Sodium chloride	526 mg
Sodium gluconate	502 mg
Sodium acetate trihydrate	368 mg
Potassium chloride	37 mg
Magnesium chloride	30 mg

The formula for sodium gluconate is $C_6H_{11}NaO_7$; for sodium acetate trihydrate, $C_2H_3NaO_2 \cdot 3H_2O$; and for magnesium chloride, $MgCl_2 \cdot 6H_2O$.
Calculate the mEq/L of Na^+ in the injection.

12.D.[a] A patient has been receiving lithium carbonate (Li_2CO_3) capsules but, due to difficulty in swallowing, needs to change to a liquid form. If the patient's dose of lithium carbonate is 300 mg three times a day, how many millimoles of lithium is the patient receiving per day? If lithium citrate syrup contains 300 mg of lithium citrate ($C_6H_5Li_3O_7$) per 5 mL, how many milliliters of syrup per day would be equivalent to the lithium in the capsules?

12.E.[a] A patient is receiving an intravenous infusion containing 40 mEq of potassium chloride in 1000 mL of dextrose 5% in half–normal saline. The infusion has been running at a rate of 80 mL/h for the past 6.5 hours. Following a lab report showing the patient's serum potassium level to be 3.5 mEq/L, the physician decides to increase the potassium dose while slowing the infusion flow rate to 40 mL/h. The physician prescribes potassium chloride injection (14.9% KCl) to be added to the IV such that the patient will receive a total of 80 mEq of potassium over the remaining time for completion of the infusion. How many milliliters of the potassium chloride injection should be added by the pharmacist?

[a]Problem courtesy of Flynn Warren, Bishop, GA.

ANSWERS TO "CASE IN POINT" AND PRACTICE PROBLEMS

Case in Point 12.1

(a) Molecular weight of $CaCl_2 \cdot 2H_2O = 40\ (Ca^{2+}) + [2 \times 35.5\ (Cl^-)] + [2 \times 18(H_2O)] = 147$

Valence = 2

$$\text{Conversion} = \frac{147\ \text{mg}}{2\ \text{mEq}}$$

$$10\ \text{mEq} \times \frac{147\ \text{mg}}{2\ \text{mEq}} \times \frac{1\ \text{g}}{1000\ \text{mg}} \times \frac{100\ \text{mL}}{10\ \text{g}} = 7.35\ \text{mL of injection}$$

Thus, 7.35 mL of the injection contains 10 mEq of calcium and should be added to the 500-mL bag of normal saline solution.

(b) Since 0.5 mEq of calcium is to be administered per hour and there are 10 mEq of calcium in 507.35 mL of fluid (500 mL of NSS + 7.35 mL of calcium chloride dihydrate injection), the volume of fluid to be administered per hour may be calculated as:

$$\frac{0.5\ \text{mEq}}{\text{h}} \times \frac{507.35\ \text{mL}}{10\ \text{mEq}} = 25.37\ \text{mL/h}$$

Finally, the drops per minute may be calculated:

$$\frac{25.37\ \text{mL}}{\text{h}} \times \frac{1\ \text{h}}{60\ \text{min}} \times \frac{12\ \text{drops}}{\text{mL}} = 5.07\ \text{drops/min} \approx 5\ \text{drops/min}$$

Case in Point 12.2

(a) Molecular weight of $Fe\,(C_6H_{11}O_7)_2 = 56\ (Fe^{2+}) + [2 \times 195\ (C_6H_{11}O_7^-)] = 446$

Valence = 2

$$\text{Conversion} = \frac{446\ \text{mg}}{2\ \text{mEq}}$$

$$\frac{0.12\ \text{mEq}}{\text{kg/day}} \times \frac{1\ \text{kg}}{2.2\ \text{lb}} \times 132\ \text{lb} \times \frac{446\ \text{mg}}{2\ \text{mEq}} = 1605.6\ \text{mg/day}$$

$$\frac{1605.6\ \text{mg}}{\text{day}} \times \frac{1\ \text{day}}{3\ \text{doses}} \times \frac{1\ \text{tsp}}{300\ \text{mg}} \times \frac{5\ \text{mL}}{1\ \text{tsp}} = 8.92\ \text{mL/dose}$$

(b) $$\frac{300\ \text{mg}}{\text{tsp}} \times \frac{1\ \text{tsp}}{5\ \text{mL}} \times \frac{29.57\ \text{mL}}{\text{fl.oz.}} \times 6\ \text{fl.oz.} \times \frac{1\ \text{g}}{1000\ \text{mg}} = 10.65\ \text{g ferrous gluconate}$$

Case in Point 12.3

(a) $$\frac{40\ \text{mEq}}{1000\ \text{mL}} \times \frac{1\ \text{mL}}{15\ \text{drops}} \times \frac{12\ \text{drops}}{\text{min}} \times \frac{60\ \text{min}}{\text{h}} \times 15\ \text{h} = 28.8\ \text{mEq KCl}$$

(b) Molecular weight of $KCl = 39\ (K^+) + 35.5\ (Cl^-) = 74.5$

$$\text{Valence} = 1$$

$$\text{Conversion} = \frac{74.5\ \text{mg}}{1\ \text{mEq}}$$

$$28.8\ \text{mEq} \times \frac{74.5\ \text{mg}}{1\ \text{mEq}} \times \frac{1\ \text{g}}{1000\ \text{mg}} = 2.15\ \text{g KCl}$$

(c) $$28.8\ \text{mEq} \times \frac{74.5\ \text{mg}}{1\ \text{mEq}} \times \frac{1\ \text{mmol}}{74.5\ \text{mg}} = 28.8\ \text{mmol}$$

(d) *Dextrose:*

$$\text{Molecular weight} = 180$$

Dextrose does not dissociate, therefore the "number of species" = 1

$$\text{Conversion} = \frac{180\ \text{mg}}{1\ \text{mOsmol}}$$

$$\frac{5\ \text{g}}{100\ \text{mL}} \times \frac{1000\ \text{mg}}{\text{g}} \times \frac{1000\ \text{mL}}{\text{L}} \times \frac{1\ \text{mOsmol}}{180\ \text{mg}} = 277.78\ \text{mOsmol/L}$$

Sodium chloride:

Molecular weight of $NaCl = 23\ (Na^+) + 35.5\ (Cl^-) = 58.5$

Number of species = 2 (Na^+ and Cl^-)

$$\text{Conversion} = \frac{58.5\ \text{mg}}{2\ \text{mOsmol}}$$

$$\frac{0.9\ \text{g}}{100\ \text{mL}} \times \frac{1000\ \text{mg}}{\text{g}} \times \frac{1000\ \text{mL}}{\text{L}} \times \frac{2\ \text{mOsmol}}{58.5\ \text{mg}} = 307.69\ \text{mOsmol/L}$$

Potassium chloride:

Molecular weight of $KCl = 39\ (K^+) + 35.5\ (Cl^-) = 74.5$

Number of species = 2 (K^+ and Cl^-)

$$\text{Conversion} = \frac{74.5\ \text{mg}}{2\ \text{mOsmol}}$$

$$\frac{40\ \text{mEq}}{1000\ \text{mL}} \times \frac{1000\ \text{mL}}{\text{L}} \times \frac{74.5\ \text{mg}}{1\ \text{mEq}} \times \frac{2\ \text{mOsmol}}{74.5\ \text{mg}} = 80\ \text{mOsmol/L}$$

Total osmolarity:

277.78 mOsmol/L (Dextrose) + 307.69 mOsmol/L (NaCl) + 80 mOsmol/L (KCl) = 665.47 mOsmol/L

NOTE: The osmolarity of serum is about 300 mOsmol/L, so this solution is *hyperosmotic*.

Practice Problems

1. 0.699 to 1.59 mcg/mL copper
2. 3.001 mmol/mL phosphate
   4.36 mEq/mL potassium
3. 4 mEq/mL potassium chloride
4. 9.42 mL ammonium chloride injection
5. 0.298% potassium chloride
6. 6.762 g calcium chloride
7. 100 mEq ammonium chloride
8. 14.73 mEq potassium
9. 180.18 g sodium chloride
10. 7.45 g potassium chloride
11. 20 mL potassium chloride solution
12. 1.37 mEq sodium
13. 2.49 mEq/mL sodium chloride
14. 74.93 g sodium bicarbonate
15. 131 mmol/L Na^+
    111 mmol/L Cl^-
    29 mmol/L $C_3H_5O_3^-$
    5 mmol/L K^+
    2 mmol/L Ca^{2+}
16. 166.67 mEq sodium lactate
17. 153.85 mEq/L sodium chloride
18. 20.13 mEq potassium chloride
19. 9.34 mEq potassium
20. 4.36 mEq/L potassium
21. 162 g potassium citrate
22. 25 mEq potassium
23. 147.01 mEq sodium
    4.03 mEq potassium
    4.49 mEq calcium
    155.53 mEq chloride
24. 2.7 mEq sodium
25. (a) 100 mEq ammonium
    (b) 0.54% ammonium chloride
26. 0.2% sodium chloride
27. 5.42 mEq potassium
28. 25 mL sodium bicarbonate injection
29. 4.65 mEq calcium
30. 20.13 mEq potassium chloride
31. 32.43 mEq lithium
32. 19.996% w/v magnesium chloride hexahydrate
33. (a) 28.08 g potassium gluconate
    (b) 60 mL syrup
34. 11.61 mEq potassium
35. 296 mg lithium carbonate per 5 mL
36. 300 mg/L magnesium sulfate
37. 30.2 mEq potassium chloride per day
38. 27.07 mEq/L sodium
    3.16 mEq/L magnesium
39. 62.4 mEq Ca^{2+}/day
    57.14 mEq Mg^{2+}/day
40. 1092 mL isotonic sodium chloride solution
41. 713 mL water
42. 120 mEq sodium
    38.27 mEq potassium
    8.87 mEq magnesium
43. 0.79 mEq/mL magnesium
44. 7.78 to 15.56 mL calcium gluceptate injection
45. 1035 mg/L sodium
    1242.5 mg/L chloride
    780 mg/L potassium
    1890 mg/L citrate
46. 108.2 mEq/L chloride
47. 138.89 mL/h potassium acetate infusion
48. 473.06 mEq sodium
    132.38 mEq chloride
49. 12.94 mEq/tab sodium
    1.14 mEq/tab potassium
    8.08 mmol/tab phosphate
50. (a) 8.75 mEq sodium
    (b) 0.27 mmol/mL magnesium chloride
51. (a) 24.9 mEq potassium chloride
    (b) 12.45 mL potassium chloride injection
    (c) 645.47 mOsmol/L
52. 14 mOsmol/L
53. 154 mOsmol/L
54. 4000 mOsmol/L
55. (a) 0.595 mEq/mL sodium bicarbonate
    (b) 297.62 mEq sodium bicarbonate
    (c) 1190.48 mOsmol/L
56. 2000 mOsmol/L
57. (a) 27.78 mL/h mannitol injection
    (b) 549.45 mOsmol mannitol
58. 500.34 mOsmol/L
59. 655.69 mOsmol/L
60. 654.98 mOsmol/L

61. (a) 3.49 mmol calcium gluconate
    (b) 6.98 mEq calcium gluconate
    (c) 10.47 mOsmol calcium gluconate
62. Yes, all labeled concentrations are correct
63. (a) 3990.93 mOsmol/L
    (b) 75.18 mEq sodium
64. 292.84 mOsmol/kg
65. 307.66 mOsmol/kg

References

1. Prince SJ. Calculations. *International Journal of Pharmaceutical Compounding* 2001;5:485.
2. Osmolality and Osmolarity. US Pharmacopeial Convention, Inc. *United States Pharmacopeia 37 National Formulary 32 [book online]*. Rockville, MD: US Pharmacopeial Convention, Inc.; 2014.
3. VAPRO *Vapor Pressure Osmometer [product literature]*. Logan, UT: Wescor, Inc.; 1997.
4. Plasma-Lyte 56 in Plastic Container [product label information]. U.S. Food and Drug Administration. Department of Health and Human Services. [U.S. Food and Drug Administration Website.] Available at: http://www.accessdata.fda.gov/scripts/cder/drugsatfda/index.cfm?fuseaction=Search.Label_ApprovalHistory#labelinfo. Accessed January 30, 2015.
5. Lewis JL. Water and sodium balance. In: Porter RS, ed. *The Merck Manual Professional Edition [book online]*. Whitehouse Station, NJ: Merck & Co., Inc.; 2014.
6. Prince SJ. Calculations. *International Journal of Pharmaceutical Compounding* 1998;2:378.
7. Prince SJ. Calculations. *International Journal of Pharmaceutical Compounding* 1999;3:311.
8. Cardioplegic solution. Available at: http://www.drugs.com/pro/cardioplegic.html. Accessed February 6, 2015.

13

Intravenous Infusions, Parenteral Admixtures, Rate-of-Flow Calculations

OBJECTIVES

Upon successful completion of this chapter, the student will be able to:

- Perform calculations for standard adult and pediatric intravenous infusions.
- Perform calculations for critical care intravenous infusions.
- Perform calculations for additives to intravenous infusions.
- Perform rate-of-flow calculations for intravenous infusions utilizing medication orders, standard tables, and nomograms.

Injections

Injections are sterile pharmaceutical solutions or suspensions of a drug substance in an aqueous or nonaqueous vehicle. They are administered by needle into almost any part of the body, including the joints (*intra-articular*), joint fluid (*intrasynovial*), spinal column (*intraspinal*), spinal fluid (*intrathecal*), arteries (*intra-arterial*), and in an emergency, even the heart (*intracardiac*). However, most injections are administered into a vein (*intravenous, I.V., IV*), muscle (*intramuscular, I.M., IM*), skin (*intradermal, I.D., ID, intracutaneous*), or under the skin (*subcutaneous, sub-Q, SQ, hypodermic*).

Depending upon their use, injections are packaged in small volumes in ***ampuls***[a] or in prefilled disposable syringes for single-dose use, in ***vials*** and pen injectors for single- or multiple-dose use, or in large-volume plastic bags or glass containers for administration by slow intravenous *infusion*.

Some injections are available as *prepared* solutions or suspensions with their drug content labeled as, for example, "10 mg/mL." Others contain dry powder for reconstitution *to form* a solution or suspension by adding a specified volume of diluent prior to use and are labeled as, for example, "10 mg/vial." In the latter case, the calculations required to determine the correct volume of diluent needed to prepare an injection of a certain concentration are provided in Chapter 17.

Small-volume injections may be administered as such or they may be used as *additives* to large-volume parenteral fluids for intravenous infusion. The term ***parenteral*** is defined as *any medication route other than the alimentary canal* and thus includes all routes of injection.

[a]An *ampul* (also *ampule* or *ampoule*) is a small hermetically sealed glass container.

Intravenous Infusions

Intravenous (IV) infusions are sterile, aqueous preparations administered intravenously in relatively large volumes. They are used to extend blood volume and/or provide electrolytes, nutrients, or medications. Most intravenous infusions are administered to critical care, infirm, dehydrated, or malnourished patients or to patients prior to, during, and/or following surgery. Intravenous infusions are widely employed in emergency care units, in hospitals and other patient care institutions, and in home care. Pharmacists participate in the preparation and administration of institutional as well as home intravenous infusion therapy. The *United States Pharmacopeia* has established requirements for the compounding of sterile preparations.[1]

Most intravenous infusions are solutions; however, some are very fine dispersions of nutrients or therapeutic agents or blood and blood products. Although some intravenous solutions are isotonic or nearly isotonic with blood, isotonicity is not absolutely necessary because the volumes of fluid usually administered are rapidly diluted by the circulating blood.[2]

Commercially prepared infusions are available in glass or plastic bottles or collapsible plastic "bags" in volumes of 50 mL (a *minibag*), 100 mL, 250 mL, 500 mL, and 1000 mL. The smaller volumes find particular application in treating pediatric patients and adults who require relatively small volumes of infusate. When a smaller IV bag is attached to the tubing of a larger IV being administered, it is referred to as an IV piggyback (IVPB). The abbreviation LVP is commonly used to indicate a *large-volume parenteral*, and SVP indicates a *small-volume parenteral*.

Some common solutions for intravenous infusion are listed in Table 13.1. Additional components or ***additives*** frequently are added to these basic solutions.

An ***administration set*** is attached to an intravenous bottle or bag to deliver the fluid into a patient's vein. The sets may be standard (macrodrip) or pediatric (microdrip). Depending on the particular set used, the drip rate can vary from 10 to 15 drops/mL for standard sets to 60 drops/mL for microdrip sets. It should be noted that in some literature, particularly that of nursing, the abbreviations ***gtt*** for drop and ***mcgtt*** for microdrop are used.

The passage of an infusion solution into a patient's vein of entry may be assisted by gravity (the solution is hung on a stand well above the portal of entry) or by electronic

Table 13.1 • SOME COMMON INTRAVENOUS INFUSION SOLUTIONS

Solution[a]	Abbreviation
0.9% sodium chloride	NS (normal saline)
0.45% sodium chloride	½NS
5% dextrose in water	D5W or D_5W
10% dextrose in water	D10W or $D_{10}W$
5% dextrose in 0.9% sodium chloride	D5NS or D_5NS
5% dextrose in 0.45% sodium chloride	D5½NS or $D_51/2NS$
Ringer's injection (0.86% sodium chloride, 0.03% potassium chloride, 0.033% calcium chloride)	RI
Lactated Ringer's injection	LR or LRI
5% dextrose in lactated Ringer's	D5LR or D_5LR

[a]All solutions are prepared in sterile water for injection (SWI), USP. In addition to the solutions listed, other concentrations of dextrose and sodium chloride are commercially available. These solutions may be administered as such or used as vehicles for therapeutic agents, nutrients, or other additives.

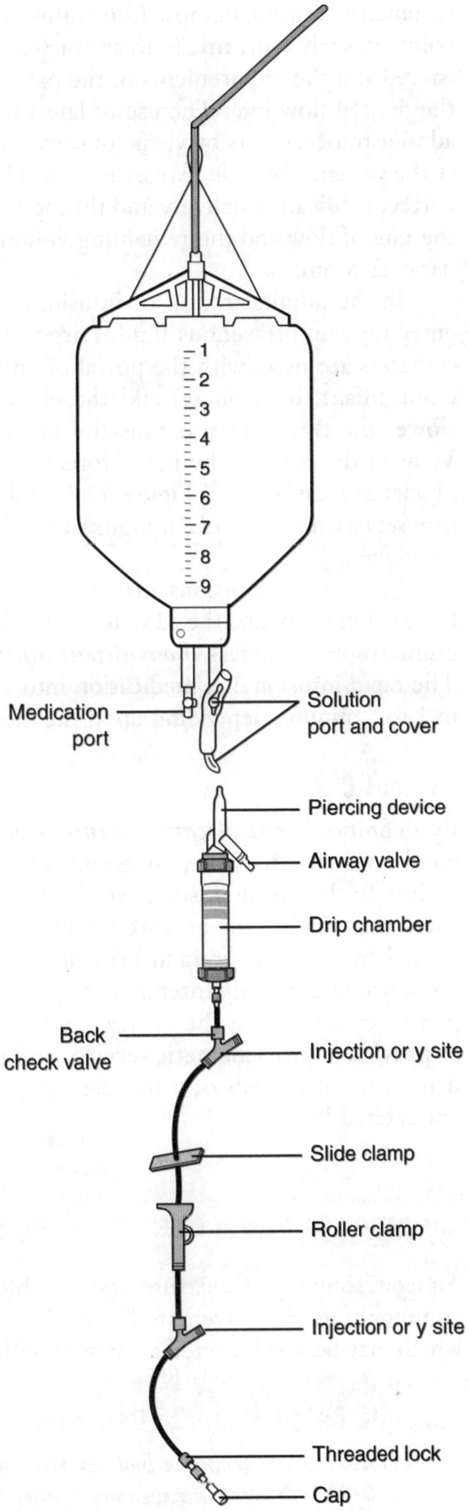

FIGURE 13.1 • A depiction of an intravenous fluid with an administration set.

volumetric infusion pumps. Some infusion pumps can be calibrated to deliver microinfusion volumes, such as 0.1 mL/h, to as much as 2000 mL/h, depending on the drug being administered and the requirements of the patient. Electronic controllers can be used to maintain the desired flow rate. The use of latest technology "smart" pumps can reduce intravenous administration errors by virtue of software that requires fewer human programming entries at the patient's bedside. Errors may also be reduced through the use of bar codes to ensure correct medication delivery and through wireless technology that allows a nurse to monitor the rate of flow and the remaining volume of an infusion when not physically present in a patient's room.

In the administration of infusions, special needles or catheters provide intravenous entry for the intravenous fluid. Large-, intermediate-, and small-gauge (bore) needles or catheters are used, with the portal of entry selected based on the patient's age (i.e., adult, child, infant, or neonate) and the clinical circumstances. The narrower the gauge, the slower the flow rate and thus the longer period required to infuse a specified volume. Veins of the back of the hand, forearm, subclavian, jugular, and scalp (e.g., in premature neonates) may be used. Figure 13.1 depicts an intravenous fluid and attached administration set (see also Fig. 14.1). Figure 13.2 shows a typical intravenous setup with a piggyback attachment.

Intravenous infusions may be continuous or intermittent. In ***continuous infusions***, large volumes of fluid (i.e., 250 to 1000 mL), with or without added drug, are run into a vein uninterrupted, whereas ***intermittent infusions*** are administered during scheduled periods.[2] The rapid infusion of a medication into a vein is termed ***IV push*** and is usually conducted in 1 to 5 minutes depending upon the medication.

Critical Care

By definition, ***critical care*** (or ***intensive care***) is the specialized care of patients whose conditions are life-threatening and who require comprehensive care and constant monitoring. In the hospital, such care is provided in an **intensive care unit (ICU)**, a **critical care unit (CCU)**, or an **intensive treatment (or therapy) unit (ITU)**. These units, staffed by specially trained critical care physicians and nurses, utilize equipment and medications expressly intended to treat critically ill pediatric and adult patients. Clinical pharmacy services in the critical care setting have expanded dramatically over the years to provide pharmacokinetic services and patient monitoring for drug efficacy and adverse drug reactions.[3] Lists of drugs used in providing critical care may be found in the references cited.[4–6]

Common Intravenous Infusion Solutions

Aqueous solutions of dextrose, sodium chloride, and lactated Ringer's injection are the most commonly used intravenous fluids. Table 13.1 describes the content of these solutions, which may be administered as such or with additional drug or nutritional components.

Example Calculations of Basic Intravenous Infusions

(1) *How many grams each of dextrose and sodium chloride are used to prepare a 250-mL bag of* D5½NS *for intravenous infusion?*

$$250 \text{ mL} \times 0.05 \ (5\% \text{ w/v}) = \mathbf{12.5 \text{ g dextrose}}$$
$$250 \text{ mL} \times 0.0045 \ (0.45\% \text{ w/v}) = \mathbf{1.125 \text{ g sodium chloride}}$$

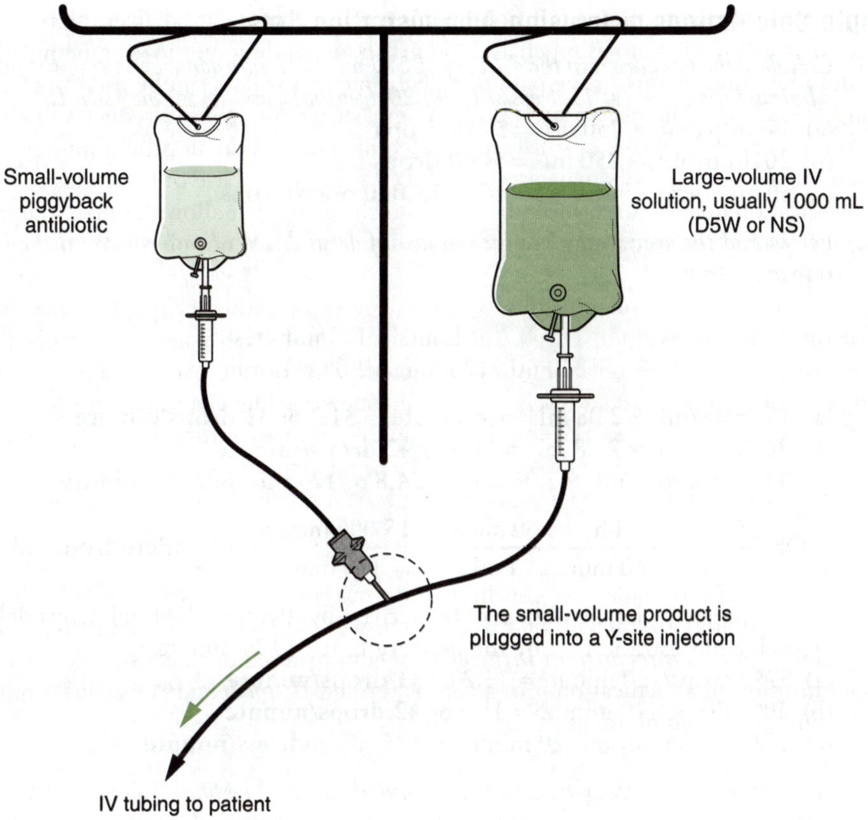

FIGURE 13.2 • A typical intravenous infusion setup with a piggybacked antibiotic. *(Courtesy of Lacher B. Pharmaceutical Calculations for the Pharmacy Technician. Baltimore, MD: Lippincott Williams & Wilkins, 2008.)*

(2) ***Calculate the milliequivalents of sodium and millimoles of dextrose in the above solution.***

Molecular weight of NaCl = 58.5 g
Equivalent weight of NaCl = 58.5 g
1 mEq NaCl = 58.5 mg
mEq in 1.125 g NaCl = 1125 mg/58.5 mg per 1 mEq = **19.2 mEq Na^+**
Molecular weight of dextrose ($C_6H_{12}O_6$) = 180.16 g
1 mmol dextrose = 180.16 mg
mmol in 12.5 g dextrose = 12,500 mg/180.16 mg per 1 mmol
= 69.38 or **69.4 mmol dextrose**

(3) ***A pharmacist prepared a liter of a 15% dextrose solution in sterile water for injection using a dextrose injection, 700 mg/mL. How many milliliters of the injection were required?***

Dextrose needed: 1000 mL × 15% - 150 g
700 mg/mL = 0.7 g/mL

$$150\ \text{g} \times \frac{1\ \text{mL}}{0.7\ \text{g}} = 214.28 \text{ or } \mathbf{214.3\ mL}$$

Example Calculations of Infusion Administration Sets

(1) *Calculate the total drops in the delivery of 250 mL of an infusion when using the following administration sets: (a) 15 drops/mL, (b) 20 drops/mL, and (c) 60 mcgtts/mL.*

(a) 15 drops/mL × 250 mL = **3750 drops**
(b) 20 drops/mL × 250 mL = **5000 drops**
(c) 60 microdrops/mL × 250 mL = **15,000 microdrops**

(2) *For each of the above, calculate the number of drops delivered each minute if the infusion is to last 2 hours.*

2 hours = 120 minutes
250 mL/120 min = 2.08 mL/min

(a) 15 drops/mL × 2.08 mL (per minute) = 31.2 or **31 drops/minute**
(b) 20 drops/mL × 2.08 mL = 41.6 or **42 drops/minute**
(c) 60 microdrops/mL × 2.08 mL = 124.8 or 125 **microdrops/minute**

$$\text{Or, } \frac{250\text{ mL}}{2\text{ h}} \times \frac{1\text{ h}}{60\text{ min}} \times \frac{60\text{ mcgtt}}{1\text{ mL}} = \frac{15{,}000\text{ mcgtt}}{120\text{ min}} = \textbf{125 microdrops/minute}$$

Alternatively, the answers may be derived by dividing the total drops delivered by each administration set by the delivery time of 120 minutes:

(a) 3750 drops/120 minute = 31.2 or **31 drops/minute**
(b) 5000 drops/120 minute = 41.6 or **42 drops/minute**
(c) 15,000 microdrops/120 minute = **125 microdrops/minute**

(3) *A rural patient is being transported by ambulance to a hospital 3 hours away. During transport, the patient is to be infused with 750 mL of normal saline injection. For each delivery set, calculate the rate of flow in drops/minute: (a) 15 gtts/mL, (b) 20 gtts/mL, and (c) 60 mcgtts/mL.*

3 hours = 180 minutes
750 mL/180 min = 4.17 mL/min

(a) 15 drops/mL × 4.17 mL/min = 62.55 or **63 drops/minute**
(b) 20 drops/mL × 4.17 mL/min = 83.4 or **83 drops/minute**
(c) 60 microdrops/mL × 4.17 mL/min = 250.2 or **250 microdrops/minute**

$$\text{Or, } \frac{750\text{ mL}}{3\text{ h}} \times \frac{1\text{ h}}{60\text{ min}} \times \frac{60\text{ mcgtt}}{1\text{ mL}} = \frac{45{,}000\text{ mcgtt}}{180\text{ min}} = \textbf{250 microdrops/minute}$$

Or,

(a) 750 mL × 15 gtts/mL = 11,250 drops
11,250/180 min = 62.5 or **63 drops/minute**
(b) 750 mL × 20 gtts/mL = 15,000 drops
15,000 drops/180 minute = 83.3 or **83 drops/minute**
(c) 750 mL × 60 mcgtts/mL = 45,000 microdrops
45,000 mcgtts/180 min = **250 microdrops/minute**

(4) *Compare (a) the number of drops and (b) the length of time, in minutes, required to deliver 50-mL of intravenous solutions when using a microdrip set, at 60 drops/mL, and a standard administration set, at 15 drops/mL, if in each case one drop is to be administered per second.*

Microdrip set:

(a) 60 drops/mL × 50 mL = **3000 drops**
(b) 3000 drops ÷ 60 drops/minute = **50 minutes**

Standard set:
(a) 15 drops/mL × 50 mL = **750 drops**
(b) 750 drops ÷ 60 drops/minute = **12.5 minutes**
Or, by dimensional analysis:

$$50\text{ mL} \times \frac{60\text{ drops}}{1\text{ mL}} \times \frac{1\text{ min}}{60\text{ drops}} = \mathbf{50\text{ minutes}}$$

$$50\text{ mL} \times \frac{15\text{ drops}}{1\text{ mL}} \times \frac{1\text{ min}}{60\text{ drops}} = \mathbf{12.5\text{ minutes}}$$

Intravenous Push (IVP) Drug Administration

The rapid injection of intravenous medications, as in emergency or critical care situations, is termed ***IV push, IVP, IV***, or sometimes a ***bolus*** dose. For the most part, drugs administered by IV push are intended to quickly control heart rate, blood pressure, cardiac output, respiration, or other life-threatening conditions. Intravenous push medications frequently are administered in a short time frame (from <1 to 5 minutes), but slowly enough so as to not cause a too rapid effect. The safe administration of a drug by IV push depends on precise calculations of dose and rate of administration. When feasible, a diluted injection rather than a highly concentrated one (e.g., 1 mg/mL versus 5 mg/mL) may be administered as an added safety precaution.[7]

The IV push may be injected directly into a vein or into a portal of an intravenous set. If the medication is administered via an administration set, a second injection of saline may be used to "flush" or help to push the medication into the bloodstream. A *flush* also may be used to clean an infusion line before and/or after use. An example of an intravenous *flush syringe* is shown in Figure 13.3.

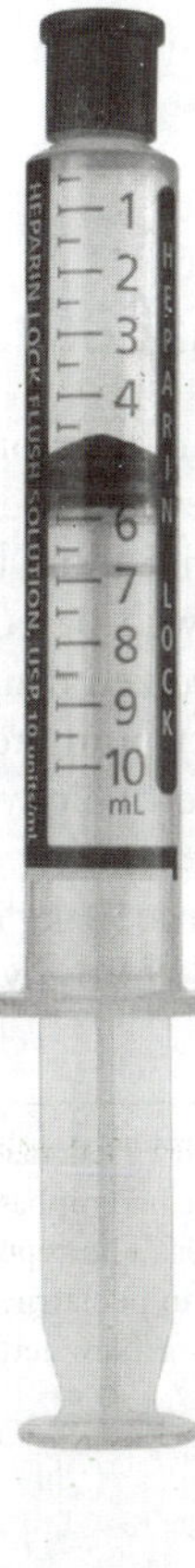

FIGURE 13.3 • An intravenous flush syringe. *(Courtesy of Becton Dickinson.)*

Example Calculations of IV Push Drug Administration

(1) *A physician orders enalaprilat (VASOTEC IV) 2 mg IVP for a hypertensive patient. A pharmacist delivers several 1-mL injections, each containing 1.25 mg of enalaprilat. How many milliliters of the injection should be administered?*

$$\frac{1.25\text{ mg}}{1\text{ mL}} = \frac{2\text{ mg}}{\text{x mL}};\ \text{x} = \mathbf{1.6\ mL}\ \text{(1 mL from one syringe and 0.6 mL from another)}$$

Or, by dimensional analysis:

$$2\text{ mg} \times \frac{1\text{ mL}}{1.25\text{ mg}} = \mathbf{1.6\ mL}$$

(2) *A physician orders midazolam hydrochloride (VERSED) 2 mg IV Stat. A pharmacist delivers a vial containing midazolam hydrochloride 5 mg/mL. How many milliliters should be administered?*

$$\frac{5\text{ mg}}{1\text{ mL}} = \frac{2\text{ mg}}{\text{x mL}};\ \text{x} = \mathbf{0.4\ mL}$$

Or, by dimensional analysis:

$$2\text{ mg} \times \frac{1\text{ mL}}{5\text{ mg}} = \mathbf{0.4\ mL}$$

(3) *General guidelines in the treatment of severe diabetic ketoacidosis include an initial bolus dose of 0.1 to 0.4 unit of insulin/kg IVP, followed by an insulin drip. Calculate the bolus dosage range for a 200-lb patient.*

$$200\text{ lb} \div 2.2\text{ lb/kg} = 90.9\text{ kg}$$
$$90.9\text{ kg} \times 0.1\text{ unit/kg} = \mathbf{9.09\ units}$$
$$90.9\text{ kg} \times 0.4\text{ unit/kg} = \mathbf{36.36\ units}$$

Special Considerations in Pediatric IV Infusion Delivery[b]

Medication error in pediatric patients is a special concern in institutional practice.[8] There is the ever-present need for weight-based dosing and highly individualized dose calculations that must be diligently performed. A reduction in errors has been achieved by the use of web-based calculators to perform infusion calculations, use of a limited number of standardized drug concentrations to prepare infusions (as noted below), and the utilization of smart-pump technology that reduces the number of human calculations required in dose and rate-of-flow determinations.

Depending on the institutional protocol, a medication order for an intravenous infusion for a 10-kg child may be stated as, for example, "dopamine 60 mg/100 mL, IV to run at 5 mL/h to give 5 mcg/kg/min." At some institutions in which *standardized drug products*

---

[b]Although *all* calculations pertaining to drug dosage and administration must be performed with 100% accuracy, it must be emphasized that pediatric patients are most vulnerable to mediation errors with often dire consequences. The report cited here underscores this point: Levine SR, et al. Guidelines for preventing medication errors in pediatrics. *Journal of Pediatric Pharmacology and Therapeutics* 2001;6:426–442. Available at: http://www.ismp.org/Newsletters/acutecare/articles/20020601.asp. Accessed May 12, 2014.

and established protocols have been developed, the same medication order may be written simply as "dopamine 5 mcg/kg/min IV" to provide equivalently accurate drug dosing of the patient.[9] This is because the standard solution of dopamine used in the institution, containing 60 mg of dopamine in each 100 mL and run at 5 mL/h, *would deliver the same dose of 5 mcg/kg/min* to the 10-kg patient. Calculate it:

$$\frac{60\text{ mg}}{100\text{ mL}} = \frac{x\text{ mg}}{5\text{ mL}};$$

$$x = 3\text{ mg or } \mathbf{3000\ mcg\ dopamine\ administered\ per\ hour}$$

$$3000\text{ mcg} \div 60\text{ min/h} = 50\text{ mcg dopamine administered per minute}$$

Since the 50 mcg/min are administered to a 10-kg child, the dose, per kg per minute, is:

$$\frac{50\text{ mcg}}{10\text{ kg}} = \frac{x\text{ mcg}}{1\text{ kg}};\ x = \mathbf{5\ mcg\ dopamine/kg/min}$$

Or, by dimensional analysis:

$$\frac{60\text{ mg}}{100\text{ mL}} \times \frac{1000\text{ mcg}}{1\text{ mg}} \times \frac{5\text{ mL}}{1\text{ h}} \times \frac{1\text{ h}}{60\text{ min}} =$$

$$50\text{ mcg/min (dose for 10-kg child)} = \mathbf{5\ mcg/kg/min}$$

All medication doses for pediatric patients, including those administered intravenously, must be carefully determined from available literature and reference sources.

In addition to medications administered by intravenous infusion to pediatric patients, fluid and electrolyte therapy is especially important in the clinical management of preterm and term neonates, particularly those with extremely low birth weights who tend to have greater loss of water through the skin, especially when they are maintained in a warm incubator.[10]

Example Calculations of Pediatric Infusions

(1) *Calculate the daily infusion volume of* D10W *to be administered to a neonate weighing 3 lb. 8 oz. on the basis of 60 mL/kg/day.*

$$3\text{ lb 8 oz.} = 3.5\text{ lb} \div 2.2\text{ lb/kg} = 1.59\text{ kg or } 1.6\text{ kg}$$

$$1.6\text{ kg} \times 60\text{ mL} = \mathbf{96\ mL}$$

(2) *Using an administration set that delivers 60 drops/mL at 20 drops/minute, calculate the total time for the above infusion.*

$$96\text{ mL} \times \frac{60\text{ drops}}{1\text{ mL}} \times \frac{1\text{ minute}}{20\text{ drops}} = \mathbf{288\ minutes,\ or\ 4\ hours\ 48\ minutes}$$

(3) *Gentamicin sulfate, 2.5 mg/kg, is prescribed for a 1.5-kg neonate. Calculate (a) the dose of the drug and, (b) when the drug is placed in a 50-mL IV bag, the flow rate, in mL/min, if the infusion is to run for 30 minutes.*

(a) 2.5 mg/kg × 1.5 kg = **3.75 mg gentamicin sulfate**

(b) 50 mL ÷ 30 minutes = **1.67 mL/minute**

(4) *A neonate born at 32 weeks' gestation weighs 2005 g and is transferred to the hospital's neonate intensive care unit with a diagnosis of sepsis. Among the physician's orders are aminophylline 5 mg/kg IV q6h, cefotaxime 50 mg/kg q12h, and vancomycin 10 mg/kg q12h.*[11]

(a) *Calculate the initial dose of each drug, in milligrams.*

$$\text{Neonate's weight} = 2005\text{ g} \times \frac{1\text{ kg}}{1000\text{ g}} = 2.005\text{ kg}$$

$$\text{Aminophylline initial dose} = 5\text{ mg/kg} \times 2.005\text{ kg} = 10.025\text{ or }\mathbf{10\text{ mg}}$$

$$\text{Cefotaxime initial dose} = 50\text{ mg/kg} \times 2.005\text{ kg} = 100.25\text{ or }\mathbf{100\text{ mg}}$$

$$\text{Vancomycin initial dose} = 10\text{ mg/kg} \times 2.005\text{ kg} = 20.05\text{ or }\mathbf{20\text{ mg}}$$

(b) *If aminophylline injection, 25 mg/mL, is available, how many milliliters of injection should be added to a 100-mL container of D10W for IV infusion?*

$$10\text{ mg} \times \frac{1\text{ mL}}{25\text{ g}} = \mathbf{0.4\text{ mL}}$$

(5) *A 4-day-old neonate born at 35 weeks' gestation and weighing 2210 g is prescribed gentamicin, 4 mg/kg, in 60 mL/kg of D10W for intravenous infusion.*[11] *If a pediatric injection contains gentamicin, 10 mg/mL, how many milliliters each of injection and D10W should be administered?*

$$\text{Neonate's weight} = 2210\text{ g} \times \frac{1\text{ kg}}{1000\text{ g}} = 2.21\text{ kg}$$

$$\text{Gentamicin dose} = 4\text{ mg/kg} \times 2.21\text{ kg} = 8.84\text{ mg}$$

$$\text{Gentamicin injection to administer} = 8.84\text{ mg} \times \frac{1\text{ mL}}{10\text{ mg}} = 0.884\text{ or }\mathbf{0.9\text{ mL}},$$

$$\text{D10W to administer} = 60\text{ mL/kg} \times 2.21\text{ kg} = \mathbf{132.6\text{ mL}}$$

(6) *A 2-year-old child weighing 30 lb is hospitalized with severe respiratory distress. Physicians' orders include aminophylline 5 mg/kg in 50-mL D5W½NS to infuse over 60 minutes. If aminophylline injection, 25 mg/mL, is available, how many milliliters should be used in the infusion?*

$$\text{Child's weight} = 30\text{ lb} \times \frac{1\text{ kg}}{2.2\text{ lb}} = 13.6\text{ kg}$$

$$\text{Aminophylline dose} = 5\text{ mg/kg} \times 13.6\text{ kg} = 68\text{ mg}$$

$$\text{Aminophylline injection to use} = 68\text{ mg} \times \frac{1\text{ mL}}{25\text{ mg}} = 2.72\text{ or }\mathbf{2.7\text{ mL}}$$

Intravenous Admixtures

The preparation of an intravenous admixture involves the transfer of one or more additives to a large-volume parenteral fluid. The additive may be incorporated into the fluid in the pharmacy or at the patient's bedside by injecting the additive into a port of the intravenous line or by administering by piggyback. Additives may include therapy-specific medications, antibiotics, electrolytes, vitamins, trace minerals, and other agents. Figure 13.4 shows the transfer of an additive to a large-volume fluid prior to administration.

Examples of calculations involving additives for *pediatric patients* are provided above and further examples are provided as follows.

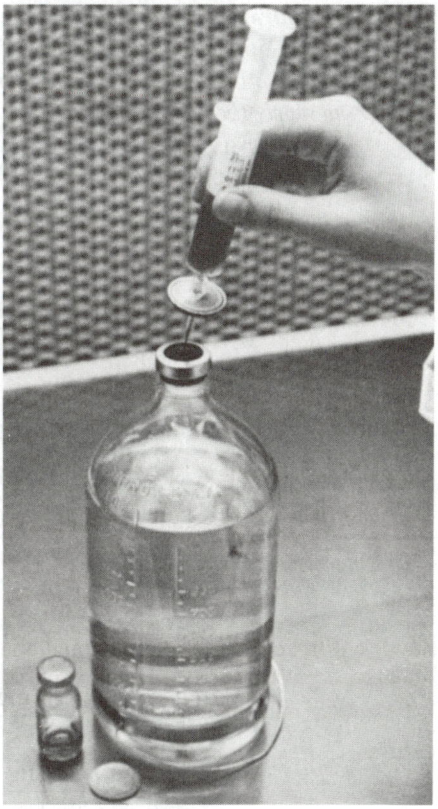

FIGURE 13.4 • The transfer of an additive to a large-volume parenteral solution. *(Millex® syringe filter courtesy of EMD Millipore Corporation. Millex® is a trademark of EMD Millipore Corporation.)*

Example Calculations of Additives to Intravenous Infusion Solutions

(1) *A medication order for a patient weighing 154 lb calls for 0.25 mg of amphotericin B per kilogram of body weight to be added to 500 mL of 5% dextrose injection. If the amphotericin B is to be obtained from a constituted injection that contains 50 mg/10 mL, how many milliliters should be added to the dextrose injection?*

$$1\text{ kg} = 2.2\text{ lb}$$

$$\frac{154\text{ (lb)}}{2.2\text{ (lb)}} = 70\text{ kg}$$

$$0.25\text{ mg} \times 70 = 17.5\text{ mg}$$

Constituted solution contains 50 mg/10 mL:

$$\frac{50\text{ (mg)}}{17.5\text{ (mg)}} = \frac{10\text{ (mL)}}{x\text{ (mL)}}$$

$$x = \mathbf{3.5\ mL}$$

Or, solving by dimensional analysis:

$$154\text{ lb} \times \frac{1\text{ kg}}{2.2\text{ lb}} \times \frac{0.25\text{ mg}}{1\text{ kg}} \times \frac{10\text{ mL}}{50\text{ mg}} = \mathbf{3.5\ mL}$$

(2) *An intravenous infusion is to contain 15 mEq of potassium ion and 20 mEq of sodium ion in 500 mL of 5% dextrose injection. Using potassium chloride injection containing 6 g/30 mL and 0.9% sodium chloride injection, how many milliliters of each should be used to supply the required ions?*

15 mEq of K^+ ion will be supplied by 15 mEq of KCl, and 20 mEq of Na^+ ion will be supplied by 20 mEq of NaCl.

$$1 \text{ mEq of KCl} = 74.5 \text{ mg}$$

$$15 \text{ mEq of KCl} = 1117.5 \text{ mg or } 1.118 \text{ g}$$

$$\frac{6 \text{ (g)}}{1.118 \text{ (g)}} = \frac{30 \text{ (mL)}}{x \text{ (mL)}}$$

$$x = 5.59 \text{ or } \mathbf{5.6\ mL}$$

$$1 \text{ mEq of NaCl} = 58.5 \text{ mg}$$

$$20 \text{ mEq of NaCl} = 1170 \text{ mg or } 1.17 \text{ g}$$

$$\frac{0.9 \text{ (g)}}{1.17 \text{ (g)}} = \frac{100 \text{ (mL)}}{x \text{ (mL)}}$$

$$x = \mathbf{130\ mL}$$

Or, solving by dimensional analysis:

$$15 \text{ mEq} \times \frac{74.5 \text{ mg}}{1 \text{ mEq}} \times \frac{1 \text{ g}}{1000 \text{ mg}} \times \frac{30 \text{ mL}}{6 \text{ g}} = 5.59 \text{ or } \mathbf{5.6\ mL}$$

$$20 \text{ mEq} \times \frac{58.5 \text{ mg}}{1 \text{ mEq}} \times \frac{1 \text{ g}}{1000 \text{ mg}} \times \frac{100 \text{ mL}}{0.9 \text{ g}} = \mathbf{130\ mL}$$

(3) *A medication order for a child weighing 44 lb calls for polymyxin B sulfate to be administered by the intravenous drip method in a dosage of 7500 units/kg of body weight in 500 mL of 5% dextrose injection. Using a vial containing 500,000 units of polymyxin B sulfate and sodium chloride injection as the solvent, explain how you would obtain the polymyxin B sulfate needed in preparing the infusion.*

$$1 \text{ kg} = 2.2 \text{ lb}$$

$$\frac{44}{2.2} = 20 \text{ kg}$$

$$7500 \text{ units} \times 20 = 150{,}000 \text{ units}$$

STEP 1. Dissolve contents of vial (500,000 units) in 10 mL of sodium chloride injection.

STEP 2. Add 3 mL of constituted solution to 500 mL of 5% dextrose injection.

Rate of Flow of Intravenous Fluids

On medication orders, the physician specifies the rate of flow of intravenous fluids in milliliters per minute, drops per minute, amount of drug (as milligrams per hour), or, more frequently, as the approximate duration of time of administration of the total volume of the infusion. Pharmacists may be called on to perform or check rate-of-flow calculations as those described in some previous problem examples as well as those in this section.

Oftentimes, the following equation finds use in rate-of-flow calculations:

$$\text{Rate of flow (drops/minute)} = \frac{\text{Volume infusion (mL)} \times \text{Drip set (drops/mL)}}{\text{Time (minutes)}}$$

In common usage are *macro sets* that deliver 10, 15, or 20 drops/milliliter and *microdrip* or *minidrip sets* that deliver 60 drops/milliliter.

Examples of Rate-of-Flow Calculations

(1) *A medication order calls for 1000 mL of D5W to be administered over an 8-hour period. Using an IV administration set that delivers 10 drops/mL, how many drops per minute should be delivered to the patient?*

$$\text{Volume of fluid} = 1000 \text{ mL}$$
$$8 \text{ hours} = 480 \text{ minutes}$$
$$\frac{1000 \text{ (mL)}}{480 \text{ (minutes)}} = 2.08 \text{ mL/min}$$
$$2.08 \text{ mL/min} \times 10 \text{ (drops/mL)} = 20.8 \text{ or } \mathbf{21 \text{ drops per minute}}$$

Or, solving by dimensional analysis:

$$\frac{10 \text{ drops}}{1 \text{ mL}} \times \frac{1000 \text{ mL}}{8 \text{ h}} \times \frac{1 \text{ h}}{60 \text{ min}} = 20.8, \text{ or } \mathbf{21 \text{ drops per minute}}$$

Or, solving by the equation:

$$\text{Rate of flow (drops/minute)} = \frac{\text{Volume infused (mL)} \times \text{Drip set (drops/mL)}}{\text{Time (minutes)}}$$
$$= \frac{1000 \text{ mL} \times 10 \text{ drops/mL}}{480 \text{ minutes}}$$
$$= 20.8 \text{ or } \mathbf{21 \text{ drops per minute}}$$

(2) *Ten (10) milliliters of 10% calcium gluconate injection and 10 mL of multivitamin infusion are mixed with 500 mL of a 5% dextrose injection. The infusion is to be administered over 5 hours. If the dropper in the venoclysis set calibrates 15 drops/mL, at what rate, in drops per minute, should the flow be adjusted to administer the infusion over the desired time interval?*

$$\text{Total volume of infusion} =$$
$$10 \text{ mL} + 10 \text{ mL} + 500 \text{ mL} = 520 \text{ mL}$$
$$\text{Dropper calibrates } 15 \text{ drops/mL}$$
$$520 \times 15 \text{ drops} = 7800 \text{ drops}$$
$$\frac{7800 \text{ (drops)}}{300 \text{ (minutes)}} = \mathbf{26 \text{ drops per minute}}$$

Or, solving by dimensional analysis:

$$\frac{15 \text{ drops}}{1 \text{ mL}} \times \frac{520 \text{ mL}}{5 \text{ hours}} \times \frac{1 \text{ h}}{60 \text{ min}} = \mathbf{26 \text{ drops per minute}}$$

Or, solving by the equation:

$$\text{Rate of flow (drops/minute)} = \frac{\text{Volume infused (mL)} \times \text{Drip set (drops/mL)}}{\text{Time (minutes)}}$$

$$= \frac{520 \text{ mL} \times 15 \text{ drops/mL}}{300 \text{ minutes}}$$

$$= \textbf{26 drops per minute}$$

(3) *An intravenous infusion contains 10 mL of a 1:5000 solution of isoproterenol hydrochloride and 500 mL of a 5% dextrose injection. At what flow rate should the infusion be administered to provide 5 μg of isoproterenol hydrochloride per minute, and what time interval will be necessary for the administration of the entire infusion?*

10 mL of a 1:5000 solution contains 2 mg.
2 mg or 2000 μg is contained in a volume of 510 mL.

$$\frac{2000\ (\mu g)}{5\ (\mu g)} = \frac{510\ (\text{mL})}{x\ (\text{mL})}$$

$$x = 1.275 \text{ or } \mathbf{1.28\ mL/minute}$$

$$\frac{1.28\ (\text{mL})}{510\ (\text{mL})} = \frac{1\ (\text{minute})}{x\ (\text{minute})}$$

$$x = 398 \text{ minutes or } \textbf{approx. 6½ hours}$$

Or, solving by dimensional analysis:

$$\frac{1 \text{ min}}{5\ \mu g} \times \frac{0.002 \text{ g}}{510 \text{ mL}} \times \frac{1{,}000{,}000\ \mu g}{1 \text{ g}} \times 510 \text{ mL} = 400 \text{ minutes} \approx \textbf{6½ hours}$$

(4) *If 10 mg of a drug is added to a 500-mL large-volume parenteral fluid:*

(a) *What should be the rate of flow, in milliliters per hour, to deliver 1 mg of drug per hour?*

$$\frac{10\ (\text{mg})}{1\ (\text{mg})} = \frac{500\ (\text{mL})}{x\ (\text{mL})}$$

$$x = \mathbf{50\ mL/hour}$$

(b) *If the infusion set delivers 15 drops/mL, what should be the rate of flow in drops per minute?*

$$15 \text{ drops/mL} \times 50 \text{ mL/h} = 750 \text{ drops/h}$$

$$\frac{750\ (\text{drops})}{x\ (\text{drops})} = \frac{60\ (\text{minutes})}{1\ (\text{minutes})}$$

$$x = \mathbf{12.5\ drops/minute}$$

Or, solving by dimensional analysis:

$$\frac{15 \text{ drops}}{1 \text{ mL}} \times \frac{50 \text{ mL}}{1 \text{ h}} \times \frac{1 \text{ h}}{60 \text{ min}} = \mathbf{12.5\ drops/minute}$$

(c) *How many hours should the total infusion last?*

$$\frac{50\ (\text{mL})}{500\ (\text{mL})} = \frac{1\ (\text{hour})}{x\ (\text{hour})}$$

$$x = \mathbf{10\ hours}$$

(5) *A physician's medication order calls for 800 mg of erythromycin to be added to 100 mL of D5W for intravenous infusion over 60 minutes. The source of erythromycin is a 1-g vial requiring dilution to 20 mL with sterile water for injection before being added to the D5W. Calculate (a) the milliliters of the erythromycin dilution that should be added to the D5W and (b) the rate of flow of the infusion, in milliliters per minute.*

(a) $\frac{1\text{ g}}{20\text{ mL}} = \frac{0.8\text{ g}}{x}$; $x = \mathbf{16\ mL}$

(b) 100 mL (D5W) + 16 mL (erythromycin dilution) = 116 mL

116 mL/60 min = **1.93 mL/min**

(6) *A physician's medication order calls for 400 mg of clindamycin to be added to 600 mL of D5W for intravenous infusion over 90 minutes. Clindamycin is available as an injection containing 600 mg/4 mL. (a) How many milliliters of the clindamycin injection should be used, (b) how many mg/mL of clindamycin will the infusion contain, and (c) how many milliliters per minute of the infusion should be delivered?*

(a) $\frac{600\text{ mg}}{4\text{ mL}} = \frac{400\text{ mg}}{x}$; $x = \mathbf{2.67\ mL}$

(b) Infusion = 600 mL (D5W) + 2.67 mL (clindamycin injection) = 602.67 mL
400 mg clindamycin/602.67 mL infusion = **clindamycin 0.66 mg/mL**

(c) 602.67 mL/90 min = 6.69 or **6.7 mL/min**

(7) *An intravenous fluid that contains 25 mg nitroglycerin in 250 mL is to be administered at 20 μg/min. Calculate the correct drip rates, in drops/minute, from administration sets that deliver (a) 15 drops/mL, (b) 20 drops/mL, and (c) 60 drops/mL.*

25 mg in 250 mL = 0.1 mg/mL = 100 μg/mL
Therefore, *20 μg/min* = 0.2 mL/min
Thus,

(a) 15 drops/mL × 0.2 mL/min = **3 drops/minute**
(b) 20 drops/mL × 0.2 mL/min = **4 drops/minute**
(c) 60 drops/mL × 0.2 mL/min = **12 drops/minute**

IV Infusion Rate Calculations for the Critical Care Patient

Many patients, including those in critical care, require both a maintenance fluid, as D5W, and a therapeutic drug additive, as an antibiotic (see Fig. 13.2). However, many critical care patients have fluid restrictions and must be maintained and treated within a stated maximum volume of fluid intake per day. Thus, consideration must be given to the *rate* and *volumes* of any infusions administered including intravenous piggybacked (IVPB) additives.

(1) *An order for a patient, with a 3-L daily IV fluid limit, calls for 3 L of D5W with a 100-mL IVPB antibiotic to be run in alone over a 1-hour period and administered every 6 hours. The administration set is calibrated to deliver 10 drops/milliliter. Calculate the following:*
(a) *The flow rate of the IVPB antibiotic*
(b) *The total flow time for the IV antibiotic*
(c) *The total volume for the IV antibiotic*
(d) *The total flow time for the D5W*
(e) *The total volume for the D5W*
(f) *The flow rate for the D5W*

Answers:

(a) $\frac{10\text{ mL} \times 10\text{ drops/mL}}{60\text{ min}} = 16.6$ or **17 drops/minute**

(b) 1 hour × 4 times a day = **4 hours** or 240 minutes
(c) 100 mL × 4 times a day = **400 mL**
(d) 24 hours – 4 hours (run time for the antibiotic) = **20 hours** or 1200 minutes
(e) 3000 mL – 400 mL (the IVPB antibiotic) = **2600 mL**

(f) $\frac{2600\text{ mL} \times 10\text{ drops/mL}}{1200\text{ min}} = 21.6$ or **22 drops/minute**

(2) *A physician's order calls for the administration of dopamine 800 mg in 500 mL of D5W to be administered at 5 mcg/kg/min using an IV pump. If the critical care patient weighs 130 lb, calculate the rate of flow of the infusion in mL/h.*

Patient's weight in kg = 130 lb/2.2 lb/kg = 59.1 kg

Rate of dopamine = 5 mcg/kg/min × 59.1 kg = 295.5 mcg/min

295.5 mcg/min × 60 min/h = 17,730 mcg/h

17,730 mcg/h ÷ 1000 mcg/mg = 17.73 mg/h

17.73 mg/h × 500 mL/800 mg = 11.08 or **11.1 mL/h**

Or,

$$\frac{500\text{ mL}}{800\text{ mg}} \times \frac{1\text{ mg}}{1000\text{ mcg}} \times \frac{5\text{ mcg}}{1\text{ kg/min}} \times \frac{60\text{ min}}{1\text{ h}} \times \frac{1\text{ kg}}{2.2\text{ lb}} \times 130\text{ lb} = 11.08 \text{ or } \mathbf{11.1\ mL/h}$$

(3) *A pharmacist prepares 250 mL of an infusion to contain 250 mg of dobutamine for administration to a 190-lb patient. The rate of flow is determined to be 34 mL/h. Calculate the rate of flow in mcg/kg/min.*

Patient's weight in kg = 190 lb/2.2 lb/kg = 86.4 kg

Rate of flow (mL/min) = 34 mL/1 h or 60 min = 0.567 mL/min

Dobutamine = 250 mg/250 mL = 1 mg/mL = 1000 mcg/mL

0.567 mL/min × 1000 mcg/mL = 567 mcg/min

Rate of flow = 567 mcg/min ÷ 86.4 kg = **6.56 mcg/kg/min**

Or,

$$\frac{250\text{ mg}}{250\text{ mL}} \times \frac{1000\text{ mcg}}{1\text{ mg}} \times \frac{34\text{ mL}}{1\text{ h}} \times \frac{1\text{ h}}{60\text{ min}} \times \frac{2.2\text{ lb}}{1\text{ kg}} \times \frac{1}{190\text{ lb}} = \mathbf{6.56\ mcg/kg/min}$$

Using a Nomogram

A nomogram, as that shown in Figure 13.5, may be used in determining the rate of flow of a parenteral fluid. Given the volume to be administered, the infusion time (duration), and the drops per milliliter delivered by the infusion set, the rate of flow, in drops per minute, may be determined directly.

If 1 L of a parenteral fluid is to be infused over a 12-hour period using an infusion set that delivers 20 drops/mL, what should be the rate of flow in drops per minute?

First, locate the intercept of the diagonal line representing an infusion time of 12 hours with the horizontal line representing 1 L of fluid. Next, follow the point of the intercept down to the drop counter scale representing "20 drops/mL" to determine the answer. In the example, the horizontal line would be crossed between 20 and 30 drops/minute—closer to the 30 or approximately 28 drops/minute.

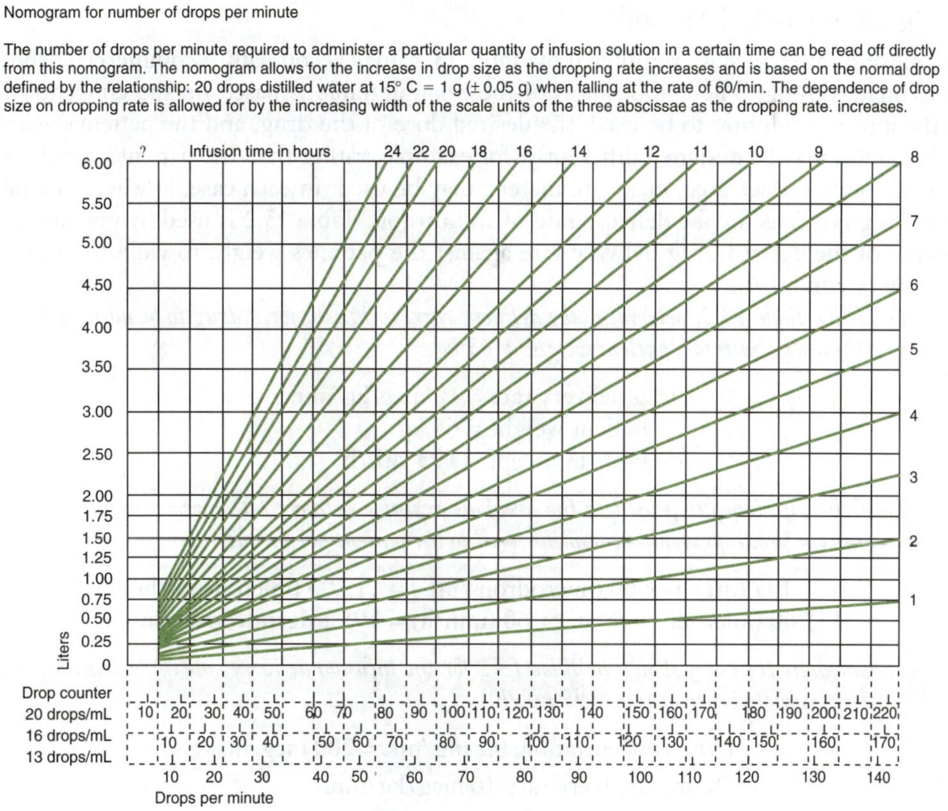

FIGURE 13.5 • Rate of flow versus quantity of infusion solution versus time nomogram. *(From Documenta Geigy Scientific Tables, 7th Ed., 1970. With permission of Ciba-Geigy Limited, Basel, Switzerland.)*

As a check to the proper use of the nomogram, the preceding example may be calculated as follows:

$$\text{Infusion time} = 12 \text{ hours} = 750 \text{ minutes}$$

$$\text{Infusion fluid} = 1 \text{ liter} = 1000 \text{ mL}$$

$$\text{Drops per milliliter} = 20$$

$$\text{Total drops in infusion liquid} = 20 \text{ drops/mL} \times 1000 \text{ mL} = 20{,}000$$

$$\frac{20{,}000 \text{ (drops)}}{720 \text{ (minutes)}} = 27.7 \text{ or } \mathbf{28 \text{ drops/minute}}$$

Or, solving by dimensional analysis:

$$\frac{20 \text{ drops}}{1 \text{ mL}} \times \frac{1000 \text{ mL}}{12 \text{ h}} \times \frac{1 \text{ h}}{60 \text{ min}} = 27.7 \text{ or } \mathbf{28 \text{ drops/minute}}$$

Or, solving by the equation:

$$\text{Rate of flow (drops/minute)} = \frac{\text{Volume infused (mL)} \times \text{Drip set (drops/mL)}}{\text{Time (minutes)}}$$

$$= \frac{1000 \text{ mL} \times 20 \text{ drops/mL}}{720 \text{ minutes}}$$

$$= 27.7 \text{ or } \mathbf{28 \text{ drops/minute}}$$

Using an Infusion Rate Table

An infusion rate table, as exemplified by Table 13.2, may accompany a commercial product to facilitate dosing. The composition of the example table is based on the concentration of the infusion solution to be used, the desired dose of the drug, and the patient's weight. Other tables may be designed differently; for example, rather than the patient's weight, the patient's body surface area, in square meters, may be used. In each case, however, the table provides guidelines for the delivery rate of an infusion. Table 13.2 is used by matching the column of the desired drug delivery rate against the patient's weight to yield the infusion delivery rate in mL/h.

(1) *Using Table 13.2, determine the delivery rate, in mL/h, for a drug to be administered at 10 mcg/kg/min to a patient weighing 65 kg.*

Drug delivery rate = 10 mcg/kg/min
Patient weight = 65 kg
Table intercept = **195 mL/h**

(2) *If the infusion pump used in the previous example delivers 60 microdrops/milliliter, how many microdrops would be administered to the patient per minute?*

195 (mL/h) × 60 (microdrops/mL) = 11,700 (microdrops/hour)
11,700 (microdrops/hour) ÷ 60 (min/h) = **195 microdrops/minute**

(3) *Calculate the entry shown in Table 13.2 for the infusion delivery rate as determined in the first example problem (i.e., 195 mL/h).*

Drug concentration: 0.2 mg/mL = 200 mcg/mL
Desired delivery rate: 10 mcg/kg/min
Patient weight: 65 kg

Table 13.2 • INFUSION RATE OF A HYPOTHETICAL DRUG FOR A CONCENTRATION OF 0.2 mg/mL

Patient Weight (kg)	Drug Delivery Rate (mcg/kg/min) 5	6	7	8	9	10	11	12	13
	Infusion Delivery Rate (mL/h)								
30	45	54	63	72	81	90	99	108	117
35	53	63	74	84	95	105	116	126	137
40	60	72	84	96	108	120	132	144	156
45	68	81	95	108	122	135	149	162	176
50	75	90	105	120	135	150	165	180	195
55	83	99	116	132	149	165	182	198	215
60	90	108	126	144	162	180	198	216	234
65	98	117	137	156	176	195	215	234	254
70	105	126	147	168	189	210	231	252	273
75	113	135	158	180	203	225	248	270	293
80	120	144	168	192	216	240	264	288	312
90	135	162	189	216	243	270	297	324	351
100	150	180	210	240	270	300	330	360	390

$$\text{Drug to be delivered} = 10\,(\text{mcg/kg/min}) \times 65\,(\text{kg}) = 650\,\text{mcg/min}$$
$$650\,(\text{mcg/min}) \times 60\,(\text{min}) = 3900\,\text{mcg/h}$$
$$\text{Infusion delivery rate} = 3900\,(\text{mcg/h}) \div 200\,(\text{mcg/h}) = \mathbf{195\ mL/h}$$

Note: For data such as these, when the patient's weight, the dose of the drug, and the drug concentration in the infusion are given or may be calculated, the infusion rate may be calculated by the following equation[9]:

$$\text{Infusion rate (mL/h)} = \frac{\text{Patient's weight (kg)} \times \text{Dose (mcg, mg, or units/kg/min)} \times 60}{\text{Drug concentration, infusion (mcg, mg, or units/mL)}}$$
$$= \frac{65\,(\text{kg}) \times 10\,(\text{mcg/kg/min}) \times 60}{200\,(\text{mcg/mL})}$$
$$= \mathbf{195\ mL/h}$$

In using this equation, the denominations for the dose and drug concentration must be the same (e.g., mcg, mg, or units). Also, if the dosage rate is stated in hours (e.g., mcg/kg/h), the 60 is not needed in the equation to arrive at flow rate per hour.

A different type of flow rate table is shown in Table 13.3. This type of table is used for determining flow rates for different doses when using a specific drug concentration. The data in the table are calculated as by the following illustration:

Drug concentration: 200 μg/mL

Dose selected: 5 μg/min

Calculation of mL of infusion providing 5 μg dose:

$$\frac{200\,\mu\text{g}}{1\,\text{mL}} = \frac{5\,\mu\text{g}}{x\,\text{mL}};\ x = 0.025\,\text{mL} = \text{dose/min}$$

Calculation, dose in mL/h:

$$0.025\,\text{mL (dose/min)} \times 60\,(\text{min/h}) = \mathbf{1.5\ mL/h}$$

(4) *Use Table 13.3 to determine the infusion administration rate, in mL/h, to deliver drug at 16 μg/min.*
For 8 μg/min, the rate is 2.4 mL/h
Thus, for 16 μg/min, the rate would be double or 4.8 mL/h
Proof: The infusion contains 200 μg/mL

$$16\,\mu\text{g (per minute)}/200\,\mu\text{g/mL} = 0.08\,\text{mL (per minute)}$$
$$0.08\,\text{mL/min} \times 60\ \text{minutes (per hour)} = 4.8\,\text{mL/h}$$

Or, note from the table that the rate in mL/h for each dose may be determined by multiplying by the factor 0.3. Thus, 16 μg/min × 0.3 = 4.8 mL/h

Table 13.3 • EXAMPLE OF A FLOW RATE TABLE FOR AN INFUSION CONTAINING DRUG IN A CONCENTRATION OF 200 μg/mL[a]

Dose, μg/min	1	2	3	4	5	6	7	8	9	10	15	20	30	40	50
RATE, mL/h	0.3	0.6	0.9	1.2	1.5	1.8	2.1	2.4	2.7	3	4.5	6	9	12	15

[a]After finding the desired dose in μg/min in the top column, the rate of flow in mL/h is found by the number below. The table may be extrapolated; for example, a dose of 80 μg/min would translate into a rate of 24 mL/h. Also, the table may be changed for a different drug concentration; for example, a drug concentration of 100 μg/mL and a dose of 5 μg/min would necessitate a flow rate of 3 mL/h.

CALCULATIONS CAPSULE

Intravenous Infusions

In certain calculations, the following equations find application.

To calculate infusion time:

$$\text{Infusion time} = \frac{\text{Volume of infusion in mL}}{\text{Flow rate in mL/h or mL/min}}$$

To calculate flow rate in drops/minute:

$$\text{Rate of flow (drops/minute)} = \frac{\text{Volume infused (mL)} \times \text{Drip set (drops/mL)}}{\text{Time (minutes)}}$$

To calculate flow rate in mL/h when based on dose[4]:

$$\text{Infusion rate (mL/h)} = \frac{\text{Patient s weight (kg)} \times \text{Dose (mcg, mg, or units/kg/min)} \times 60}{\text{Drug concentration, infusion (mcg, mg, or units/mL)}}$$

In using this equation, the denominations for the dose and drug concentration must be the same (e.g., mcg, mg, or units). Also, if the dosage rate is stated in hours (e.g., mcg/kg/h), the 60 is not needed in the equation to arrive at flow rate per hour.

CASE IN POINT 13.1 A physician prescribes amiodarone HCl IV (CORDARONE) for a patient with ventricular fibrillation. The prescribing information is:

Loading infusions:

Rapid infusion over first 10 minutes:	15 mg/min
Slow infusion over the next 6 hours:	1 mg/min

Maintenance infusion:

Slow infusion over the remaining 18 hours:	0.5 mg/min

Amiodarone HCl IV is available in 3-mL ampuls containing 50 mg/mL.

The pharmacist uses a 100-mL bag of D5W for the rapid infusion and 250-mL bottles of D5W for the slow infusions.

(a) How many milliliters from an amiodarone HCl IV ampul should be placed in the 100-mL bag for the rapid infusion?

(b) What is the drug concentration in the rapid infusion, in mg/mL?

(c) If the pharmacist added the contents of 3 ampuls to each 250-mL bottle of D5W needed for the slow infusions, calculate the drug concentration in mg/mL.

(d) What rate of administration, in mL/h, should the pharmacist have recommend during the 6-hour infusion segment?

(e) Calculate the rate of administration in (d) in drops/minute with an administration set that delivers 15 drops/mL.

(f) Calculate the milligrams of drug administered by slow infusion over the 6-hour segment.

(g) Make the same calculation as that in (f) but over the 18-hour segment.

Monoclonal Antibodies (mAbs) Infusion Calculations

Monoclonal antibodies (mAbs) are used in the diagnosis and treatment of various diseases. In general, mAbs are dosed on the basis of body weight or body surface area and are administered by injection or infusion. Table 13.4 presents some examples of mAb infusions.

(1) *In preparing an infusion of the drug trastuzumab, a pharmacist adds 20 mL of bacteriostatic water for injection to a vial containing 440 mg of the mAb. The resulting solution contains trastuzumab, 21 mg/mL. Using the information from Table 13.4, (a) calculate the milliliters of solution required for the loading dose for a 165-lb patient. The pharmacist then transfers the calculated volume into an infusion bag containing 250 mL of sodium chloride injection. Calculate (b) the quantity of trastuzumab administered in mg/min and (c) the drip rate, in drops/minute, using an administration set that delivers 20 drops/mL.*

(a) Weight of patient: 165 lb/2.2 lb/kg = 75 kg
Loading dose in mg: 75 kg × 4 mg/kg = 300 mg

$$\text{Volume of injection (dose): } \frac{21\text{ mg}}{1\text{ mL}} = \frac{300\text{ mg}}{x\text{ mL}};\ x = 14.29 \text{ or } \mathbf{14.3\ mL}$$

(b) 300 mg/90 min = **3.33 mg/min**
(c) Volume of infusion: 250 mL + 14.3 mL = 264.3 mL
Drops in infusion: 264.3 mL × 20 drops/mL = 5286 drops
Drops per minute: 5286 drops/90 min = 58.7 or **59 drops/minute**

Example Calculations Derived from a Product Label

The following calculations are derived from the product label for CLEOCIN PHOSPHATE, shown in Figure 13.6.

(1) *According to the package insert, a solution of clindamycin for intravenous infusion should not exceed a concentration of 18 mg/mL. On this basis, calculate the minimal volume of infusion, which may be prepared from the entire contents of the vial.*

$$\frac{18\text{ mg}}{1\text{ mL}} = \frac{600\text{ mg}}{x} = \mathbf{33.33\ mL}$$

(2) *If the contents of the vial are added to 50 mL of D5W and an infusion administered over a 20-minute period of time, calculate the clindamycin administered in (a) mg/mL and (b) mg/min.*

(a) 4 mL (vial) + 50 mL D5W = 54 mL, total volume
600 mg/54 mL = **11.11 mg/mL**
(b) 600 mg/20 min = **30 mg/min**

Table 13.4 • EXAMPLES OF MONOCLONAL ANTIBODIES (MABS) ADMINISTERED BY INTRAVENOUS INFUSION

mAb	Primary Use	Usual Adult Dose and Infusion Rate[a]
Cetuximab	Agent or coagent in the treatment of colorectal and head and neck cancer	400 mg/m^2 (120-minute infusion); then 250 mg/m^2 (60-minute infusion) weekly
Natalizumab	Monotherapy in treatment of relapsing forms of multiple sclerosis and in Crohn's disease	300 mg (60-minute infusion)
Tocilizumab	Rheumatoid arthritis	4 mg/kg once every 4 wk (60-minute infusion)
Trastuzumab	Sole or coagent in treatment of breast cancer	4-mg/kg loading dose (90-minute infusion) 2-mg/kg/wk maintenance dose (30-minute infusion)

[a]Stated usual doses/rates are for illustration; actual clinical doses/rates are determined based on individual patient parameters.

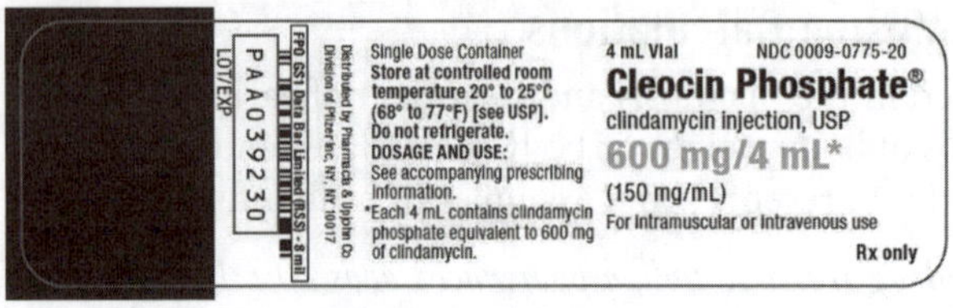

FIGURE 13.6 • Label of product used in intramuscular and intravenous solutions. *(Source: http://dailymed.nlm.nih.gov/dailymed/about.cfm. Courtesy of Pfizer, Inc.)*

(3) *If a pediatric patient weighing 12 lb is to receive clindamycin at the rate of 20 mg/kg/day in three equally divided doses, calculate the contents of the vial, in milliliters, which may be used as an additive for a single dose.*

$$12 \text{ lb}/2.2 \text{ lb/kg} = 5.45 \text{ kg}$$
$$5.45 \text{ kg} \times 20 \text{ mg/kg/day} = 109 \text{ mg/day}$$
$$109 \text{ mg/day} \div 3 \text{ doses/day} = 36.3 \text{ mg/dose}$$
$$36.5 \text{ mg} \div 150 \text{ mg/mL} = \mathbf{0.24 \text{ mL}}$$

PRACTICE PROBLEMS

Calculations of Basic Intravenous Infusion Solutions

1. How many grams each of sodium chloride and dextrose are present in a 1000-mL IV bag of 0.18% sodium chloride and 4% dextrose?
2. A medication calls for 1000 mL of D5W½NSS to be administered over 8 hours. Calculate the quantity, in grams, each of dextrose and sodium chloride administered in a 20-minute period.

Calculations of Infusion Time

3. If a standard *microdrop* infusion set is used to administer 100 mL of an infusion over a 2-hour period, calculate the rate of delivery, in drops/min.
4. A patient was administered 150 mL of D_5W at a rate of 25 mL/h. If the infusion was begun at 8 AM, at what time was it completed?
5. A patient received 500 mL of D_5W½NS at a rate of 15 drops/min. If the administration set used delivered 15 drops/mL, calculate the infusion time in hours, minutes.
6. A pediatric patient received 50 mL of an infusion at 10 drops/min with an administration set that delivered 60 drops/mL. Calculate the duration of the infusion in minutes.
7. An intravenous drip contains 2 g of lidocaine HCl (XYLOCAINE) and is administered at a rate of 4 mg/min. Calculate the total time, in minutes, for the complete infusion.

Calculations of Intravenous Infusions with Additives

8. Daptomycin (CUBICIN), 4 mg/kg, is recommended for administration over a 30-minute period by intravenous infusion in 0.9% sodium chloride. How many milliliters of a vial containing 500 mg of daptomycin in 10 mL should be added to a 100-mL bag of normal saline in treating a 165-lb patient?
9. An emergency syringe contains lidocaine, 1 g/5 mL. How many milliliters should be used in preparing 250 mL of an infusion to contain 4 mg/mL of lidocaine in D5W?

10. A fluconazole injection contains 400 mg of fluconazole in 200 mL of normal saline injection for infusion. Calculate the concentration of fluconazole in mg/mL.
11. Intravenous immunoglobulin (IVIG) has been administered in the pretransplantation of organs at a rate of 0.08 mL/kg/min. Calculate the number of milliliters administered to a 154-lb patient over a period of 4 hours.
12. If 200 mg of dopamine in 250 mL D5W is administered to a 145-lb patient, at 15 mL/h, how many mcg/kg/min is the patient receiving?
13. A pharmacist receives a medication order for 300,000 units of penicillin G potassium to be added to 500 mL of D5W. The directions on the 1,000,000-unit vial state that if 1.6 mL of solvent is added, the solution will measure 2 mL. How many milliliters of the solution must be withdrawn and added to the D5W?
14. A physician orders 2 g of an antibiotic to be placed in 1000 mL of D5W. Using an injection that contains 300 mg of the antibiotic per 2 mL, how many milliliters should be added to the dextrose injection in preparing the medication order?
15. An intravenous infusion for a patient weighing 132 lb calls for 7.5 mg of amikacin sulfate per kilogram of body weight to be added to 250 mL of 5% dextrose injection. How many milliliters of an amikacin sulfate injection containing 500 mg/2 mL should be used in preparing the infusion?
16. Lidocaine injection may be administered by continuous intravenous infusion to treat cardiac arrhythmias at a dose of 2 mg/min. Solutions for intravenous infusion may be prepared by the addition of 1 g of lidocaine hydrochloride to 1 L of 5% dextrose in water. Calculate the maximum duration of this infusion in minutes.
17. A medication order calls for acyclovir, 355 mg, to be administered by intravenous infusion over 60 minutes. A 500-mg vial of acyclovir is available that must be mixed with sterile water for injection to prepare 10 mL of injection. The proper amount is then admixed with 100 mL of normal saline solution. Calculate (a) the volume to be taken from the vial of mixed acyclovir, (b) the rate of infusion in mL/min, and (c) the drops/minute if using an intravenous set that delivers 20 drops/mL.
18. A medication order for a 20-lb pediatric patient calls for vancomycin, 10 mg/kg, to be administered by intravenous infusion. The pharmacy has a 10-mL injection containing 500 mg of vancomycin. The pharmacist adds the correct amount to a 100-mL bag of normal saline solution. (a) How many milliliters of the injection were added and (b) what is the content of vancomycin in the infusion, in mg/mL?

Various Calculations of Infusions Including Drip Rates

19. A medication order calls for a dopamine drip at 5 μg/kg/min for a 185-lb patient. The pharmacy adds 400 mg dopamine in 250 mL of D5W. Calculate the drip rates per minute when using administration sets delivering (a) 15 drops/mL, (b) 20 drops/mL, and (c) 60 drops/mL.
20. A physician orders 4 L of intravenous fluids for a dehydrated patient to be administered over a period of 24 hours using an intravenous set that delivers 15 drops/mL. Calculate the drip rate in (a) drops per minute and in (b) milliliters per hour.
21. How many milliliters of an injection containing 1 g of drug in 4 mL should be used in filling a medication order requiring 275 mg of the drug to be added to 500 mL of D5W solution? If the solution is administered at the rate of 1.6 mL/min, how many milligrams of the drug will the patient receive in 1 hour?

22. A physician orders a 2-g vial of a drug to be added to 500 mL of D5W. If the administration rate is 125 mL/h, how many milligrams of the drug will a patient receive per minute?
23. The drug labetalol has a dose of 300 mg and is administered in 300 mL of an intravenous infusion at a rate of 2 mg/min. Using an infusion set that delivers 20 drops/mL, calculate the required drip rate in drops/minute.
24. A physician orders 35 mg of amphotericin B and 25 units of heparin to be administered intravenously in 1000 mL of D5W over an 8-hour period. In filling the medication order, the available sources of the additives are a vial containing 50 mg of amphotericin B in 10 mL and a syringe containing 10 units of heparin per milliliter.
    (a) How many milliliters of each additive should be used in filling the medication order?
    (b) How many milliliters of the intravenous fluid per minute should the patient receive?
25. A solution containing 500,000 units of polymyxin B sulfate in 10 mL of sterile water for injection is added to 250 mL of 5% dextrose injection. The infusion is to be administered over 2 hours. If the administration set delivers 15 drops/mL, at what rate, in drops per minute, should the flow be adjusted to administer the infusion over the designated time interval?
26. Five hundred milliliters of a 2% sterile solution of a drug are to be administered by intravenous infusion over a period of 4 hours. If the administration set delivers 20 drops/mL, at what rate, in drops per minute, should the infusion flow? Solve the problem by calculation *and* by using the nomogram in this chapter.
27. An 8-kg infant requires a continuous infusion of a drug to run at 1 mL/h to deliver 4 mcg of drug/kg/min. Calculate the milligrams of drug that must be added to a 100-mL intravenous infusion solution.
28. Five hundred milliliters of an intravenous solution contains 0.2% of succinylcholine chloride. At what flow rate should the infusion be administered to provide 2.5 mg of succinylcholine chloride per minute?
29. A hospital pharmacist prepared thirty 100-mL epidural bags containing 0.125% of bupivacaine hydrochloride and 1 μg/mL of fentanyl citrate in 0.9% sodium chloride injection. How many (a) 30-mL vials of 0.5% bupivacaine hydrochloride, (b) 20-mL vials of 50 μg/mL of fentanyl citrate, and (c) 1-L bags of 0.9% sodium chloride were required?
30. An intravenous fluid of 1000 mL of lactated Ringer's injection was started in a patient at 8 AM and was scheduled to run for 12 hours. At 3 PM, 800 mL of the fluid remained in the bottle. At what rate of flow should the remaining fluid be regulated using an IV set that delivers 15 drops/mL to complete the administration of the fluid in the scheduled time?
31. If a physician orders 5 units of insulin to be added to a 1-L intravenous solution of D5W to be administered over 8 hours, (a) how many drops per minute should be administered using an IV set that delivers 15 drops/mL, and (b) how many units of insulin would be administered in each 30-minute period?
32. A patient is to receive 3 μg/kg/min of nitroglycerin from a solution containing 100 mg of the drug in 500 mL of D5W. If the patient weighs 176 lb and the infusion set delivers 60 drops/mL, (a) how many milligrams of nitroglycerin would be delivered per hour, and (b) how many drops per minute would be delivered?

33. Using the nomogram in Figure 13.5, determine the approximate rate of infusion delivery, in drops per minute, based on 1.5 liters of fluid to be used over a period of 8 hours with an infusion set calibrated to deliver 16 drops/mL.
34. The drug alfentanil hydrochloride is administered by infusion at the rate of 2 μg/kg/min for anesthesia induction. If a total of 0.35 mg of the drug is to be administered to a 110-lb patient, how long should be the duration of the infusion?
35. The recommended maintenance dose of aminophylline for children is 1 mg/kg/h by injection. If 10 mL of a 25-mg/mL solution of aminophylline is added to a 100-mL bottle of dextrose injection, what should be the rate of delivery, in milliliters per hour, for a 40-lb child?
36. A patient is to receive an infusion of a drug at the rate of 5 mg/h for 8 hours. The drug is available in 10-mL vials containing 8 mg of drug per milliliter. If a 250-mL bottle of D5W is used as the vehicle, (a) how many milliliters of the drug solution should be added, and (b) what should be the flow rate in milliliters per minute?
37. A patient is receiving 500 mL of an intravenous drip containing 25,000 units of sodium heparin in sodium chloride injection. Calculate (a) the administration rate, in mL/h, to deliver 1200 units of sodium heparin per hour and (b) the administration rate, in drops/minute, with an IV set that delivers 15 drops/mL.
38. A 50-mL vial containing 1 mg/mL of the drug alteplase is added to 100 mL of D5W and administered intravenously with an infusion set that delivers 15 drops/mL. How many drops per minute should be given to administer 25 mg of the drug per hour?
39. If the loading dose of phenytoin in children is 20 mg/kg of body weight to be infused at a rate of 0.5 mg/kg/min, over how many minutes should the dose be administered to a 32-lb child?
40. A pharmacist prepares an intravenous infusion containing 1 g dobutamine in 250 mL of D5W. An IV pump is programmed to deliver 10 mcg/kg/min to a 209-lb patient. Calculate the flow rate in mL/h.
41. If a medication order calls for a dobutamine drip, 5 μg/kg/min, for a patient weighing 232 lb, what should be the drip rate, in drops per minute, if the 125-mL infusion bag contains 250 mg of dobutamine and a microdrip chamber is used that delivers 60 drops/mL?
42. At what rate, in drops per minute, should a dose of 20 μg/kg/min of dopamine be administered to a 65-kg patient using a solution containing dopamine, 1200 μg/mL, and a drip set that delivers 60 drops/mL?
43. A pharmacist places 5 mg/mL of acyclovir sodium in 250 mL of D5W for parenteral infusion into a pediatric patient. If the infusion is to run for 1 hour and the patient is to receive 500 mg/m^2 BSA, what would be the rate of flow in milliliters per minute for a patient measuring 55 cm in height and weighing 10 kg?
44. Aminophylline is not to be administered in pediatric patients at a rate greater than 25 mg/min to avoid excessive peak serum concentrations and possible circulatory failure. What should be the maximum infusion rate, in milliliters per minute, for a solution containing 10 mg/mL of aminophylline in 100 mL of D5W?
45. An intravenous infusion contains 5 mg of zoledronic acid (RECLAST) in 100 mL. If the infusion is to be administered in 15 minutes, how many (a) milligrams of zoledronic acid and (b) milliliters of infusion must be administered per minute? And (c), using a drip set that delivers 20 drops/milliliter, how many drops per minute must be infused?

46. Abatacept (ORENCIA), used to treat rheumatoid arthritis, is available in vials, each containing 250 mg of powdered drug, intended to be reconstituted to 10 mL with sterile water for injection. The dose of abatacept depends on a patient's body weight: <60 kg, 500 mg; 60 to 100 kg, 750 mg; and >100 kg, 1 g. The contents of the appropriate number of vials are aseptically added to a 100-mL infusion bag or bottle of sodium chloride injection *after* the corresponding volume of sodium chloride injection has been removed. The concentration of abatacept in an infusion for a 200-lb patient would be:
    (a) 5.8 mg/mL
    (b) 6.25 mg/mL
    (c) 6.8 mg/mL
    (d) 7.5 mg/mL
47. Temsirolimus (TORISEL), for use in advanced renal cell carcinoma, is prepared for infusion by adding 1.8 mL of special diluent to the drug vial resulting in 3 mL of injection containing 10 mg/mL of temsirolimus. The required quantity is then added to a 250-mL container of sodium chloride injection for infusion. The recommended dose of temsirolimus is 25 mg infused over 30 to 60 minutes. The quantity of drug delivered, in mg/mL, and the rate of infusion, in mL/min, for a 30-minute infusion are:
    (a) 0.099 mg/mL and 8.42 mL/min
    (b) 0.099 mg/mL and 8.33 mL/min
    (c) 1 mg/mL and 8.42 mL/min
    (d) 1 mg/mL and 8.33 mL/min
48. Nicardipine hydrochloride (CARDENE IV) is administered in the short-term treatment of hypertension by slow intravenous infusion at a concentration of 0.1 mg/mL. A 10 mL containing 25 mg of nicardipine hydrochloride should be added to what volume of D5W to achieve the desired concentration of infusion?
    (a) 80 mL
    (b) 100 mL
    (c) 240 mL
    (d) 250 mL

Calculations of Monoclonal Antibody (mAb) Infusions

49. The mAb eculizumab is available in 30-mL vials containing 300 mg of drug. Prior to administration by intravenous infusion, the solution is diluted with sodium chloride injection to a concentration of 5 mg/mL. The dose of eculizumab is 600 mg infused over a 35-minute period. Calculate the rate of infusion in drops/minute using an administration set that delivers 15 drops/mL.
50. Using Table 13.4 and Figure 8.2 as references, (a) calculate the initial dose of cetuximab for a 140-lb patient measuring 65 inches in height. If cetuximab is available in vials containing 200 mg/100 mL, (b) calculate the volume to be used in an infusion. If the infusion is delivered over 120 minutes and the package insert states that rate of delivery of cetuximab should not exceed 10 mg/min, calculate whether or not that standard is being met.
51. The mAb natalizumab is available in vials containing 300 mg/15 mL. Prior to infusion, the contents are added to 100 mL of normal saline injection. Refer to Table 13.4 as needed, and calculate (a) the concentration of natalizumab in the infusion, in mg/mL, and (b) the rate of infusion, in mL/min.

52. Cetuximab (ERBITUX) injection is used by intravenous infusion in the treatment of certain cancers. It has a recommended initial dose of 400 mg/m^2 to be administered over 120 minutes with a maximum infusion rate of 10 mg/min. The injection is supplied in single-use vials containing cetuximab, 100 mg/50 mL. (a) Using the BSA equation, calculate the dose for a patient weighing 154 lb and measuring 5 feet 8 inches in height. (b) How many milliliters of cetuximab injection will provide the dose required? (c) If the calculated dose is administered over 120 minutes, what would be the rate of flow in mg/min?
53. The dose of ofatumumab (ARZERRA) for a patient is 300 mg. In preparing an intravenous infusion, a pharmacist draws a calculated volume of ofatumumab injection from a 50-mL vial containing 1 g of ofatumumab. This quantity is then added to a 1-L bag of sodium chloride injection for the intravenous infusion. The infusion is programmed to flow at a rate of 3.6 mg of atumumab/hour. Calculate (a) the volume, in milliliters, of ofatumumab injection to use, (b) the rate of flow of the infusion in mL/min, and (c) the total flow time, in hours, for completion of the infusion.

Critical Care Calculations

54.[12] A medication order calls for dopamine, 400 mg in 500 mL of D5W, to run initially at 4 mcg/kg/min and then titrated to 12 mcg/kg/min to stabilize blood pressure in a 140-lb patient. Calculate the (a) initial infusion rate in mL/h and (b) titrated rate in mL/h.

55.[12] A medication order calls for esmolol hydrochloride, 5 g/500 mL of D5W, for the rapid control of ventricular rate in a 143-lb patient. The infusion is programmed to run at 50 mcg/kg/min. Calculate the infusion rate in mL/h.

56.[12] Sodium nitroprusside is ordered at 0.3 mcg/kg/min for a 220-lb patient. A vial containing 50 mg of sodium nitroprusside in 2 mL is diluted to 250 mL with NSI and ordered to run at 14 mL/h. Is this run rate correct? If not, what should be the correct infusion rate?

57.[12] Procainamide 0.5 g in 250 mL of D5W is ordered to run at 2 mg/min. Calculate the flow rate in mL/h.

58. A pharmacist prepared a dopamine HCl solution to contain 400 mg/250 mL D5W. Calculate:
(a) the concentration of dopamine HCl in the infusion, in mg/mL, and (b) the infusion flow rate, in mL/h, for a 150-lb patient, based on a dose of 5 mcg/kg/min.

59.[12] The following was ordered for a critical care patient: 2 L D5W/0.45%NS to run over 24 hours with a 2000-mL IV fluid daily limit. An IVPB antibiotic is ordered to run every 6 hours separately in 50 mL of D5W over 30 minutes. The drop factor is 60 drops/mL. Calculate the flow rates, in drops/minute, of the (a) IVPB and (b) D5W/0.45% NS.

Miscellaneous Calculations

60. NIMBEX injection contains 2 mg cisatracurium besylate/mL in 5-mL single-dose vials. The contents of the vial are diluted in dextrose injection to a drug concentration of 0.1 mg/mL prior to infusion. How many milliliters of dextrose injection are required to prepare the infusion?
61. If the NIMBEX infusion, as described above, is administered to a 70-kg patient at the rate of 1.5 mcg/kg/min, calculate the delivery rate in mL/h.

62. How many minutes will the NIMBEX infusion, as described above, run until empty?
63. If the infusion delivery set for the NIMBEX infusion, as described above, delivers 60 microdrops/milliliter, how many microdrops/minute would be delivered?
64. If the infusion rate for epoprostenol sodium (FLOLAN) at a concentration of 3,000 ng/mL is prescribed as 10 ng/kg/min, calculate the infusion delivery rate, in mL/h, for a patient weighing 132 lb.
65. If the infusion, as described in the previous problem, runs for 15 minutes, how many mcg of epoprostenol sodium will have been infused?
66. Eptifibatide (INTEGRILIN) injection, for intravenous infusion, is a platelet aggregation inhibitor. The usual dose is 180 mcg/kg as an intravenous bolus followed by infusion at 2 mcg/kg/min. Calculate, for a 220-lb patient, the (a) bolus dose, in mL, from a single-use vial containing eptifibatide, 2 mg/mL, and (b) infusion rate, in mL/h, using an infusion containing eptifibatide, 0.75 mg/mL.
67. The dose of an antimicrobial drug for pediatric patients ≤ 3 months of age and weighing ≥ 1500 g is given as:

    <1 week of age: 25 mg/kg every 12 hours
    1 to 4 weeks of age: 25 mg/kg every 8 hours
    4 weeks to 3 months of age: 25 mg/kg every 6 hours

    Doses of 500 mg or less should be administered by intravenous infusion over 15 to 30 minutes.

    Doses greater than 500 mg should be infused over 40 to 60 minutes. If the infusion is prepared to contain 250 mg of drug/100 mL of solution, calculate (a) the dose, in milligrams/__hours, for a patient who is 2 months old and weighs 3.76 kg and (b) the rate of the infusion, in mL over ____ minutes.
68. The following questions relate to the product label shown here (Fig. 13.7).
    (a) Pharmacy directions: The contents of the vial are added to 5% dextrose injection to prepare an intravenous infusion to have a drug concentration in the range of 0.12 mg/mL to 2.8 mg/mL. How many milliliters of infusion may be prepared for each concentration extreme?
    (b) If a drug concentration of 2.8 mg/mL is prepared and the dose for a patient is 125 mg/m^2 infused over 90 minutes, what should be the rate of flow in mL/min for the patient having a BSA of 0.8 m^2?

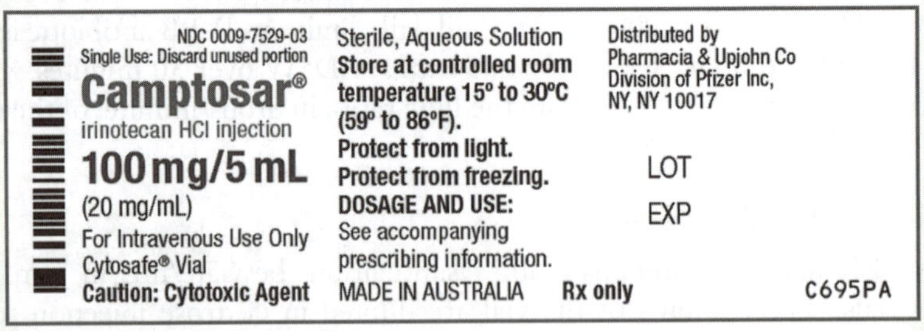

FIGURE 13.7 • Drug product label. *(Source: http://dailymed.nlm.nih.gov/dailymed/about.cfm. Courtesy Pfizer, Inc.)*

CALCQUIZ

13.A.[a] A hospital pharmacy receives a medication order for 500 mg aminophylline in 250 mL normal saline solution for a 132-lb patient. The aminophylline is to be administered at a dose of 300 μg/kg/h using an IV set that delivers 60 drops/mL. The pharmacy has 20-mL vials of injection containing aminophylline, 25 mg/mL. Calculate the following:

(a) The milliliters of aminophylline injection that should be added to the normal saline solution
(b) The total volume of the intravenous infusion
(c) The milligrams of aminophylline administered per hour
(d) The duration, in hours, for the complete infusion
(e) The number of milliliters of infusion delivered per hour (flow rate, mL/h)
(f) The number of drops administered per minute (flow rate, drops/minute)

13.B.[a] A hospitalized patient is receiving an intravenous infusion containing 40 mEq of potassium chloride in a liter of fluid. The IV set being used is calibrated to deliver 15 drops/mL with a flow rate of 12 drops/minute. How many (a) milligrams, (b) milliequivalents, and (c) millimoles of potassium chloride are delivered each hour?

13.C. A physician submits a medication order for a 110-lb patient calling for an intravenous drip containing 400 mg of dopamine in a 250-mL bag of normal saline solution. The drip is to be run at 5 μg/kg/min with an IV set that delivers 15 drops/mL. Calculate the following:

(a) The milliliters of a dopamine injection, 40 mg/mL, to use in the infusion
(b) The concentration of dopamine in the infusion in mg/mL
(c) The drip rate in drops/minute
(d) The infusion rate in mL/h

13.D. A medication order for a patient in the critical care unit of a hospital calls for a continuous intravenous infusion of isoproterenol, 5 μg/min. The standard protocol is to add the contents of a 5-mL ampule of a 1:5000 isoproterenol injection to 250 mL of dextrose 5% in water. The critical care nurse uses an IV set programmed to deliver 12 drops/mL. Calculate the following:

(a) The quantity of isoproterenol, in μg/mL, in the 5-mL ampule of isoproterenol injection
(b) The concentration of isoproterenol, in μg/mL, in the infusion
(c) The flow rate of the intravenous infusion in drops/minute
(d) The duration of the completed infusion in minutes

13.E. A hospital pharmacy received an order for 250 mL of a premixed injection containing 50 mg of nitroglycerin in D5W. The initial infusion rate was prescribed at 5 μg/min to be increased by 5 μg/min every 5 minutes as needed up to a maximum of 20 μg/min. An infusion set delivering 60 microdrops/mL was used. Calculate the following:

(a) The concentration of nitroglycerin in the infusion in μg/mL
(b) The initial rate of infusion in mL/h
(c) The maximum rate of infusion (20 μg/min) in microdrops/min *and* in mL/h

[a]Problem courtesy of Flynn Warren, Bishop, GA.

ANSWERS TO "CASE IN POINT" AND PRACTICE PROBLEMS

Case in Point 13.1

(a) 15 mg/min × 10 min = 150 mg amiodarone HCl needed for the rapid infusion.
Ampul contains 50 mg/mL, so 3 mL is needed = one 3-mL ampul.
(b) 150 mg amiodarone in 103 mL; 150 mg ÷ 103 mL = 1.46 mg/mL
(c) 3 (ampuls) × 3 mL = 9 mL × 50 mg/mL = 450 mg amiodarone HCl
450 mg ÷ 259 mL = 1.74 mg/mL amiodarone HCl
(d) 60 minutes × 1 mg/min = 60 mg amiodarone HCl
60 mg ÷ 1.74 mg/mL = 34.5 mL/h
(e) 34.5 mL × 15 drops/mL = 517.5 drops in 1 hour
517.5 drops ÷ 60 = 8.625 or about 9 drops/minute
(f) 1 mg/min × 60 min/h × 6 h = 360 mg
(g) 0.5 mg/min × 60 min/h × 18 h = 540 mg

Practice Problems

1. 1.8 g sodium chloride
   40 g dextrose
2. 2.083 g dextrose
   0.187 g sodium chloride
3. 50 drops/minute
4. 2:00 PM
5. 8 hours, 20 minutes
6. 300 minutes
7. 500 minutes
8. 6 mL daptomycin injection
9. 5 mL lidocaine injection
10. 2 mg/mL fluconazole
11. 1344 mL IVIG
12. 3.03 mcg/kg/min dopamine HCl
13. 0.6 mL
14. 13.33 mL
15. 1.8 mL amikacin sulfate injection
16. 500 minutes
17. (a) 7.1 mL
    (b) 1.785 or 1.8 mL/min
    (c) 35.7 or 36 drops/minute
18. (a) 1.8 mL
    (b) 0.89 mg/mL vancomycin
19. (a) 3.9 or 4 drops/minute
    (b) 5.25 or 5 drops/minute
    (c) 15.7 or 16 drops/minute
20. (a) 41.7 or 42 drops/minute
    (b) 166.7 mL/h
21. 1.1 mL
    52.8 mg
22. 8.33 mg
23. 40 drops/minute
24. (a) 7 mL amphotericin B
    2.5 mL heparin
    (b) 2.08 mL/min
25. 32.6 or 33 drops/minute
26. 41.7 or 42 drops/minute
27. 192 mg
28. 1.25 mL/min
29. (a) 25
    (b) 3
    (c) 3
30. 40 drops/minute
31. (a) 31.25 or 31 drops/minute
    (b) 0.3 unit
32. (a) 14.4 mg/h
    (b) 72 drops/minute
33. Approximately 50 drops/minute
34. 3.5 minutes
35. 8 mL/h
36. (a) 5 mL
    (b) 0.53 mL/min
37. (a) 24 mL/h
    (b) 6 drops/minute
38. 18.75 or 19 drops/minute
39. 40 minutes
40. 14.25 mL/h
41. 15.82 or 16 drops/minute
42. 66 drops/minute
43. 0.58 mL/min
44. 2.5 mL/min
45. (a) 0.33 mg zoledronic acid
    (b) 6.67 mL
    (c) 133 drops/minute

46. (d) 7.5 mg/mL
47. (a) 0.099 mg/mL and 8.42 mL/min
48. (c) 240 mL
49. 51.4 or 51 drops/minute
50. (a) 680 mg cetuximab
    (b) 340 mL
    (c) 5.7 mg/min, yes
51. (a) 2.6 mg/mL natalizumab
    (b) 1.9 mL/min
52. (a) 733 mg cetuximab dose
    (b) 366.5 mL cetuximab injection
    (c) 6.1 mg/min
53. (a) 15 mL of atumumab injection
    (b) 0.203 mL/min
    (c) 83.33 hours
54. (a) 19.08 or 19 mL/h
    (b) 57.24 or 57 mL/h
55. 19.5 mL/h
56. No; 9 mL/h
57. 60 mL/h
58. (a) 1.6 mg/mL
    (b) 12.78 mL/h
59. (a) 100 drops/minute IVPB
    (b) 83 drops/minute D5W/0.45NS
60. 95 mL dextrose injection
61. 63 mL/h delivery rate of infusion
62. 95.2 minutes
63. 63 microdrops/minute
64. 12.0 mL/h
65. 9 mcg epoprostenol sodium
66. (a) 9 mL, bolus dose
    (b) 15.99 or 16 mL/h
67. (a) 94 mg drug every 6 hours
    (b) 37.6 mL infused over 15 to 30 minutes.
68. (a) 35.7 mL (at 2.8 mg/mL) to 833.3 mL (at 0.12 mg/mL)
    (b) 0.396 or 0.4 mL/min

References

1. *Pharmaceutical Compounding—Sterile Preparations. United States Pharmacopeia 32 National Formulary* 27. Rockville, MD: The United States Pharmacopeial Convention; 2009;1:318–354.
2. Boh L. *Pharmacy Practice Manual: A Guide to the Clinical Experience*. Baltimore, MD: Lippincott Williams & Wilkins; 2001:418.
3. Papadopoulos J, Rebuck JA, Lober C, et al. The critical care pharmacist: an essential intensive care practitioner. Pharmacotherapy 2002;22(11). Available at http://www.medscape.com/viewarticle/444371. Accessed May 10, 2014.
4. Critical Care Drugs. Available at: http://quizlet.com/12905842/critical-care-drugs-flash-cards/. Accessed May 10, 2014.
5. Critical Care Drug Manual. Available at: http://lifeinthefastlane.com/book/critical-care-drugs/. Accessed May 10, 2014.
6. Commonly Used Critical Care Infusions. Available at: http://workplacenurses.com/id69.html. Accessed May 10, 2014.
7. Institute for Safe Medication Practices. ISMP medication safety alert: how fast is too fast for IV push medications? May 15, 2003. Available at: https://www.ismp.org/Newsletters/acutecare/articles/20030515.asp. Accessed September 1, 2014.
8. Larsen GY, Howard PB, Cash J, et al. Standard drug concentrations and smart-pump technology reduce continuous-medication-infusion errors in pediatric patients. *Pediatrics* 2005;116:e21–e25. Available at: http://pediatrics.aappublications.org/content/116/1/e21.full. Accessed September 1, 2014.
9. Mitchell A, Sommo P, Mocerine T, et al. A standardized approach to pediatric parenteral medication delivery. *Hospital Pharmacy* 2004;39:433–459.
10. Gomella TL, Cunningham MD, Eyal FG, et al. *Neonatology: Management Procedures, On-Call Problems, Diseases, and Drugs*. New York, NY: Lange Medical Books; 2004:69–73.
11. Craig GP. *Clinical Calculations Made Easy*. 2nd Ed. Philadelphia, PA: Lippincott Williams & Wilkins; 2001:225–228.
12. Lacher B. *Pharmaceutical Calculations for the Pharmacy Technician*. Baltimore, MD: Lippincott Williams & Wilkins; 2008:287.

14

Assessment of Nutritional Status, Enteral and Parenteral Nutrition, and the Food Nutrition Label

OBJECTIVES

Upon successful completion of this chapter, the student will be able to:

- Assess a patient's nutritional status based on calculation of body mass index (BMI) and ideal body weight (IBW).
- Perform basic calculations for enteral and parenteral nutrition.
- Apply the food nutrition label in related calculations.

Assessment of Nutritional Status

In community pharmacies, pharmacists routinely counsel patients on matters of nutrition. It is well recognized that poor dietary choices contribute to obesity and many chronic conditions, including hypertension, coronary heart disease, sleep apnea, and type 2 diabetes mellitus.[1–3] Furthermore, being *extremely* overweight, or *obese*, predisposes one to an even greater risk of disease, disease complications, and mortality. Community pharmacists frequently advise patients on general dietary requirements for the maintenance of good health, provide counseling with regard to weight control, help patients understand the nutritional labeling on food products, and explain the use and composition of various dietary supplements. In addition to diet, other factors that can result in obesity include behavioral, cultural, metabolic, and genetic disposition.

Body Mass Index

The initial phase in managing the overweight or obese patient is an assessment of the degree of excessive weight. ***Body mass index (BMI)*** is accepted as the clinical standard for judging excessive weight and obesity. BMI is defined as body weight in kilograms divided by the square of height measured in meters. According to the National Institutes of Health (NIH),[2] individuals with a BMI (kg/m^2)

- ≤18.5 (kg/m^2) is considered underweight
- 18.5 to 24.9 (kg/m^2) is considered normal
- 25.0 to 29.9 (kg/m^2) is considered overweight
- 30.0 to 39.9 (kg/m^2) is considered obese
- ≥40 (kg/m^2) is considered extremely obese

For an elderly person, a BMI of less than 21 can be a sign of malnutrition.[4] BMI in *most people* is an indicator of high body fat; however, this may not be the case for persons who are especially muscular such as some athletes.

Determining BMI from a Standardized Table

BMI may be determined by using a standardized table like that shown in Table 14.1, in which the intercept of a person's height and weight indicates the BMI. Many of the standardized tables available are in units of the common systems of measurement (i.e., feet/inches and pounds) to facilitate ease of use by the general public. Others are available in metric or dual scale.

(1) *Using Table 14.1, determine the BMI for a person measuring 5 feet 8 inches and weighing 160 lb.*

The intercept of 5 feet 8 inches and 160 lb shows a BMI of **24**.

(2) *Using Table 14.1, determine the BMI for a person 183 cm in height and weighing 96 kg.*

$$183 \text{ cm} \times \frac{1 \text{ inch}}{2.54 \text{ cm}} = 72.05 \text{ inches} \approx 72 \text{ inches}$$

$$96 \text{ kg} \times \frac{2.2 \text{ lb}}{\text{kg}} = 211.2 \text{ lb} \approx 210 \text{ lb}$$

The intercept of 72 inches, or 6 feet 0 inches in height and 210 lb, shows a BMI of **28**.

Table 14.1 • DETERMINING BODY MASS INDEX (BMI, kg/m²)

WEIGHT

HEIGHT	100	110	120	130	140	150	160	170	180	190	200	210	220	230	240	250
5'0"	20	21	23	25	27	29	31	33	35	37	39	41	43	45	47	49
5'1"	19	21	23	25	26	28	30	32	34	36	38	40	42	43	45	47
5'2"	18	20	22	24	26	27	29	31	33	35	37	38	40	42	44	46
5'3"	18	19	21	23	25	27	28	30	32	34	35	37	39	41	43	44
5'4"	17	19	21	22	24	26	27	29	31	33	34	36	38	39	41	43
5'5"	17	18	20	22	23	25	27	28	30	32	33	35	37	38	40	42
5'6"	16	18	19	21	23	24	26	27	29	31	32	34	36	37	39	40
5'7"	16	17	19	20	22	23	25	27	28	30	31	33	34	36	38	39
5'8"	15	17	18	20	21	23	24	26	27	29	30	32	33	35	36	38
5'9"	15	16	18	19	21	22	24	25	27	28	30	31	32	34	35	37
5'10"	14	16	17	19	20	22	23	24	26	27	29	30	32	33	34	36
5'11"	14	15	17	18	20	21	22	24	25	26	27	28	30	32	33	35
6'0"	14	15	16	18	19	20	22	23	24	26	27	28	30	31	33	34
6'1"	13	15	16	17	18	20	21	22	24	25	26	28	29	30	32	33
6'2"	13	14	15	17	18	19	21	22	23	24	26	27	28	30	31	32
6'3"	12	14	15	16	17	19	20	21	22	24	25	26	27	29	30	31
6'4"	12	13	15	16	17	18	19	21	22	23	24	26	27	28	29	30

BMI interpretation

- Underweight: under 18.5
- Normal: 18.5–24.9
- Overweight: 25–29.9
- Obese: 30–39.9
- Extremely obese ≥ 40

Determining BMI by Calculation

If a person's height and weight are outside the range of a BMI table, or if a BMI table is unavailable, BMI may be determined by the formula:

$$\text{BMI} = \frac{\text{Weight (kg)}}{[\text{Height (m)}]^2}$$

(1) *Calculate the BMI of a person 4 feet 11 inches in height and weighing 98 lb.*

$$98 \text{ lb} \times \frac{1 \text{ kg}}{2.2 \text{ lb}} = 44.55 \text{ kg}$$

$$4 \text{ feet } 11 \text{ inches} = 59 \text{ inches} \times \frac{2.54 \text{ cm}}{\text{inch}} \times \frac{1 \text{ m}}{100 \text{ cm}} = 1.5 \text{ m}$$

$$\text{BMI} = \frac{44.55 \text{ kg}}{(1.5 \text{ m})^2} = \mathbf{19.83}$$

(2) *Calculate the BMI of a person 6 feet 0 inches in height weighing 210 lb.*

$$210 \text{ lb} \times \frac{1 \text{ kg}}{2.2 \text{ lb}} = 95.45 \text{ kg}$$

$$6 \text{ feet} = 72 \text{ inches} \times \frac{2.54 \text{ cm}}{\text{inch}} \times \frac{1 \text{ m}}{100 \text{ cm}} = 1.83 \text{ m}$$

$$\text{BMI} = \frac{95.45 \text{ kg}}{(1.83 \text{ m})^2} = \mathbf{28.54}$$

An Alternative Formula for the Calculation of BMI

BMI may be calculated by the formula:

$$\text{BMI} = \frac{\text{Weight (lb)}}{[\text{Height (inch)}]^2} \times 704.5$$

NOTE: The factor 704.5, used by the NIH, is derived by dividing the square of 39.37 (inches/m) by 2.2 (lb/kg).

Calculate the BMI for a person weighing 210 lb and standing 72 inches in height.

$$\text{BMI} = \frac{210 \text{ lb}}{(72 \text{ inches})^2} \times 704.5 = \mathbf{28.54}$$

Ideal Body Weight

As presented in Chapter 10, a patient's IBW may be calculated through the use of the following formulas based on height and gender:

For males:

IBW = 50 kg + 2.3 kg for each inch of patient height over 5 feet

or, in pounds

110 lb + 5 lb for each inch over 5 feet

For females:

IBW = 45.5 kg + 2.3 kg for each inch of patient height over 5 feet *or*, in pounds

100 lb + 5 lb for each inch over 5 feet

A patient's actual body weight (ABW) can be compared with his or her IBW to assess nutritional status as shown below[5]:

- ABW ≤89% IBW are considered underweight.
- ABW 90 to 120% IBW are considered normal.
- ABW >120 to <150% IBW are considered overweight.
- ABW ≥150 to <200% are considered obese.
- ABW ≥200% are considered extremely obese.

Calculation of IBW and Comparison of ABW

(1) *Calculate the IBW (in pounds) for a male patient who is 6 feet tall and weighs 210 lb, determine the percentage of his ABW compared to his IBW, and indicate the nutritional category into which he falls according to his weight.*

IBW = 110 lb + (12 × 5 lb) = 110 lb + 60 lb = **170 lb**

$$\frac{210\text{ lb}}{170\text{ lb}} \times 100 = \mathbf{123.53\%}$$

Since his ABW is between 120% and 150% of his IBW, he falls into the "**overweight**" category.

(2) *Calculate the weight range in pounds for a female patient who is 5 feet 4 inches tall to fall within the "normal" nutritional category based on her IBW.*
IBW = 100 lb + (4 × 5 lb) = 100 lb + 20 lb = 120 lb
120 lb × 90% = 108 lb
120 lb × 120% = 144 lb
Range = **108–144 lb**

Considerations in Parenteral and Enteral Nutrition

Pharmacists are increasingly involved in providing enteral and parenteral nutrition services in the institutional as well as in the home care setting. In this role, pharmacists may take part in the selection of the nutritional formula, prepare the product for use, and/or participate in its administration. Figure 14.1 depicts the three routes of nutrition: oral, enteral, and parenteral.

The content provided in this chapter is *introductory*. Pharmacists' actual participation in providing parenteral and enteral nutrition services requires a comprehensive understanding of all aspects of this specialized field. Practice guidelines and critical reports are provided by the *American Society for Parenteral and Enteral Nutrition (ASPEN)*; its publication, *Journal of Parenteral and Enteral Nutrition*; and its Web site, http://www.nutritioncare.org.

The following points are emphasized within the context of the limited scope of this chapter:

- The order form for parenteral nutrition (PN) presented by Figure 14.2 is an *example*. Such forms and their content vary between institutions.
- Nutritional orders are individualized for each patient based on age, metabolic condition, organ function, disease state, and medication usage.
- Calculations are often performed to provide the "targets" for nutritional components, which then may be rounded or modified based on individual patient requirements.

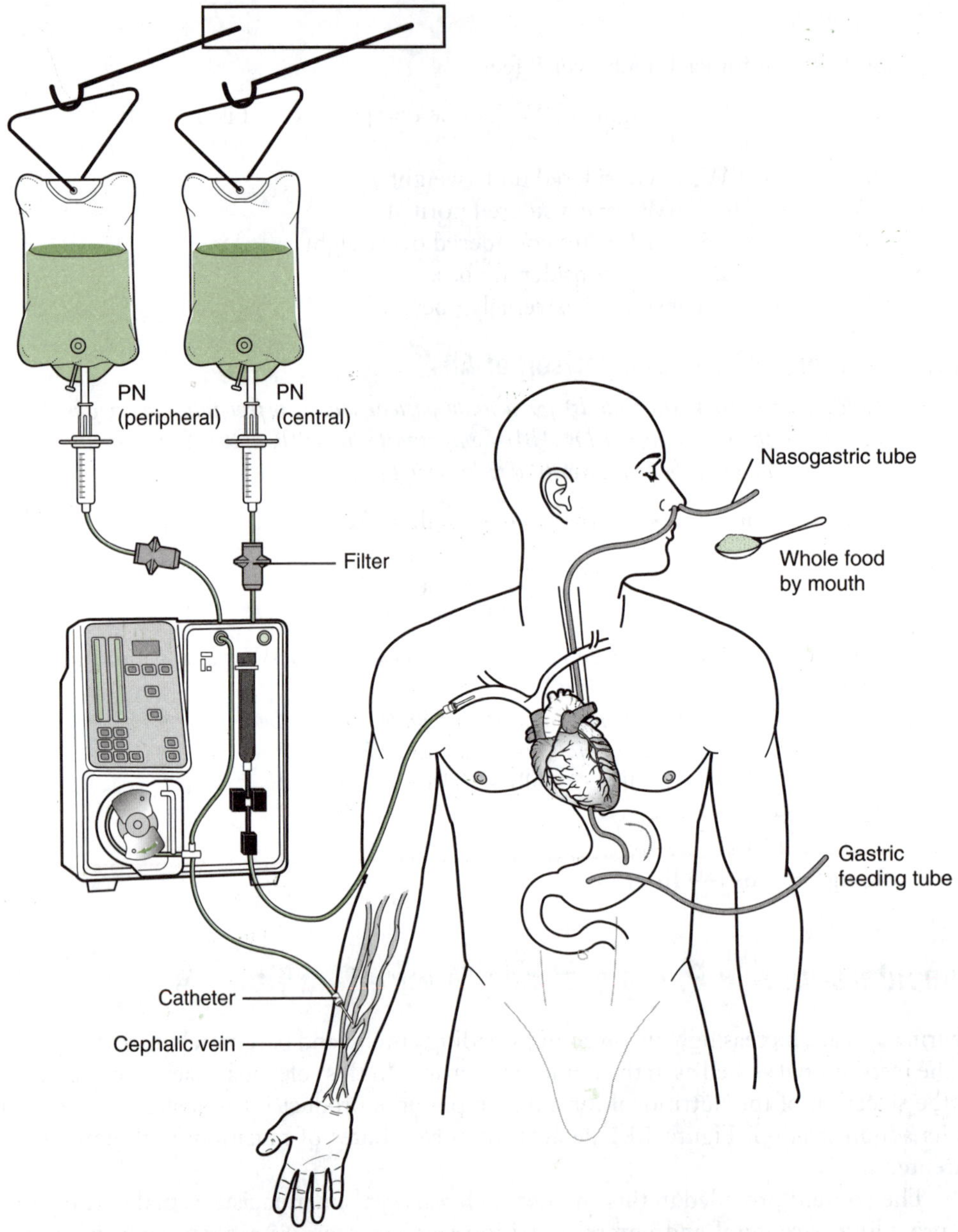

FIGURE 14.1 • Routes of nutrition: oral, enteral, and parenteral.

- The most common errors associated with PN involve dosage formulation, dosage calculations, and infusion rates.[6]
- Standard units of measure used are *grams* for the base components (i.e., dextrose, amino acids, and lipids), *milliequivalents* for electrolytes, and *millimoles* for phosphate, all in a specified volume, as per *liter*, or volume for a 24-hour infusion. The rate of flow is stated in *milliliters per hour* for a designated period of time, usually 24 hours.
- Parenteral and enteral nutrition orders should be clearly labeled with all *identifiers* of the patient, formula and quantity, route and rate of administration, infusion time, expiration date, and, for enteral preparations, the statement "Not for I.V. Use."[6]

Patient Information

ADULT PARENTERAL NUTRITION ORDERS

Primary Diagnosis:		PN Indication:
Dosing Wt: kg	Height:	Allergies:

Administration Route: ☐ CVC or PICC (proper tip placement must be confirmed) ☐ Peripheral IV

STANDARD FORMULATIONS

☐ **Peripheral formula: Amino Acids 4.25%/ Dextrose 5%** Total Calories/L 340 Amino Acid **42.5** g/L Dextrose **50** g/L	☐ **Central line only: Amino Acids 5%/ Dextrose 20%** Total Calories/L 880 Amino Acid **50** g/L Dextrose **200** g/L

☐ Standard electrolytes	☐ Custom electrolytes (fill out below)	☐ Standard electrolytes	☐ Custom electrolytes (fill out below)
Sodium 35 mEq/L Potassium 30 mEq/L Magnesium 5 mEq/L Calcium 4.5 mEq/L Phosphate 15 mmol/L Acetate 70 mEq/L Chloride 39 mEq/L	NaCl ________ mEq/L KCl ________ mEq/L Mg Sulf ________ mEq/L Ca Gluc ________ mEq/L K Phos ________ mmol/L	Sodium 35 mEq/L Potassium 30 mEq/L Magnesium 5 mEq/L Calcium 4.5 mEq/L Phosphate 15 mmol/L Acetate 80 mEq/L Chloride 39 mEq/L	NaCl ________ mEq/L KCl ________ mEq/L Mg Sulf ________ mEq/L Ca Gluc ________ mEq/L K Phos ________ mmol/L

ADDITIVES:
☐ Adult Multivitamin 10mL per day
☐ Trace Elements (Multitrace 4 concentrate 1mL) per bag
☐ Regular Insulin ________units per bag (minimum of 20 units per bag due to absorption)
☐ **Other** ________________________________
☐ **Other** ________________________________

☐ **Fat Emulsion: 20% Lipid (2 kcal/mL) 250mL 3 in 1 bag** ☐ **Fat Emulsion 10% Lipid (1.1 kcal/mL) 500mL bag to run in IV separately daily over 12 hours**

Select Administration Rate: Infuse at__________mL/hour

***When discontinuing, reduce rate by 25% for one hour X3 rate reductions, then discontinue.

Monitoring guidelines: (Please check all that apply)
☐ Dietary consult
☐ Weigh patient daily
☐ Monitor intake and output
☐ Baseline Laboratory tests: Comprehensive metabolic panel, Pre-albumin, Magnesium, Phosphorus & Triglycerides
☐ Routine Laboratory test: Comprehensive metabolic panel, Pre-albumin, Magnesium, Phosphorus & Triglycerides every Monday
Basic metabolic profile every Thursday.
☐ Fingerstick Blood Glucose every 6 hours for two days, then every 48 hours **OR** every ________hours thereafter.
☐ Insulin Sliding Scale (use standard insulin order form)

PHYSICIAN SIGNATURE DATE / TIME

FIGURE 14.2 • Example of part of an order form for adult parenteral nutrition.

Enteral Nutrition

Enteral nutrition is a method of providing nutritional support via tubes inserted into the stomach or small intestine. It finds application in patients who have an inability or decreased ability to ingest nutrients by mouth. As shown in Figure 14.1, nasogastric tubes may be used, or tubes may be inserted through surgical openings into the stomach, duodenum, or jejunum.[7] Surgical insertions generally are reserved for the relatively long-term feeding requirements of patients (e.g., more than 4 weeks). Enteral nutrition may be used for total nutrition, for supplemental nutrition, or as a transitional phase for patients transitioning from parenteral nutrition. Tube feedings may be intermittent or continuous, and in addition to nutritional requirements, they address the need to replace water lost daily through urination, bowel function, respiration, and perspiration.

Enteral nutrition takes into account a patient's caloric requirements and his or her need for protein, carbohydrate and fat, vitamins and minerals, dietary fiber, electrolytes, and fluids. Commercial formulas for enteral feeding are multiple and varied. Some are designed specifically for pediatric or adult patients. Some provide a balanced or general requirement; others are high in calories, protein, fat, and/or fiber; and still others are low in carbohydrate, sodium, or cholesterol. Some commercial formulas are designed to meet the disease-specific requirements of certain patients, such as those with renal or hepatic disease or those who are diabetic, lactose intolerant, or allergic to specific foods. As required, additions may be made to commercial formulas to meet the needs of a specific patient.

The osmolality of an enteral formula is an important consideration. Some patients exhibit intolerance to a hyperosmolar formula, resulting in vomiting, osmotic diarrhea, abdominal distention, and other symptoms.[8] Most infant formulas have osmolalities between 150 and 380 mOsmol/kg, and adult formulas from about 270 to 700 mOsmol/kg. It should be recalled that the osmolality of extracellular fluid is considered to be 285 to 295 mOsmol/kg.

When necessary, medications can be administered through the enteral feeding tubes, preferably as liquid dosage forms. As required, well-diluted slurries can be prepared and administered from the solid contents of tablets or capsules. Liquid medications with high osmolalities (some are greater than 1000 mOsmol/kg) can be diluted with 10 to 30 mL of sterile water prior to administration.[7,9]

Medications generally are administered separately from the nutrient formulas, with care taken not to conflict with the feeding schedule, to avoid drug incompatibilities with other medications and nutritional components, to consider a medication's possible gastrointestinal effects (e.g., diarrhea or constipation), and to make certain that no residual medication remains in the feeding tubes after medication delivery.[7,9]

Parenteral Nutrition

Parenteral nutrition (PN) or ***intravenous hyperalimentation (IVH*** or ***HAL)*** is the feeding of a patient by the intravenous infusion of fluids and basic nutrients. ***Partial parenteral nutrition (PPN)*** is nutritional support that *supplements* oral intake and provides only part of daily nutritional requirements. ***Total parenteral nutrition (TPN)*** provides *all* the patient's daily nutritional requirements.

Parenteral nutrition is used for patients who cannot obtain adequate nutrition by oral means. This includes patients who are severely malnourished, those whose critical illness temporarily precludes their receiving oral or enteral nutrition and there is need to *prevent* starvation-induced complications, those whose gastrointestinal tracts are unavailable or malfunctioning, those with a demonstrated or assessed probability of ineffective nourishment by enteral feeding, and patients in renal or hepatic failure, among others.[10,11]

Figure 14.2 is an example of a hospital adult parenteral nutrition form. Note that the prescribing physician may select the standard formulas or modifications for central or peripheral administration. In the example, the quantities of the basic components, amino acids (protein), dextrose (carbohydrate), and lipid (fat), are expressed in percent strength; however, other such forms may express these quantities in grams per stated volume. Added electrolytes are expressed in milliequivalents and phosphorous in millimoles. The patient's *dosing weight* (the actual, ideal, or adjusted body weight) is used to determine the component doses. Central administration lines are inserted into the superior vena cava, whereas peripheral lines are inserted into veins of the arm or hand (see Fig. 14.1). Because concentrated dextrose solutions are hypertonic and may be damaging to veins, central lines are preferred over peripheral lines for higher concentrations of dextrose (e.g., 25%). Nutritional formulas for peripheral parenteral nutrition generally are isotonic or near isotonic.

Typically, parenteral nutrition formulas contain the following:

- *Macronutrients:*
  - Carbohydrate (e.g., dextrose)
  - Protein (e.g., amino acids)
  - Fat (e.g., lipid emulsions)
- *Micronutrients:*
  - Electrolytes
  - Vitamins
  - Trace elements
- *Sterile water for injection*

Parenteral nutrition formulas can be obtained commercially or they may be prepared in the pharmacy, often through the use of automated compounding devices that mix the basic as well as additive ingredients according to input managed by computer software. Nutritional requirements and thus formulations differ based on age groups (e.g., neonates, general pediatrics, adults) as well as patient-specific diseases (e.g., renal, liver, pulmonary). In preparing formulas for parenteral nutrition, pharmacists use calculated quantities of small-volume parenterals (ampuls and vials) as the source of electrolytes, vitamins, and minerals, and large-volume parenterals (LVPs) as the source of amino acids, dextrose, lipids, and sterile water for injection.

Typically, infusion rates are begun at about 25 to 50 mL/h and adjusted every 8 to 12 hours as dictated by the patient's condition and fluid and nutritional status.[11] TPN solutions may be administered continuously over a 24-hour period or cyclically, depending on a patient's requirements. Infusions may be administered by gravity flow or through the use of automated, high-speed multichannel pumping devices.

In many instances, parenteral nutrition begun in a hospital is continued in a long-term care or rehabilitation facility or in home care.

Nutritional Requirements

Nutritional requirements are the quantities of macronutrients and micronutrients needed for a patient to obtain or maintain the desired nutritional status. The quantitative amounts of fluid and specific nutrients required vary with an individual's age, gender, physical parameters, disease state, and current nutritional status. The purpose of this section is to provide only *general* considerations. More detailed and patient-specific considerations are presented in other resources, including those referenced.[5,6,9 15]

Fluid Requirements

Total body water in adult males normally ranges between 50% and 70% of body weight depending on the proportion of body fat. The greater the proportion of fat, the lesser the proportion of water. Values for adult women are about 10% less than those for men. Of the adult body's water content, up to two-thirds is intracellular and one-third is extracellular. For an adult, approximately 2500 mL of daily water intake (from ingested liquids and foods and from oxidative metabolism) is needed to balance the daily water output.[16]

A factor of 30 to 35 mL/kg of body weight, 1500 mL per square meter of body surface area, or 1 mL/kcal of nutrition required is among the methods used to estimate an adult patient's daily fluid or water requirement. On a case-by-case basis, these values may be increased (e.g., for patients who are dehydrated) or decreased (e.g., for patients with renal failure or congestive heart failure). A daily requirement of between 2 and 3 L per day is usual for adults.

Examples:

(1) *Calculate the daily fluid requirement range for a patient weighing 162 lb*

$$\frac{30\text{ mL}}{\text{kg/day}} \times \frac{1\text{ kg}}{2.2\text{ lb}} \times 162\text{ lb} = 2209.09\text{ mL/day}$$

$$\frac{35\text{ mL}}{\text{kg/day}} \times \frac{1\text{ kg}}{2.2\text{ lb}} \times 162\text{ lb} = 2577.27\text{ mL/day}$$

Range = **2209.09 – 2577.27 mL/day**

(2) *Calculate the daily fluid requirement for a patient who is 5 feet 2 inches tall and weighs 114 lb. Use the equation in Chapter 8 to determine BSA.*

$$5\text{ feet 2 inches} = 62\text{ inches} \times \frac{2.54\text{ cm}}{\text{inches}} = 157.48\text{ cm}$$

$$114\text{ lb} \times \frac{1\text{ kg}}{2.2\text{ lb}} = 51.82\text{ kg}$$

$$\text{BSA} = \sqrt{\frac{157.48\text{ cm} \times 51.82\text{ kg}}{3600}} = \sqrt{2.27} = 1.51\text{ m}^2$$

$$\frac{1500\text{ mL}}{\text{m}^2\text{/day}} \times 1.51\text{ m}^2 = \mathbf{2258.36\text{ mL/day}}$$

Caloric Requirements

The ***kilocalorie*** (*kcal*) is the unit used in metabolism studies. By definition, the kilocalorie (or large Calorie, C, or Cal.) is the amount of heat required to raise the temperature of 1 kg of water by 1°C. The caloric requirements for patients vary, depending on their physical state and medical condition. The Harris-Benedict equations,[17] which follow, are commonly used to estimate the *daily basal energy expenditure* (*BEE*) requirements for nonprotein calories. The BEE is also referred to as the *resting metabolic energy* (*RME*) or the *resting energy expenditure* (*REE*).

For males:

$$\text{BEE} = 66.5 + [13.75 \times \text{Weight (kg)}] + [5 \times \text{Height (cm)}] - [6.78 \times \text{Age (y)}]$$

For females:

$$\text{BEE} = 655.1 + [9.56 \times \text{Weight (kg)}] + [1.85 \times \text{Height (cm)}] - [4.68 \times \text{Age (y)}]$$

The *total daily expenditure* (*TDE*) of energy, as calculated, may be adjusted for activity and stress factors[5,10]:

$$\text{TDE} = \text{BEE} \times \text{activity factors} \times \text{stress factors}$$

Activity factors	Confined to bed: 1.2
	Ambulatory: 1.3
Stress factors	Surgery: 1.2
	Infection: 1.4 to 1.6
	Trauma: 1.3 to 1.5
	Burns: 1.5 to 2.0

As an alternative to the use of the Harris-Benedict equations, clinicians can estimate the BEE for adults as 20 to 25 kcal/kg/day for otherwise healthy patients with mild illness, 25 to 30 kcal/kg/day for nonobese patients with moderate illness, and 30 kcal/kg/day or greater for severely burned patients.[5] Energy requirements for infants, children, and teenagers are different than those for adults and vary according to age, growth rate, and clinical/metabolic status.

Examples:

(1) *Using the Harris-Benedict equation, calculate the BEE for a 78-year-old male patient, measuring 5 feet 8 inches in height and weighing 160 lb.*

$$5 \text{ feet } 8 \text{ inches} = 68 \text{ inches}; 68 \text{ inches} \times 2.54 \text{ cm/inches} = 172.72 \text{ cm}$$

$$160 \text{ lb} \div 2.2 \text{ lb/kg} = 72.73 \text{ kg}$$

$$\begin{aligned} \text{BEE} &= 66.5 + (13.75 \times \text{weight, kg}) + (5 \times \text{height, cm}) - (6.78 \times \text{age, y}) \\ &= 66.5 + (13.75 \times 72.73\,[\text{kg}]) + (5 \times 172.72\,[\text{cm}]) - (6.78 \times 78\text{ y}) \\ &= 66.5 + 1000 + 863.6 - 528.84 \\ &= \mathbf{1401.26\ kcal} \end{aligned}$$

(2) *Calculate the TDE for the patient in example problem 1 factoring in an activity factor of 1.2 (confined to bed) and a stress factor of 1.2 (surgery).*

$$\begin{aligned} \text{TDE} &= \text{BEE} \times \text{activity factor} \times \text{stress factor} \\ &= 1401.26 \text{ kcal} \times 1.2 \times 1.2 = \mathbf{2017.81\ kcal} \end{aligned}$$

(3) *Calculate the BEE for the above patient using the alternative method of 25 kcal/kg/day.*

$$25 \text{ kcal/kg/day} \times 72.73 \text{ kg} = \mathbf{1818.18\ kcal}$$

Carbohydrate Requirements

Carbohydrates are the primary source of cellular energy. In formulas for parenteral nutrition, dextrose provides 3.4 kcal of energy per gram; for example, each 100 mL of a 25% dextrose injection provides 85 kcal of energy. For enteral nutrition, the factor used is 4 kcal/g.

Protein Requirements

In TPN, protein is provided as amino acids. The purpose of the protein support is not to produce energy, although energy is produced by proteins by a factor of 4 kcal/g, but rather to build tissues and body strength.[15] Therefore, a patient's caloric needs should be provided by *nonprotein calories*, and the contribution of protein calories to the daily expenditure is optional and may be omitted. The daily quantity of protein required in adults is generally estimated to be[5]:

- 0.8 g/kg/day in an unstressed patient
- 1 to 1.5 g/kg/day for most patients over 60 years old
- 1.5 to 2 g/kg/day for a patient with a critical illness, infection, or trauma
- 0.5 g/kg/day for a patient with liver failure

Lipid (Fat) Requirements

Lipids may be used to provide energy when the body cannot obtain all the necessary energy requirement from carbohydrates. The proportion of calories provided by lipids is usually restricted to 20% to 40% of the total daily calories. Lipids provide 9 kcal of energy per gram. Lipids are generally administered parenterally in the form of an emulsion containing carbohydrate-based emulsifying agents, which also contribute to the caloric content. It has been determined that a 10% lipid emulsion provides 11 kcal/g of total energy or 1.1 kcal/mL, and a 20% to 30% lipid emulsion provides 10 kcal/g of total energy (2 kcal/mL and 3 kcal/mL, respectively).[12] The abbreviation *IVFE*, for *intravenous fat emulsion*, is often used to indicate the lipid component of a parenteral nutritional formula.

Fiber Requirements

Dietary guidelines generally recommend a daily intake of 14 g of fiber for each 1000 calories consumed. This translates to approximately 21 to 25 g of daily fiber for women and between 30 and 38 g for men. *Insoluble* fiber reaches the large intestine after ingestion and is associated with good bowel function, whereas *soluble* fiber partially dissolves in the upper gastrointestinal tract and is associated with reduced absorption of dietary fat and cholesterol.[18]

Electrolytes

As shown in Figure 14.2, the standard quantities of electrolytes may be used or modified by the following parameter, or other.[6]

Sodium 1 to 2 mEq/kg/day
Potassium 1 to 2 mEq/kg/day
Calcium 10 to 15 mEq/day
Magnesium 8 to 20 mEq/day
Phosphorus 20 to 40 mmol/day

Enteral and Parenteral Nutrition Calculations

Example Calculations of Enteral Nutrition

The nutritional requirements for a 76-year-old male who is 6 feet 2 inches tall and weighs 201 lb have been determined to be as follows:

Protein: 73.09 g/day
Lipids: 81.23 g/day
Carbohydrates: 266.34 g/day
Water: 2088.82 to 2740.91 mL/day
Total calories: 2088.82 kcal/day

A ready-to-drink nutritional liquid product is selected for this patient. A one-quart container provides 37 g protein, 143 g carbohydrates, 37 g lipids, and 1.06 kcal/mL.

(a) *How many milliliters of the product should this patient receive daily to meet his caloric requirements?*

$$\frac{2088.82\text{ kcal}}{1\text{ day}} \times \frac{1\text{ mL}}{1.06\text{ kcal}} = \mathbf{1970.58\ mL/day}$$

(b) *How many grams each of protein, carbohydrates, and lipids would this volume provide?*

$$\text{Protein: } \frac{1970.58\text{ mL}}{1\text{ day}} \times \frac{1\text{ qt}}{946\text{ mL}} \times \frac{37\text{ g}}{1\text{ qt}} = \mathbf{77.07\ g/day}$$

$$\text{Carbohydrates: } \frac{1970.58\text{ mL}}{1\text{ day}} \times \frac{1\text{ qt}}{946\text{ mL}} \times \frac{143\text{ g}}{1\text{ qt}} = \mathbf{297.88\ g/day}$$

$$\text{Lipids: } \frac{1970.58\text{ mL}}{1\text{ day}} \times \frac{1\text{ qt}}{946\text{ mL}} \times \frac{37\text{ g}}{1\text{ qt}} = \mathbf{77.07\ g/day}$$

(c) *If the product contains 85% free water, does it meet the patient's daily water requirement?*

$$1970.58 \text{ mL/day} \times 85\% = 1675 \text{ mL/day}$$

Therefore, the amount of water provided by 1970.58 mL of the formula would ***not*** fully meet the patient's daily water requirement.

(d) *If the formula is to be delivered continuously over a 24-hour period, what would be the flow rate in mL/h?*

$$\frac{1970.58 \text{ mL}}{1 \text{ day}} \times \frac{1 \text{ day}}{24 \text{ h}} = 82.11 \text{ mL/h} \approx \mathbf{82 \text{ mL/h}}$$

(e) *If the patient is to continue receiving this formula at home by intermittent feedings over 40 minutes every 4 hours, what volume would be administered with each feeding, and what would be the flow rate in mL/h?*

$$\frac{1970.58 \text{ mL}}{1 \text{ day}} \times \frac{1 \text{ day}}{24 \text{ h}} \times \frac{4 \text{ h}}{1 \text{ dose}} = \mathbf{328.43 \text{ mL/dose}}$$

$$\frac{328.43 \text{ mL}}{40 \text{ min}} \times \frac{60 \text{ min}}{1 \text{ h}} = 492.65 \text{ mL/h} \approx \mathbf{493 \text{ mL/h}}$$

Example Calculations of Parenteral Nutrition

The following basic steps may be used as a guide in TPN calculations:

STEP 1. Calculate the TDE required using the Harris-Benedict equations, and apply the appropriate stress or activity factors.

STEP 2. Calculate the daily quantity (g) of amino acids (protein) required based on 0.8 g/kg of body weight, or use one of the other values listed on page 279 to accommodate for various disease states.

STEP 3. Calculate the number of calories supplied by the amino acids (from STEP 2) at 4 kcal/g. This step may be omitted if protein calories are not included in the TDE.

STEP 4. Calculate the kcal of lipids required at 20% to 40% of the TDE.

STEP 5. Calculate the volume of lipid emulsion required (from STEP 4) based on 1.1 kcal/mL (10% lipid emulsion), 2 kcal/mL (20% lipid emulsion), or 3 kcal/mL (30% lipid emulsion).

STEP 6. Calculate the quantity of carbohydrate required based on 3.4 kcal/g after accounting for the contribution of the lipids.

STEP 7. Calculate the daily fluid requirement using 30 to 35 mL/kg/day or one of the other methods described earlier in the text.

NOTES: In some clinical practices (a), a patient's actual body weight, the ideal body weight, or adjusted body weight may be used in the calculations (in STEP 1), and (b) in STEP 6, the energy provided by the protein, in addition to that from lipids, may or may not be taken into account. In addition to STEPS 1 through 7, TPN calculations also can include:

- Determination of the quantities of the pharmaceutical sources of the macronutrients (e.g., LVPs) and micronutrients (e.g., vials) to use to obtain the required components
- Determination of the total TPN volume, the number of TPN bags to be prepared, and the rate of flow

(1) *Calculate the parenteral nutrition and fluid requirements for a 58-year-old woman who is 5 feet 3 inches tall and weighs 140 lb. She is ambulatory (activity factor = 1.3) and has undergone surgery (stress factor = 1.2). The solutions to be used for the macronutrients are 8.5% w/v amino acid solution, 20% w/v lipid emulsion, and 70% w/v dextrose solution.*

STEP 1. Total daily kcal required by Harris-Benedict equation:

$$5 \text{ feet } 3 \text{ inches} = 63 \text{ inches} \times \frac{2.54 \text{ cm}}{\text{inches}} = 160.02 \text{ cm}$$

$$140 \text{ lb} \times \frac{1 \text{ kg}}{2.2 \text{ lb}} = 63.64 \text{ kg}$$

$$\text{BEE} = 655.1 + (9.56 \times 63.64 \text{ kg}) + (1.85 \times 160.02 \text{ cm}) - (4.68 \times 58 \text{ y})$$
$$= 1288.06 \text{ kcal/day}$$

$$\text{TDE} = 1288.06 \text{ kcal/day} \times 1.3 \times 1.2 = 2009.37 \text{ kcal/day}$$

STEP 2. Protein required (grams):

$$\frac{0.8 \text{ g}}{\text{kg/day}} \times 63.64 \text{ kg} = 50.91 \text{ g/day}$$

$$\text{Volume of 8.5\% amino acid solution needed} = \frac{50.91 \text{ g}}{\text{day}} \times \frac{100 \text{ mL}}{8.5 \text{ g}}$$
$$= 598.93 \text{ mL/day}$$

STEP 3. Protein (kcal):

$$\frac{50.91 \text{ g}}{1 \text{ day}} \times \frac{4 \text{ kcal}}{1 \text{ g}} = 203.64 \text{ kcal/day}$$

STEP 4. Lipids required (kcal), using 30% of TDE:

$$2009.37 \text{ kcal/day} \times 30\% = 602.81 \text{ kcal/day}$$

STEP 5. Lipids required (mL), using a 20% lipid emulsion:

$$\frac{602.81 \text{ kcal}}{\text{day}} \times \frac{1 \text{ mL}}{2 \text{ kcal}} = 301.41 \text{ mL/day}$$

STEP 6. Carbohydrates (dextrose) required (grams), accounting for kcal from both protein and lipids:

$$2009.37 \text{ kcal/day} - 203.64 \text{ kcal/day (protein)} - 602.81 \text{ kcal/day (lipids)}$$
$$= 1202.93 \text{ kcal/day}$$

$$\frac{1202.93 \text{ kcal}}{\text{day}} \times \frac{1 \text{ g}}{3.4 \text{ kcal}} = 353.802 \text{ g/day}$$

$$\text{Volume of 70\% dextrose solution needed} = \frac{353.802 \text{ g}}{\text{day}} \times \frac{100 \text{ mL}}{70 \text{ g}}$$
$$= 505.43 \text{ mL/day}$$

STEP 7. Fluid required (milliliters):
Based on 30 mL/kg/day:

$$\frac{30 \text{ mL}}{\text{kg/day}} \times 63.64 \text{ kg} = 1909.09 \text{ mL/day}$$

Based on 1 mL/kcal required/day:

$$\frac{2009.37 \text{ kcal}}{\text{day}} \times \frac{1 \text{ mL}}{\text{kcal}} = 2009.37 \text{ mL/day}$$

Total volume provided by macronutrient solutions:
598.93 mL/day (protein) + 301.41 mL/day (lipids) + 505.43 mL/day (dextrose) = 1405.77 mL/day

The patient should receive 598.93 mL of 8.5% amino acid solution, 301.41 mL of 20% lipid emulsion, 505.43 mL of 70% dextrose solution, and approximately 500 mL of additional fluids per day.

(2) *The following is a formula for a desired parenteral nutrition solution. Using the source of each drug as indicated, calculate the amount of each component required in preparing the solution.*

Formula	Component Source
(*a*) Sodium chloride 35 mEq	Vial, 5 mEq per 2 mL
(*b*) Potassium acetate 35 mEq	Vial, 10 mEq per 5 mL
(*c*) Magnesium sulfate 8 mEq	Vial, 4 mEq per mL
(*d*) Calcium gluconate 9.6 mEq	Vial, 4.7 mEq per 10 mL
(*e*) Potassium chloride 5 mEq	Vial, 40 mEq per 20 mL
(*f*) Folic acid 1.7 mg	Ampul, 5 mg per mL
(*g*) Multiple vitamin infusion 10 mL	Ampul, 10 mL

To be added to:
Amino acid infusion (8.5%) 500 mL
Dextrose injection (50%) 500 mL

(a) $35 \text{ mEq} \times \frac{2 \text{ mL}}{5 \text{ mEq}} = 14 \text{ mL}$

(b) $35 \text{ mEq} \times \frac{5 \text{ mL}}{10 \text{ mEq}} = 17.5 \text{ mL}$

(c) $8 \text{ mEq} \times \frac{1 \text{ mL}}{4 \text{ mEq}} = 2 \text{ mL}$

(d) $9.6 \text{ mEq} \times \frac{10 \text{ mL}}{4.7 \text{ mEq}} = 20.43 \text{ mL}$

(e) $5 \text{ mEq} \times \frac{20 \text{ mL}}{40 \text{ mEq}} = 2.5 \text{ mL}$

(f) $1.7 \text{ mg} \times \frac{1 \text{ mL}}{5 \text{ mg}} = 0.34 \text{ mL}$

(g) 10 mL

(3) *The formula for a TPN solution calls for the addition of 2.7 mEq of Ca^{2+} and 20 mEq of K^+ per liter. How many milliliters of an injection containing 20 mg of calcium chloride dihydrate per milliliter and how many milliliters of a 15% (w/v) potassium chloride injection should be used to provide the desired additives?*

$$\text{Molecular weight of } CaCl_2 \cdot 2H_2O = 40\ (Ca^{2+}) + [2 \times 35.5\ (Cl^-)] + [2 \times 18\ (H_2O)] = 147$$

$$\text{Valence} = 2$$

$$\text{Conversion} = \frac{147 \text{ mg}}{2 \text{ mEq}}$$

$$2.7 \text{ mEq } Ca^{2+} = 2.7 \text{ mEq } CaCl_2 \cdot 2H_2O$$

$$2.7 \text{ mEq} \times \frac{147 \text{ mg}}{2 \text{ mEq}} \times \frac{1 \text{ mL}}{20 \text{ mg}} = \mathbf{9.92 \text{ mL of } CaCl_2 \cdot 2H_2O \text{ solution}}$$

$$\text{Molecular weight of KCl} = 39\ (K^+) + 35.5\ (Cl^-) = 74.5$$

$$\text{Valence} = 1$$

$$\text{Conversion} = \frac{74.5 \text{ mg}}{1 \text{ mEq}}$$

$$20 \text{ mEq } K^+ = 20 \text{ mEq KCl}$$

$$20 \text{ mEq} \times \frac{74.5 \text{ mg}}{1 \text{ mEq}} \times \frac{1 \text{ g}}{1000 \text{ mg}} \times \frac{100 \text{ mL}}{15 \text{ g}} = \mathbf{9.93 \text{ mL of KCl solution}}$$

(4) *A potassium phosphate injection contains a mixture of 224 mg of monobasic potassium phosphate (KH_2PO_4) and 236 mg of dibasic potassium phosphate (K_2HPO_4) per milliliter. If 10 mL of the injection are added to a TPN solution containing 500 mL each of 7% amino acid solution and D10W (10% dextrose in water for injection), (a) how many milliequivalents of K^+ and (b) how many millimoles of total phosphate are represented in the prepared solution?*

$$\text{Molecular weight of } KH_2PO_4 = 39\ (K^+) + 97\ (H_2PO_4^-) = 136$$

$$\text{Conversion} = \frac{136 \text{ mg}}{1 \text{ mEq}} \text{ and } \frac{136 \text{ mg}}{1 \text{ mmol}}$$

$$\text{Molecular weight of } K_2HPO_4 = [2 \times 39\ (K^+)] + 96\ (HPO_4^{2-}) = 174$$

$$\text{Conversion} = \frac{174 \text{ mg}}{2 \text{ mEq}} \text{ and } \frac{174 \text{ mg}}{1 \text{ mmol}}$$

(a) $\frac{224 \text{ mg}}{\text{mL}} \times 10 \text{ mL} \times \frac{1 \text{ mEq}}{136 \text{ mg}} = 16.47 \text{ mEq } K^+$

$\frac{236 \text{ mg}}{\text{mL}} \times 10 \text{ mL} \times \frac{2 \text{ mEq}}{174 \text{ mg}} = 27.13 \text{ mEq } K^+$

Total K^+ = 16.47 mEq + 27.13 mEq = **43.6 mEq**

(b) $\frac{224 \text{ mg}}{\text{mL}} \times 10 \text{ mL} \times \frac{1 \text{ mmol}}{136 \text{ mg}} = 16.47 \text{ mmol phosphate}$

$\frac{236 \text{ mg}}{\text{mL}} \times 10 \text{ mL} \times \frac{1 \text{ mmol}}{174 \text{ mg}} = 13.56 \text{ mmol phosphate}$

Total phosphate = 16.47 mmol + 13.56 mmol = **30.03 mmol**

CASE IN POINT 14.1 A hospital pharmacist is asked to provide TPN for a 75-year-old female patient who is 5 feet 2 inches in height and weighs 120 lb. The patient is confined to bed but has no stress factors. The pharmacist reviews the patient's laboratory records and based on experience decides to prepare a 2000 mL TPN, utilizing a 10% amino acid injection as the protein source, D50W as the source of dextrose, and a 20% lipid emulsion as the fat source, with a standard mixture of electrolytes, minerals, and vitamins. The pharmacist asks a student on a pharmacy practice experience program to perform these basic calculations:

(a) Target amount of the patient's daily fluid requirement
(b) Target amount of daily protein requirements (g/day)
(c) Volume of amino acid injection that may be required
(d) Target amount of nonprotein calories (kcal)
(e) The volume of D50W that could supply the nonprotein calories

The Nutrition Label

The *Dietary Guidelines for Americans 2010*,[19] issued by the U.S. Department of Agriculture (USDA) and Health and Human Services (HHS), provide guidance aimed at improving health and reversing obesity and related diseases. The document includes basic nutritional information and dietary recommendations while the Web site offers interactive tools to assist consumers in meeting dietary objectives. The familiar "Nutrition Facts" (Fig. 14.3) that accompanies packaged foods is a labeling requirement of the FDA and provides direct guidance to the consumer.[19–21] Through knowledge of dietary requirements and the nutrition label, pharmacists have a unique opportunity to counsel patients.

Percent Daily Value

As is depicted in Figure 14.3, nutrition labeling includes a listing of daily values (DVs) based on a 2000-calorie diet (most labels also include values based on a 2500-calorie diet). These values allow consumers to ascertain the amount of a particular nutrient in a food product and to compare the nutritional content between products.

Required labeling includes the *percent daily value* (% DV) for certain nutritional components. In order to calculate the % DV, the quantity of a nutrient in a serving is compared to its daily value and expressed as a percent. For example, in Figure 14.3, the total fat per serving is 13 g and the total DV for total fat (on the bottom of label, based on a 2000-calorie diet) is 65 g. Thus, 13 g/65 g × 100% = 20%, the labeled % DV for total fat.

Serving Size and Servings per Container

The labeled ***serving size*** reflects the amount that people generally eat at one time and is indicated in common household units (e.g., 1 cup) and approximate corresponding metric measure (e.g., 228 g). Items of discrete size, such as cookies, are listed in both units and metric equivalent, for example, "2 cookies (26 g)." The ***servings per container*** indicate the number of servings in the package.

Calories

On the nutrition label, ***calories per serving*** and the number of ***calories derived from fat*** are of special importance to many consumers. High-calorie and high-fat diets are linked to overweight and obesity and the consequent illnesses.

A ***calorie*** (spelled with a small *c*) is the amount of energy needed to raise the temperature of 1 g of water 1°C. A ***kilocalorie (kcal)*** equals 1000 calories. The kilocalorie, or

Nutrition Facts

Serving Size 1 cup (228g)
Servings Per Container 2

Amount Per Serving

Calories 260 Calories from Fat 120

	% Daily Value*
Total Fat 13g	20%
Saturated Fat 5g	25%
Trans Fat 2g	
Cholesterol 30mg	10%
Sodium 660mg	28%
Total Carbohydrate 31g	10%
Dietary Fiber 0g	0%
Sugars 5g	
Protein 5g	
Vitamin A	4%
Vitamin C	2%
Calcium	15%
Iron	4%

*Percent Daily Values are based on a 2,000 calorie diet. Your Daily Values may be higher or lower depending on your calorie needs:

	Calories:	2,000	2,500
Total Fat	Less than	65g	80g
Sat Fat	Less than	20g	25g
Cholesterol	Less than	300mg	300mg
Sodium	Less than	2,400mg	2,400mg
Total Carbohydrate		300g	375g
Dietary Fiber		25g	30g

Calories per gram:
Fat 9 • Carbohydrate 4 • Protein 4

FIGURE 14.3 • Example of a nutrition label.

Calorie (spelled with a capital *C*), is the unit used in metabolism studies and in nutrition to describe the energy provided by various foods. In common usage, the "small C" *calorie* is often used interchangeably (albeit incorrectly).

According to the *Dietary Guidelines for Americans 2010*,[19] the caloric requirements as stated in Table 14.2 generally are suitable for most persons.

For the calculations in this section, it is important to note that:

- **Carbohydrates yield 4 kcal/g**
- **Protein, 4 kcal/g**
- **Fat, 9 kcal/g**

Macronutrients: Carbohydrates, Protein, and Fats

The recommended *relative proportions* of daily dietary calories between carbohydrate, protein, and fat for age groups are shown in Table 14.3.[19]

Carbohydrates are important components of a healthy diet providing the fuel for energy and organ function. Dietary fiber (a carbohydrate) is a food component providing valuable "roughage" to the digestive tract. The generally recommended daily amount of carbohydrate intake for adults is about 300 g based on a 2000-calorie diet. Daily fiber requirements were stated previously in this chapter.

Protein intake is not considered a general health concern for adults and children over 4 years of age.[19] Consequently, a labeled percent of the daily value *is not* required unless a protein claim is made for the product or if the product is intended for use by infants or

Table 14.2 • ESTIMATED DAILY CALORIE REQUIREMENTS[a]

	Sedentary[b]		Moderately active[c]		Active[d]	
Age (years)	Female	Male	Female	Male	Female	Male
2	1100	1100	1200	1200	1200	1200
6	1300	1300	1500	1500	1600	1800
11	1500	1800	1800	2000	2000	2300
16	1800	2200	2000	2600	2400	3000
19–30	1900	2500	2100	2700	2400	3000
31–50	1800	2300	2000	2500	2200	2900
51+	1600	2100	1800	2300	2100	2600

[a]Adapted with modification from *Dietary Guidelines for Americans 2010*.[19]

[b]*Sedentary* includes only light physical activity associated with daily life.

[c]*Moderately active* includes walking 1.5 to 3 miles/day at 3 to 4 miles/h or equivalent other activity in addition to light physical activity associated with daily life.

[d]*Active* includes walking more than 3 miles/day at 3 to 4 miles/h or equivalent other activity in addition to light physical activity associated with daily life.

children under 4 years of age. Guidelines suggest a daily protein requirement of 0.8 g/kg or 50 g for adults and children 4 or more years of age, 16 g for children less than 4 years of age, 14 g for infants, 60 g for pregnant women, and 65 g for lactating women.

In addition to the listing requirement for *total fat*, the nutrition label also is required to contain the content of *saturated fat* and *trans fat*. Intake of these components increases the body's low-density lipoprotein (LDL) cholesterol and the risk of developing coronary heart disease. Guidelines suggest total dietary fat of less than 65 g/day with less than 20 g being saturated fat. It is recommended that the intake of cholesterol be less than 300 mg daily.

Sodium and Potassium

The labeling of sodium and potassium content is required. Guidelines suggest that sodium intake should be less than 2400 mg daily and reduced to 1500 mg for persons who are 51 years of age and older and for persons of any age who are African American or have hypertension, diabetes, or chronic kidney disease.[19] Presently, the daily 1500-mg recommendation applies to about half of the US population, including children, and the majority of adults.

The adult requirement of potassium is considered to be about 4 g/day.

Micronutrients: Vitamins and Minerals

The nutrition label must specify the content of vitamins A and C and the minerals, calcium and iron. Any additional content of vitamins and minerals must appear in a food's general ingredient list.

Use of Special Terms on the Nutrition Label

Descriptive terms as "*lite, free, low, and reduced*," as used with reference to calories, fat, saturated fat, cholesterol, sodium, and sugars, are defined and regulated by the FDA. The qualifying definitions are found in the reference.[22]

Table 14.3 • RECOMMENDED MACRONUTRIENT PROPORTIONS OF DAILY DIETARY CALORIES BY AGE[19]

	Carbohydrate (%)	Protein (%)	Total Fat (%)[a]
Young children (1–3 y)	45–65	5–20	30–40
Older children and adolescents (4–18 y)	45–65	10–30	25–35
Adults (19 y and older)	45–65	10–35	20–35

[a]Saturated fat, less than 10% of daily calories.

Example Calculations Involving the Nutrition Label

NOTE: In calculations of the labeled "% daily values," the FDA allows latitude in rounding.

(1) *Based on the "Nutrition Facts" depicted in Figure 14.3, for a 2500-calorie intake and with the consumption of one serving size, calculate the percent daily value (% DV) for (a) total fat, (b) cholesterol, and (c) sodium.*

(a) 13 g/80 g × 100% = **16% total fat** (rounded)

(b) 30 mg/300 mg × 100% = **10% cholesterol**

(c) 660 mg/2400 mg × 100% = **28% sodium** (rounded)

(2) *For a person on a sodium-reduced diet (i.e., 1500 mg/day), recalculate the % DV in the above problem.*

660 mg/1500 mg × 100% = **44% sodium**

(3) *Using the data from Tables 14.2 and 14.3, calculate the caloric intake of each macronutrient by a moderately active 20-year-old female who consumes 45% carbohydrate, 35% protein, and 20% fat.*

Total daily intake = 2100 calories (Table 14.2)

Carbohydrate: 2100 calories × 45% = **945 calories**

Protein: 2100 calories × 35% = **735 calories**

Fat: 2100 calories × 20% = **420 calories**

(4) *For the previous problem, calculate the intake in grams for each macronutrient.*

$$\text{Carbohydrate: } 945 \text{ calories} \times \frac{1 \text{ g}}{4 \text{ calories}} = \mathbf{236.25\ g}$$

$$\text{Protein: } 735 \text{ calories} \times \frac{1 \text{ g}}{4 \text{ calories}} = \mathbf{183.75\ g}$$

$$\text{Fat: } 420 \text{ calories} \times \frac{1 \text{ g}}{9 \text{ calories}} = \mathbf{46.67\ g}$$

(5) *For a diet of 3000 calories, calculate the dietary grams of fat for an adult based on the daily reference values for this substance in Table* 14.3.

According to Table 14.3, the recommended proportion of fat is 20% to 35%.

3000 calories × 20% = 600 calories

3000 calories × 35% = 1050 calories

$$600 \text{ calories} \times \frac{1 \text{ g}}{9 \text{ calories}} = 66.67 \text{ g}$$

$$1050 \text{ calories} \times \frac{1 \text{ g}}{9 \text{ calories}} = 116.67 \text{ g}$$

Range = **66.67 – 116.67 g fat per day**

(6) *How many food calories would be provided by a diet of 65 g of fat, 500 g of carbohydrate, and 180 g of protein?*

65 g fat × 9 calories/g = 585 calories

500 g carbohydrate × 4 calories/g = 2000 calories

180 g protein × 4 calories/g = 720 calories

3305 calories

(7) *A multiple vitamin tablet contains 7500 international units of vitamin A. If this amount represents a % DV of 150%, what is the 100% daily requirement of vitamin A?*

$$\frac{150\%\ \text{DV}}{100\%\ \text{DV}} = \frac{7500\ \text{I.U.}}{\text{x I.U.}};\ \text{x} = \mathbf{5000\ international\ units}$$

(8) *A multiple vitamin and mineral tablet contains 162 mg of calcium. If the minimum daily value for calcium is 1000 mg, what percentage of the minimum daily value of calcium is contained in each tablet?*

$$\frac{162\ \text{mg}}{1000\ \text{mg}} \times 100 = \mathbf{16.2\%}$$

CALCULATIONS CAPSULE

Adult Nutrition

Basal energy expenditure (BEE):

The Harris-Benedict equations may be used to approximate the BEE, in kcal:

$$BEE_{males} = 66.5 + [13.75 \times \text{Weight (kg)}] + [5 \times \text{Height (cm)}] - [6.78 \times \text{Age (y)}]$$

$$BEE_{females} = 655.1 + [9.56 \times \text{Weight (kg)}] + [1.85 \times \text{Height (cm)}] - [4.68 \times \text{Age (y)}]$$

The BEE is adjusted by activity and stress factors to yield the estimated total daily energy expenditure (TDE).

Macronutrient values:

Carbohydrates: Enteral = 4 kcal/g, parenteral = 3.4 kcal/g
Proteins: Enteral and parenteral = 4 kcal/g
Fats (lipids): Enteral = 9 kcal/g; parenteral = 1.1 kcal/mL (10%), 2 kcal/mL (20%), and 3 kcal/mL (30%)

Fluid requirement:

30 to 35 mL/kg patient weight, or
1 mL/kcal, nutrition provided, or
1500 mL/m^2 BSA

CASE IN POINT 14.2 A parent asks a pharmacist to explain the nutritional content of PEDIASURE Enteral Formula, which has been recommended for her 12-year-old child. The label indicates that 1500 mL of the product, taken daily, provides complete nutrition for children 9 to 13 years of age. The product is packaged in 237-mL cans containing 7.1 g protein, 9.4 g fat, 31.4 g carbohydrate, 202 g water, and over 30 vitamins and minerals. Calculate:

(a) The kilocalories per milliliter of product
(b) The grams each of protein, fat, and carbohydrate, consumed from a daily intake of 1500 mL of product
(c) The proportion, expressed in percentage, of daily kilocalories derived from each of protein, fat, and carbohydrate
(d) Whether or not the answers in (c) compare favorably with the recommended parameters as stated in Table 14.3

PRACTICE PROBLEMS

Calculations of Body Mass Index and Percent of Ideal Body Weight

1. Using Table 14.1, determine the body mass index for a person measuring 62 inches in height and weighing 150 lb.
2. Calculate the body mass index for a person measuring 1.7 meters in height and weighing 87 kilograms (round answer).
3. An investigational drug for obesity is being dosed at either of two protocols: (a) 7.6 mg/0.5 BMI for persons with a BMI over 25 but less than 30 or (b) 9.6 mg/0.5 BMI for persons with a BMI of 30 or greater. In each protocol, the dose is equally divided and administered "t.i.d. a.c." What would be the divided dose for a male standing 5 feet 8 inches and weighing 230 lb?
4. Calculate the weight in pounds for a male patient who is 5 feet 10 inches tall to be considered "extremely obese" based on his IBW.
5. Calculate the IBW (in pounds) for a female patient who is 5 feet 5 inches tall and weighs 106 lb, determine the percentage of her ABW compared to her IBW, and indicate the nutritional category into which she falls according to her weight.

Calculations of Nutritional Requirements

6. From the information in this chapter, calculate the estimated daily protein requirement, in g/day, for a 141-lb patient with liver failure.
7. A nutritional formula calls for 500 g of dextrose. How many milliliters of a 70% w/v dextrose injection are needed to provide the required amount of dextrose?
8. A patient requires 1800 kcal/day, including 60 g of protein. How many kilocalories would be provided by the protein?
9. If the source of the protein in problem 8 is a 5% amino acid solution, how many milliliters of the solution would be needed to provide the requirement?
10. Calculate the following for enteral nutrition:
    (a) Grams of dextrose needed to supply 1400 kcal
    (b) Grams of protein needed to supply 800 kcal
    (c) Grams of lipid needed to supply 1000 kcal
11. Calculate the approximate daily water requirement for a/an:
    (a) 165-lb patient
    (b) Adult patient with a BSA of 1.6 m^2
    (c) Patient receiving 1500 kcal by TPN
12. JF is a 73-year-old male patient who is 6 feet 1 inch tall and weighs 155 lb. He is ambulatory (activity factor = 1.3) and has a severe infection (stress factor = 1.6). Calculate (a) TDE, (b) grams of protein (1.25 g/kg/day), (c) grams of lipid (30% TDE), (d) grams of carbohydrate, and (e) milliliters of fluid (32 mL/kg) required for enteral nutrition.
13. A TPN order calls for a liter of solution to contain 3.5% of amino acids and 15% of dextrose. How many milliliters each of 8.5% amino acid injection, 70% dextrose injection, and sterile water for injection should be used to prepare the solution?
14. If a 50% dextrose injection provides 170 kcal in each 100 mL, how many milliliters of a 70% dextrose injection would provide the same caloric value?
15. Using the Harris-Benedict equation, calculate the TPN caloric requirement for a hospitalized, bedridden, 60-year-old male surgical patient, weighing 160 lb and measuring 5 feet 8 inches in height.

16. RJ is a 55-year-old female patient who is 5 feet 4 inches tall and weighs 112 lb. She is bedridden (activity factor = 1.2) and has a fractured pelvis due to an automobile accident (stress factor = 1.4). For this patient, determine (a) TDE, (b) milliliters of 8.5% amino acid solution, (c) milliliters of 20% lipid emulsion (30% TDE), (d) milliliters of 50% dextrose solution, and (e) milliliters of fluid (1 mL/kcal) required for a TPN regimen to supply a balanced caloric daily intake for this patient.
17. If amino acids have a caloric value of 4 kcal/g and the daily protein requirement is 0.8 g/kg, calculate the kilocalories administered to a patient weighing 180 lb.
18. A medication order for a TPN solution calls for additives as indicated in the following formula. Using the sources designated below, calculate the amount of each component required in filling the medication order.

TPN Solution Formula	*Component Source*
Sodium chloride 40 mEq	10-mL vial of 30% solution
Potassium acetate 15 mEq	20-mL vial containing 40 mEq
Vitamin B_{12} 10 μg	Vial containing 1 mg in 10 mL
Insulin 8 units	Vial of insulin U-100

To be added to:
500 mL of 50% dextrose injection
500 mL of 7% amino acid injection

19. A solution of potassium phosphate contains a mixture of 164 mg of monobasic potassium phosphate and 158 mg of dibasic potassium phosphate per milliliter.
    (a) If a TPN fluid calls for the addition of 45 mEq of K^+, how many milliliters of the solution should be used to provide this level of potassium?
    (b) How many millimoles of total phosphate will be represented in the calculated volume of potassium phosphate solution?
20. Using the component sources as indicated, calculate the amount of each component required in preparing 1000 mL of the following parenteral nutrition solution:

Parenteral Nutrition Solution Formula	*Component Source*
(a) Amino acids 2.125%	500 mL of 8.5% amino acids injection
(b) Dextrose 20%	500 mL of 50% dextrose injection
(c) Sodium chloride 30 mEq	20-mL vial of 15% solution
(d) Calcium gluconate 2.5 mEq	10-mL vial containing 4.6 mEq
(e) Insulin 15 units	Vial of U-100 insulin
(f) Heparin 2500 units	5-mL vial containing 1000 units/mL
(g) Sterile water for injection to make 1000 mL	500 mL of sterile water for injection

21. If the parenteral nutrition solution in problem 20 is infused continuously at a rate of 85 mL/h, how many kilocalories would the patient receive in a 24-hour period? (Note: The electrolytes and medications do not contribute significant calories.)

Calculations of Nutrition Label Information

22. If a person consumes 1800 calories per day, calculate the intake of fat, in grams, based on dietary fat being 30% of caloric intake.
23. A high-fiber cereal contains 13 g of dietary fiber in each 30 g of cereal. Calculate the % DV of dietary fiber from the nutrition label example (Fig. 14.3), based on a 2000-calorie diet.
24. A sweetened cereal contains 14 g of sugar (carbohydrate) per 30 g serving size of cereal. Calculate the % DV based on a 2000-calorie diet.

25. How many grams of fat are contained in a 2500-calorie diet if 450 of those calories are derived from fat?
26. If an 8-oz container of yogurt contains 300 mg of calcium, calculate the percent daily requirement for a young adult met by consuming half the contents of the container. The daily requirement of calcium is listed as 1000 mg.
27. If a food serving contains 240 mg of potassium, listed as 6% of the daily value, calculate 100% of the daily value of potassium in milligrams.
28. Using the information in Figure 14.3, calculate the % DV for sodium if a different product contained 140 mg of sodium.

CALCQUIZ

14.A. A pharmacist is providing TPN for hospitalized patients. One patient is a 75-year-old female weighing 115 lb and measuring 5 feet 1 inch in height. She is confined to her bed and is somewhat stressed following a surgical procedure. Another patient is an 80-year-old male weighing 162 lb and measuring 5 feet 10 inches in height. He is ambulatory but stressed due to a severe infection. The pharmacist uses the Harris-Benedict equations adjusted for activity and stress factors to determine patients' daily energy requirements. Perform the same calculations.

14.B.[a] A TPN formula is as follows:

Dextrose injection, 50%	1000 mL
Amino acids, 10%	400 mL
Electrolyte/vitamin mix	200 mL
Sterile water for injection	800 mL

If the TPN fluid is to be administered over 24 hours, (a) how many calories will be administered per hour, and (b) what would be the flow rate, in drops/min, when using an IV set that delivers 10 drops/mL?

14.C.[a] A TPN formula is as follows:

Dextrose	15%
Amino acids	4%
Sodium chloride	0.75%
Potassium chloride	0.2%
Multivitamin injection	10 mL
Sterile water for injection, ad	1000 mL

(a) How many milliliters of each of the following will be needed to prepare the formula?

Dextrose injection	700 mg/mL
Amino acid injection	10%
Sodium chloride injection	4 mEq/mL
Potassium chloride injection	2 mEq/mL

(b) If the flow rate for the TPN is prescribed at 1 mL/kg/h, how many total calories will a 187-lb patient receive in 24 hours?

14.D. Compare a 152-lb 5-feet 8-inch patient's target daily fluid requirement based on (a) weight, (b) body surface area, and (c) a daily nutritional requirement of 2000 kcal.

CALCQUIZ (*Continued*)

14.E. A high-protein oral nutritional drink has the following label content based on a 2000-calorie diet. For each item with a question mark (?), fill in the missing number.

Nutrition Facts		**Calories 210**	
Serving size: 1 bottle (14 fl. oz.)		Calories from fat: (?)	
Amount per serving	% DV	Amount per serving	% DV
Total fat 2.5 g	(?)	Potassium 440 mg	(?)
Saturated fat 0.5 g	(?)	Total carbohydrates (?) g	8%
Trans fat 0 g		Dietary fiber 3 g	12%
Cholesterol (?) mg	7%	Sugars 5 g	
Sodium 280 mg	(?)	Protein 25 g	(?)

[a]Problem courtesy of Flynn Warren, Bishop, GA.

ANSWERS TO "CASE IN POINT" AND PRACTICE PROBLEMS

Case in Point 14.1

(a) The patient weighs 120 lb × 1 kg/2.2 lb = 54.55 kg.
The patient's height is 5 feet 2 inches = 62 inches × 2.54 cm/inches = 157.48 cm.
Daily fluid requirement:
Based on 30 to 35 mL/kg/day:

54.55 kg × 30 mL/kg/day = 1636.36 mL
54.55 kg × 35 mL/kg/day = 1909.09 mL

Thus, the target is between 1636.36 and 1909.09 mL/day and the predetermined TPN volume of 2000 mL would suffice.

(b) Since this patient is over 60 years old, a target protein requirement may be based on 1 to 1.5 g/kg/day:

54.55 kg × 1 g/kg/day = 54.55 g/day
54.55 kg × 1.5 g/kg/day = 81.82 g/day

Thus, the acceptable target for protein would be between 54.55 g and 81.82 g/day

(c) The 10% amino acid injection that would be required:

100 mL/10 g × 54.55 g = 545.45 mL, and
100 mL/10 g × 81.82 g = 818.18 mL.

Thus, the target for protein would be met by between 545.45 and 818.18 mL of the 10% amino acid injection.

(d) The target of the patient's nonprotein caloric requirements (BEE) is determined by the Harris-Benedict equation:

655.1 + (9.56 × weight, kg) + (1.85 × height, cm) – (4.68 × age, y) =
655.1 + (9.56 × 54.55 kg) + (1.85 × 157.48 cm) – (4.68 × 75) =
655.1 + 521.45 + 291.34 – 351 = 1116.89 kcal/day × 1.2 (activity factor) = 1340.27 kcal/day

(e) 1340.27 kcal/day × 1 g/3.4 kcal = 394.2 g/day dextrose required
D50W = 50 g dextrose/100 mL;
100 mL/50 g × 394.2 g dextrose = 788.39 mL D50W

(NOTE: In practice, the quantities may be rounded and individualized based on clinical factors.)

Case in Point 14.2

(a) Protein: 7.1 g × 4 kcal/g = 28.4 kcal
Fat: 9.4 g × 9 kcal/g = 84.6 kcal
Carbohydrate: 31.4 g × 4 kcal/g = 125.6 kcal
Total kcal = 28.4 + 84.6 + 125.6 = 238.6 kcal
kcal/mL = 238.6 kcal/237 mL = 1.007 kcal/mL

(b) Protein: 7.1 g/237 mL × 1500 mL = 44.94 g protein
Fat: 9.4 g/237 mL × 1500 mL = 59.49 g fat
Carbohydrate: 31.4 g/237 mL × 1500 mL = 198.73 g carbohydrate

(c) Daily kcal: Protein, 44.94 g × 4 kcal/g = 179.75 kcal
Fat, 59.49 g × 9 kcal/g = 535.44 kcal
Carbohydrate, 198.73 g × 4 kcal/g = 794.94 kcal
Total daily kcal = 179.75 + 535.44 + 794.94 = 1510.13 kcal
% kcal from protein = 179.75 kcal/1510.13 kcal × 100% = 11.9%
% kcal from fat = 535.44 kcal/1510.13 kcal × 100% = 35.46%
% kcal from carbohydrate = 794.94 kcal/1510.13 kcal × 100% = 52.64%

(d) Yes, they compare favorably.

Practice Problems

1. 27 BMI
2. 30.1 BMI
3. 224.28 mg/dose
4. ≥320 lb
5. IBW = 125 lb
   84.8%, underweight
6. 32.05 g/day
7. 714.29 mL
8. 240 kcal
9. 1200 mL
10. (a) 350 g dextrose
    (b) 200 g protein
    (c) 111.11 g lipid
11. (a) 2250 to 2625 mL
    (b) 2400 mL
    (c) 1500 mL
12. (a) 3052.21 kcal/day
    (b) 88.07 g protein/day
    (c) 101.74 g lipids/day
    (d) 446.07 g dextrose/day
    (e) 2254.55 mL fluids/day
13. 411.76 mL amino acids injection
    214.29 mL dextrose injection
    373.95 mL sterile water for injection
14. 71.43 mL dextrose injection
15. 2193.55 kcal/day
16. (a) 1991.01 kcal/day
    (b) 479.14 mL amino acids solution/day
    (c) 298.65 mL lipid emulsion/day
    (d) 724 mL dextrose solution/day
    (e) 1991.01 mL fluids/day
17. 261.82 kcal
18. 7.8 mL sodium chloride solution
    7.5 mL potassium acetate solution
    0.1 mL vitamin B_{12}
    0.08 mL insulin
19. (a) 14.89 mL
    (b) 31.48 mmol
20. (a) 250 mL amino acids injection
    (b) 400 mL dextrose injection
    (c) 11.7 mL sodium chloride solution
    (d) 5.43 mL calcium gluconate solution
    (e) 0.15 mL insulin
    (f) 2.5 mL heparin
    (g) 330.22 mL sterile water
21. 1560.6 kcal
22. 60 g fat/day
23. 52% DV
24. 4.67% DV
25. 50 g fat
26. 15%
27. 4000 mg potassium
28. 5.83% DV

References

1. Dombrowski SR. Pharmacist counseling on nutrition and physical activity—part 1 of 2: understanding current guidelines. *Journal of the American Pharmacists Association* 1999;39:479–491.
2. National Heart Lung and Blood Institute, National Institutes of Health. Management of Overweight and Obesity in Adults: Systematic Evidence Review from the Expert Panel, 2013. Available at: http://www.nhlbi.nih.gov/sites/www.nhlbi.nih.gov/files/obesity-evidence-review.pdf. Accessed March 16, 2015.
3. Continuing Education Monograph. *Managing Obesity as a Chronic Disease*. Washington, DC: American Pharmacists Association; 2001.
4. Zagaria MAE. Nutrition in the elderly. *U.S. Pharmacist* 2000;25:42–44.
5. Chessman KH, Kumpf VJ. Assessment of nutrition status and nutrition requirements. In: DiPiro JT, Talbert RL, Yee GC, et al., eds. *Pharmacotherapy: A Pathophysiologic Approach*, 9th ed. [book online]. New York, NY: McGraw-Hill; 2014.
6. Mirtallo J, Canada T, Johnson D, et al. Safe practices for parenteral nutrition. *Journal of Parenteral and Enteral Nutrition* 2004;28:S39–S70. Available at: http://pen.sagepub.com/content/28/6/S39.full.pdf+html. Accessed March 16, 2015.
7. Beckwith MC, Feddema SS, Barton RG, et al. A guide to drug therapy in patients with enteral feeding tubes: dosage form selection and administration methods. *Hospital Pharmacy* 2004;39:225–237.
8. Davis A. Indications and techniques for enteral feeds. In: Baker SB, Baker RD Jr, Davis A, eds. *Pediatric Enteral Nutrition*. New York, NY: Chapman Hall; 1994:67–94.
9. Wolf TD. Enteral nutrition. In: Boh LE, ed. *Pharmacy Practice Manual: A Guide to the Clinical Experience*. Baltimore, MD: Lippincott Williams & Wilkins; 2001:431–459.
10. Whitney J. Parenteral nutrition. In: Boh LE, ed. *Pharmacy Practice Manual: A Guide to the Clinical Experience*. Baltimore, MD: Lippincott Williams & Wilkins; 2001:460–506.
11. Wallace JI. Malnutrition and enteral/parenteral alimentation. In: Hazzard WR, Blass JP, Halter JB, et al., eds. *Principles of Geriatric Medicine and Gerontology*. New York, NY: McGraw-Hill; 2003:1179–1192.
12. Mattox TW, Crill CM. Parenteral nutrition. In: DiPiro JT, Talbert RL, Yee GC, et al., eds. *Pharmacotherapy: A Pathophysiologic Approach*, 9th ed. [book online]. New York, NY: McGraw-Hill; 2014.
13. Kumpf VJ, Chessman KH. Enteral nutrition. In: DiPiro JT, Talbert RL, Yee GC, et al., eds. *Pharmacotherapy: A Pathophysiologic Approach*, 9th ed. [book online]. New York, NY: McGraw-Hill; 2014.
14. Craig SB, Dietz WH. Nutritional requirements. In: Baker SB, Baker RD Jr, Davis A, eds. *Pediatric Enteral Nutrition*. New York, NY: Chapman Hall; 1994:67–94.
15. O'Sullivan TA. Parenteral nutrition calculations. In: *Understanding Pharmacy Calculations*. Washington, DC: American Pharmacists' Association; 2002:143–237.
16. Lewis JL. Water and sodium balance. In: Porter RS, ed. *The Merck Manual Professional Edition* [book online]. Whitehouse Station, NJ: Merck & Co., Inc.; 2014.
17. Basal Energy Expenditure: Harris Benedict Equation. Available at: http://www-users.med.cornell.edu/~spon/picu/calc/beecalc.htm. Accessed March 16, 2015.
18. Dlugosz C. Pharmacist's guide to fiber and digestive health. *Pharmacy Today* 2008;14.
19. United States Department of Agriculture, Center for Nutrition Policy and Promotion. Dietary Guidelines for Americans, 2010. Available at: http://www.health.gov/dietaryguidelines/dga2010/DietaryGuidelines2010.pdf. Accessed March 17, 2015.
20. Department of Health and Human Services, Food and Drug Administration. How to Understand and Use the Nutrition Facts Label. Available at: http://www.fda.gov/food/ingredientspackaginglabeling/labelingnutrition/ucm274593.htm. Accessed March 17, 2015.
21. Department of Health and Human Services, Food and Drug Administration. Food Labeling Guide. Available at: http://www.fda.gov/food/guidanceregulation/guidancedocumentsregulatoryinformation/labelingnutrition/ucm2006828.htm. Accessed March 17, 2015.
22. Department of Health and Human Services, Food and Drug Administration. Guidance for Industry: A Food Labeling Guide (9. Appendix A: Definitions of Nutrient Content Claims). Available at: http://www.fda.gov/food/guidanceregulation/guidancedocumentsregulatoryinformation/labelingnutrition/ucm064911.htm. Accessed March 17, 2015.

15

Altering Product Strength, Use of Stock Solutions, and Problem Solving by Alligation

OBJECTIVES

Upon successful completion of this chapter, the student will be able to:

- Perform calculations for altering product strength through dilution or fortification.
- Perform calculations for the preparation and use of stock solutions.
- Apply *alligation medial* and *alligation alternate* in problem solving.

The strength of a pharmaceutical preparation may be increased or decreased by changing the proportion of active ingredient to the whole. A preparation may be strengthened or made more concentrated by the addition of active ingredient, by admixture with a like preparation of greater strength, or through the evaporation of its vehicle, if liquid. The strength of a preparation may be decreased or diluted by the addition of diluent or by admixture with a like preparation of lesser strength.

In the course of pharmacy practice, the *reduction* in the strength of a commercially available pharmaceutical product may be desired to treat a particular patient, based on the patient's age (e.g., pediatric or elderly) or medical status, or to assess a patient's initial response to a new medication. The *strengthening* of a product may be desired to meet the specific medication needs of an individual patient.

Various methods of calculation for the alteration of the strength of pharmaceutical preparations are presented in this chapter.

Relationship between Strength and Total Quantity

The strength of a pharmaceutical preparation is based on its content of active ingredient relative to the whole.

Guidance: *If the amount of active ingredient remains constant, a change in the total quantity (volume or weight) of a preparation will alter the strength inversely; that is, the strength decreases as the total quantity increases, and vice versa.*

For instance, 1 g in 10 mL = 10% w/v, whereas 1 g in 20 mL = 5% w/v. Thus, by doubling the volume, the strength is halved.

Problems in this section generally may be solved by any of the following methods:

(1) Inverse proportion

(2) The equation: (1st quantity) × (1st concentration) = (2nd quantity) × (2nd concentration), or **Q1 × C1 = Q2 × C2**

NOTE: Many students prefer this method.

(3) Traditional calculations, by determining the quantity of active ingredient present and relating that amount to the quantity of the total preparation

Dilution of Liquids

Example Calculations of Dilution of Liquids

(1) *If 500 mL of a 15% v/v solution are diluted to 1500 mL, what is the percent strength (v/v) of the dilution?*

Solving by inverse proportion:

$$\frac{1500\ (\text{mL})}{500\ (\text{mL})} = \frac{15\ (\%)}{x\ (\%)}$$

$$x = \mathbf{5\%\ v/v}$$

Or solving by equation:

$$\text{Q1 (quantity)} \times \text{C1 (concentration)} = \text{Q2 (quantity)} \times \text{C2 (concentration)}$$

$$500\ (\text{mL}) \times 15\ (\%) = 1500\ (\text{mL}) \times x\ (\%)$$

$$x = \mathbf{5\%\ v/v}$$

Or solving by traditional calculations:

$$500\ \text{mL} \times 15\% = 75\ \text{mL of solute}$$

$$\frac{75\ (\text{mL})}{1500\ (\text{mL})} \times 100\% = \mathbf{5\%\ v/v}$$

(2) *How many milliliters of a 1:5000 w/v solution of the preservative lauralkonium chloride can be made from 125 mL of a 0.2% w/v solution of the preservative?*

NOTE: It is often simpler to convert a given ratio strength to the corresponding percent strength in solving certain problems.

Solving by inverse proportion:

$$1{:}5000 = 0.02\%\ \text{w/v}$$

$$\frac{0.02\ (\%)}{0.2\ (\%)} = \frac{125\ (\text{mL})}{x\ (\text{mL})}$$

$$x = \mathbf{1250\ mL}$$

Or solving by equation:

$$\text{Q1 (quantity)} \times \text{C1 (concentration)} = \text{Q2 (quantity)} \times \text{C2 (concentration)}$$

$$125\ (\text{mL}) \times 0.2\ (\%) = x\ (\text{mL}) \times 0.02\ (\%)$$

$$x = \mathbf{1250\ mL}$$

Or solving by traditional calculations:

$$125\ \text{mL} \times 0.2\%\ \text{w/v} = 0.25\ \text{g lauralkonium chloride}$$

$$\frac{0.25\ \text{g} \times 100\ \text{mL}}{0.02\ \text{g}} = \mathbf{1250\ mL}$$

(3) *How many milliliters of water should be added to 80 mL of a 20% w/v aqueous solution to prepare a 3% w/v solution?*
<u>*Solving by traditional calculations:*</u>

$$80 \text{ mL} \times 20\% \text{ w/v} = 16 \text{ g solute}$$

$$\frac{3 \text{ g}}{100 \text{ mL}} = \frac{16 \text{ g}}{\text{x mL}}$$

x = 533.3 mL (quantity of a 3% w/v solution that 16 g of solute will prepare)

533.3 mL − 80 mL = **453.3 mL of water** to add

<u>*Or solving by equation:*</u>

$$\text{Q1 (quantity)} \times \text{C1 (concentration)} = \text{Q2 (quantity)} \times \text{C2 (concentration)}$$

$$80 \text{ (mL)} \times 20 \text{ (\%)} = \text{x (mL)} \times 3 \text{ (\%)}$$

$$\text{x} = 533.3 \text{ mL} - 80 \text{ mL} = \mathbf{453.3 \text{ mL of water}} \text{ to add}$$

(4) *If an injection containing a medication, 50 mg/10 mL, is diluted to 1 L, calculate the percent strength of the resulting solution.*
<u>*Solving by traditional calculations:*</u>

$$50 \text{ mg} = 0.05 \text{ g}$$

$$\frac{0.05 \text{ g}}{1000 \text{ mL}} \times 100\% = \mathbf{0.005\%}$$

(5) *Dopamine HCl injection is available in 5-mL vials each containing 40 mg of dopamine HCl per milliliter. The injection must be diluted before administration by intravenous infusion. If a pharmacist dilutes the injection by adding the contents of one vial to 250 mL of 5% dextrose injection, calculate the percent concentration of dopamine HCl in the infusion.*
<u>*Solving by traditional calculations:*</u>
Dopamine HCl per vial:

$$5 \text{ mL} \times 40 \text{ mg/mL} = 200 \text{ mg (0.2 g)}$$

Total infusion volume:

5 mL (dopamine HCl injection) + 250 mL (5% dextrose injection) = 255 mL

Percent concentration calculation:

$$\frac{0.2 \text{ g}}{255 \text{ mL}} \times 100\% = \mathbf{0.078\% \text{ w/v}}$$

<u>*Or solving by equation:*</u>

$$\text{Q1 (quantity)} \times \text{C1 (concentration)} = \text{Q2 (quantity)} \times \text{C2 (concentration)}$$

$$5 \text{ mL} \times 4\% \text{ (40 mg/mL)} = 255 \text{ mL} \times \text{x}$$

$$\text{x} = \mathbf{0.078\% \text{ w/v}}$$

(6) *If a pharmacist reconstitutes a vial to contain 1 g of cefazolin in 3 mL of injection (see* Fig. 15.1*), and then dilutes 1.6 mL of the injection with sodium chloride injection to prepare 200 mL of intravenous infusion, calculate the concentration of cefazolin in the infusion in percent and in mg/mL.*
<u>*Solving by the traditional calculations:*</u>
Quantity of cefazolin in the infusion:

$$1 \text{ g} \times 1.6 \text{ mL/3 mL} = 0.53 \text{ g cefazolin}$$

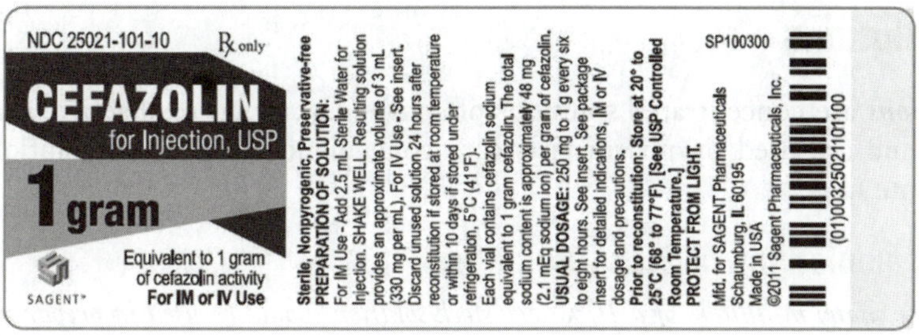

FIGURE 15.1 • Product label for cefazolin for injection. *(Courtesy Sagent Pharmaceuticals.)*

Percent calculation:

$$0.53\ \text{g}/200\ \text{mL} \times 100\% = \mathbf{0.27\%\ w/v\ cefazolin}$$

mg/mL calculation:

$$0.27\%\ \text{w/v} = 0.27\ \text{g}/100\ \text{mL} = 270\ \text{mg}/100\ \text{mL} = \mathbf{2.7\ mg/mL\ cefazolin}$$

<u>*Or solving by equation:*</u>

$$\text{Q1 (quantity)} \times \text{C1 (concentration)} = \text{Q2 (quantity)} \times \text{C2 (concentration)}$$

$$1.6\ \text{mL} \times 33.3\%\ (1\ \text{g}/3\ \text{mL}) = 200\ \text{mL} \times x$$

$$x = \mathbf{0.27\%\ w/v\ cefazolin}$$

$$0.27\%\ \text{w/v} = 0.27\ \text{g}/100\ \text{mL} = 270\ \text{mg}/100\ \text{mL} = \mathbf{2.7\ mg/mL\ cefazolin}$$

Strengthening of a Pharmaceutical Product

Strengthening an existing pharmaceutical product may be accomplished by the addition of active ingredient or by the admixture with a calculated quantity of a like product of greater concentration. The latter type of calculation is presented later in this chapter under the discussion of *alligation alternate*.

If a cough syrup contains in each teaspoonful 1 mg of chlorpheniramine maleate and if a pharmacist desired to double the strength, how many milligrams of that ingredient would need to be added to a 60-mL container of the syrup. Assume no increase in volume.

$$\frac{1\ \text{mg}}{5\ \text{mL}} \times 60\ \text{mL} = \mathbf{12\ mg\ chlorpheniramine\ maleate}\ \text{in original syrup}$$

To double the strength, 12 mg of additional chlorpheniramine maleate would be required.

CASE IN POINT 15.1 A pharmacist received a prescription for 100 mL of a cefuroxime axetil suspension to contain 300 mg of drug in each 5 mL. The pharmacist has 100 mL of a suspension containing 250 mg/5 mL and also has 250-mg scored tablets of the drug. How many tablets should be pulverized and added to the suspension to achieve the desired strength? Assume no increase in the volume of the suspension.

A Second Look

The pharmacist observed that after adding the pulverized tablets, the suspension measured 102 mL in volume. Calculations revealed that rather than the prescribed drug strength of 300 mg/5 mL, there were 294.1 mg/5 mL. What could the pharmacist do to bring the suspension to the desired strength?

Stock Solutions

Stock solutions are concentrated solutions of active (e.g., drug) or inactive (e.g., colorant) substances and are used by pharmacists as a convenience to prepare solutions of lesser concentration.

Example Calculations of Stock Solutions

(1) *How many milliliters of a 10% w/v stock solution should be used in preparing 1 gallon of a 0.05% w/v solution?*

$$1 \text{ gallon} = 3785 \text{ mL}$$
$$3785 \text{ mL} \times 0.05 \text{ g}/100 \text{ mL} = 1.89 \text{ g}$$
$$1.89 \text{ g} \times \frac{100 \text{ mL}}{10 \text{ g}} = \mathbf{18.9 \text{ mL}}$$

<u>Or by solving by equation:</u>

$$\text{Q1 (quantity)} \times \text{C1 (concentration)} = \text{Q2 (quantity)} \times \text{C2 (concentration)}$$
$$3785 \text{ mL} \times 0.05\% = \text{x mL} \times 10\% = \mathbf{18.9 \text{ mL}}$$

(2) *How many milliliters of a 1% w/v stock solution of a certified red dye should be used in preparing 4000 mL of a mouthwash that is to contain 1:20,000 w/v of the certified red dye as a coloring agent?*

$$1{:}20{,}000 \text{ w/v} = 0.005\% \text{ w/v}$$
$$\text{Q1} \times \text{C1} = \text{Q2} \times \text{C2}$$
$$4000 \text{ mL} \times 0.005\% \text{ w/v} = \text{x mL} \times 1\% \text{ w/v}$$
$$\text{x} = \mathbf{20 \text{ mL}}$$

Some interesting calculations are used in pharmacy practice in *which the strength of a diluted portion of a solution is defined, but the strength of the concentrated stock solution used to prepare it must be determined*. This may be further explained by the need of a pharmacist to prepare and dispense a concentrated solution of a drug and direct the patient to use a specific household measure of a solution (e.g., 1 teaspoonful) in a specified volume of water (e.g., a pint) to make the solution of the desired concentration (e.g., for irrigation or soaking). This permits the dispensing of a relatively small volume of liquid, enabling a patient to prepare relatively large volumes as needed, rather than carrying home large volumes of a diluted solution from a pharmacy.

(3) *How much drug should be used in preparing 50 mL of a stock solution such that 5 mL diluted to 500 mL will yield a 1:1000 w/v solution?*

$$1{:}1000 \text{ w/v} = 1 \text{ g of drug in } 1000 \text{ mL of solution}$$
$$500 \text{ mL} \times \frac{1 \text{ g}}{1000 \text{ mL}} = 0.5 \text{ g}$$

Thus, 0.5 g of drug would be in the 500 mL of the 1:1000 w/v diluted solution, and importantly, the source of that 0.5 g of drug is the 5 mL of the stock solution. If 0.5 g of drug is in each 5 mL of the stock solution, calculate the grams of drug needed to prepare the 50 mL of stock solution:

$$50 \text{ mL} \times \frac{0.5 \text{ g}}{5 \text{ mL}} = \mathbf{5 \text{ g}}$$

The accompanying diagrammatic sketch demonstrates the problem.

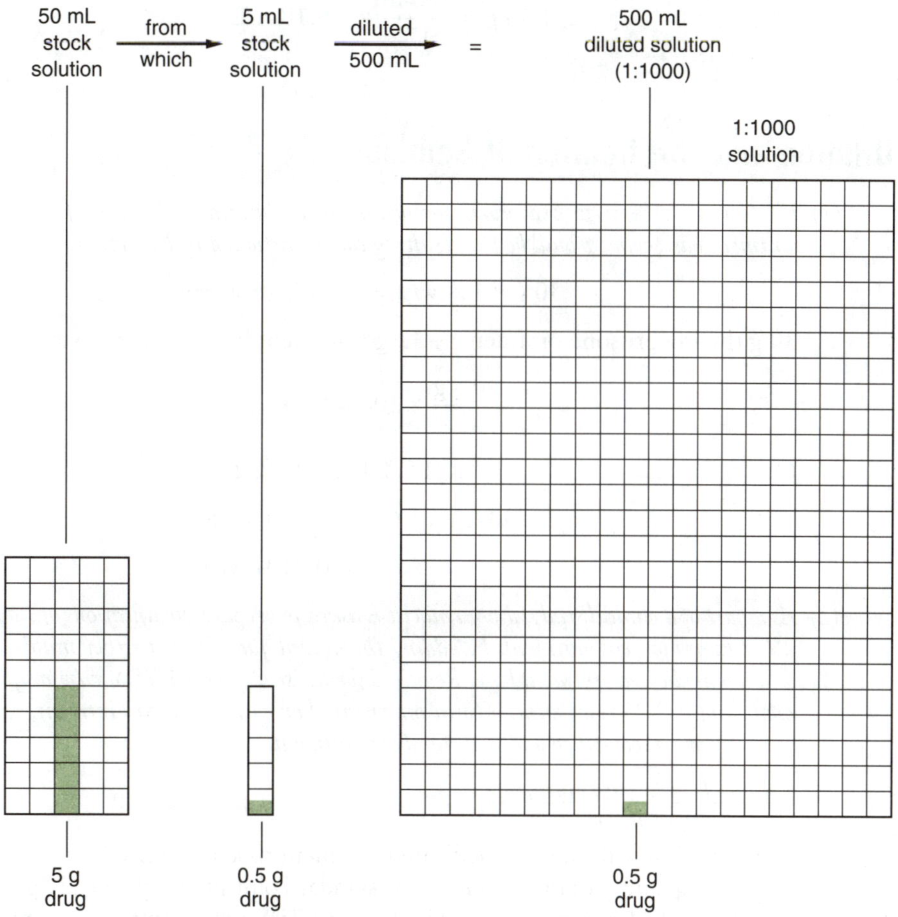

(4) *How many grams of sodium chloride should be used in preparing 500 mL of a stock solution such that 50 mL diluted to 1000 mL will yield a 0.3% w/v solution for irrigation?*

$$1000 \text{ mL} \times 0.3\% \text{ w/v} = 3 \text{ g of sodium chloride in } 1000 \text{ mL},$$

which is also the amount in 50 mL of the stock solution.

Thus, the amount of sodium chloride in 500 mL of the stock solution is:

$$3 \text{ g} \times \frac{500 \text{ mL}}{50 \text{ mL}} = \mathbf{30\ g}$$

(5) *How many milliliters of a 17% w/v concentrate of benzalkonium chloride should be used in preparing 100 mL of a stock solution such that 5 mL diluted to 60 mL will yield a 0.13% w/v solution of benzalkonium chloride?*

$$60 \text{ mL} \times 0.13\% \text{ w/v} = 0.078 \text{ g of benzalkonium chloride in } 60 \text{ mL},$$

which is also the amount in 5 mL of the stock solution.

Thus, the amount of benzalkonium chloride in 100 mL of the stock solution is:

$$0.078 \text{ g} \times \frac{100 \text{ mL}}{5 \text{ mL}} = 1.56 \text{ g}$$

And the amount of the 17% w/v concentrate to use is:

$$1.56\ g \times \frac{100\ mL}{17\ g} = \mathbf{9.18\ mL}$$

Dilution and Fortification of Semisolids

(1) *If 30 g of a 1% w/w hydrocortisone ointment are mixed with 12 g of a nonmedicated ointment base, what would be the resulting concentration of hydrocortisone in the mixture?*

$$30\ g \times 1\%\ w/w = 0.3\ g\ \text{hydrocortisone}$$

30 g (hydrocortisone ointment) + 12 g (ointment base) = 42 g mixture

$$\frac{0.3\ g}{42\ g} \times 100 = \mathbf{0.71\%\ w/w}$$

Or,

$$Q1 \times C1 = Q2 \times C2$$

$$30\ (g) \times 1\ (\%) = 42\ (g) \times x\ (\%)$$

$$x = \mathbf{0.71\%\ w/w}$$

(2) *As a part of a clinical study, a pharmacist is asked to prepare modifications of standard 22 g 2% w/w mupirocin ointments by adding the needed quantities of either mupirocin powder or a nonmedicated ointment base. Required for the study are a 1.75% w/w mupirocin ointment and a 2.25% w/w mupirocin ointment. For each modified ointment, calculate the quantity of component to add to a standard ointment.*

<u>*For the 1.75% w/w ointment:*</u>
Consider the following:

- Dilution with the nonmedicated ointment base is required.
- The quantity of mupirocin in the standard ointment is 0.44 g (22 g × 2% w/w).
- From 0.44 g of mupirocin, 25.14 g of a 1.75% w/w mupirocin ointment may be prepared (0.44 g × 100 g/1.75 g = 25.14 g).
- Since the standard ointment weighs 22 g, the addition of 3.14 g of nonmedicated ointment base is required (25.14 g – 22 g = 3.14 g).

Proof: 0.44 g (mupirocin) in 25.14 g (diluted ointment) = 1.75% w/w

<u>*For the 2.25% w/w ointment:*</u>
Consider the following:

- Fortification with mupirocin powder is required.
- 22 g of the 2% w/w mupirocin ointment contains 0.44 g of mupirocin (22 g × 2% w/w).
- The remainder, 21.56 g (22 g – 0.44 g), is the nonmedicated portion (ointment base) of the standard ointment.
- If the fortified ointment is to contain 2.25% w/w mupirocin, the nonmedicated portion, or 21.56 g, would then represent 97.75% of the whole.
- If 21.56 g is equal to 97.75% of the whole, 100% would be equal to 22.056 g (21.56 g × 100%/97.75%), and the difference, 0.496 g (22.056 g – 21.56 g), is the total required mupirocin in the final product.
- Since the original ointment contains 0.44 g of mupirocin, the addition of 0.056 g of mupirocin is required.

Proof: 0.496 g (mupirocin) in 22.056 g (fortified ointment) = 2.249% ≈ 2.25% w/w

NOTE: This problem should be reworked later in the chapter using the alligation alternate method.

Alligation

Alligation is an arithmetical method of solving problems that involves the mixing of solutions or mixtures of solids of different percentage strengths.

Alligation Medial. This is a method by which the "weighted average" strength of a mixture of two or more substances of known quantity and concentration may be calculated.

Example Calculations Using Alligation Medial

(1) *What is the percentage of zinc oxide in an ointment prepared by mixing 200 g of 10% ointment, 50 g of 20% ointment, and 100 g of 5% ointment?*

$$0.10 \times 200 \text{ g} = 20 \text{ g}$$
$$0.20 \times 50 \text{ g} = 10 \text{ g}$$
$$0.05 \times \underline{100} \text{ g} = \underline{5} \text{ g}$$
$$\text{Total: } 350 \text{ g} \quad 35 \text{ g}$$
$$35 \text{ (g)} \div 350 \text{ (g)} = 0.10 \times 100 = \mathbf{10\%\ w/w}$$

In some problems, the addition of a diluent or vehicle must be considered and treated as zero percent strength, as in the following example.

(2) *What is the percentage strength of alcohol in a mixture of 500 mL of a solution containing 40% v/v alcohol, 400 mL of a second solution containing 21% v/v alcohol, and a sufficient quantity of a nonalcoholic third solution to make a total of 1000 mL?*

$$0.40 \times 500 \text{ mL} = 200 \text{ mL}$$
$$0.21 \times 400 \text{ mL} = 84 \text{ mL}$$
$$0 \times \underline{100} \text{ mL} = \underline{0} \text{ mL}$$
$$\text{Totals: } 1000 \text{ mL} \quad 284 \text{ mL}$$
$$284 \text{ (mL)} \div 1000 \text{ (mL)} = 0.284 \times 100 = \mathbf{28.4\%\ v/v}$$

(3) A pharmacist–herbalist wishes to consolidate the following assayed batches of *Gingko biloba* leaves: 200 g containing 22% w/w glycosides, 150 g containing 26% w/w glycosides, and 80 g containing 27% w/w glycosides. Calculate the percent of glycosides in the combined mixture.

$$0.22 \times 200 \text{ g} = 44 \text{ g}$$
$$0.26 \times 150 \text{ g} = 39 \text{ g}$$
$$0.27 \times \underline{80} \text{ g} = \underline{21.6} \text{ g}$$
$$\text{Totals: } 430 \text{ g} \quad 104.6 \text{ g}$$
$$104.6 \text{ (g)} \div 430 \text{ (g)} = 0.243 \times 100 = \mathbf{24.3\%\ w/w}$$

Alligation Alternate. This is a method used to determine the quantities of ingredients of differing strengths needed to make a mixture of a desired strength. *It involves matching pairs of ingredients, one higher in strength and one lower in strength than the desired strength, which lies* *somewhere in between.* As shown in the example below, the desired strength is placed in the center of the working diagram.

Example Calculations Using Alligation Alternate

(1) *In what proportion should alcohols of 95% and 50% strengths be mixed to make 70% alcohol?*

Note that the difference between the *strength of the stronger component* (95%) and the *desired strength* (70%) indicates the *number of parts of the weaker* to be used (25 parts), and the difference between the *desired strength* (70%) and the *strength of the weaker component* (50%) indicates the *number of parts of the stronger* to be used (20 parts).

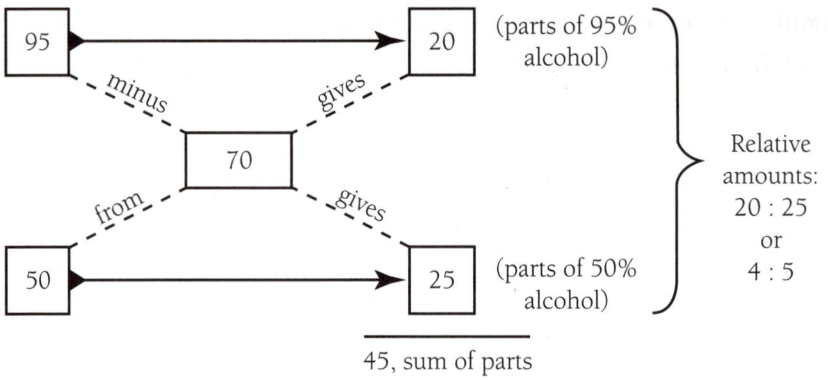

The mathematical validity of this relationship can be demonstrated.

Percent given	Percent desired	Proportional parts required
a		*x*
	c	
b		*y*

Given these data, the ratio of x to y may be derived algebraically as follows:

$$ax + by = c\,(x + y)$$
$$ax + by = cx + cy$$
$$ax - cx = cy - by$$
$$x\,(a - c) = y\,(c - b)$$
$$\frac{x}{y} = \frac{c - b}{a - c}$$

Given a = 95%, b = 50%, and c = 70%, we may therefore solve the problems as follows:

$$0.95x + 0.50y = 0.70(x + y)$$

Or

$$95x + 50y = 70x + 70y$$
$$95x - 70x = 70y + 50y$$
$$x(95 - 70) = y(70 - 50)$$
$$\frac{x}{y} = \frac{70 - 50}{95 - 70} = \frac{20}{25} = \frac{\mathbf{4\ (parts)}}{\mathbf{5\ (parts)}}$$

The result can be shown to be correct by *alligation medial*:

$$95 \times 4 = 380$$
$$50 \times 5 = 250$$
$$\text{Total: } 9 \quad 630$$
$$630 \div 9 = 70\%$$

The customary layout of *alligation alternate*, used in the subsequent examples, is a convenient simplification of the preceding diagram.

(2) *In what proportion should 20% benzocaine ointment be mixed with an ointment base to produce a 2.5% benzocaine ointment?*

Note that an "ointment base" has no drug content and thus is represented by a zero in the scheme.

20%	2.5%	2.5 parts of 20% ointment
0%		17.5 parts of ointment base

(3) *A hospital pharmacist wants to use three lots of zinc oxide ointment containing, respectively, 50%, 20%, and 5% of zinc oxide. In what proportion should they be mixed to prepare a 10% zinc oxide ointment?*

Note that *pairs* must be used in each determination, one lower and one greater in strength than the desired strength.

50%		5 parts of 50% ointment
20%	10%	5 parts of 20% ointment
5%		10 + 40 = 50 parts of 5% ointment

Other answers are possible, of course, by using alternate pairings.

(4) *In what proportions may a manufacturing pharmacist mix 20%, 15%, 5%, and 3% zinc oxide ointments to produce a 10% ointment?*

Each of the weaker lots is paired with one of the stronger to give the desired strength, and because we may pair them in two ways, we may get two sets of correct answers.

20%		7 parts of 20% ointment
15%	10%	5 parts of 15% ointment
5%		5 parts of 5% ointment
3%		10 parts of 3% ointment

(5) *How many milliliters each of a 50% w/v dextrose solution and a 5% w/v dextrose solution is required to prepare 4500 mL of a 10% w/v solution?*

50%	10%	5 parts of 50% solution
5%		40 parts of 5% solution

There is a *total* of 45 parts to prepare the 4500 mL mixture, or 100 mL per part (4500 mL/45 parts). And the amount of each component may be calculated by:

5 (parts) × 100 mL = **500 mL of the 50% w/v dextrose solution**

40 (parts) × 100 mL = **4000 mL of 5% w/v dextrose solution**

(6) *How many grams of 2.5% w/w hydrocortisone cream should be mixed with 360 g of 0.25% w/w cream to make a 1% w/w hydrocortisone cream?*

2.5%	1%	0.75 parts of 2.5% cream
0.25%		1.5 parts of 0.25% cream

The 0.25% w/w hydrocortisone cream is 1.5 parts of the whole with a given weight of 360 g. This means that each part is equivalent to 240 g [360 g/1.5 (parts)]. Thus, the quantity of the 2.5% w/w hydrocortisone cream required would be **180 g** [(240 g/0.75 part)].

(7) *How many grams of zinc oxide powder should be added to 3200 g of a 5% w/w zinc oxide ointment to prepare a 20% w/w zinc oxide ointment?*

NOTE: In the allegation alternate diagram, the zinc oxide powder is 100% zinc oxide.

100%	20%	15 parts of the zinc oxide powder
5%		80 parts of the 5% zinc oxide ointment

Since each of the 80 parts (of the 5% zinc oxide ointment) is equal to 40 g [3200 g/80 (parts)], the value of 15 parts of the zinc oxide powder would be calculated by 40 g × 15 (parts) = **600 g.**

Proof: 3200 g × 5% w/w = 160 g zinc oxide content

+600 g zinc oxide powder

760 g zinc oxide total

760 g/3800 g (3200 g + 600 g) × 100% = 20% w/w zinc oxide

Specific Gravity of Mixtures

The methods of alligation medial and alligation alternate may be used in solving problems involving the specific gravities of liquids as demonstrated below.

(1) *What is the specific gravity of a mixture of 1000 mL of syrup with a specific gravity of 1.300, 400 mL of glycerin with a specific gravity of 1.250, and 1000 mL of an elixir with a specific gravity of 0.950?*

$$1.300 \times 1000\,\text{mL} = 1300\,\text{g}$$
$$1.250 \times 400\,\text{mL} = 500\,\text{g}$$
$$0.950 \times \underline{1000\,\text{mL}} = \underline{950\,\text{g}}$$
$$\text{Totals:}\ 2400\,\text{mL} \quad 2750\,\text{g}$$
$$2750\,\text{g} \div 2400\,\text{mL} = \mathbf{1.146}$$

(2) *In what proportion must glycerin with a specific gravity of 1.25 and water be mixed to prepare a liquid having a specific gravity of 1.10?*

1.25	0.10	0.10 parts of glycerin
1.00		0.15 parts of water

Relative amounts: 0.10:0.15 or **2:3**

(3) *How many milliliters of each of two liquids with specific gravities of 0.950 and 0.875 should be used to prepare 1500 mL of a liquid having a specific gravity of 0.925?*

0.950	0.925	0.050, or 50 parts of liquid with specific gravity of 0.95
0.875		0.025, or 25 parts of liquid with specific gravity of 0.875

Relative amounts: 50:25, or 2:1, with a total of three parts:

$$\frac{3\ (\text{parts})}{2\ (\text{parts})} = \frac{1500\ (\text{mL})}{x\ (\text{mL})}$$

x = **1000 mL of liquid with specific gravity of 0.950**

$$\frac{3\ (\text{parts})}{1\ (\text{parts})} = \frac{1500\ (\text{mL})}{y\ (\text{mL})}$$

y = **500 mL of liquid with specific gravity of 0.875**

CASE IN POINT 15.2[a] A pharmacist received the following prescription:

℞	Clindamycin phosphate	1.5%
	Alcohol (52% v/v) q.s. ad	120 mL
	Sig: apply daily for acne.	

The pharmacist has no clindamycin phosphate powder but does have clindamycin phosphate sterile solution, 150 mg/mL, in vials. From the label, the pharmacist learns that the solution is aqueous.

(a) How many milliliters of the clindamycin phosphate sterile solution should the pharmacist use in filling the prescription?
(b) How many milliliters of 95% v/v of alcohol are required?
(c) How many milliliters of water should be added to make 120 mL?

[a]Problem courtesy of Warren Beach, College of Pharmacy, The University of Georgia Athens, GA.

CASE IN POINT 15.3 A pharmacist received the following prescription:

℞	Hydrocortisone	0.6%
	AQUAPHOR q.s. ad	15 g
	Sig: apply to child's affected area t.i.d.	

The pharmacist has no hydrocortisone powder but does have a hydrocortisone cream, 1%. How many grams each of hydrocortisone cream and AQUAPHOR should be used in filling the prescription?

PRACTICE PROBLEMS

Altering Strength, Stock Solutions, and Alligation Calculations

1. A farm product contains a 12.5% w/v concentrate of tiamulin hydrogen fumarate, used to treat swine dysentery when diluted as a medicated drinking water. How many gallons of medicated water may be prepared from a liter of concentrate if the final product is to contain 227 mg of tiamulin hydrogen fumarate per gallon?
2. If a pharmacist added 12 g of azelaic acid to 50 g of an ointment containing 15% azelaic acid, what would be the final concentration of azelaic acid in the ointment?
3. If 400 mL of a 20% w/v solution were diluted to 2 L, what would be the final percentage strength?
4. BACTROBAN ointment contains 2% w/w mupirocin. How many grams of a polyethylene glycol ointment base must be mixed with the contents of a 22-g tube of the BACTROBAN ointment to prepare one having a concentration of 5 mg/g?
5. How many grams of an 8% w/w progesterone gel must be mixed with 1.45 g of a 4% w/w progesterone gel to prepare a 5.5% w/w gel?
6. Chlorhexidine gluconate is available in different products in concentrations of 4% w/v and 0.12% w/v. How many milliliters of the more dilute product may be prepared from each fluidounce of the more concentrated product?
7. A pharmacist fills a prescription for 30 g of a 0.1% w/w hydrocortisone cream by combining a 1% w/w hydrocortisone cream and a cream base. How many grams of each were used?
8. How many milliliters of water should be added to 1.5 L of a 20% w/v solution to prepare one containing 12% w/v of solute?
9. If two tablespoonfuls of a 10% w/v povidone–iodine solution were diluted to 1 quart with purified water, what would be the ratio strength of the dilution?
10. How many milliliters of a 1:50 w/v boric acid solution can be prepared from 500 mL of a 5% w/v boric acid solution?
11. How many milliliters of water must be added to 250 mL of a 25% w/v stock solution of sodium chloride to prepare a 0.9% w/v sodium chloride solution?
12. How many milliliters of undecylenic acid should be added to 30 mL of a 20% v/v undecylenic acid topical solution to change its concentration to 25% v/v?
13. A pharmacy intern is asked to prepare 3 L of a 30% w/v solution. The pharmacy stocks the active ingredient in 8-ounce bottles of 70% w/v strength. How many bottles will be needed as the source of the active ingredient?
14. How many milliliters of a 10% w/v stock solution are needed to prepare 120 mL of a solution containing 10 mg of the chemical per milliliter?
15. How many milliliters of a 2.0 molar sodium chloride solution would be needed to prepare 250 mL of 0.15 molar sodium chloride solution?
16. NEORAL oral solution contains 100 mg/mL of cyclosporine. If a pharmacist prepares 30 mL of an oral solution containing 10% w/v cyclosporine, how many milliliters of diluent should be used?
17. The formula for a buffer solution contains 1.24% w/v of boric acid. How many milliliters of a 5% w/v boric acid solution should be used to obtain the boric acid needed in preparing 1 L of the buffer solution?
18. In filling a hospital order, a pharmacist diluted 1 mL of an amphotericin B injection containing 50 mg/10 mL with a 5% w/v dextrose injection to prepare an intravenous infusion containing amphotericin B, 0.1 mg/mL. How many milliliters of infusion did the pharmacist prepare?

19. What would be the concentration of a solution prepared by diluting 45 mL of a 4.2-molar solution to a volume of 250 mL?
20. A pharmacist combines the contents of a 30-g tube of a 0.5% ointment and a 90-g tube of a 1.5% ointment of the same active ingredient. What is the concentration of the mixture?
21.[1] ℞ Rhus toxicodendron extract 10 mg/mL
Sterile water for injection q.s. 100 mL
Sig: as directed

How many milliliters of a 100 mg/mL concentrate of Rhus toxicodendron extract should be used in preparing the prescription?
22. If a pharmacist fortified 10 g of a 0.1% w/w tacrolimus (PROTOPIC) ointment by adding 12.5 g of an ointment containing 0.03% w/w of the same drug, what would be the percentage strength of the mixture?
23. A physician prescribes an ophthalmic suspension to contain 100 mg of cortisone acetate in 8 mL of normal saline solution. The pharmacist has on hand a 2.5% w/v suspension of cortisone acetate in normal saline solution. How many milliliters of this and how many milliliters of normal saline solution should be used in preparing the prescribed suspension?
24. ℞ Benzalkonium chloride solution 240 mL
Make a solution such that 10 mL diluted
to a liter equals a 1:5000 w/v solution.
Sig: 10 mL diluted to a liter for external use

How many milliliters of a 17% w/v stock solution of benzalkonium chloride should be used in preparing the prescription?
25. A pharmacist–herbalist mixed 100 g lots of St. John's wort containing the following percentages of the active component hypericin: 0.3%, 0.7%, and 0.25%. Calculate the percent strength of hypericin in the mixture.
26. How many milliliters of a lotion base must be added to 30 mL of oxiconazole nitrate (OXISTAT) lotion 1% w/v, to reduce its concentration to 6 mg/mL?
27.[2] ℞ Lactic acid 10% w/v
Salicylic acid 10% w/v
Flexible collodion q.s. 15 mL
Sig: for wart removal. Use externally as directed.

How many milliliters of an 85% w/w solution of lactic acid with a specific gravity of 1.21 should be used in preparing the prescription?
28. A pharmacist receives a prescription for 60 g of a 0.75% w/w bexarotene gel. How many grams each of a 1% w/w bexarotene gel and gel base must be used?
29. As a part of a clinical study, a pharmacist is asked to prepare a modification of a standard 22 g package of a 2% mupirocin ointment by adding the needed quantity of mupirocin powder to prepare a 3% w/w mupirocin ointment. How many milligrams of mupirocin powder are required?
30. A pharmacist receives an order for 60 mL of an oral solution containing memantine hydrochloride (NAMENDA) 1.5 mg/mL. She has on hand a 360-mL bottle of oral solution containing memantine hydrochloride, 10 mg/5 mL, and a diluent of sorbitol solution. How many milliliters each of the available oral solution and sorbitol solution may be used to fill the order?
31. If a pharmacist added each of the following to 22-g packages of 2% mupirocin ointment, what would be the percentage strengths of the resulting ointments: (a) 0.25 g mupirocin powder and (b) 0.25 g of nonmedicated ointment base? (answer to two decimal places).

32. A physician prescribes an ophthalmic suspension to contain 100 mg of cortisone acetate in 8 mL of normal saline solution. The pharmacist has on hand a 2.5% suspension of cortisone acetate in normal saline solution. How many milliliters each of the 2.5% suspension and of normal saline solution should be used?
33. If 1 mL of a 0.02% w/v isoproterenol hydrochloride solution is diluted to 10 mL with sodium chloride injection before intravenous administration, calculate the percent concentration of the diluted solution.
34. A 1:750 w/v solution of benzalkonium chloride diluted with purified water in a ratio of 3 parts of the benzalkonium solution and 77 parts of purified water is recommended for bladder and urethral irrigation. What is the ratio strength of benzalkonium chloride in the final dilution?
35. How many milliliters of a suspension base must be mixed with 250 mL of a paroxetine (PAXIL) oral suspension, 10 mg/5 mL, to change its concentration to 0.1% w/v?
36. A standing institutional order for a 25% w/w topical antibiotic ointment has been changed to one for a 12.5% w/w ointment. How many grams of white petrolatum must be mixed with each 120-g package of the 25% w/w preparation to make the new 10% w/w preparation?
37. How many grams of a 2.5% w/w benzocaine ointment can be prepared by diluting 1 lb of a 20% w/w benzocaine ointment with white petrolatum?
38. How many grams of salicylic acid should be added to 75 g of a polyethylene glycol ointment to prepare an ointment containing 6% w/w of salicylic acid?
39. How many grams of an ointment base must be added to 45 g of clobetasol (TEMOVATE) ointment, 0.05% w/w, to change its strength to 0.03% w/w?
40. ℞ Hydrocortisone acetate ointment 0.25% 10 g
Sig: apply to the eye.

How many grams of 2.5% ophthalmic hydrocortisone acetate ointment and how many grams of ophthalmic base (diluent) should be used in preparing the prescription?
41. How many milliliters of a nonmedicated, flavored syrup base must be added to 1 pint of ranitidine (ZANTAC) syrup, 15 mg/mL, to change its concentration to 5 mg/mL?
42. ℞

Zinc oxide	1.5
Hydrophilic petrolatum	2.5
Purified water	5
Hydrophilic ointment ad	30

Sig: apply to affected areas.

How much zinc oxide should be added to the product to make an ointment containing 10% of zinc oxide?
43. If equal portions of tretinoin gel (RETINA MICRO), 0.1% w/w and 0.04% w/w, are combined, what would be the resultant percentage strength?
44. A vaginal douche powder concentrate contains 2% w/w of active ingredient. What would be the percentage concentration of the resultant solution after a 5-g packet of powder is dissolved in enough water to make 1 quart of solution?
45.[3] How many milliliters of a 0.2% solution of a skin test antigen must be used to prepare 4 mL of a solution containing 0.04 mg/mL of the antigen?
46. How many milligrams of sodium fluoride are needed to prepare 100 mL of a sodium fluoride stock solution such that a solution containing 2 ppm of sodium fluoride results when 0.5 mL is diluted to 250 mL with water?

47.[4] ℞ Cyclosporine 2%
Corn oil q.s.
Sig: use as directed.

(a) How many milliliters each of corn oil and a 10% solution of cyclosporine would be needed to prepare 30 mL of the prescription? (b) If you then wished to dilute the prescription to a concentration of 1.5% cyclosporine, how many additional milliliters of corn oil would be required?

48. A hospital pharmacist is to prepare three doses of gentamicin 0.6 mg/2 mL. In stock is gentamicin 20 mg/mL. How many milliliters each of the gentamicin on hand and appropriate diluent would be needed?

49. A hospital worker combined 2 fluidounces of a povidone–iodine cleaner, 7.5% w/v, with 4 fluidounces of a povidone–iodine topical solution, 10 % w/v. Calculate the resulting strength of the povidone–iodine mixture.

50. If 60 mL of a combination gel of hydrocortisone acetate, 1% w/w, and pramoxine, 1% w/w, is mixed with 12.5 mL of a gel containing hydrocortisone acetate, 2.5% w/w, and pramoxine, 1% w/w, calculate the percentage strength of each of the two drugs in the mixture.

51. A drug is commercially available in capsules each containing 12.5 mg of drug and 37.5 mg of diluent. How many milligrams of additional diluent must be added to the contents of one capsule to make a dilution containing 0.5 mg of drug in each 100 mg of powder?

52. In what proportion should 5% and 1% hydrocortisone ointments be mixed to prepare a 2.5% ointment?

53. In what proportion should a 20% zinc oxide ointment be mixed with white petrolatum (diluent) to produce a 3% zinc oxide ointment?

54. A parent diluted 1-mL ibuprofen oral drops (Infant's MOTRIN Concentrated Drops) with 15 mL of water prior to administering the medication. The concentrated drops contain ibuprofen, 50 mg/1.25 mL. Calculate the concentration of ibuprofen in the dilution in (a) mg/mL and (b) as a percentage strength.

55. How many milliliters of a 2.5% w/v chlorpromazine hydrochloride injection and how many milliliters of 0.9% w/v sodium chloride injection should be used to prepare 500 mL of a 0.3% w/v chlorpromazine hydrochloride injection?

56. How many milliliters of a 2% w/v solution of lidocaine hydrochloride should be used in preparing 500 mL of a solution containing 4 mg of lidocaine hydrochloride per milliliter of solution?

57. Dopamine hydrochloride injection is available in 5-mL ampuls containing 40 mg of dopamine hydrochloride per milliliter. The injection must be diluted before administration. If a physician wishes to use sodium chloride injection as the diluent and wants a dilution containing 0.04% w/v of dopamine hydrochloride, how many milliliters of sodium chloride injection should be added to 5 mL of the injection?

58. A pharmacist is to prepare 10 mL of amikacin sulfate in a concentration of 0.4 mg/0.1 mL for ophthalmic use. Available is an injection containing amikacin sulfate, 250 mg/mL. How many milliliters of this injection and of sterile normal saline solution as the diluent should be used?

59.[5] How many milliliters of sterile water for injection should be added to a vial containing 5 μg/mL of a drug to prepare a solution containing 1.5 μg/mL of the drug?

60. How many milligrams of a 1:10 w/w powdered dilution of colchicine should be used by a manufacturing pharmacist in preparing 100 capsules for a clinical drug study if each capsule is to contain 0.5 mg of colchicine?

Specific Gravity Calculations of Mixtures

61. What is the specific gravity of a mixture containing 1000 mL of water, 500 mL of glycerin having a specific gravity of 1.25, and 1500 mL of alcohol having a specific gravity of 0.81? (Assume no contraction occurs when the liquids are mixed.)
62. If a pharmacist mixed 1 pint of propylene glycol having a specific gravity of 1.20 with 500 mL of water, how many milliliters additional of propylene glycol should be added to change the specific gravity to 1.15?
63. How many milliliters of a syrup having a specific gravity of 1.350 should be mixed with 3000 mL of a syrup having a specific gravity of 1.250 to obtain a product having a specific gravity of 1.310?
64. How many grams of sorbitol solution having a specific gravity of 1.285 and how many grams (milliliters) of water should be used in preparing 500 g of a sorbitol solution having a specific gravity of 1.225?

CALCQUIZ

15.A.[a] A pharmacist receives a special request from an ophthalmologist to prepare a fortified tobramycin ophthalmic solution. The available solution contains tobramycin, 3 mg/mL. How many milliliters of a tobramycin injection containing 40 mg/mL must be aseptically added to a 5-mL container of the ophthalmic solution to prepare one 0.5% in concentration?

15.B. How many milliliters of water must be added to 15 mL of a 23.4% solution of sodium chloride to dilute the concentration to 0.06 mEq/mL?

15.C.[a] A pharmacy receives a medication order for 1 L of a 3% sodium chloride injection. The pharmacy stocks 0.9% sodium chloride injection in 1-L bags and sodium chloride injection, 23.4% in 50-mL vials. How many milliliters of the latter should be added to the 1-L bag of normal saline solution to fill the order?

15.D. A 60-mL bottle of an oral solution contains a drug in a concentration of 15 mg/mL. A medication order requests that the drug concentration be reduced to 5 mg/mL by using three parts water to one part polyethylene glycol 400. How many milliliters of each of these two agents should be used?

15.E. How many milliliters of a 17% solution of benzalkonium chloride should a pharmacist use in preparing 120 mL of a prescription such that when a patient adds 15 mL of the dispensed medication to a gallon of water, as a foot soak, the resulting benzalkonium chloride concentration will be 1:5000?

[a]Problem courtesy of Flynn Warren, Bishop, GA.

ANSWERS TO "CASE IN POINT" AND PRACTICE PROBLEMS

Case in Point 15.1

Cefuroxime axetil present in original suspension:

$$100 \text{ mL} \times \frac{250 \text{ mg}}{5 \text{ mL}} = 5000 \text{ mg}$$

Cefuroxime axetil required in strengthened suspension:

$$100 \text{ mL} \times \frac{300 \text{ mg}}{5 \text{ mL}} = 6000 \text{ mg}$$

Cefuroxime axetil to add:

$$6000 \text{ mg} - 5000 \text{ mg} = 1000 \text{ mg}$$

Tablets required:

$$1000 \text{ mg} \times \frac{1 \text{ tablet}}{250 \text{ mg}} = 4 \text{ tablets}$$

A Second Look

There are a number of ways in which this problem could be addressed. One way would be to add another 250-mg pulverized tablet, calculate the volume of suspension that could be prepared at a concentration of 300 mg/5 mL, dispense 100 mL of that, and discard the remaining volume.

Cefuroxime axetil in strengthened suspension plus another tablet:

$$6000 \text{ mg} + 250 \text{ mg} = 6250\text{-mg cefuroxime axetil}$$

Volume of suspension that could be prepared at a concentration of 300 mg/5 mL:

$$\frac{5 \text{ mL}}{300 \text{ mg}} \times 6250 \text{ mg} = 104.17 \text{ mL}$$

Volume to dispense:

100 mL

Volume to discard:

4.17 mL

Proof: "If there are 6250 mg of cefuroxime axetil in 104.17 mL, how many milligrams would be present in each 5 mL?"

$$6250 \text{ mg} \times \frac{5 \text{ mL}}{104.17 \text{ mL}} = 299.99 \text{ or } 300 \text{ mg}$$

Case in Point 15.2

(a) 120 mL × 0.15 (1.5%) = 1.8 g
1.8 g = 1800 mg

$$1800 \text{ mg} \times \frac{1 \text{ mL}}{150 \text{ mg}} = 12 \text{ mL},$$

clindamycin phosphate sterile solution

(b) *If* the pharmacist had had clindamycin phosphate powder with which to fill the prescription, 1.8 g would have been used, and that quantity would have taken up a negligible volume on solution in the 52% v/v alcohol. Thus, the interpretation of the prescription is that the 120 mL (not 120 mL – 12 mL) of 52% v/v alcohol should be used.

120 mL × 0.52 (52% v/v) = 62.4 mL of solute (100% v/v alcohol)

$$\frac{62.4 \text{ mL}}{x \text{ mL}} = \frac{95 \text{ mL}}{100 \text{ mL}}; \ x = 65.68 \text{ mL } 95\% \text{ v/v alcohol}$$

(c) Due to contraction when alcohol and water are mixed, the volume of water cannot be determined by subtracting 65.68 mL from 120 mL; thus, a sufficient volume of water is used (q.s.) to make 120 mL.

Case in Point 15.3

15 g × 0.006 (0.6% w/w) = 0.09 g hydrocortisone
1% hydrocortisone cream = 1 g hydrocortisone/100 g

$$\text{Thus, } \frac{0.09 \text{ g}}{x \text{ g}} = \frac{1 \text{ g}}{100 \text{ g}};$$

x = 9 g hydrocortisone cream
15 g – 9 g = 6 g AQUAPHOR

NOTE: The problem also may be solved by alligation alternate.

Practice Problems

1. 550.6 gallons
2. 31.5% w/w
3. 4% w/v
4. 66 g polyethylene glycol ointment base
5. 0.87 g progesterone gel (8% w/w)
6. 985.67 mL
7. 3 g hydrocortisone cream (1% w/w)
   27 g cream base
8. 1000 mL water
9. 1:315 w/v
10. 1250 mL boric acid solution
11. 6694.4 mL water
12. 2 mL undecylenic acid
13. 6 bottles
14. 12 mL stock solution
15. 18.75 mL of the 2.0-molar solution
16. 0 mL diluent
17. 248 mL boric acid solution
18. 50 mL infusion
19. 0.76 molar
20. 1.25% w/w
21. 0.01 mL concentrate
22. 0.06% w/w
23. 4 mL cortisone acetate suspension
    4 mL normal saline solution

24. 28.2 mL stock solution
25. 0.42% hypericin
26. 20 mL lotion base
27. 1.46 mL lactic acid solution
28. 45 g bexarotene gel
    15 g gel base
29. 227 mg mupirocin powder
30. 45 mL memantine oral solution
    15 mL sorbitol solution
31. (a) 3.10% w/w
    (b) 1.98% w/w
32. 4 mL of each
33. 0.002% w/v
34. 1:20,000 w/v
35. 250 mL suspension base
36. 180 g white petrolatum
37. 3632 g benzocaine ointment, 2.5%
38. 4.787 g salicylic acid
39. 30 g ointment base
40. 1 g hydrocortisone acetate ointment, 2.5%
    9 g ophthalmic base
41. 946 mL syrup base
42. 1.667 g zinc oxide
43. 0.07% w/w
44. 0.011% w/v
45. 0.08 mL antigen, 0.2%
46. 100 mg sodium fluoride
47. (a) 24 mL corn oil
    6 mL cyclosporine solution
    (b) 10 mL corn oil
48. 0.09 mL gentamicin solution and 5.91 mL diluent
49. 9.17% w/v
50. 1% w/w pramoxine
    1.26% w/w hydrocortisone
51. 2450 mg diluent
52. 3:5
53. 3:17
54. (a) 2.5 mg/mL ibuprofen
    (b) 2.5% w/v ibuprofen
55. 60 mL chlorpromazine hydrochloride injection
    440 mL sodium chloride injection
56. 100 mL lidocaine hydrochloride injection
57. 495 mL sodium chloride injection
58. 0.16 mL amikacin injection and 0.84 mL normal saline solution
59. 2.33 mL sterile water for injection
60. 500 mg colchicine dilution
61. 0.947
62. 1031.38 mL propylene glycol
63. 4500 mL syrup
64. 394.737 g sorbitol solution
    105.263 mL water

References

1. Karolchyk S. Treating patients allergic to poison ivy. *International Journal of Pharmaceutical Compounding* 1998;2:421.
2. Prince SJ. Calculations. *International Journal of Pharmaceutical Compounding* 1998;2:310.
3. Prince SJ. Calculations. *International Journal of Pharmaceutical Compounding* 1998;2:453.
4. Prince SJ. Calculations. *International Journal of Pharmaceutical Compounding* 2000;4:393.
5. Prince SJ. Calculations. *International Journal of Pharmaceutical Compounding* 1999;3:145.

16

Reducing and Enlarging Formulas

OBJECTIVES

Upon successful completion of this chapter, the student will be able to:

- Perform calculations by various methods to reduce or enlarge formulas for pharmaceutical preparations.

Pharmacists may have to reduce or enlarge formulas for pharmaceutical preparations in the course of their professional practice or manufacturing activities. Formulas in the *United States Pharmacopeia–National Formulary* generally are based on the preparation of 1000 mL or 1000 g of product. Formulas from other sources may be based on other quantities.

The need to prepare different quantities of a pharmaceutical product depends on the nature of the practice. Whereas only small quantities may be required in a community pharmacy, modest quantities in a hospital pharmacy, and larger quantities in outsourcing facilities, very large quantities are prepared in the pharmaceutical manufacturing industry. In the latter case, hundreds of thousands of dosage units may be prepared in a single production batch.

The important criterion is that irrespective of the quantity prepared, the *correct proportion of one ingredient to the other* in a given formula must be maintained.

Methods to Reduce or Enlarge Formulas

As demonstrated below, the methods of *ratio and proportion*, *dimensional analysis*, and the *factor method* may be used to reduce or enlarge a pharmaceutical formula. For many, the *factor method* is the simplest to use.

Example Calculations

From the following standard formula for Calamine Compounded Topical Suspension, USP,[1] *calculate the quantity of each ingredient required to prepare 240 mL of product.*

Calamine	80 g
Zinc oxide	80 g
Glycerin	20 mL
Bentonite magma	250 mL
Calcium hydroxide	
Topical solution, qs ad	1000 mL

SOLVING BY *RATIO AND PROPORTION:*

$$\frac{80\text{ g}}{1000\text{ mL}} = \frac{\text{x g}}{240\text{ mL}};\ \text{x} = \mathbf{19.2\ g,\ calamine}$$

$$\frac{80\text{ g}}{1000\text{ mL}} = \frac{\text{x g}}{240\text{ mL}};\ \text{x} = \mathbf{19.2\ g,\ zinc\ oxide}$$

$$\frac{20\text{ mL}}{1000\text{ mL}} = \frac{\text{x mL}}{240\text{ mL}};\ \text{x} = \mathbf{4.8\ mL,\ glycerin}$$

$$\frac{250\text{ mL}}{1000\text{ mL}} = \frac{\text{x mL}}{240\text{ mL}};\ \text{x} = \mathbf{60\ mL,\ bentonite\ magma}$$

and calcium hydroxide topical solution, to make **240 mL**

SOLVING BY *DIMENSIONAL ANALYSIS:*

$$240\text{ mL} \times \frac{80\text{ g}}{1000\text{ mL}} = \mathbf{19.2\ g\ calamine}$$

and so forth for each ingredient, arriving at the same answers as shown above.

SOLVING BY THE *FACTOR METHOD:*

The *factor method* is based on the *relative quantity* of the total formula to be prepared. For instance, in the problem example, 240 mL of a 1000-mL standard formula are to be prepared. The *factor* is derived as follows:

$$\frac{240\text{ mL (to be prepared)}}{1000\text{ mL (standard formula)}} = 0.24\text{ (factor)}$$

Then, by multiplying the quantity of *each ingredient* in the standard formula by the factor, the correct quantity of that ingredient is determined. Thus,

80 g × 0.24 = **19.2 g calamine**, and so forth for each ingredient, arriving at the same answers as shown above.

(1) *From the following formula for artificial tears,*[2] *calculate the quantity of each ingredient required to prepare a dozen 30-mL containers.*

Polyvinyl alcohol	1.4 g
Povidone	0.6 g
Chlorobutanol	0.5 g
Sterile sodium chloride solution 0.9%, ad	100 mL

$$30\text{ mL} \times 12 = 360\text{ mL}$$

$$\frac{360\text{ mL}}{100\text{ mL}} = 3.6\text{ (factor)}$$

Using the factor *3.6*, the quantity of each ingredient is calculated:

Polyvinyl alcohol	= 1.4 g × 3.6 = **5.04 g**
Povidone	= 0.6 g × 3.6 = **2.16 g**
Chlorobutanol	= 0.5 g × 3.6 = **1.8 g**

Sterile sodium chloride solution 0.9%, ad **360 mL**

(2) *From the following formula for an estradiol vaginal gel,*[3] *calculate the quantity of each ingredient required to prepare 1 lb of gel.*

Estradiol	200 g
Polysorbate 80	1 g
Methylcellulose Gel, 2%	95 g

$$1 \text{ lb} = 454 \text{ g}$$

$$\text{Formula weight} = 200 \text{ g} + 1 \text{ g} + 95 \text{ g} = 296 \text{ g}$$

$$\frac{454 \text{ g}}{296 \text{ g}} = 1.534 \text{ (factor)}$$

Using the factor *1.534*, the quantity of each ingredient is calculated:

Estradiol	$= 200 \text{ g} \times 1.534 =$ **306.8 g**
Polysorbate 80	$= 1 \text{ g} \times 1.534 =$ **1.534 g**
Methylcellulose Gel, 2%	$= 95 \text{ g} \times 1.534 =$ **145.73 g**

(3) *From the following formula for a dexamethasone ophthalmic ointment,*[4] *calculate the quantity of each ingredient needed to prepare 7.5 g of ointment.*

Dexamethasone sodium phosphate	55 mg
Lanolin, anhydrous	5 g
Mineral oil	10 g
White petrolatum, ad	100 g

$$\frac{7.5 \text{ g}}{100 \text{ g}} = 0.075 \text{ (factor)}$$

Using the factor *0.075*, the quantity of each ingredient is calculated:

Dexamethasone sodium phosphate	$= 55 \text{ mg} \times 0.075 =$ **4.125 mg**
Lanolin, anhydrous	$= 5 \text{ g} \times 0.075 =$ **0.375 g**
Mineral oil	$= 10 \text{ g} \times 0.075 =$ **0.75 g**
White petrolatum, ad	**7.5 g**

Formulas That Specify Proportional Parts

On a rare occasion, a pharmacist may encounter an old formula that indicates the ingredients in "parts" rather than in measures of weight or volume. The parts indicate the relative proportion of each of the ingredients in the formula. A formula for solid or semisolid ingredients may be considered in terms of *grams*, whereas a formula of liquids may be considered in terms of *milliliters*.

Example Calculation of a Formula Expressed in Parts

From the following formula, calculate the quantity of each ingredient required to make 1000 g of the ointment.

Coal tar	5 parts
Zinc oxide	10 parts
Hydrophilic ointment	50 parts

Total number of parts (by weight) = 65
1000 g will contain 65 parts

$$\frac{65 \text{ (parts)}}{5 \text{ (parts)}} = \frac{1000 \text{ (g)}}{x \text{ (g)}}$$

$$x = \mathbf{76.92\ g\ of\ Coal\ Tar}$$

and

$$\frac{65 \text{ (parts)}}{10 \text{ (parts)}} = \frac{1000 \text{ (g)}}{y \text{ (g)}}$$

$$y = \mathbf{153.85\ g\ of\ Zinc\ Oxide}$$

and

$$\frac{65 \text{ (parts)}}{50 \text{ (parts)}} = \frac{1000 \text{ (g)}}{z \text{ (g)}}$$

$$z = \mathbf{769.23\ g\ of\ Hydrophilic\ Ointment}$$

(Check total: 1000 g)

An alternative method at solution would be to determine that there are 15.385 g per part (1000 g/65 parts) and thus

Coal tar: 5 parts × 15.385	= **76.92 g**
Zinc oxide: 10 parts × 15.385 g/part	= **153.85 g**
Hydrophilic ointment: 50 parts × 15.385	= **769.25 g**

PRACTICE PROBLEMS

1. From the following formula for 40 sertraline hydrochloride capsules,[5] calculate the quantity of each ingredient needed to prepare 250 such capsules.

Sertraline hydrochloride	300 mg
Silica gel	6 g
Calcium citrate	4 g

2. From the following formula for a progesterone nasal spray,[6] calculate the quantity of each ingredient needed to prepare twenty-four 15-mL containers of the spray.

Progesterone	20 mg
Dimethyl-β-cyclodextrin	62 mg
Purified water, ad	1 mL

3. From the following formula, calculate the quantities required to make 5 lb of hydrophilic ointment.

Methylparaben	0.25 g
Propylparaben	0.15 g
Sodium lauryl sulfate	10 g
Propylene glycol	120 g
Stearyl alcohol	250 g
White petrolatum	250 g
Purified water, ad	1000 g

4. The formula, by weight, for a tube of an ophthalmic ointment is as follows:

Sulfacetamide sodium	10%
Prednisolone acetate	0.2%
Phenylmercuric acetate	0.0008%
Mineral oil	1%
White petrolatum, ad	3.5 g

How much of each ingredient would be needed to manufacture 2000 such tubes of ointment?

5. Calculate the quantity of each ingredient needed to prepare 15 mL of the following ophthalmic solution.[7]

Erythromycin lactobionate	500 mg
Dexamethasone sodium phosphate	100 mg
Glycerin	2.5 mL
Sterile water for injection, ad	100 mL

6. According to the literature, the biotechnology product pegfilgrastim (NEULASTA) contains the following in 0.6 mL pre-filled syringes[8]:

Pegfilgrastim	6 mg
Sorbitol	30 mg
Polysorbate 20	0.02 mg
Water for injection, ad	0.6 mL

How much of the first three ingredients would be needed to manufacture 100,000 such syringes?

7. From the following formula, calculate the quantity of each ingredient required to make 1500 g of the powder.

Calcium carbonate	5 parts
Magnesium oxide	1 part
Sodium bicarbonate	4 parts
Bismuth subcarbonate	3 parts

8. The following is a formula for 100 triple estrogen capsules.[9] Calculate the quantities of the first three ingredients, in grams, and the last two ingredients, in kilograms, required to prepare 5000 such capsules.

Estriol	200 mg
Estrone	25 mg
Estradiol	25 mg
Polyethylene glycol 1450	20 g
Polyethylene glycol 3350	20 g

9. The formula for a ciprofloxacin otic drop is given in the literature as follows[10]:

Ciprofloxacin	1 g
Propylene glycol	50 mL
Glycerin, ad	100 mL

How many grams of ciprofloxacin would be required to prepare two hundred 15-mL bottles of the ear drop?

10. The formula for a sports rub cream is given in the literature as follows[11]:

Methyl salicylate	15 mL
Menthol	10 g
Eucalyptus oil	1 g
Hydrophilic ointment, ad	100 g

If the specific gravity of methyl salicylate is 1.18, how many grams of each ingredient would be needed to prepare a dozen 30-g tubes of ointment?

CALCQUIZ

16.A. An ophthalmic solution has the following formula[12]:

Tobramycin sulfate	300 mg
Diclofenac sodium	100 mg
Sodium chloride	806 mg
Sterile water for injection, ad	100 mL

Calculate the quantities of each ingredient required to prepare twenty-four 7.5-mL containers of the ophthalmic solution.

16.B. The formula for "Lubow's Solution" is as follows[13]:

Progesterone	1 g
Hydrocortisone	500 mg
Propylene glycol	2 g
Ethanol (95%) ad	100 mL

(a) Calculate the quantities of each ingredient required to prepare 2.5 mL of solution.
(b) How many milliliters of propylene glycol (sp. gr. 1.04) are needed to prepare a liter of the formula?

16.C. An ophthalmic solution for veterinary use has the following formula[14]:

Miconazole	1 g
PEG 40 castor oil	1.5 mL
Lactic acid 88% solution	0.4 mL
Sterile water for injection qs ad	100 mL

(a) Calculate the quantities of each ingredient required to prepare twelve 1.5-mL drop-containers of the medication.
(b) If the PEG 40 castor oil has a specific gravity of 1.1, calculate the grams present in (a).
(c) Calculate the quantity, in milliliters, of pure (100%) lactic acid in the formula.

16.D. A vial for injection contains 0.6 mL of solution. The dose is 0.5 mL, which contains 7.5 mg of drug. How many grams of drug is needed to manufacture 5000 vials of the product?

ANSWERS TO PRACTICE PROBLEMS

1. 1.875 g sertraline hydrochloride
   37.5 g silica gel
   25 g calcium citrate
2. 7.2 g progesterone
   22.32 g dimethyl-β-cyclodextrin
   ad 360 mL, purified water
3. 0.568 g methylparaben
   0.341 g propylparaben
   22.7 g sodium lauryl sulfate
   272.4 g propylene glycol
   567.5 g stearyl alcohol
   567.5 g white petrolatum
   ad 2270 g or 5 lb purified water
4. 700 g sulfacetamide sodium
   14 g prednisolone acetate
   56 mg phenyl mercuric acetate
   70 g mineral oil
   6215.944 g white petrolatum
5. 75 mg erythromycin lactobionate
   15 mg dexamethasone sodium phosphate
   0.375 mL glycerin
   qs ad 15 mL sterile water for injection
6. 600 g pegfilgrastim
   3000 g sorbitol
   2 g polysorbate 20
7. 576.923 g calcium carbonate
   115.385 g magnesium oxide
   461.539 g sodium bicarbonate
   346.154 g bismuth subcarbonate
8. 10 g estriol
   1.25 g estrone
   1.25 g estradiol
   1 kg polyethylene glycol 1450
   1 kg polyethylene glycol 3350
9. 30 g ciprofloxacin
10. 63.72 g methyl salicylate
    36 g menthol
    3.6 g eucalyptus oil
    256.68 g hydrophilic ointment

References

1. *USP–NF Monographs for Compounded Preparations*. Rockville, MD: United States Pharmacopeial Convention, 2014. Available at: http://www.usp.org/usp-healthcare-professionals/compounding/compounding-monographs/usp-nf-monographs-compounded-preparations. Accessed September 13, 2014.
2. Allen LV Jr. Artificial tears for dry eyes. *International Journal of Pharmaceutical Compounding* 2000;4:376.
3. Allen LV Jr. Estradiol vaginal gel (0.2%). *International Journal of Pharmaceutical Compounding* 1998;2:51.
4. Allen LV Jr. Dexamethasone phosphate 0.05% ophthalmic ointment. *International Journal of Pharmaceutical Compounding* 2003;7:215.
5. Allen LV Jr. Sertraline 7.5-mg capsules. *International Journal of Pharmaceutical Compounding* 1998;2:443.
6. Allen LV Jr. Progesterone nasal spray (2%). *International Journal of Pharmaceutical Compounding* 1998;2:56.
7. Allen LV Jr. Erythromycin and dexamethasone ophthalmic solution. *International Journal of Pharmaceutical Compounding* 2002;6:452.
8. NEULASTA (pegfilgrastim). *Product Literature*. Thousand Oaks, CA: Amgen, Inc., 2011.
9. Allen LV Jr. Triple estrogen 2.5-mg semisolid-filled hard-gelatin capsules. *International Journal of Pharmaceutical Compounding* 1997;1:187.
10. Allen LV Jr. Ciprofloxacin 1% otic drops. *International Journal of Pharmaceutical Compounding* 2002;8:47.
11. Allen LV Jr. Compounding for sports injuries. Available at: http://www.ijpc.com/rxtriad/pdf/RxTriad_V10_N08_Sample.pdf. Accessed October 31, 2015.
12. Allen LV Jr. Tobramycin sulfate 0.3% and diclofenac sodium 0.1% ophthalmic solution. *International Journal of Pharmaceutical Compounding* 2010;14:74.
13. Allen LV Jr. Lubow's solution. *International Journal of Pharmaceutical Compounding* 2009;13:558.
14. Allen LV Jr. Miconazole 1% ophthalmic solution, veterinary. *International Journal of Pharmaceutical Compounding* 2009;13:559.

17

Selected Calculations in Contemporary Compounding

OBJECTIVES

Upon successful completion of this chapter, the student will be able to:

- Differentiate between traditional in-pharmacy compounding and compounding in outsourcing facilities.
- Perform calculations for the constitution of dry powders for oral solution or suspension.
- Perform calculations for the constitution of dry powders for parenteral use.
- Perform calculations for the use of prefabricated dosage forms in compounding procedures.
- Perform calculations applied to the filling of capsules.
- Perform calculation applied to the preparation of suppositories by molding.
- Perform calculations applicable to specialized formulas and their methods of preparation.

Traditional pharmaceutical compounding is the process by which pharmacists combine therapeutically active ingredients with pharmaceutical materials in the preparation of *customized* prescriptions and medication orders to meet the specific needs of *individual patients*. This is in contrast to compounding, which occurs in ***outsourcing facilities*** in which large volumes of product are compounded, *without individual prescriptions or medication orders*, for distribution to inpatient and outpatient pharmacies. Differentiated further is ***pharmaceutical manufacturing,*** which is the large-scale production of pharmaceutical products by the pharmaceutical research and manufacturing industry.

The *Authors' Extra Point* at the end of this chapter encapsulates the regulation of pharmacy compounding under the federal Drug Quality and Security Act of 2013.[1] This section also provides a listing of the USP-NF chapters relevant to the compounding of both sterile and nonsterile products.[2]

Compounding is an activity for which pharmacists are uniquely qualified by virtue of their education, training, and experience. Many pharmacists have developed *specialized practices* in compounding in order to provide customized medications for their patients. In support of these practices, a Pharmacy Compounding Accreditation Board and a number of pharmacy compounding associations and organizations have been established.[a]

[a]The Pharmacy Compounding Accreditation Board (http://www.pcab.org/) develops and maintains standards to improve the quality of pharmacy compounding; other pharmacy compounding organizations include Professional Compounding Centers of America (http://www.pccarx.com/), Association of Compounding Pharmacists of Canada (http://acpcrx.org/), and the International Academy of Compounding Pharmacists (http://www.iacprx.org/).

The Need for Compounding

Compounded prescriptions and medication orders may be desired for a number of reasons, including[3,4]:

- The need to adjust the strength or dose of a commercially available product to meet the specific requirements of a patient (e.g., a pediatric patient)
- The need to provide a product more organoleptically acceptable (e.g., taste) to a pediatric or veterinary patient
- The need to prepare a different dosage form (e.g., a liquid) than the commercially available product (e.g., a tablet) to meet the requirements of a patient unable to swallow the existing dosage form (e.g., a pediatric or elderly patient)
- The need to prepare a dosage form free of an agent (e.g., sugar, preservatives) in the commercially available product that cannot be tolerated by a patient
- The need to provide a patient with a specifically designed formulation of an approved drug or drug combination, which is unavailable as a commercial product

Constitution of Dry Powders

Constitution of Dry Powders for Oral Solution or Suspension

Some drugs, most notably antibiotics, lose their potency in a relatively short period when prepared in a liquid dosage form. To enhance the shelf-life of these drugs, manufacturers provide products to the pharmacy in dry powder form for *constitution* (or *reconstitution*) with purified water or special diluent at the time a prescription or medication order is received. Depending on the product, the dry powder may be stable for about 24 months. After constitution, the resultant solution or suspension is stable in the quantities usually dispensed for the treatment period.

Dry powders for constitution are packaged in self-contained bottles of sufficient size to accommodate the addition of the required volume of diluent (Fig. 17.1). In addition to the quantitative amount of therapeutic agent, the powder contains such pharmaceutical ingredients as solubilizing or suspending agents, stabilizers, colorants, sweeteners, and flavorants.

On receipt of a prescription order, the pharmacist follows the label instructions for constitution, adding the proper amount of purified water or other diluent to prepare the liquid form. Figure 17.2 presents an example of such a label. Depending on the product's formulation, constitution results in the preparation of a clear *solution* (often called a *syrup*) or a *suspension*. The final volume of product is the sum of the volume of solvent or diluent added and the volume occupied by the dissolved or suspended powder mixture. These products generally are intended for infants and children but also can be used by adults who have difficulty swallowing counterpart solid dosage form products.

Manufacturer's products generally are formulated to provide the usual dose by teaspoon or calibrated dropper. Pharmacists may customize products for individual patients, as demonstrated by the calculations that follow.

Example Calculations for the Constitution of Dry Powders for Oral Use

(1) *The label for a dry powder package of cefprozil (CEFZIL) for oral suspension directs the pharmacist to add 72 mL of purified water to prepare 100 mL of suspension. If the package contains 2.5 g of cefprozil, how many milligrams of the drug would be contained in each teaspoonful dose of the constituted suspension?*

$$2.5 \text{ g} = 2500 \text{ mg}$$

$$\frac{2500 \text{ mg}}{100 \text{ mL}} = \frac{\text{x mg}}{5 \text{ mL}}$$

$$\text{x} = \mathbf{125\ mg\ cefprozil}$$

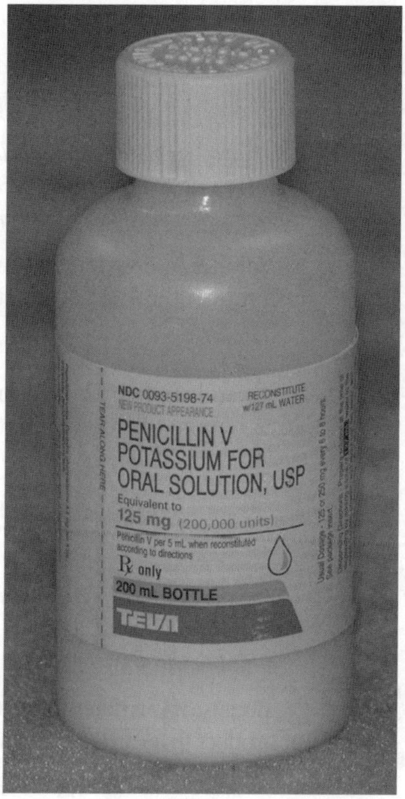

FIGURE 17.1 • Example of a dry powder for reconstitution to prepare an oral solution. The label calls for the addition of 127 mL of water to prepare 200 mL of solution having a concentration of 125 mg or 200,000 units of penicillin V per 5 mL of solution.

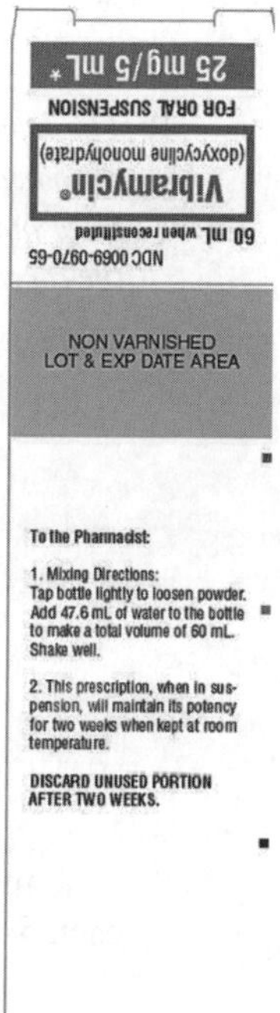

FIGURE 17.2 • Outer carton panel indicating the mixing directions for the pharmacist in the reconstitution of an oral suspension. *(Courtesy of Pfizer, Inc. Source: http://dailymed.nlm.nih.gov/dailymed/index.cfm.)*

Or solving by dimensional analysis:

$$\frac{1000\text{ mg}}{1\text{ g}} \times \frac{5\text{ mL}}{1\text{ tsp}} \times \frac{2.5\text{ g}}{100\text{ mL}} = \mathbf{125\text{ mg cefprozil}}$$

(2) *Label instructions for an ampicillin product call for the addition of 78 mL of water to make 100 mL of constituted suspension such that each 5 mL contains 125 mg of ampicillin. Calculate the volume represented by the suspended powder in the product and the total content of ampicillin.*

Volume of powder: Because the addition of 78 mL of water results in the preparation of 100 mL of product, the volume occupied by the powder is:

$$100\text{ mL} - 78\text{ mL} = \mathbf{22\text{ mL}}$$

Total drug (ampicillin) present: If, in the constituted product, each 5 mL contains 125 mg of ampicillin, the total amount of ampicillin in the 100-mL product is:

$$\frac{5\text{ mL}}{125\text{ mg}} = \frac{100\text{ mL}}{\text{x}}$$

$$\text{x} = \mathbf{2500\text{ mg}}$$

(3) *Using the product in the previous example, if a physician desires an ampicillin concentration of 100 mg/5 mL (rather than 125 mg/5 mL), how many milliliters of water should be added to the dry powder?*

Because it was determined that 2500 mg of ampicillin is in the dry product, the volume of product that can be made with a concentration of 100 mg/5 mL may be calculated by:

$$\frac{2500\text{ mg}}{\text{x mL}} = \frac{100\text{ mg}}{5\text{ mL}} \quad \text{x} = \mathbf{125\text{ mL}}$$

Then, because it had been determined that the dry powder occupies 22 mL of volume, it is possible to determine the amount of water to add:

$$125\text{ mL} - 22\text{ mL} = \mathbf{103\text{ mL}}$$

(4) *The label of a dry powder for oral suspension states that when 111 mL of water is added to the powder, 150 mL of a suspension containing 250 mg of ampicillin per 5 mL is prepared. How many milliliters of purified water should be used to prepare, in each 5 mL of product, the correct dose of ampicillin for a 60-lb child based on the dose of 8 mg/kg of body weight?*

The dose of ampicillin may be determined by:

$$\frac{8\text{ mg}}{2.2\text{ lb}} = \frac{\text{x mg}}{60\text{ lb}}$$

$$\text{x} = 218\text{ mg}$$

Then, the amount of ampicillin in the container is determined by:

$$\frac{250\text{ mg}}{5\text{ mL}} = \frac{\text{x mg}}{150\text{ mL}}$$

$$\text{x} = 7500\text{ mg}$$

Thus, the amount of product that can be made from 7500 mg of drug such that each 5 mL contains 218 mg of drug may be found by:

$$\frac{218\text{ mg}}{5\text{ mL}} = \frac{7500\text{ mg}}{\text{x mL}}$$

$$\text{x} = 172\text{ mL}$$

Finally, because the volume of powder occupies 39 mL (150 mL – 111 mL), the amount of water to add is determined by:

$$172 \text{ mL} - 39 \text{ mL} = \mathbf{133 \text{ mL}}$$

(5) *The label of a dry powder for constitution into pediatric drops states that when 12 mL of purified water is added to the powder, 15 mL of a pediatric suspension containing 50 mg of amoxicillin per milliliter results. How many milliliters of water should be added to prepare the dose of amoxicillin in each 10 drops if the dropper delivers 20 drops/mL, the child has a body surface area (BSA) of 0.4 m², and the dose of the drug is based on 50 mg/m² of* BSA?

The dose of amoxicillin may be determined by:

$$\frac{50 \text{ mg}}{1 \text{ m}^2 \text{ BSA}} = \frac{\text{x mg}}{0.4 \text{ m}^2 \text{ BSA}}$$
$$\text{x} = 20 \text{ mg}$$

The volume of product to contain the 20-mg dose is determined by:

$$\frac{10 \text{ drops}}{\text{x mL}} = \frac{20 \text{ drops}}{1 \text{ mL}}$$
$$\text{x} = 0.5 \text{ mL}$$

The amount of amoxicillin in the package is determined by:

$$\frac{50 \text{ mg}}{1 \text{ mL}} = \frac{\text{x mg}}{15 \text{ mL}}$$
$$\text{x} = 750 \text{ mg}$$

The amount of product of the desired dose that may be prepared is determined by:

$$\frac{750 \text{ mg}}{\text{x mL}} = \frac{20 \text{ mg}}{0.5 \text{ mL}}$$
$$\text{x} = 18.75 \text{ mL}$$

Subtracting the volume accounted for by the dry powder (15 mL – 12 mL = 3 mL), the volume of water to add is determined by:

$$18.75 \text{ mL} - 3 \text{ mL} = \mathbf{15.75 \text{ mL}}$$

CASE IN POINT 17.1[a] A pediatrician telephones a pharmacist asking that the concentration of an antibiotic suspension be changed. The pediatrician wants the child–patient to take 200 mg of amoxicillin per teaspoonful dose. The label for amoxicillin powder for oral suspension indicates that the addition of 68 mL of purified water will result in a final volume of 100 mL with a concentration of 250 mg amoxicillin per 5 mL of suspension.

How many milliliters of water should the pharmacist add to the amoxicillin powder to produce a concentration of 200 mg/teaspoonful?

[a]Problem courtesy of Flynn Warren, Bishop, GA.

Constitution of Dry Powders for Parenteral Solution

Some medications intended for injection are provided as dry powder in vials to be constituted with sterile water for injection or other designated solvent or diluent immediately before use. Generally, these medications are small-volume products intended for use by injection or as additives to large-volume parenterals.

In contrast to the dry powders intended for oral use after constitution, injectable products may contain only limited amounts of specified added ingredients to increase the stability and effectiveness of the drug (obviously, no colorants, flavorants, or sweeteners are added). So, in effect, the bulk volume of the dry contents of a vial is largely or entirely the medication.

If the quantity of the dry drug powder is small and does not contribute significantly to the final volume of the constituted solution, the volume of solvent used will approximate the final volume of solution. For example, if 1000 units of a certain antibiotic in dry form is to be dissolved, and if the powder does not account for any significant portion of the final volume, the addition of 5 mL of solvent will produce a solution containing 200 units/mL. If the dry powder, however, because of its bulk, contributes to the final volume of the constituted solution, the increase in volume produced by the drug must be considered, and this factor must then be used in calculating the amount of solvent needed to prepare a solution of a desired concentration. For example, the package directions for making injectable solutions of piperacillin sodium specify that 4 mL of sterile solvent should be added to 2 g of the dry powder to produce 5 mL of a solution that is to contain 400 mg/mL. The drug, in this case, accounts for 1 mL of the final volume.

Example Calculations for the Constitution of Dry Powders for Parenteral Use

(1) *When a vial containing 3.5 mg of a sterile powder of the monoclonal antibody bortezomib (VELCADE) is reconstituted with 3.5 mL of 0.9% sodium chloride injection, a drug concentration of 1 mg/mL results. Calculate the volume of injection occupied by the bortezomib powder.*

1 mg/mL is equivalent to 3.5 mg/3.5 mL; thus, the volume occupied by bortezomib may be considered negligible.

(2) *When a vial is reconstituted to a volume of 1.2 mL with sterile water for injection, the resulting solution contains 20 mg/mL of drug. Calculate the drug content of the vial.*

$$\frac{20\text{ mg}}{1\text{ mL}} = \frac{\text{x mg}}{1.2\text{ mL}}; \text{ x} = \mathbf{24\text{ mg}}$$

(3) *Label instructions for the reconstitution of a 500-mg vial of ceftazidime for intramuscular injection (FORTAZ) call for the addition of 1.5 mL of diluent to prepare 1.8 mL of injection. Calculate (a) the volume occupied by the dry drug; (b) the concentration of ceftazidime in the injection, in mg/mL; and (c) the volume of injection to provide a dose of 250 mg of ceftazidime.*

(a) 1.8 mL − 1.5 mL = **0.3 mL**, volume of ceftazidime
(b) 500 mg/1.8 mL = **277.8 mg/mL**
(c) 250 mg × 1.8 mL/500 mg = **0.9 mL**

(4) *Using a vial containing 200,000 units of penicillin G potassium, how many milliliters of solvent should be added to the dry powder in preparing a solution having a concentration of 25,000 units/mL?*

$$\frac{25{,}000\ (\text{units})}{200{,}000\ (\text{units})} = \frac{1\ (\text{mL})}{x\ (\text{mL})}$$

$$x = \mathbf{8\ mL}$$

(5) *Using a vial containing 200,000 units of penicillin G sodium and sodium chloride injection as the solvent, explain how you would obtain the penicillin G sodium needed in preparing the following prescription.*

℞	Penicillin G sodium		15,000 units/mL
	Sodium chloride injection	ad	10 mL
	Sig. for IM injection		

15,000 units × 10 = 150,000 units of penicillin G sodium needed

Because the dry powder represents 200,000 units of penicillin G sodium or $^4/_3$ *times* the number of units desired, ¾ of the powder will contain the required number of units.

Step 1. Dissolve the dry powder in 4 mL of sodium chloride injection.

Step 2. Use **3 mL** of the constituted solution.

Or solving by dimensional analysis:

$$10\ \text{mL} \times \frac{15{,}000\ \text{units}}{1\ \text{mL}} \times \frac{4\ \text{mL}}{200{,}000\ \text{units}} = \mathbf{3\ mL}$$

(6) *The package information enclosed with a vial containing 5,000,000 units of penicillin G potassium (buffered) specifies that when 23 mL of a sterile solvent is added to the dry powder, the resulting concentration is 200,000 units/mL. On the basis of this information, how many milliliters of sterile water for injection should be used in preparing the following solution?*

℞	Penicillin G potassium (buffered)	5,000,000 units
	Sterile water for injection	q.s.
	Make solution containing 500,000 units/mL	
	Sig. one mL = 500,000 units of penicillin G potassium	

The package information states that the constituted solution prepared by dissolving 5,000,000 units of the dry powder in 23 mL of sterile solvent has a final volume of 25 mL. The dry powder, then, accounts for 2 mL of this volume.

Step 1. The final volume of the prescription is determined as follows:

$$\frac{500{,}000\ (\text{units})}{5{,}000{,}000\ (\text{units})} = \frac{1\ (\text{mL})}{x\ (\text{mL})}$$

$$x = \mathbf{10\ mL}$$

Step 2. 10 mL – 2 mL (dry powder accounts for this volume) = **8 mL.**

(7) *Piperacillin sodium is available in 2-gram vials, and the dry powder accounts for 1 mL of the volume of the constituted solution. Using a 2-gram vial of piperacillin sodium and sodium chloride injection as the solvent, explain how you could fill the following medication order:*

Piperacillin sodium		250 mg
Sodium chloride injection	ad	15 mL

Step 1. Dissolve the 2 g of dry powder in 9 mL of sodium chloride injection to prepare 10 mL of solution. Each milliliter will contain 200 mg of piperacillin sodium.

Step 2. Use 1.25 mL of the constituted solution and 13.75 mL of sodium chloride injection.

CASE IN POINT 17.2 A hospital pharmacist received the following order for a patient[5]:

Medication Order: Staphcillin, 750 mg IV every 4 hours

The following product and procedures were followed:

Product: 6-g vial Staphcillin

Pharmacy Operations: Reconstitute vial with sterile water for injection to yield Staphcillin, 500 mg/mL. For the infusion, add the calculated dose to 100 mL of sodium chloride injection.

Administer: 30-minute IV infusion.

(a) How many milliliters of solution from the reconstituted solution (vial) should be added to the sodium chloride injection for the infusion?

(b) What should be the infusion rate in milliliters per hour?

(c) With a drop factor of 10 drops per milliliter, calculate the infusion rate in drops per minute.

Use of Prefabricated Dosage Forms in Compounding

Pharmacists frequently find that bulk supplies of certain proprietary drug substances are not available for extemporaneous compounding and that prefabricated tablets, capsules, injections, and other dosage forms provide the only available source of the medicinal agents needed.

When using commercially prepared dosage forms as the source of a medicinal agent, the pharmacist selects products that are of the most simple, economic, and convenient form. For example, uncoated tablets or capsules are preferred over coated tablets or sustained-release dosage forms. For both convenience and economy, use of the fewest dosage units is preferred, for example, five 100-mg tablets rather than one hundred 5-mg tablets. An injection often provides a convenient source of medicinal agent when the volume of injection required is small and it is compatible with the physical characteristics of the dosage form being prepared (e.g., an oral liquid).

Occasionally, when of the prescribed strength, small whole tablets or broken *scored* (grooved) tablets may be placed within capsule shells when capsules are prescribed. In most instances, however, tablets are crushed in a mortar and reduced to a powder. When capsules are used as the drug source, the capsule shells are opened and their powdered contents are expelled. The correct quantity of powder is then used to fill the prescription or medication order.

It is important to understand that in addition to the medicinal agent, most solid dosage forms contain additional materials, such as fillers, binders, and disintegrants. These ingredients may need to be considered in the required calculations. For example, a tablet labeled to contain 10 mg of a drug may actually weigh 200 mg or more because of the added ingredients. Calculations involved in the use of injections generally are simplified because injections are labeled according to quantity of drug per unit volume, for example, milligrams per milliliter (mg/mL).

A factor to consider when using manufacturer's dosage forms in compounding is the uncertainty of the *precise* content of active therapeutic agent. This is because there are legally allowable variances that, in some cases, may be 90% to 110% of labeled drug content. Thus, whenever possible, use of the bulk chemical in compounding procedure provides better assurance of drug content.

Example Calculations for the Use of Prefabricated Dosage Forms in Compounding

(1) *Only capsules, each containing 25 mg of indomethacin, are available. How many capsules should be used to obtain the amount of indomethacin needed in preparing the following prescription?*

℞	Indomethacin		2 mg/mL
	Cherry syrup	ad	150 mL
	Sig. 5 mL b.i.d.		

Because 2 mg/mL of indomethacin is prescribed, 300 mg is needed in preparing the prescription. Given that each capsule contains 25 mg of indomethacin, then 300 (mg) ÷ 25 (mg) = **12 capsules** are needed.

(2) *The drug metoprolol tartrate (LOPRESSOR) is available as 50-mg tablets. Before preparing the following prescription, a pharmacist determined that each tablet weighed 120 mg. Explain how to obtain the proper quantity of LOPRESSOR.*

℞	LOPRESSOR		15 mg
	Lactose, qs	ad	300 mg
	Prepare 24 such capsules.		
	Sig. one cap. 2 × a day		

15 (mg) × 24 = 360 mg of LOPRESSOR needed
Crush 8 tablets, which contain:
400 mg (8 × 50 mg) of LOPRESSOR
960 mg (8 × 120 mg) of total powder

$$\frac{400 \text{ mg LOPRESSOR}}{360 \text{ mg LOPRESSOR}} = \frac{960 \text{ mg total}}{x \text{ mg total}}$$

x = **864 mg** quantity of powder to use

(3) *How many milliliters of an injection containing 40 mg of triamcinolone per milliliter may be used in preparing the following prescription?*

℞	Triamcinolone		0.05%
	Ointment base	ad	120 g
	Sig. apply to affected area		

120 g × 0.0005 = 0.06 g = 60 mg triamcinolone needed

$$\frac{40 \text{ mg}}{60 \text{ mg}} = \frac{1 \text{ mL}}{x \text{ mL}}$$

x = **1.5 mL**

(4) *A pharmacist receives the following prescription*[a]:

℞	Diazepam	0.75 mg
	Ft. charts #30	

In filling the prescription, the pharmacist chooses to use 10-mg unscored diazepam tablets.

(a) How many tablets must be used?
(b) If the tablets in answer (a) are powdered and weigh a total of 345 mg, how many milligrams of the powder would provide the diazepam required?
(c) If the desired total weight for the contents of each divided powder is 250 mg, how much lactose should be used as diluent?

---

[a]Problem courtesy of Deborah Elder, Pharmaceutical and Biomedical Sciences, College of Pharmacy, The University of Georgia, Athens, GA.

Calculations:

(a) 0.75 mg × 30 = 22.5 mg diazepam required.
22.5 mg/10 mg per tablet = 2.25 tablets, so **3 tablets** must be used.

(b) $345 \text{ mg} \times \frac{2.25 \text{ tablets}}{3 \text{ tablets}} = \mathbf{258.75\ mg}$

(c) 250 mg × 30 = 7500 mg (total weight) – 258.75 mg (tablet powder weight) = **7241.25 mg lactose**

(5) *A pharmacist receives the following prescription*[b]:

℞ Baby Stephanie Jones (22 lb)
Reserpine liquid: 0.1 mg/mL
Dispense: 60 mL
Sig: 0.01 mg/kg/b.i.d.

In filling the prescription, the pharmacist chooses to use 0.25-mg reserpine tablets.

(a) How many reserpine tablets are required to compound the prescription?
(b) What volume of reserpine liquid will be required per dose?
(c) Using a calibrated dropper that delivers 12 drops/0.5 mL, how many drops would constitute a single dose?
(d) If the medication is taken as directed, how many days will the medication last?

Calculations:

(a) 0.1 mg/mL × 60 mL = 6 mg of reserpine required.
6 mg/0.25 mg per tablet = **24 tablets**

(b) 22 1b/2.2 lb/kg = 10 kg
0.01 mg/kg × 10 kg = 0.1 mg reserpine required

$$\frac{6 \text{ mg}}{60 \text{ mL}} = \frac{0.1 \text{ mg}}{\text{x mL}}; \text{ x} = \mathbf{1\ mL}$$

(c) $\frac{12 \text{ drops}}{0.5 \text{ mL}} = \frac{\text{x drops}}{1 \text{ mL}}; \text{ x} = \mathbf{24\ drops}$

(d) 60 mL/2 mL per day = **30 days**

CASE IN POINT 17.3 Following FDA-approved directions for the emergency compounding of an oral suspension from oseltamivir phosphate (TAMIFLU) capsules,[6] a pharmacist determined that:

- The suspension should have a drug concentration of 6 mg/mL
- The volume to compound is based on the patient's weight, that is,
  ≤33 lb = 30 mL
  33 to 51 lb = 40 mL
  51 to 88 lb = 50 mL
  >88 lb = 60 mL
- 75-mg TAMIFLU capsules are to be used
- Cherry Syrup or Ora-Sweet SF may be used as the vehicle
- Specific compounding procedures as outlined in the reference should be employed.[6]

(a) How many 75-mg TAMIFLU capsules should be used in compounding a suspension for a 30-kg patient?
(b) If the prophylactic dose for a 30-kg patient is listed as 60 mg once daily, how many milliliters of the compounded oral suspension would constitute a dose?

[b]Problem courtesy of Flynn Warren, Bishop, GA.

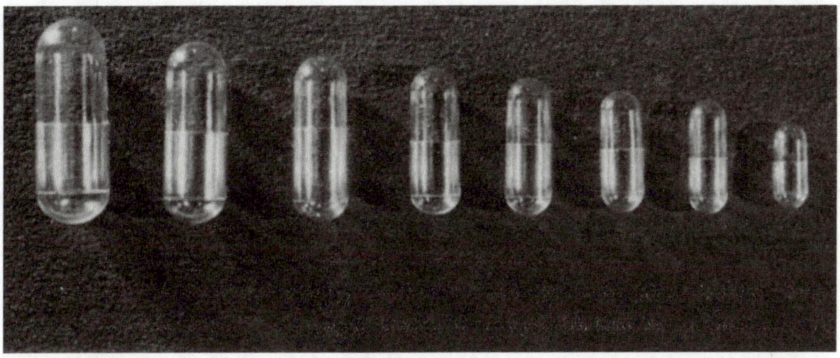

FIGURE 17.3 • Hard gelatin capsule sizes, from left to right: 000, 00, 0, 1, 2, 3, 4, and 5.

Special Calculations: Capsule Filling and Suppository Molding

Capsule Filling[7]

The extemporaneous filling of capsules enables the pharmacist to prepare patient-specific doses of drugs in a conveniently administrated form. Empty capsule shells, made of gelatin, are readily available in a variety of sizes, as shown in Figure 17.3, with size 000 being the largest and size 5 the smallest.

Filled capsules should be neither underfilled nor overfilled but should hold the ingredients snugly. Different drug powders have different densities, and thus, different weights can be packed into a given size capsule (see Table 17.1). In filling a prescription or medication order, a pharmacist should select a capsule size that accommodates the fill and will be easy for the patient to swallow.

Most oral drugs have relatively small doses; thus, a diluent, like lactose, commonly is added to provide the necessary bulk to completely fill the prescribed capsules.

The steps used in calculating the proper capsule fill may be described as follows:

STEP 1. Select an appropriate capsule size.

STEP 2. Fill the capsule shell separately with each drug and diluent, and record the weights of each.

STEP 3. Calculate the *diluent displacement weight* for each drug, as demonstrated in the following example problem.

STEP 4. Calculate the amount of diluent required per capsule.

STEP 5. Calculate the total quantities of each drug and the diluent needed to fill all of the capsules prescribed.

Table 17.1 • CAPSULE SIZES AND APPROXIMATE FILL CAPACITIES

Capsule Size	Approximate Volume	Approximate Powder Weight
000	1.4 mL	430 mg–1.8 g
00	0.95 mL	390 mg–1.3 g
0	0.68 mL	325–900 mg
1	0.5 mL	227–650 mg
2	0.37 mL	200–520 mg
3	0.3 mL	120–390 mg
4	0.21 mL	100–260 mg
5	0.13 mL	65–130 mg

NOTE: Some pharmacists calculate for an extra capsule or two so as not to run short of fill due to any powder residue remaining in the mortar after the mixing process; this may not be done for "accountable" drugs, such as narcotics.

Example Calculation to Determine a Capsule Fill

Determine the total quantities of each drug and lactose required to fill the following prescription:

℞ Drug A	20 mg
Drug B	55 mg
Lactose, q.s.	
M. ft. caps #20	

STEP 1. For the purpose of this example, assume the pharmacist selected a size 1 capsule.

STEP 2. The pharmacist filled a capsule individually with each ingredient, weighed them, and found:

Capsule filled with drug A weighed	620 mg
Capsule filled with drug B weighed	470 mg
Capsule filled with lactose weighed	330 mg

STEP 3. The ***diluent displacement weights*** for drugs A and B are calculated by ratio and proportion as follows:

For drug A:

$$\frac{620 \text{ mg (drug A in filled capsule)}}{330 \text{ mg (lactose in filled capsule)}} = \frac{20 \text{ mg (drug A per capsule)}}{\text{x (lactose displacement)}}$$

$$\text{x} = 10.65 \text{ mg (diluent displacement by 20 mg of drug A)}$$

For drug B:

$$\frac{470 \text{ mg}}{330 \text{ mg}} = \frac{55 \text{ mg}}{\text{x}}$$

$$\text{x} = 38.62 \text{ mg (diluent displacement by 55 mg of drug B)}$$

STEP 4. The diluent required per capsule:

$$330 \text{ mg} - 49.27 \text{ mg } (10.65 \text{ mg} + 38.62 \text{ mg}) = 280.73 \text{ mg lactose}$$

STEP 5. The total quantities of each drug and diluent needed to fill all the capsules prescribed:

Drug A = 20 mg × 20 (capsules) = **400 mg**
Drug B = 55 mg × 20 (capsules) = **1100 mg**
Lactose = 280.73 mg × 20 (capsules) = **5614.6 mg**

Suppository Molding[7]

Pharmacists extemporaneously prepare suppositories by using a mold, such as that shown in Figure 17.4. The drug(s) prescribed and a suppository base are the components of any suppository.

As defined in Appendix B, ***suppositories*** are solid dosage forms intended for insertion into body orifices where they soften, melt, or dissolve, releasing their medications to the surrounding tissues. Any of a number of suppository bases can be used as vehicles for the medication; in extemporaneous compounding, cocoa butter (also termed theobroma oil) is commonly used. Cocoa butter is a solid at room temperature but melts at body temperatures.

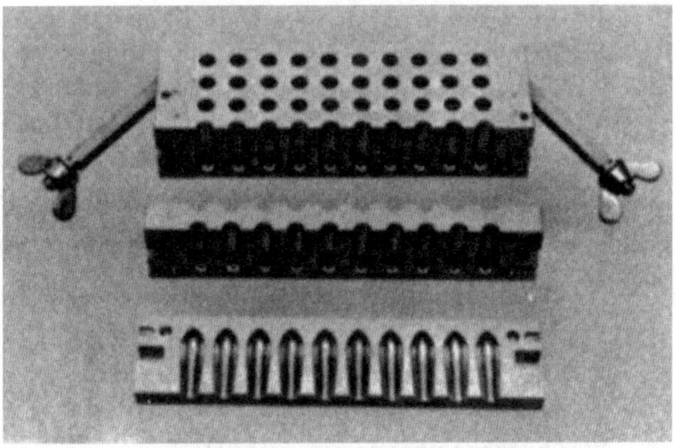

FIGURE 17.4 • An opened aluminum suppository mold that prepares twelve 2-g suppositories in a universal shape for rectal or vaginal use. When assembled, the threaded posts and wingnuts secure the mold in precise alignment to receive the liquid fill. When the fill is solidified, the mold is opened for easy removal of the formed suppositories. *(Courtesy of Total Pharmacy Supply.)*

The calculations involved in preparing suppositories by molding are described by the following steps. Other methods are used and may be found in the cited reference.[8]

To calibrate the suppository mold:

STEP 1. Fill all the cells of the suppository mold with melted base. After allowing time to cool and harden, extract the formed suppositories, weigh them, and determine the total and average suppository weights.

STEP 2. Divide the total and average suppository weights by the density of the suppository base to determine the volume capacity of the suppository mold and the average volume of each cell.

To calculate and prepare medicated suppositories:

STEP 1. Weigh the active ingredient for the preparation of a single suppository.

STEP 2. Mix the single dose of active ingredient with a portion of melted base *insufficient* to fill one cell of the mold (based on information obtained by previously calibrating the mold).

STEP 3. Pour the drug–base mixture into a cell, and add additional melted base to completely fill the cell.

STEP 4. After the suppository cools and hardens, extract and weigh it.

STEP 5. The weight of the base is determined by subtracting the amount of the drug from the weight of the molded suppository.

STEP 6. The individual weights of the drug and base required to prepare the prescribed number of suppositories may then be determined by multiplying the amounts for a single suppository. The volume of base required may also be calculated, if desired, by the use of its known density.

Example Calculation to Prepare Suppositories by Molding

Calculate the quantities of drug A and cocoa butter needed to fill the following prescription:

℞ Drug A 350 mg
Cocoa butter q.s.
M. ft. rectal suppos. #12

STEP 1. 350 mg of drug A is weighed.

STEP 2. Since a rectal suppository mold prepares suppositories weighing approximately 2 g, the amount of cocoa butter to use that would be *insufficient* to fill one cell may be estimated by:

2 g – 0.35 g (drug A) = 1.65 g (cocoa butter)

1.65 g ÷ 0.86 g/mL (density of cocoa butter) = 1.92 mL (approximate volume of melted cocoa butter, when added to drug A, to *completely* fill the cell)

By mixing the drug with 1 mL of melted cocoa butter, the pharmacist knows that this volume is *insufficient* to fill a cell.

STEP 3. The mixture of 350 mg of drug A and 1 mL of melted cocoa butter is placed in a cell, and sufficient additional melted cocoa butter is used to completely fill the cell.

STEP 4. The cooled and hardened suppository is extracted and is found to weigh 1.95 g.

STEP 5. The weight of the cocoa butter in one suppository is calculated:

$$1.95 \text{ g} - 0.35 \text{ g (drug A)} = 1.6 \text{ g cocoa butter}$$

STEP 6. The total quantities of drug A and cocoa butter needed to fill the prescription are:

$$0.35 \text{ g} \times 12 \text{ (suppositories)} = \mathbf{4.2 \text{ g drug A}}$$

$$1.6 \text{ g} \times 12 \text{ (suppositories)} = \mathbf{19.2 \text{ g cocoa butter}}$$

NOTE: Some pharmacists calculate for an extra suppository or two so as not to run short of fill mixture. In filling the mold, each cell should be slightly overfilled to allow for contraction on cooling.

Compounding Specialized Formulas

Not all commercially available products are suitable for every patient. On occasion, a pharmacist must modify an existing product or prepare an original formulation to meet the requirements of a patient.

In their compounding practices, pharmacists may develop their own formulas, or they may refer to contemporary formulas developed and published by colleagues.[9] In order to facilitate pharmacy compounding, some specialty companies and professional associations make available instructional programs, resource materials, compounding equipment, bulk active therapeutic agents, and compounding vehicles for the preparation of a range of dosage forms.[10]

Example Calculations of Specialized Formulas

(1) *Calculate the number of tablets containing the combination of spironolactone 25 mg and hydrochlorothiazide 25 mg that must be used to prepare the following formula using Ora-Plus as the oral suspending vehicle.*[11]

Spironolactone	5 mg/mL
Hydrochlorothiazide	5 mg/mL
Ora-Plus ad	120 mL

Spironolactone/hydrochlorothiazide:

$$5 \text{ mg of each drug/mL} \times 120 \text{ mL} = 600 \text{ mg of each drug}$$

$$600 \text{ mg (of each drug)} \div 25 \text{ mg (of each drug/tablet)} = \mathbf{24 \text{ tablets}}$$

(2) *Calculate the amount of FATTIBASE, a suppository base, required to prepare 200 suppositories from the following formula for one progesterone vaginal suppository*[12]:

Progesterone, micronized	25 mg
Silica gel, micronized	20 mg
FATTIBASE ad	2 g

25 mg (progesterone) + 20 mg (silica gel) = 45 mg

2 g − 0.045 g = 1.955 g

1.955 g × 200 (suppositories) = **391 g FATTIBASE**

CASE IN POINT 17.4[a] A pharmacist receives a telephone call from a pediatrician who has an 8.8-lb 1-month-old patient with an acid reflux condition. The infant was started on ranitidine (ZANTAC) syrup, 15 mg/mL, at a dose of 10 mg/kg/day, and has shown improvement. However, because of the flavor (peppermint) and alcohol content (7.5%), the baby frequently rejects the medication.

The pharmacist suggests preparing a sugar-free and alcohol-free syrup/suspension with a fruity odor and taste. The physician agrees and prescribes ranitidine syrup/suspension, 60 mL, at a dose of 10 mg/kg/day, divided into two 0.5-mL doses.

The pharmacist uses finely crushed 75-mg ranitidine tablets as the source of the drug and Ora-Sweet SF as the vehicle.

How many 75-mg ranitidine tablets are required?

[a]Problem courtesy of Warren Beach, Department of Pharmaceutical and Biomedical Sciences, College of Pharmacy, The University of Georgia, Athens, GA.

PRACTICE PROBLEMS

Calculations for the Constitution of Dry Powders for Oral Administration

1. After constitution of a dry powder, each 5 mL of ampicillin for oral suspension contains 250 mg of ampicillin in package sizes to prepare 100 mL, 150 mL, or 200 mL of suspension. Which package size should be dispensed for a 20-kg child who is to take 50 mg/kg/day total, q.i.d., in equally divided and spaced doses for 10 days?
2. From the information in Figure 17.2, calculate the following: (a) the volume of the original contents of the package upon dissolution; (b) the content of doxycycline monohydrate, in mg; (c) the volume of water to add to the original container if a doxycycline monohydrate concentration of 10 mg/mL is desired; and (d) the concentration of doxycycline monohydrate, in mg/5 mL, if 50 mL of water were used rather than the directed 47.6 mL?
3. The label on a bottle of dry powder mix for constitution states that when 128 mL of water is added, 150 mL of an oral suspension containing 250 mg of ampicillin in each 5 mL results.
   (a) How many milliliters of water should be added to the dry powder mix if a strength of 150 mg of ampicillin per 5 mL is desired?
   (b) If the dose of ampicillin is 5 mg/kg of body weight, how many milliliters of water should be added to the dry powder mix so that a child weighing 66 lb would receive the proper dose in each 5 mL of the suspension?
4. Amoxicillin/clavulanate potassium (AUGMENTIN) powder for oral suspension is prepared prior to dispensing by adding 134 mL of purified water to the contents of the container to prepare 150 mL of suspension. If each teaspoonful of suspension contains 125 mg of amoxicillin and 31.25 mg of clavulanate potassium, how much of each of these agents is contained in the dry powder prior to reconstitution?

5. If, in the above problem, a pharmacist wished to use the dry product to prepare an oral suspension containing 200 mg of amoxicillin and 50 mg of clavulanate potassium/5 mL of suspension, how many milliliters of purified water should be used for reconstitution?
6. Clarithromycin for oral suspension is available in bottles containing dry granules intended for constitution with water to prepare a suspension. The package insert instructs a pharmacist to add 27 mL of water to prepare 50 mL of suspension for a clarithromycin concentration of 125 mg/5 mL. Calculate (a) the weight, in milligrams, of the dry clarithromycin in the product. If the pediatric dose is 7.5 mg/kg every 12 hours, calculate the dose, in milliliters, for (b) a child weighing 16.7 kg and (c) another child weighing 55 lb.

Calculations Applied to Compounding for Parenteral Administration

7. A vial contains 5 g of a powdered drug for reconstitution prior to use in an infusion. The label states that when 9.6 mL of diluent is added, the solution that results contains a drug concentration of 500 mg/mL. A medication order calls for a drug concentration of 200 mg/mL. How many milliliters of diluent should be added to the vial?
8. A hospital pharmacist constitutes a vial containing 2 g of piperacillin sodium to 10 mL with sterile water for injection. This solution is then diluted by adding it to 100 mL of 5% dextrose injection for administration by infusion. What is the concentration, in milligrams per milliliter (mg/mL), of piperacillin sodium in the infusion solution?
9. A vial of cefazolin injection contains 1 g of drug. When 2.5 mL of diluent is added, 3 mL of injection is prepared. If 1.6 mL of the injection is diluted to 200 mL with sodium chloride injection, how many milliliters of the dilution should be administered daily to a child weighing 40 lb if the daily dose is 25 mg/kg of body weight?
10.[7] Medication Order: Piperacillin, 1500 mg every 6 hours.
Product: 3-g vial, piperacillin.
Pharmacy operations: Reconstitute vial with 14 mL of sterile water for injection to prepare 15 mL of injection. Add portion required to 50 mL of sodium chloride injection.
Administer: 20-minute IV infusion.
(a) How many milliliters of solution from the reconstituted vial should be used?
(b) What should be the infusion rate in milliliters per hour?
(c) With a drop factor of 20 drops per milliliter, calculate the infusion rate in drops per minute.
11. A medication order calls for 400 mg of cefazolin sodium to be administered IM to a patient every 12 hours. Vials containing 500 mg, 1 g, and 10 g of cefazolin sodium are available. According to the manufacturer's directions, dilutions may be made as follows:

Vial Size	*Solvent to Be Added*	*Final Volume*
500 mg	2 mL	2.2 mL
1 g	2.5 mL	3 mL
10 g	45 mL	51 mL

Explain how the prescribed amount of cefazolin sodium could be obtained.

12. Using the vial sizes in Problem 11 as the source of cefazolin sodium, how many milliliters of the diluted 500-mg vial should be administered to a 40-lb child who is to receive 8 mg of cefazolin sodium per kilogram of body weight?
13. Using cefazolin sodium injection in a concentration of 125 mg/mL, complete the following table representing a *Pediatric Dosage Guide:*

Weight		*Dose (25 mg/kg/d divided into 3 doses)*	
lb	*kg*	*Approximate single dose (mg/q8h)*	*mL of dilution (125 mg/mL) needed*
10	4.5	37.5 or 38 mg	0.3 mL
20	______	______	______
30	______	______	______
40	______	______	______
50	______	______	______

14. A vial contains 1 g of ceftazidime. Express the concentrations of the drug, in milligrams per milliliter, following constitution with sterile water for injection to the following volumes: (a) 2.2 mL, (b) 4.5 mL, and (c) 10 mL.
15. Acetazolamide sodium is available in 500-mg vials to be constituted to 5 mL with sterile water for injection before use. The dose of the drug for children is 5 mg/kg of body weight. How many milliliters of the injection should be administered to a child weighing 25 lb?
16. An intravenous infusion for a child weighing 60 lb is to contain 20 mg of vancomycin hydrochloride per kilogram of body weight in 200 mL of sodium chloride injection. Using a 10-mL vial containing 500 mg of vancomycin hydrochloride (dry powder), explain how you would obtain the amount needed in preparing the infusion.

Calculations for the Use of Prefabricated Dosage Forms in Compounding

17. ℞ Potassium permanganate solution 1:10,000 — 500 mL
    Sig. use as directed
    Using tablets, each containing 0.3 g of potassium permanganate, explain how you would obtain the amount of potassium permanganate needed for the prescription.
18. ℞ Estropipate — 0.0125% w/w
    Cream base ad — 60 g
    Sig. vaginal cream
    How many 0.75-mg tablets of estropipate may be used to prepare the prescription?
19.[a] ℞ Testosterone — 10 mg/0.25 mL
    Sucralose — 0.15 g
    BHT — 0.01 g
    Flavor — 0.3 mL
    Almond oil, ad — 30 mL
    How many 30-mg tablets of testosterone are needed to fill the prescription?
20. ℞ Phenacaine hydrochloride solution (1%) — 7.5 mL
    Scopolamine hydrobromide solution (0.2%) — 7.5 mL
    Sig. for the eye
    How many tablets, each containing 600 μg of scopolamine hydrobromide, should be used in preparing the prescription?

---

[a] Problem courtesy of Deborah Elder, Department of Pharmaceutical and Biomedical Sciences, College of Pharmacy, The University of Georgia, Athens, GA.

21. ℞ Hexachlorophene
    Hydrocortisone aa 0.25%
    Coal tar solution 30 mL
    Hydrophilic ointment ad 120 g
    Sig. apply

    How many tablets, each containing 20 mg of hydrocortisone, should be used in preparing the prescription?

22. How many milliliters of an injection containing 40 mg of a drug per milliliter would provide the amount of the drug needed to prepare 120 mL of a 0.2% suspension?

23. ℞ Allopurinol 65 mg/5 mL
    Cologel 40 mL
    Syrup ad 150 mL
    M. ft. susp.
    Sig. as directed

    How many scored 100-mg allopurinol tablets may be used in preparing the prescription?

24. ℞ Enalapril 7.5 mg
    Lactose ad 200 mg
    DTD Caps #40
    Sig. take one capsule each morning

    How many 20-mg tablets of enalapril, each weighing 120 mg, and how many grams of lactose would be needed to prepare the prescription?

25. How many tablets for topical solution, each containing 300 mg of potassium permanganate, should be added to 1 gallon of purified water to provide a concentration of 0.012% w/v?

26. A prescription for 240 mL of a cough mixture calls for 2 mg of hydrocodone bitartrate per teaspoonful. How many tablets, each containing 5 mg of hydrocodone bitartrate, should be used in preparing the cough mixture?

27. ℞ Dantrolene sodium 5 mg/mL
    Citric acid 150 mg
    Purified water 10 mL
    Syrup ad 125 mL
    M. ft. susp.
    Sig. as directed

    If the only source of dantrolene sodium is 100-mg capsules, each containing 200 mg of drug–diluent powder mix, (a) how many capsules must be opened and (b) how many milligrams of the powder mix should be used in preparing the prescription?

28.[13] ℞ Ketorolac tromethamine 7.5 mg/5 mL
    Suspension vehicle ad 120 mL
    Sig. 1 tsp q6h

    How many 10-mg ketorolac tromethamine (TORADOL) tablets may be used to prepare this prescription?

29. How many DANTRIUM capsules, each containing 25 mg of dantrolene, are needed to prepare 100 mL of a pediatric suspension containing 5 mg of dantrolene per milliliter?

30. The following is a formula for a diazepam rectal gel.[14] How many 10-mL vials of VALIUM injection containing 5 mg/mL of diazepam would be needed to compound the formula?

Diazepam	100 mg
Methylcellulose (1500 cps)	2.5 g
Methylparaben	100 mg
Glycerin	5 g
Purified water ad	100 mL

31. How many tablets, each containing 25 mg of spironolactone, are needed to prepare 200 mL of a pediatric suspension to contain 5 mg of spironolactone per milliliter?
32. A physician prescribes 30 capsules, each containing 300 mg of ibuprofen, for a patient. The pharmacist has on hand 400-mg and 600-mg ibuprofen tablets. How many each of these tablets could be used to obtain the amount of ibuprofen needed in preparing the prescription?
33. ℞

Indomethacin powder	1%
Carbopol 941 powder	2%
Purified water	10%
Alcohol ad	90 mL

Sig. use as directed

How many 75-mg capsules of indomethacin should be used in preparing the prescription?

34. ℞

Minoxidil	0.3%
Vehicle/N ad	50 mL

Sig. apply to affected areas of the scalp b.i.d.

Tablets containing 2.5 mg and 10 mg of minoxidil are available. Explain how you would obtain the amount of minoxidil needed in preparing the prescription, using the available sources of the drug.

35. If a pharmacist used one 50-mg tablet of a drug to prepare 30 mL of an otic suspension in sweet oil, calculate the percentage strength of the preparation.
36. ℞

Aminophylline	500 mg
Sodium pentobarbital	75 mg
Carbowax base ad	2 g

Ft. suppos. no. 12
Sig. insert one at night

How many capsules, each containing 100 mg of sodium pentobarbital, should be used to provide the sodium pentobarbital needed in preparing the prescription?

37. A starting pediatric dose of phenytoin sodium (DILANTIN) is 6 mg/kg/day, administered in three equally divided doses. Using tablets containing 50 mg of phenytoin sodium, a pharmacist prepared a suspension such that each 1 mL, delivered from a calibrated dropper, contained a single dose for a 44-lb child. How many tablets should be used to prepare 30 mL of the suspension?
38. ℞

CARAFATE	400 mg/5 mL
Cherry syrup	40 mL
Sorbitol solution	40 mL
Flavor	q.s.
Purified water ad	125 mL

Sig. 5 mL t.i.d.

How many 1-g CARAFATE tablets should be used in preparing the prescription?

Calculations Used in Capsule Filling and Suppository Molding

39.[7] A pharmacist needs to prepare 50 capsules, each containing 4 mg of estriol and 1 mg of estradiol. A size 3 capsule is selected for use. Capsule shells are individually filled with each drug and lactose and the weights recorded as follows:

Estriol	250 mg
Estradiol	190 mg
Lactose	320 mg

(a) How many milligrams of each component will be needed to fill all the capsules?
(b) How many milligrams should the content of each capsule weigh?

40.[7] A pharmacist prepares six suppositories using a polyethylene glycol base, density 1.18 g/mL. The total weight of the suppositories is found to be 13.81 g. Calculate the volume of the mold per cell.

41.[7,15] ℞ Fluconazole 200 mg
PEG base, q.s.
M. ft. suppos #20
(a) How many grams of fluconazole are needed?
(b) If a trial molded suppository weighs 2.4 g, how many grams of PEG base are needed to compound the prescription?

Calculations of Specialized Formulas

42. The following is a formula for an oral ulceration mouthwash.[16]

Hydrocortisone	55.2 mg
Lidocaine HCl	2.4 g
Erythromycin stearate	1.5 g
Diphenhydramine HCl	150 mg
Nystatin	2,000,000 units
Xanthan gum	240 mg
Stevia powder extract	280 mg
Sodium saccharin	120 mg
Flavor	1 mL
Simple syrup or sorbitol solution (70%) ad	120 mL

(a) Calculate the percentage strength of hydrocortisone in the formula.
(b) If nystatin is available as a powder containing 5225 units/mg, calculate the quantity required, in milligrams, to compound the formula.
(c) Calculate the concentration of erythromycin stearate, in mg/mL, in the formula.

43. Misoprostol and lidocaine in glycerin mouth paint[17]

Misoprostol 200-mcg tablets	12 tablets
Lidocaine HCl	1 g
Glycerin qs ad	100 mL

How many micrograms of misoprostol would be present in each milliliter of mouth paint?

44. Progesterone liquid fill capsules.[18]

Progesterone, micronized	10 g
Sesame oil qs ad	30 mL
To make 100 capsules	

How many (a) micrograms of progesterone and (b) microliters of the formula would be contained in each capsule?

45. Tri-Est aqueous injection[19]

Estriol	200 mg
Estrone	25 mg
Estradiol	25 mg
Polysorbate 80	0.2 mL
Benzyl alcohol	1 mL
Sterile water for injection ad	100 mL

How many milliliters of the injection should be used to deliver 1.75 mg of total estrogens?

46. Intracavernosal injection[20]

Prostaglandin E	5.9 μg/mL
Papaverine HCl	17.6 mg/mL
Phentolamine mesylate	0.6 mg/mL
Sterile water for injection ad	1.5 mL

How many milligrams of each ingredient should be used in preparing 12 syringes, each containing 1.5 mL of injection?

47. Progesterone nasal spray[21]

Progesterone	20 mg
Dimethyl-β-cyclodextrin	62 mg
Purified water ad	1 mL

How many milligrams each of progesterone and dimethyl-β-cyclodextrin would be delivered in each 0.05 mL spray of solution?

48. Triple estrogen slow-release capsules[22]

For 100 capsules:

Estriol	200 mg
Estrone	25 mg
Estradiol	25 mg
Methocel E4M	10 g
Lactose	23.75 g

Calculate the weight, in milligrams, of the formula in each capsule.

49. Nail fungus solution[23]

NIZORAL, 200-mg tablets	10 tablets
Clotrimazole	900 mg
Ethyl alcohol, 95%	5 mL
Polyethylene glycol 300	67 mL
Dimethylsulfoxide	23 mL

If the formula prepares 98 mL, what is the percent concentration of NIZORAL in the solution?

50.[a] ℞

Menthol	2% w/w
Camphor	1% w/w
Urea	10% w/w
Potassium sorbate	0.1% w/w
Absorbent ointment base, ad	30 g

[a]Problem courtesy of Deborah Elder, Department of Pharmaceutical and Biomedical Sciences, College of Pharmacy, The University of Georgia, Athens, GA.

If a 1% w/v potassium sorbate solution (sp. gr. 0.96) is used as the source of potassium sorbate, how many grams of the absorbent ointment base are required to fill the prescription?

51.[a] A pharmacist compounds 45 g of a transdermal gel to contain 50 mg/g of promethazine hydrochloride. The promethazine hydrochloride is dissolved in a sufficient quantity of 20% Pluronic F-127 in water, representing 80% w/w of the gel (aqueous phase), with the remainder being lecithin-isopropyl palmitate (oil phase). How many grams of each of the three ingredients are required?

52. Migraine headache suppositories[24]

Ergotamine tartrate	2 mg
Caffeine	100 mg
Hyoscyamine sulfate	0.25 mg
Pentobarbital sodium	60 mg
FATTIBASE ad	2 g

The formula is for one suppository. If the specific gravity of FATTIBASE is 0.89, how many milliliters of the melted base (assuming no volume change due to heat) may be used to prepare 36 suppositories?

53. Veterinary dexamethasone ophthalmic ointment[25]

Dexamethasone sodium phosphate	39.6 mg
Bacteriostatic water for injection	0.4 mL
Polysorbate 80	0.3 mL
Lacri-Lube qs	30 g

Calculate the percentage strength of dexamethasone (base) in the formula if 1 mg of dexamethasone (base) is equivalent to 1.32 mg of dexamethasone sodium phosphate.

54. The following is a formula for a captopril oral liquid.[26]

℞	Captopril	100-mg tablet
	Ora-Sweet ad	134 mL

How many milliliters of the oral liquid would provide 0.75 mg of captopril?

55. The following is a formula for a rifampin oral liquid.[26]

℞	Rifampin	25 mg/mL
	Ora-Plus ad	120 mL

How many 300-mg tablets of rifampin should be used?

56. The following is a formula for fluconazole topical cream.[26]

℞	Fluconazole	10 g
	Glycerin	18.75 g
	DERMABASE ad	100 g

How many milliliters of glycerin should be used (sp. gr. 1.25)?

57. The following is a formula for a clotrimazole topical preparation.[26]

℞	Clotrimazole, powder	1%
	DERMABASE ad	30 g

How many grams of DERMABASE are required?

58.[a] A pharmacist receives a prescription for 45 mL of a 50% castor oil emulsion. A mixture of two emulsifying agents is used, 5.4 parts of Tween 80 and 1 part of Span 20. If a total of 5% emulsifying agents is used in compounding the prescription, how many grams each of Tween 80 and Span 20 are used?

Miscellaneous Compounding Calculations with Methods of Preparation[b]

NOTE: Examples of methods of compounding are included with practice problems (59 to 63) for the purpose of demonstration.

59.[27] Fluconazole 2% topical microemulsion

Fluconazole	2 g
Lauryl alcohol	10 g
Labrasob alcohol (50%)	20 g
Purified water qs, ad	100 mL

Method of Preparation:

1. *Calculate the required quantity of each ingredient for the total amount to be prepared.*
2. *Weigh and/or measure each ingredient accurately.*
3. *Mix the lauryl alcohol with the labrasob alcohol mixture until uniform.*
4. *Incorporate the fluconazole slowly and mix well.*
5. *Incorporate sufficient purified water slowly with continuous stirring to volume.*

Calculate:

(a) Lauryl alcohol has a specific gravity of 0.83. Calculate the milliliters of lauryl alcohol to use.

(b) Lauryl alcohol dissolves about 14.25 mg of fluconazole per milliliter. Calculate the fluconazole to lauryl alcohol ratio (mg/mL) in the formula.

(c) Based on (b), would fluconazole be in suspension or solution?

60.[28] Rufinamide 40 mg/mL oral suspension

Rufinamide	4 g
Ora-Plus	50 mL
Ora-Sweet, ad	100 mL

Method of Preparation:

1. *Calculate the required quantity of each ingredient for the total amount to be prepared.*
2. *Weigh and/or measure each ingredient accurately.*
3. *Pulverize the required number of rufinamide tablets to a fine powder.*
4. *Add about 25 mL of Ora-Plus (suspending agent) and mix to form a smooth paste.*
5. *Add the remainder of the Ora-Plus and mix well.*
6. *Add sufficient Ora Sweet (flavoring vehicle) to final volume and mix well.*

Calculate:

(a) How many 200-mg rufinamide tablets would be required to compound the formula?

(b) If treatment with rufinamide is initiated for a 55-lb child at a daily dose of 10 mg/kg/day and increased by 10 mg/kg/day on the third day, how many milliliters of the formula would remain after the first week of treatment if 100 mL were dispensed?

---

[a]Problem courtesy of Deborah Elder, Department of Pharmaceutical and Biomedical Sciences, College of Pharmacy, The University of Georgia, Athens, GA.

[b]Formulas and methods of preparation reproduced with permission of Loyd V. Allen Jr, Editor- in-Chief, *International Journal of Pharmaceutical Compounding*. Edmond, OK.

61.[29] Topiramate 6 mL/mL oral suspension

Topiramate	600 mg
Ora-Plus	50 mL
Ora-Sweet, ad	100 mL

Method of Preparation:

1. *Calculate the required quantity of each ingredient for the total amount to be prepared.*
2. *Weigh and/or measure each ingredient accurately.*
3. *Obtain the topiramate as the 100-mg tablets and pulverize to a fine powder.*
4. *Incorporate the Ora-Plus (suspending agent) slowly and mix until uniform and smooth.*
5. *Incorporate sufficient Ora-Sweet (flavoring vehicle) slowly to volume and mix well.*

Calculate:

(a) Calculate the number of topiramate tablets needed to prepare the formula.

(b) For adult prophylaxis of migraine headache, the dose is gradually increased from 25 mg/day during week 1, to 25 mg twice a day during week 2, to 25 mg in the AM and 50 in the PM each day during the third week. How many milliliters of the formula would be required for the first 3 weeks of treatment?

62.[30] Acyclovir 200 mg/5 mL oral suspension (from the injection)

Acyclovir sodium	4 g
Ora-Plus	50 mL
Ora-Sweet, ad	100 mL

Method of Preparation:

1. *Calculate the required quantity of each ingredient for the total amount to be prepared.*
2. *Weigh and/or measure each ingredient accurately.*
3. *Reconstitute the acyclovir sodium vial with the smallest quantity of purified water required to allow withdrawal from the vial. Note: It does not have to all be in solution.*
4. *Place in a suitable calibrated container.*
5. *Add the Ora-Plus geometrically and mix well.*
6. *Add sufficient Ora-Sweet to volume and mix well.*

Calculate:

(a) Acyclovir sodium is available as a sterile lyophilized powder for reconstitution with sterile water for injection in vials containing 1000 mg of acyclovir. If a pharmacist used 6 mL of diluent to prepare 7 mL of injection from each vial required, how many milliliters of Ora-Sweet would be needed to compound the formula?

(b) If the dose prescribed for a 60-lb child for the treatment of chickenpox was 20 mg/kg per dose orally, four times daily for 5 days, what volume of formula would be needed?

63.[31] Dexpanthenol 5% gel cream

Dexpanthenol	5 g
Mineral oil, light	10 mL
Polyethylene glycol 400	15 mL
Pluronic F-127	20 g
Purified water, ad	100 g

Method of Preparation:

1. *Calculate the required quantity of each ingredient for the total amount to be prepared.*
2. *Weigh and/or measure each ingredient accurately.*
3. *Dissolve the dexpanthenol in the polyethylene glycol 400.*

4. *Add the mineral oil and stir, heating to 60°C to 70°C.*
5. *Incorporate the Pluronic F-127 slowly and stir until dissolved.*
6. *Cool to room temperature.*
7. *Add sufficient purified water to final weight and mix well.*

Calculate:

(a) If the mineral oil has a specific gravity of 0.82 and the polyethylene glycol has a specific gravity of 1.14, what would be the expected weight of the mixture in above steps 3 and 4?

(b) How many milliliters of purified water is needed to compound the formula?

CALCQUIZ

17.A. Due to incompletely developed renal function in neonates and infants less than 3 months old, which affects the elimination of amoxicillin, the upper dose is considered 30 mg/kg/day, divided and administered every 12 hours. A pharmacist receives a medication order for a 12-week-old infant weighing 15 lb with a mild upper respiratory infection. A bottle of amoxicillin pediatric drops is prescribed. When this is reconstituted with the addition of 23 mL of water, a 30-mL suspension of amoxicillin, 50 mg/mL, is prepared. Calculate (a) the volume occupied by the dry amoxicillin content, (b) the daily dose of amoxicillin for the infant at 20 mg/kg/day in two divided doses, (c) the daily dose of suspension required, and (d) the single dose, in drops, using a calibrated dropper delivering 20 drops/mL.

17.B. A package contains 1250 mg of the antibiotic clarithromycin. When reconstituted with 27 mL of water, 50 mL of oral suspension may be prepared. The pediatric dose for a 20-lb child is determined to be 62.5 mg. How many milliliters of water should be used to reconstitute the antibiotic such that the dose may be administered by 5 mL of oral suspension?

17.C. A vial contains 1 g of capreomycin in a 10-mL vial for reconstitution prior to injection. According to the package insert, when 2.15 mL of diluent is added, 2.85 mL of injection is prepared and when 3.3 mL of diluent is added, 4 mL of injection is prepared. How many milliliters of diluent should be added to prepare an injection containing capreomycin, 300 mg/mL?

17.D. An injection of epoprostenol sodium (FLOLAN) is prepared by dissolving the contents of one 0.5 mg vial with 5 mL of the copackaged sterile diluent. Then, prior to intravenous infusion, 3 mL is withdrawn from the vial to prepare 100 mL of injection. Calculate (a) the concentration of epoprostenol sodium in ng/mL in the injection, and (b) if the injection is to infused at a rate of 8 ng/kg/min, calculate the infusion delivery rate in mL/h for a patient weighing 176 lb.

17.E.[a] A compounding pharmacist receives a prescription for 14 medicated chewable gummy bears for a pediatric patient. Each gummy bear is to contain 10 mg of hydroxyzine. The pharmacist decides to use three 50-mg capsules of hydroxyzine as the drug source and determines their combined contents to weigh 625 mg. If each cell of the gummy bear mold holds a calibrated 1.56 g, and if the gummy gel base has the following general formula,[32] how much of each ingredient is required to fill the prescription?

Gelatin	43.4 g
Glycerin	155 mL (sp. gr. 1.25)
Purified water	21.6 mL

[a] Problem courtesy of Deborah Elder, Department of Pharmaceutical and Biomedical Sciences, College of Pharmacy, The University of Georgia, Athens, GA.

ANSWERS TO "CASE IN POINT" AND PRACTICE PROBLEMS

Case in Point 17.1

Calculate the amount of amoxicillin in container:

$$\frac{250 \text{ mg (amoxicillin)}}{5 \text{ mL}} = \frac{\text{x mg (amoxicillin)}}{100 \text{ mL}}$$

$$\text{x} = 5000 \text{ mg amoxicillin in container}$$

Calculate volume that can be prepared from 5000 mg at 200 mg/5 mL:

$$\frac{200 \text{ mg}}{5 \text{ mL}} = \frac{5000 \text{ mg}}{\text{x ml}};$$

$$\text{x} = 125 \text{ mL of oral suspension can be prepared}$$

Calculate volume of amoxicillin powder in container:

100 mL – 68 mL (water added by label instructions) = 32 mL (volume of powder)

Calculate water requirement for new concentration:

125 mL – 32 mL = 93 mL of water required

Proof: 5000 mg amoxicillin per 125 mL = 200 mg amoxicillin per 5 mL

Case in Point 17.2

(a) $750 \text{ mg} \times \frac{1 \text{ mL}}{500 \text{ mg}} = 1.5 \text{ mL of reconstituted solution.}$

(b) Infusion time: 30 minutes
Infusion volume: 101.5 mL
Infusion rate per hour:

$$60 \text{min} \frac{101.5 \text{ mL}}{30 \text{ min}} = 203 \text{ mL, infusion rate per hour}$$

(c) 101.5 mL (infusion volume)

$$\times \frac{10 \text{ drops}}{1 \text{ mL}} = 1015 \text{ drops}$$

$$\frac{1015 \text{ drops}}{30 \text{min}} = 33.8 \text{ or } 34 \text{ drops per minute}$$

Case in Point 17.3

(a) A 30-kg patient weighs 66 lb (30 kg × 2.2 lb/kg)
According to the guideline, a 66-lb patient should receive 50 mL of oral suspension.
According to the specification, the oral suspension should have a drug concentration of 6 mg/mL.
6 mg/mL × 50 mL (oral suspension) = 300 mg TAMIFLU needed.
300 mg/75 mg per capsule = 4 TAMIFLU capsules required

(b) 60 mg (dose)/6 mg per mL = 10 mL daily dose

Case in Point 17.4

Calculate milligrams of ranitidine required per 0.5-mL dose:

$$\frac{8.8 \text{ lb}}{2.2 \text{ lb/kg}} = 4 \text{ kg (weight of child)}$$

$$4 \text{ kg} \times 10 \text{ mg/kg/day} = 40 \text{ mg/day}$$

$$40 \text{ mg} \div 2 \text{ doses/day} = 20 \text{ mg/doses; thus,}$$

$$20 \text{ mg/0.5} - \text{mL dose}$$

Calculate milligrams of ranitidine required in 60-mL prescription:

$$\frac{20 \text{ mg}}{0.5 \text{ mL}} = \frac{x \text{ mg}}{60 \text{ mL}};$$

$$x = 2400 \text{ mg ranitidine required}$$

Calculate number of 75-mg ranitidine tablets needed to provide 2400 mg
2400 mg ÷ 75 mg/tablet = 32 tablets

Practice Problems

1. 200 mL
2. (a) 12.4 mL
   (b) 300 mg doxycycline monohydrate
   (c) 17.6 mL water
   (d) 24 mg/5 mL
3. (a) 228 mL water
   (b) 228 mL water
4. 3750 mg amoxicillin
   937.3 mg clavulanate potassium
5. 77.75 mL purified water
6 (a) 1.25 g clarithromycin
   (b) 5-mL dose
   (c) 7.5-mL dose
7. 24.6 mL diluent
8. 18.18 mg/mL piperacillin
9. 170.5 mL
10. (a) 7.5 mL
    (b) 172.5 mL/h
    (c) 57.5 or 58 drops/min
11. Dilute and use 1.767 mL of the 500-mg vial, or
    dilute and use 1.2 mL of the 1-g vial, or
    dilute and use 2.04 or 2 mL of the 10-g vial
12. 0.64 mL
13.

20	9.1 kg	75.8 mg	0.61 mL
30	13.6 kg	113.3 mg	0.91 mL
40	18.2 kg	151.7 mg	1.21 mL
50	22.7 kg	189.2 mg	1.51 mL

14. (a) 454.55 mg/mL
    (b) 222.22 mg/mL
    (c) 100 mg/mL
15. 0.57 mL acetazolamide sodium injection
16. 545 mg needed. Use l vial + 10 mL of sterile diluent to a second vial to make 10 mL, and use 0.9 mL of the dilution.
17. Dissolve 1 tablet in enough distilled water to make 60 mL, and take 10 mL of the dilution.
18. 10 tablets estropipate
19. 40 tablets testosterone
20. 25 tablets scopolamine hydrobromide
21. 15 tablets hydrocortisone
22. 6 mL injection
23. 19.5 tablets allopurinol
24. 15 tablets enalapril
    6.2 g lactose
25. 1.5 tablets potassium permanganate

26. 19.2 tablets hydrocodone bitartrate
27. (a) 7 capsules dantrolene sodium
    (b) 1250 mg powder
28. 18 tablets TORADOL
29. 20 capsules DANTRIUM
30. 2 vials VALIUM injection
31. 40 tablets spironolactone
32. 22.5 tablets (400 mg each) ibuprofen, or 15 tablets (600 mg each) ibuprofen
33. 12 capsules indomethacin
34. 60 tablets (2.5 mg each) minoxidil, or 15 tablets (10 mg each) minoxidil
35. 0.167%
36. 9 capsules sodium pentobarbital
37. 24 tablets phenytoin sodium
38. 10 tablets CARAFATE
39. (a) 200 mg estriol
    50 mg estradiol
    15,660 mg lactose
    (b) 318.2 mg
40. 1.95 mL
41. (a) 4 g fluconazole
    (b) 44 g PEG base
42. (a) 0.046% hydrocortisone
    (b) 382.78 mg nystatin
    (c) 12.5 mg/mL erythromycin stearate
43. 24 μg misoprostol
44. (a) 100,000 μg progesterone
    (b) 300 μL
45. 0.7 mL injection
46. 0.106 mg prostaglandin E
    316.8 mg papaverine HCl
    10.8 mg phentolamine mesylate
47. 1 mg progesterone
    3.1 mg dimethyl-β-cyclodextrin
48. 340 mg
49. 2.04% NIZORAL
50. 23.22 g absorbent ointment base
51. 2.25 g promethazine hydrochloride
    33.75 g Pluronic F-127 in water (20%)
    9 g lecithin-isopropyl palmitate
52. 74.34 mL FATTIBASE
53. 0.1% dexamethasone
54. 1 mL oral liquid
55. 10 tablets rifampin
56. 15 mL glycerin
57. 29.7 g DERMABASE
58. 1.89 or 1.9 g Tween 80
    0.35 g Span 20
59. (a) 12.05 mL lauryl alcohol
    (b) 165.9 mg/mL fluconazole/lauryl alcohol
    (c) suspension
60. (a) Twenty 200-mg rufinamide tablets
    (b) 25 mL
61. (a) Six 100-mg topiramate tablets
    (b) 175 mL
62. (a) 22 mL Ora-Sweet
    (b) 272.73 mL
63. (a) 30.3 g
    (b) 49.7 mL purified water

AUTHORS' EXTRA POINT

REGULATION OF PHARMACY COMPOUNDING

The federal Drug Quality and Security Act of 2013 distinguishes between traditional compounding pharmacies, which are regulated by state boards of pharmacy, and large-scale compounding pharmacies, known as *outsourcing facilities.*[a,b] Whereas traditional pharmacies compound prescriptions and medication orders for individual patients, outsourcing facilities compound large quantities of product without reference to individual patients. Outsourcing facilities may engage in both sterile and nonsterile compounding and provide their products to pharmacies, which, in turn, provide them to patients in the filling of prescriptions or medication orders. The Drug Quality and Security Act provides for the registration and regulation of outsourcing facilities through the federal Food and Drug Administration. This legislation also differentiates outsourcing facilities from the large-scale industrial manufactures of pharmaceuticals, which have long been guided by FDA regulations including Good Manufacturing Practice Standards (GMPs).

It should be noted that legislation and regulations governing outsourcing facilities are presently being developed at state levels under the aegis of boards of pharmacy.[c]

The *United States Pharmacopeia—National Formulary* has developed standards for compounding that are intended to assist pharmacy practitioners in adhering to generally recognized scientific methods and established practices.[d] The relevant USP-NF chapters are:

<797> Pharmaceutical Compounding—Sterile Preparations

<795> Pharmaceutical Compounding—Nonsterile Preparations

<1160> Pharmaceutical Calculations in Prescription Compounding

<1163> Quality Assurance in Pharmaceutical Compounding

<1176> Prescription Balances and Volumetric Apparatus

USP-NF standards are enforceable in the United States by the Food and Drug Administration and thus are considered requirements for practice.

[a]Drug Quality and Security Act, 2013. Available at: https://www.govtrack.us/congress/bills/113/hr3204/text. Accessed September 17, 2014.

[b]American Pharmacists Association. Available at: http://www.pharmacist.com/hr-3204-drug-quality-and-security-act-signed-law. Accessed September 17, 2014.

[c]Collins S. Two years after meningitis outbreak, *Massachusetts passes compounding overhaul. Pharmacy Today* 2014;20:61.

[d]U.S. Pharmacopeia National Formulary. USP Compounding Standards & Resources. Available at: http://www.usp.org/usp-healthcare-professionals/compounding. Accessed September 17, 2014.

References

1. Drug Quality and Security Act, 2013. Available at: https://www.govtrack.us/congress/bills/113/hr3204/text. Accessed September 17, 2014.
2. United States Pharmacopeia National Formulary. USP compounding standards & resources. Available at: http://www.usp.org/usp-healthcare-professionals/compounding. Accessed September 17, 2014.
3. Pharmacy Compounding Accreditation Board. Available at: http://pcab.org. Accessed October 3, 2014.
4. International Academy of Compounding Pharmacists. Available at: http://www.iacprx.org. Accessed October 3, 2014.
5. Craig GP. *Clinical Calculations Made Easy*. Baltimore, MD: Lippincott Williams & Wilkins; 2001:196.
6. Directions for the emergency compounding of an oral suspension from TAMIFLU capsules. Available at: http://www.tamiflu.com/hcp/resources/hcp_resources_pharmacists.jsp. Accessed October 3, 2014.
7. Ansel HC, Prince SJ. *Pharmaceutical Calculations: The Pharmacist's Handbook*. Baltimore, MD: Lippincott Williams & Wilkins; 2004:96–105.
8. Allen LV Jr, Ansel HC. *Pharmaceutical Dosage Forms and Drug Delivery Systems*. 10th Ed. Baltimore, MD: Lippincott Williams & Wilkins; 2014:379–382.
9. Allen LV Jr. *Allen's Compounded Formulations*. 2nd Ed. Washington, DC: American Pharmacist's Association, 2004.
10. PCCA, Professional Compounding Centers of America. Available at: http://www.pccarx.com/pcca-products Accessed October 1, 2014.
11. Allen LV Jr. Spironolactone 5-mg/mL with hydrochlorothiazide 5-mg/mL oral liquid. *International Journal of Pharmaceutical Compounding* 1997;1:183.
12. Allen LV Jr. Progesterone vaginal suppositories (fatty acid base). *International Journal of Pharmaceutical Compounding* 1998;2:65.
13. Prince SJ. Calculations. *International Journal of Pharmaceutical Compounding* 1998;2:164.
14. Allen LV Jr. Diazepam dosed as a rectal gel. *US Pharmacist* 2000;25:98.
15. Allen LV Jr. *The Art, Science, and Technology of Pharmaceutical Compounding*. Washington, DC: American Pharmacist's Association; 1997:140.
16. Allen LV Jr. Oral ulceration mouthwash. *International Journal of Pharmaceutical Compounding* 1999;3:10.
17. Ford PR. Misoprostol 0.0024% and lidocaine 1% in glycerin mouth paint. *International Journal of Pharmaceutical Compounding* 1999;3:48.
18. Allen LV Jr. Progesterone liquid fill capsules. *International Journal of Pharmaceutical Compounding* 1999;3:294.
19. Allen LV Jr. Tri-est 2.5 mg/mL aqueous injection. *International Journal of Pharmaceutical Compounding* 1999;3:304.
20. Preckshot J. Medication combinations for penile injections. *International Journal of Pharmaceutical Compounding* 1999;3:81.
21. Allen LV Jr. Progesterone nasal spray (2%). *International Journal of Pharmaceutical Compounding* 1998;2:56.
22. Allen JV Jr. Triple estrogen 2.5 mg slow-release capsules. *International Journal of Pharmaceutical Compounding* 1998;2:56.
23. Nelson JL. Nail fungus solution. *International Journal of Pharmaceutical Compounding* 1998;2:277.

24. Allen LV Jr. Ergotamine tartrate, caffeine, hyoscyamine sulfate and pentobarbital sodium suppositories. *International Journal of Pharmaceutical Compounding* 1998;2:151.
25. Allen LV Jr. Veterinary dexamethasone ophthalmic ointment. *International Journal of Pharmaceutical Compounding* 1998;2:206.
26. Paddock Laboratories. Compounding. Available at: http://www.paddocklabs.com. Accessed August 8, 2011.
27. Allen LV Jr, Editor-in-Chief. Fluconazole 2% topical microemulsion. *International Journal of Pharmaceutical Compounding* 2009;13:555.
28. Allen LV Jr, Editor-in-Chief. Rufinamide 40-mg/mL oral suspension. *International Journal of Pharmaceutical Compounding* 2010;14:426.
29. Allen LV Jr, Editor-in-Chief. Topiramate 6-mg/mL oral suspension. *International Journal of Pharmaceutical Compounding* 2009;13:560.
30. Allen LV Jr, Editor-in-Chief. Acyclovir 200 mg/5-mL oral suspension (from the injection). *International Journal of Pharmaceutical Compounding* 2010;14:151.
31. Allen LV Jr, Editor-in-Chief. Dexpanthenol 5% gel-cream. *International Journal of Pharmaceutical Compounding* 2010;14:155.
32. Allen LV Jr, Editor-in-Chief. Pediatric chewable gummy gel base. *International Journal of Pharmaceutical Compounding* 1997;1:106.

18

Selected Calculations Involving Veterinary Pharmaceuticals

OBJECTIVES

Upon successful completion of this chapter, the student will be able to:

- Calculate doses applicable to pharmaceuticals used in veterinary medicine.
- Calculate doses for cats and dogs based on weight conversion to body surface area.

Veterinary medicine, like human medicine, uses pharmaceuticals of various dosage forms and strengths in the diagnosis, prevention, and treatment of disease and illness. Animals suffer from many of the same medical conditions as humans, such as cardiovascular disease, infectious disease, and cancer.[1,2] Thus, many of the medications used in human medicine also are used in veterinary medicine. In addition, however, there are diseases that are specific to various animal species that require medications developed expressly for veterinary use.[2,3]

Veterinary drugs gain approval for specified uses in an animal species through the Center for Veterinary Medicine (CVM) of the Food and Drug Administration (FDA).[4,5] A product label for a veterinary drug product is shown in Figure 18.1. It should be noted that the label states "For Use in Animals Only."

Veterinarians are permitted to prescribe both human- and animal-approved drugs for ***extralabel*** uses—that is, for uses *not* specified in the approved labeling, so long as the drug is used within the context of a "veterinarian–client–patient relationship."[6,7] This permits use of a wide range of approved drugs in animal care.

The dosage forms used in veterinary medicine are like those used in human medicine, that is, compressed and chewable tablets, capsules, oral liquids, injections, eyedrops, and topical applications. However, specialized drug delivery devices commonly are used to administer the dosage forms. This includes esophageal syringes, drench guns, and oral tubes designed to deliver medication directly into an animal's stomach; pole-mounted syringes and projectile delivery systems, which allow injections to be administered from a safe distance; mastitis syringes, for inserting a drug formulation directly into the mammary gland; and others.[8]

The most obvious and striking difference between veterinary medicine and human medicine is the nature of the patient. Whereas humans *do* differ from one another in many respects, the differences are relatively minor compared with the wide-ranging differences among veterinary patients. The various species of animals differ quite dramatically in their size, physical appearance, physiologic and biochemical makeup, intelligence, temperament, and natural habitat. There are about 62,300 identified vertebrates, including 31,300 fish, 6,400 amphibians, 9,100 reptiles, 10,000 birds, and 5,500 mammals.[9]

Of special importance in veterinary practice is the calculation of a drug's dose based on the animal's weight, weight being an important variable among animals. Consider this contrast: a pet cockatiel may weigh less than 100 g, a kitten several pounds, a race horse 1,000 pounds, and an elephant 12,000 pounds or more. Even among pet dogs, the range is dramatic, from the small "toy" dogs—the Chihuahua that may weigh 2 pounds—to one of the heaviest dogs, the Saint Bernard that may weigh up to 180 pounds. In some instances, an animal's body surface area (BSA) is the factor used in determining drug dosage (Table 18.1).

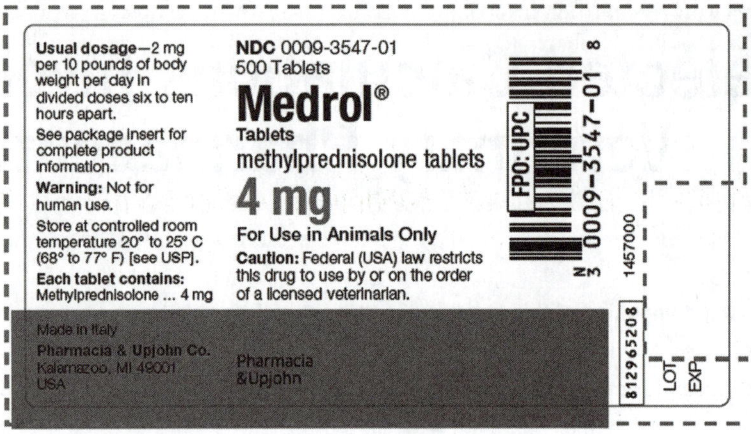

FIGURE 18.1 • Product label for a drug used in veterinary medicine. *(Courtesy Pharmacia & Upjohn. Source http://dailymed.nlm.nih.gov/dailymed/index.cfm)*

Table 18.1 • WEIGHT TO BODY SURFACE AREA CONVERSION FOR DOGS AND CATS

Body Surface Area (BSA) in Square Meters = K × (Body Weight in Grams$^{2/3}$) × 10^{-4}
K = Constant (10.1 for Dogs and 10.0 for Cats)

Dogs				Cats	
Body Wt (kg)	BSA (m^2)	Body Wt (kg)	BSA (m^2)	Body Wt (kg)	BSA (m^2)
0.5	0.06	26	0.88	0.5	0.06
1	0.10	27	0.90	1	0.10
2	0.15	28	0.92	1.5	0.12
3	0.20	29	0.94	2	0.15
4	0.25	30	0.96	2.5	0.17
5	0.29	31	0.99	3	0.20
6	0.33	32	1.01	3.5	0.22
7	0.36	33	1.03	4	0.24
8	0.40	34	1.05	4.5	0.26
9	0.43	35	1.07	5	0.28
10	0.46	36	1.09	5.5	0.29
11	0.49	37	1.11	6	0.31
12	0.52	38	1.13	6.5	0.33
13	0.55	39	1.15	7	0.34
14	0.58	40	1.17	7.5	0.36
15	0.60	41	1.19	8	0.38
16	0.63	42	1.21	8.5	0.39
17	0.66	43	1.23	9	0.41
18	0.69	44	1.25	9.5	0.42
19	0.71	45	1.26	10	0.44
20	0.74	46	1.28		
21	0.76	47	1.30		
22	0.78	48	1.32		
23	0.81	49	1.34		
24	0.83	50	1.36		
25	0.85				

Adapted from Rosenthal RC. Chemotherapy. In: Ettinger SJ, Feldman EC, eds. *Textbook of Internal Medicine, Diseases of the Dog and Cat.* 4th Ed. Philadelphia, PA: W.B. Saunders Company; 1995, with permission.

Species variation is another important consideration in drug dosing, as each species has unique physiologic and pharmacokinetic characteristics.[10] There are many sources for animal dosing information including product labels, package inserts, and references as those cited here.[2,11]

Veterinarians specialize in small- and large-animal medicine as well as in various subspecialties, such as avian, poultry, equine, zoological medicine, and in further defined areas as anesthesiology, surgery, cardiology, radiology, oncology, and so forth.

Veterinary Pharmacy Practice

A number of pharmacists have established practice sites within veterinary clinics and hospitals and thus routinely fill the prescription and medication orders of veterinarians. Additionally, many community pharmacists have created a veterinary component to their practices and dispense both prefabricated pharmaceuticals and customized compounded preparations.

As is the case for human drugs, pharmacists are obliged to report incidents of adverse drug experiences (ADE), which occur through the use of veterinary drugs. This may be done by contacting the drug manufacturer directly or the federal FDA in the United States[12] and in Canada, Health Canada.[13] Other countries have comparable requirements.

Pharmacists who have an interest in the practice of veterinary pharmacy commonly belong to organizations as the American College of Veterinary Pharmacists (ACVP)[14] and the Society of Veterinary Hospital Pharmacists (SVHP).[15]

Special Considerations in Compounding Veterinary Pharmaceuticals

Compounded prescriptions for veterinary use have the same benefits and restrictions as do compounded prescriptions for human use. The primary benefit is the provision of a customized preparation that meets the specific needs of an animal patient (as strength, dosage form, or other feature, such as flavor) when a counterpart commercial product is unavailable. Specific restrictions and guidance for veterinary compounding may be found in the cited references.[16–19] In essence, the following apply:

- A valid veterinarian–client patient relationship must exist.
- Failure to treat may result in adverse consequences to the animal.
- The compounded prescription must meet standards of safety, effectiveness, and stability.
- No FDA-approved human or animal drug in desired dosage form and/or strength is commercially available.
- The compounded dosage form must be prepared from an FDA-approved commercially available human or animal drug.
- The product must be compounded by a licensed pharmacist upon order from a licensed veterinarian or by a veterinarian within the scope of professional practice.
- The scale of the compounding must be commensurate with the need of the individual client–patient.
- Compounded products intended for food animals must address special concerns of food safety including the avoidance of remaining tissue residues of drug, and all relevant federal and state laws relating to the compounding of drugs for use in animals must be followed including the regulations of the state Board of Pharmacy having jurisdiction.

Table 18.2 • EXAMPLES OF THERAPEUTIC AGENTS COMPOUNDED INTO CUSTOMIZED VETERINARY MEDICATIONS[a]

Drug Category	Therapeutic Agent	Customized Forms[b]
Anticonvulsant, neuropathic pain analgesic	Gabapentin	Flavored oral liquid, capsules, soft chewables
Oral antidiabetic	Acarbose	Flavored oral liquid, flavored chewable
Behavior-modifying agent	Amitriptyline HCl	Transdermal gel, flavored oral liquid, flavored chewables
Antiviral (herpes)	Acyclovir	Flavored oral liquid, ophthalmic ointment
Miotic	Demecarium bromide	Ophthalmic drops
Antiemetic	Ondansetron HCl	Flavored oral liquid, flavored chewables
Sympathomimetic	Phenylpropanolamine	Transdermal gel, capsules, flavored oral liquid, flavored chewables

[a]Source: Specialty Veterinary Compounding Pharmacy at http://www.svpmeds.net/home.html
[b]Compounded into customized dosage strengths.

Therapeutic agents commonly compounded into customized veterinary medications may be found in the cited reference,[20] with some examples from this source provided in Table 18.2.

CALCULATIONS CAPSULE

Veterinary Dosing

While most veterinary dosing parallels that for human dosing in considerations of age, weight, pathological condition, and concomitant therapy, species variation is a special consideration in the treatment of animals. In addition, there is a unique equation for the determination of the BSA in dosage calculations for dogs and cats[21]:

$$\text{BSA (m}^2) = \text{K} \times (\text{Body weight [grams]})^{2/3} \times 10^{-4}$$

where K is the constant 10.1 for dogs and 10.0 for cats.

CASE IN POINT 18.1 A pharmacist received a prescription for the drug allopurinol for a pet parakeet in the treatment of gout. The veterinarian prescribed 0.5 mg to be administered by oral drops four times a day.

The pharmacist has 100-mg tablets and a dropper that has been calibrated to deliver 20 drops/mL. The pharmacist decides to crush a tablet, mix it with a sufficient quantity of water, and make a suspension such that the pet's owner can conveniently administer the doses to the parakeet.

(a) How many milliliters of suspension should be prepared from the crushed 100-mg allopurinol tablet?

(b) How many drops should be administered to the parakeet per dose?

PRACTICE PROBLEMS

NOTE: The doses and treatments used in the following Practice Problems were derived from the referenced sources.[2,3,20–26] The prescription abbreviation "sid," meaning "once a day," finds particular application in veterinary prescriptions.

1. The drug pimobendan (VETMEDIN) is used in the treatment of CHF in dogs at a daily dose of 0.5 mg/kg. Scored, chewable tablets are commercially available containing 1.25 mg and 5 mg/tablet. Which of the following would best approximate the daily dose for a 16.5-lb dog?
   (a) one-half 5-mg tablet
   (b) two 1.25-mg tablets
   (c) two and a half 1.25-mg tablets
   (d) three 1.25-mg tablets
2. A 0.12% solution of chlorhexidine gluconate may be used as an oral cleansing solution to clean pets' teeth. Calculate the quantity of a 2% concentrate required to prepare a pint of the diluted solution.
3. Albuterol sulfate is administered orally to horses for bronchospasm at a dose of 8 mcg/kg. Calculate the number of milliliters of a 0.083% solution of albuterol sulfate to administer to a 900-lb horse.
4.[22] A veterinarian writes a prescription for metronidazole, 20 mg/kg, for a 1100-lb horse to be administered every 8 hours for 10 days. The pharmacist has 250-mg metronidazole tablets. How many tablets should be (a) administered per dose and (b) dispensed?
5. What fraction of a 50-mg aspirin suppository should be administered as an antipyretic to a 5.5-lb cat if the veterinary dose is 10 mg/kg?
6. The dose of methotrexate sodium for neoplastic disease in cats is 2.5 mg/m^2 PO twice weekly. If a 2-kg cat is determined to have a BSA of 0.15 m^2, calculate the single dose.
7. Phenylbutazone, an anti-inflammatory agent, may be administered to horses by intravenous injection at an average dose of 1.5 g/450 kg for 5 consecutive days. The usual injection contains phenylbutazone 200 mg/mL. How many milliliters of injection would be required in treating a 990-lb horse?
8.[22] How many milliliters of a gentamicin injection, 100 mg/mL, should be administered to a 1250-lb horse for a dose of 6.6 mg/kg?
9. The maximum dose of doxorubicin in canine chemotherapy is 200 mg/m^2. Using Table 18.1, calculate the maximum dose for a dog weighing 20 kg.
10. Furosemide in the treatment of CHF in animals is used as a maintenance dose of 0.5 mg/kg sid. Calculate the dose for a 15-lb dog.
11. Which strength tablets of enalapril maleate (ENACARD) would be most convenient to dispense in the treatment of an 11-lb dog at a daily dose of 0.5 mg/kg?
    (a) 1-mg tablets
    (b) 2.5-mg tablets
    (c) 5-mg tablets
    (d) 10-mg tablets
    (e) 20-mg tablets
12. The dose of digoxin in dogs is 0.005 to 0.01 mg/kg PO. Calculate the dosage range for a dog weighing 15 lb

13. For large dogs, the dose of digoxin is 0.22 mg/m^2. Using Table 18.1, calculate the dose for a dog weighing 22 kg.
14. A cockatiel may be given 6 mg of ketamine intramuscularly for anesthesia. Calculate the dose, on a mg/kg basis, for an 85-g cockatiel.
15. Some veterinarians treat seizures in dogs with potassium bromide, administering a loading dose of 90 mg/kg/day for 5 days concurrently with a maintenance dose of 30 mg/kg/day, the latter continued after the initial 5-day period. Calculate (a) the daily dose (each day for days 1 to 5) for a 12-lb dog, (b) the maintenance dose, (c) the quantity of potassium bromide needed to prepare one pint of a solution containing 250 mg of potassium bromide per milliliter, and (d) the number of milliliters of the solution needed to provide the maintenance dose.
16.[22] A veterinarian is treating a 66-lb dog for ascarids with fenbendazole, 50 mg/kg/day orally for 3 days. How many milliliters of a 10% w/v suspension of fenbendazole should the pharmacist dispense?
17.[23] Cimetidine may be administered in the treatment of feline stomatitis at a dose of 5 to 10 mg/kg by mouth every 6 to 8 hours. Calculate (a) the dosage range for a cat weighing 9.4 lb and (b) the corresponding dosage range for an oral solution containing cimetidine, 300 mg/5 mL.
18. The product label for CONVENIA (cefovecin sodium) includes the following information:
    - Reconstitute with 10 mL of sterile water for injection.
    - Reconstituted product contains 80 mg/mL.
    - Dose for dogs and cats = 3.6 mg/lb administered subcutaneously
    - Minimum pet age for use is 4 months.

    Calculate the dose in milligrams of cefovecin sodium and the corresponding milliliters of CONVENIA for animals weighing the following:
    (a) 5.5 lb
    (b) 2.3 kg
    (c) 15 lb
    (d) 15 kg
19. ANTIROBE AQUADROPS contain in each milliliter clindamycin hydrochloride equivalent to 25 mg of clindamycin. The medication is used in cats and dogs to treat infections. If a 3-kg dog is treated every 12 hours for 10 days at a dose of 10 mg clindamycin/lb, how many 20-mL bottles of medication should be dispensed?
20. A pharmacist wishes to compound a topical aerosol spray to treat abraded skin lesions in dogs. The spray is to deliver 0.4 mg of gentamicin sulfate and 0.2 mg of betamethasone valerate in each 0.7 mL of spray. Calculate the quantity, in milligrams, of each drug to use in preparation of a 50-mL container of the preparation.

CALCQUIZ

18.A. Actinomycin is one of the chemotherapeutic agents used in veterinary medicine. The dose used is generally 0.7 to 1 mg/m^2 intravenously every 2 to 3 weeks. The drug is available as a lyophilized powder, 500 μg per vial, for reconstitution with sterile water for injection prior to use.

(a) Using the information in this chapter for conversion of weight to body surface area, and a 0.85 mg/m^2 dose of actinomycin, calculate the dose, in milligrams, for a 33-lb dog.

(b) If the drug in the vial results in a drug concentration of 0.5 mg/mL when reconstituted, calculate the volume of injection prepared.

(c) Calculate the dose of injection, in milliliters, applicable to the dog described in (a).

18.B.[24] Amlodipine besylate, an antihypertensive agent, has been administered orally to cats at a once-daily dose of 0.625 mg by the formula:

℞	Amlodipine besylate	100 mg
	Fish flavor, qs	
	Cod liver oil, ad	100 mL

Calculate the daily dose of amlodipine besylate for a 5.5-lb cat on the basis of:

(a) mg/kg

(b) mg/BSA in m^2

(c) milliliters of prescription

18.C.[25] A method of producing intravenous anesthesia in large animals utilizes an intravenous injection of diazepam (0.05 to 0.1 mg/kg) immediately prior to an intravenous infusion of the following:

Ketamine	2.2 mg/kg
Xylazine	500 mg
Guaifenesin	5%
D5W, ad	1000 mL

The infusion is administered at a rate of 1 mL/kg/h.

For a horse weighing 980 lb, calculate:

(a) The dosage range for diazepam

(b) The quantity of ketamine, in milligrams, to use in the infusion

(c) The quantity of xylazine administered in milligrams per minute

(d) The quantity, in milliliters, of infusion remaining after 60 minutes

18.D.[26] Captopril is used in dogs to treat hypertension and congestive heart failure at an initial dose of 1 mg/kg orally, three times daily. The pharmacist plans to prepare a 30-day supply of a suspension for a 12-lb dog such that a teaspoonful provides each dose. The source of captopril is 50-mg tablets.

(a) How many milligrams of captopril are required?

(b) How many milliliters of suspension are required?

(c) How many whole captopril tablets are required?

(d) If the required tablets are crushed and weigh a total of 1.2 g, what weight of the powder would be used in the suspension?

ANSWERS TO "CASE IN POINT" AND PRACTICE PROBLEMS

Case in Point 18.1

(a) For the pet owner's convenience, the pharmacist arbitrarily decided that the 0.5-mg dose of allopurinol should be contained in each drop of the suspension. Working backward in the calculation:

$$\frac{0.5\text{ mg}}{1\text{ drop}} = \frac{\text{x mg}}{20\text{ drops}} \quad \text{x} = 10\text{ mg}$$

allopurinol (in 20 drops or 1 mL)

$$\text{then, } \frac{10\text{ mg}}{1\text{ mL}} = \frac{100\text{ mg (tablet)}}{\text{x mL}}$$

$$\text{x} = 10\text{ mL suspension}$$

(b) 1 drop/dose (predetermined)

Practice Problems

1. (d) Three 1.25-mg tablets pimobendan
2. 28.4 mL chlorhexidine gluconate concentrate
3. 3.94 mL albuterol sulfate solution
4. (a) 40 metronidazole tablets
   (b) 1200 metronidazole tablets
5. ½ aspirin suppository
6. 0.375 mg methotrexate sodium
7. 37.5-mL phenylbutazone injection
8. 37.5-mL gentamicin injection
9. 148 mg doxorubicin
10. 3.4 mg furosemide
11. (b) 2.5-mg enalapril maleate tablets
12. 0.034 to 0.06 mg digoxin
13. 0.17 mg digoxin
14. 70.6 mg/kg ketamine
15. (a) 655 mg
    (b) 164 mg
    (c) 118.25 g potassium bromide
    (d) 0.66 mL
16. 45 mL fenbendazole
17. (a) 21.36 to 42.73 mg cimetidine
    (b) 0.36 to 0.71 mL
18. (a) 19.8 mg cefovecin sodium and 0.25 mL CONVENIA
    (b) 18.2 mg cefovecin sodium and 0.23 mL CONVENIA
    (c) 54 mg cefovecin sodium and 0.68 mL CONVENIA
    (d) 118.8 mg cefovecin sodium and 1.49 mL CONVENIA
19. 3 bottles of ANTIROBE AQUADROPS
20. 28.6 mg gentamicin sulfate and 14.3 mg betamethasone valerate

References

1. Kahn CM, Editor. *The Merck Veterinary Manual.* 10th Ed. Whitehouse Station, NJ: Merck Sharp & Dohme; 2010.
2. Plumb DC. *Plumb's Veterinary Drug Handbook.* 8th Ed. Hoboken, NJ: Wiley-Blackwell; 2015.
3. Drugs.com. *Veterinary Product Database.* Available at: http://www.drugs.com/vet/. Accessed October 14, 2014.
4. U.S. Food and Drug Administration. *Animal Drug Applications.* Available at: http://www.accessdata.fda.gov/scripts/cdrh/cfdocs/cfcfr/CFRSearch.cfm?CFRPart=514. 4. Accessed October 20, 2014.
5. Center for Veterinary Medicine, Food and Drug Administration. Available at: http://www.fda.gov/AboutFDA/CentersOffices/CVM/default.htm. Accessed October 20, 2014.

6. Food and Drug Administration, Health and Human Services. Extralabel drug use in animals. Federal Register. 1996;61:57731–57746.
7. U.S. Food and Drug Administration. The Ins and Outs of Extra-Label Drug Use in Animals: A Resource for Veterinarians. Available at: http://www.fda.gov/animalveterinary/resourcesforyou/ucm380135.htm. Accessed October 20, 2014.
8. Allen LV, Jr, ed. Animal drug delivery systems. *International Journal of Pharmaceutical Compounding* 1997;1:229. Adapted from: Blodinger J. *Formulation of Veterinary Dosage Forms*. New York: Marcel Dekker; 1983.
9. Current Results. Available at: http://www.currentresults.com/Environment-Facts/Plants-Animals/number-species.php. Accessed October 14, 2014.
10. Allen LV, Jr, ed. Compounding for veterinary patients: pharmaceutical, biopharmaceutical, and physiologic considerations. *International Journal of Pharmaceutical Compounding* 1997;1:233–234. Adapted from: Blodinger J. *Formulation of Veterinary Dosage Forms*. New York: Marcel Dekker; 1983.
11. Veterinary Product Database. Available at: http://www.drugs.com/vet/. Accessed October 10, 2014.
12. Veterinary Adverse Event Voluntary Reporting. Available at: http://www.fda.gov/AnimalVeterinary/SafetyHealth/ReportaProblem/ucm055305.htm. Accessed October 14, 2014.
13. Health Canada. Available at: http://clf2-nsi2.hc-sc.gc.ca/dhp-mps/vet/index-eng.php. Accessed October 14, 2014.
14. American College of Veterinary Pharmacists (ACVP). Available at: http://acavetmeds.acainfo.org/. Accessed October 14, 2014.
15. Society of Veterinary Hospital Pharmacists (SVHP). Available at: http://svhp.org/svhp/. Accessed October 14, 2014.
16. Lust E. Compounding for animal patients: contemporary issues. *Journal of the American Pharmacists Association* 2004;44:375–386.
17. Veterinary Compounding. Available at: http://avda.net/newsletter/0704/compounding.pdf Accessed October 15, 2014.
18. Compounding. The American Veterinary Medical Association. Available at: https://www.avma.org/KB/Resources/Reference/Pages/Compounding.aspx. Accessed October 15, 2014.
19. The Society of Veterinary Hospital Pharmacists Position on Compounding Drugs for Use in Animals. Available at: http://www.lawofcompoundingmedications.com/2012/06/society-of-veterinary-hospital.htm. Accessed October 15, 2014.
20. Specialty Veterinary Compounding Pharmacy. Available at: http://www.svpmeds.net/home.html. Accessed October 15, 2014.
21. Rosenthal RC. Chemotherapy. In: Ettinger SJ, Feldman EC, eds. *Textbook of Internal Medicine, Diseases of the Dog and Cat*. 4th Ed. Philadelphia, PA: W.B. Saunders; 1995.
22. Lindell H. *Veterinary Teaching Hospital Pharmacy*. Athens, GA: University of Georgia.
23. Stockton SJ. Calculations. *International Journal of Pharmaceutical Compounding* 2010;14:419.
24. Allen LV Jr. *Editor-in-Chief. International Journal of Pharmaceutical Compounding* 2009;13:429.
25. Davidson G. Equine anesthesia: TRIPLE DRIP. *International Journal of Pharmaceutical Compounding* 2008;5:402.
26. Prince SJ. Calculations. *International Journal of Pharmaceutical Compounding* 1999;3:234.

19

Selected Calculations Associated with Plant Extractives

OBJECTIVES

Upon successful completion of this chapter, the student will be able to:

- Calculate the difference in drug content between botanic *extracts, fluidextracts, and tinctures.*
- Perform dosage calculations based on the drug content of extracted botanicals.

The public has demonstrated an ever-expanding interest in the use of herbal remedies and other dietary supplements as a part of *alternative medicine* or *complementary medicine* therapies.[a,b] Many of the herbal remedies used have their origins in *traditional or cultural medicine* and have not been studied by rigorous scientific methods. However, a systematic effort is presently underway in the United States and in other countries to study and establish the health benefits and risks associated with the use of herbal remedies and to develop reliable quality standards. It should be borne in mind that the effects of herbal remedies are due to their content of pharmacologically active components, which are usually alkaloids, glycosides, or other complex organic molecules.

The *United States Pharmacopeia–National Formulary* includes monographs, general tests, assays, and standards for botanical drugs. Included among them are currently popular herbals as echinacea, ginkgo, ginseng, Saint John's wort, saw palmetto, and valerian. The USP also publishes the *Herbal Medicines Compendium* and the *Dietary Supplements Compendium*.[2–4]

Dosage forms, as tablets and capsules, may be prepared directly from cleaned, dried, and pulverized plant parts (e.g., leaves). Other products are prepared by *extraction*—that is, by the removal of desired constituents from plant materials through the use of select solvents. The plant materials, termed *crude drugs*, may be seeds, leaves, bark, and/or other plant parts known to contain the desired active constituents.

The process of extraction has two components, *maceration* and *percolation*. The term *maceration* comes from the Latin *macerare*, meaning "to soak." By this process, ground crude drug is placed in a suitable vessel and allowed to soak in a solvent or mixture of solvents, termed the *menstruum*, for a sufficient period of time in order to soften the botanic material and allow the extraction of the soluble constituents. The menstruum is selected based on the solubility of the desired constituents. Hydroalcoholic mixtures commonly are employed. The dissolved constituents are separated from the exhausted crude drug by straining or filtration.

The term *percolation* is derived from the Latin *per*, meaning "through," and *colare*, meaning "to strain." By this process, ground crude drug is extracted of its soluble constituents by the slow passage of a menstruum through a column of the botanic material.

---

[a] The FDA defines a dietary supplement as *a product intended for ingestion that contains a "dietary ingredient" intended to add further nutritional value to the diet. A "dietary ingredient" may be one or any combination of the following substances: a vitamin, a mineral, an herb or other botanical, an amino acid, or a concentrate, metabolite, or extract.*[1]

[b] The *Authors' Extra Point* at the end of this chapter defines *alternative and complementary medicine.*

The crude drug is carefully packed in an extraction apparatus, termed a *percolator*, and allowed to macerate for a prescribed period of time prior to percolation. Percolators are of various sizes and construction. Small glass percolators for laboratory use are cone or cylindrical shaped, several inches in diameter, and about 12 inches in height. Percolators for industrial use are generally constructed of stainless steel and measure about 8 feet in diameter and 12 to 18 feet in height. An orifice at the bottom of a percolator permits the convenient removal of the extractive, termed the *percolate*.

The primary dosage forms of plant extractives are *extracts, fluidextracts, and tinctures*, as defined below. In some instances, the active therapeutic ingredients (ATIs) are isolated from the extractive, then purified and assayed, and used as the therapeutic component in manufactured dosage forms. Chemical replicas of the active therapeutic components of plants are oftentimes synthesized and used in the same manner as the naturally occurring agent.

Extracts, Fluidextracts, and Tinctures[a]

Extracts are concentrated preparations of vegetable (or animal) drugs. Most extracts are prepared by percolation followed by the evaporation of all or nearly all the menstruum, yielding a powdered or ointment-like product of extracted drug in concentrated form. On a weight-for-weight basis, extracts commonly are two to six times as potent as their crude drug source. In other words, 1 g of extract may be equivalent in active constituents to 2 to 6 g of the crude drug. Thus, an extract may be described as a "2×" (or other multiple) or as a "200%" (or other %) extract.

Fluidextracts are liquid extractives of plant materials adjusted for drug content so that each milliliter of fluidextract is equivalent in constituents to 1 g of the crude drug from which it is derived.

Botanic *tinctures* are alcoholic or hydroalcoholic solutions of plant extractives, and although there is no set strength for tinctures, the following quantities of crude drug have traditionally been used in the preparation of each 100 mL of tincture:

Potent drug (e.g., belladonna leaf)	10 g crude drug
Nonpotent drug (e.g., tolu balsam)	20 g crude drug
Fruit/flavor (e.g., sweet orange peel)	50 g crude drug

The relative strengths of extracts, fluidextracts, and tinctures are depicted in Figure 19.1, which shows an example of the quantity of each that may be prepared from the same quantity of crude drug. In terms of equivalency:

100 g =	100 mL =	25 g =	1000 mL
crude drug	fluidextract	"400%" extract	"potent drug" tincture

Examples of calculations pertaining to plant extractives are as follows.

Example Calculations of Extracted Botanicals

(1) *If 1 mg of active ingredient (AI) is present in each gram of a crude drug, determine the concentration, in mg/g or mg/mL, of AI in the corresponding (a) fluidextract, (b) "400%" extract, and (c) potent tincture.*

---

[a]The definitions and concentrations of extracts, fluidextracts, and tinctures described in this section conform with traditional pharmacy practice and USP-NF standards. Commercial herbal remedies available in the marketplace may meet these standards and be so labeled, or they may differ.

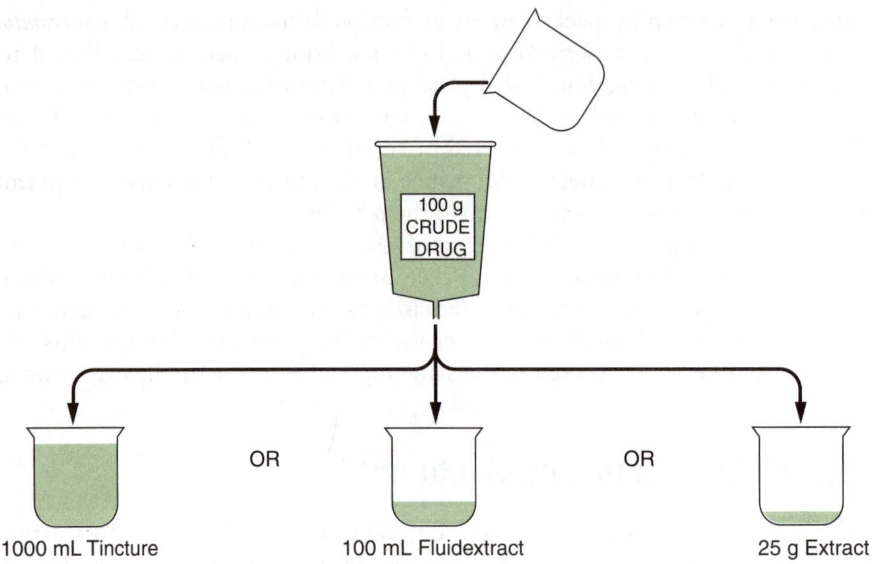

FIGURE 19.1 • Depiction of the relative concentrations of a potent tincture, a fluidextract, and an extract using as the example a "10%" tincture and a "400%" extract (see text for further explanation).

(a) Since, by definition, 1 mL of fluidextract is equivalent in active ingredient to 1 g of crude drug, 1 mg of active ingredient would be present in 1 mL of fluidextract.

1 mg AI/mL fluidextract

(b) A "400%" extract represents, in each gram, 4 g of crude drug. Thus:

$$\frac{1\text{ g crude drug}}{4\text{ g crude drug}} = \frac{1\text{ mg AI}}{x\text{ mg AI}};\ x = \mathbf{4\ mg\ AI/g\ extract}$$

(c) Since a "potent tincture" represents in each 100 mL, the AI from 10 g of crude drug, 0.1 g of crude drug would be needed to prepare 1 mL of tincture. Thus:

$$\frac{1\text{ g crude drug}}{0.1\text{ g crude drug}} = \frac{1\text{ mg AI}}{x\text{ mg AI}};\ x = \mathbf{0.1\ mg\ AI/mL\ tincture}$$

(2) *If the dose of belladonna tincture is 0.6 mL, determine the equivalent corresponding dose of (a) belladonna leaf, (b) belladonna fluidextract, and (c) an extract (400%) of belladonna.*

(a) Since a potent tincture contains in each 100 mL, the AI from 10 g of crude drug is:

$$\frac{100\text{ mL tr.}}{0.6\text{ mL tr.}} = \frac{10\text{ g crude drug}}{x\text{ g crude drug}};\ x = \mathbf{0.06\ g}$$

(b) Since 1 mL of fluidextract contains the AI from 1 g of crude drug:

$$\frac{1\text{ g crude drug}}{0.06\text{ g crude drug}} = \frac{1\text{ mL fluidextract}}{x\text{ mL fluidextract}};\ x = \mathbf{0.06\ mL\ fluidextract}$$

Or since a fluidextract is 10 times as concentrated as a potent tincture, its dose would be $\frac{1}{10}$ that of a corresponding tincture:

$$\tfrac{1}{10}\text{ of }0.6\text{ mL} = \mathbf{0.06\ mL}$$

(c) Since a "400%" extract has four times the AI content as the crude drug, and since the dose of the crude drug as calculated above is 0.06 g, the dose of the extract would be ¼ of that dose:

$$0.06 \text{ g} \times 1/4 = 0.015 \text{ g or } \mathbf{15\ mg}$$

CASE IN POINT 19.1 An industrial pharmacist is charged with preparing a "400%" extract of cascara sagrada from 100 kg of crude drug.

(a) How many kilograms of the extract would be expected to be prepared?
(b) If the crude drug is assayed to contain 11% hydroxyanthracenes, what would be the expected percentage strength of the resultant extract?

Herbal Standards

An example of a descriptive portion of a monograph for a herbal agent is:

"St. John's Wort consists of the dried flowering tops or aerial parts of Hypericum perforatum Linné (Fam. Hypericaceae), gathered shortly before or during flowering. It contains not less than 0.04 percent of the combined total of hypericin ($C_{30}H_{16}O_8$) and pseudohypericin ($C_{30}H_{16}O_9$) and not less than 0.6 percent of hyperforin ($C_{35}H_{52}O_4$)."[2]

Examples of standards for active constituents in some herbal drugs are[2–4]:

Asian ginseng, powdered	NLT 0.3% ginsenosides
American ginseng, powdered	NLT 4% ginsenosides
Black cohosh	NLT 0.4% triterpene glycosides
Echinacea pallida	NLT 0.5% caftaric acid, chicoric acid, chlorogenic acid, and echinacoside
Eleuthero	NLT 0.08% eleutheroside B and eleutheroside E
Ginkgo extract, powdered	NLT 5.4% and NMT 12% terpene lactones, and NLT 22% and NMT 27% flavonol glycosides
Milk thistle extract, powdered	NLT 20% and NMT 45% silydianin and silychristin
Garlic	NLT 0.5% alliin
Goldenseal	NLT 2% hydrastine NLT 2.5% berberine
Saint John's wort	NLT 0.3% hypericin extract
Valerian	NLT 0.17% valeric acids

Example Calculations of Herbals

(1) *A batch of garlic is determined to contain 10 mg of allicin in a 4-g sample. How many micrograms of allicin would be present in a 500-mg dose of garlic from this batch?*

$$10 \text{ mg} = 10{,}000 \ \mu\text{g}$$

$$500 \text{ mg} = 0.5 \text{ g}$$

$$\frac{4 \text{ g}}{0.5 \text{ g}} = \frac{10{,}000 \ \mu g}{x \ \mu g};\ x = \mathbf{1250\ \mu g}$$

(2) *The herb feverfew, when standardized as a powdered leaf, contains 0.2% of the agent parthenolide. How many milligrams of parthenolide would be present in a capsule containing 125 mg of powdered feverfew?*

$$125 \text{ mg} \times 0.2\% = \mathbf{0.25 \text{ mg}}$$

PRACTICE PROBLEMS

1. How many milliliters of a fluidextract would be equivalent in active ingredient to the following?
   (a) 10 g of crude drug
   (b) 10 mL of a "potent" tincture
   (c) 10 g of a "300%" extract
2. How many milliliters of a "potent" tincture may be prepared from the following?
   (a) 10 mL of a fluidextract
   (b) 10 g of a "400%" extract
   (c) 10 g of a "2×" extract
3. Cascara sagrada bark contains 7% of hydroxyanthracene derivatives, whereas the cascara sagrada extract contains 11 g of hydroxyanthracene derivatives in each 100 g. Calculate the "%" of the extract relative to the crude drug (e.g., "250%").
4. How many milliliters of a cascara sagrada fluidextract can be prepared from a pound of cascara sagrada bark?
5. Powdered opium contains 10.25% of anhydrous morphine. How many grams of powdered opium should be used to prepare 100 mL of opium tincture, which contains 10 mg/mL of anhydrous morphine?
6. If senna leaves contain 25 mg of sennosides per gram of leaves, how many milligrams of sennosides would be contained in a formula for 1000 mL of a senna syrup that contains 250 mL of senna fluidextract?
7. SENOKOT syrup, a laxative, contains 1.7 mg standardized sennosides per milliliter. The maximum adult dose is 15 mL twice daily. How many milligrams of sennosides would a patient receive by taking the maximum dose?
8. If ginkgo biloba contains 24% of ginkgo heterosides, and if 120 mg are taken daily in three divided doses, how many milligrams of the ginkgo heterosides are contained in each of the divided doses?
9. If a milk thistle sample contains 35% of silymarin, how many milligrams of this substance are contained in a 200-mg dose of milk thistle?
10. If Saint John's wort is standardized to contain 0.3% of hypericin extract, how many milligrams of the extract would be taken daily when Saint John's wort is administered as a 300-mg capsule taken three times a day?
11. If valerian extract contains 0.8% valeric acid, how many milligrams of valeric acid would be contained in each 300-mg dose of valerian extract?
12. The USP-NF states that "Powdered Asian Ginseng Extract is prepared from Asian Ginseng by maceration, percolation, or both processes performed at room temperature with suitable solvents such as alcohol, methanol, water, or mixtures of these solvents, and by concentrating the fluidextract. It contains not less than 3.0 percent of ginsenosides."[1] Using the information in this chapter, characterize the concentration of this extract in terms of a multiple (as "__ ×") compared to the powdered crude drug.
13. If the dose of the extract described in the previous problem is 200 mg, what would be the approximate comparable dose of the fluidextract in milliliters?

14. If black cohosh extract contains 2.5% triterpene glycosides, calculate the concentration of the extract, in %, compared to the crude drug. Use the information in this chapter as needed.
15. If the dose of black cohosh is 40 mg, calculate the comparable dose of the extract described in problem 14. Use the information in this chapter as needed.
16. If goldenseal root has a dose of 500 mg and contains 2% of the active constituent hydrastine, what would be the expected percent concentration of hydrastine in goldenseal root extract, which has a dose of 30 mg?
17. The USP-NF states that "Tomato Extract produced from the pulp of ripe fruits of *Lycopersicon esculentum* contains not less than 4.7 percent and not more than 12.0 percent of lycopene ($C_{40}H_{56}$)." Calculate the quantity of lycopene, as a range, in milligrams, in each gram of extract.

CALCQUIZ

19.A.[5] Belladonna and opium rectal suppositories each weigh 2 g and contain 16.2 mg of powdered belladonna extract and 30 mg of powdered opium.

(a) If powdered belladonna extract contains, in each 100 g, between 1.15 and 1.35 g of the alkaloids of belladonna leaf, calculate the range of alkaloids in each suppository.

(b) Calculate the average percent concentration of belladonna alkaloids in the suppositories.

(c) If the powdered opium used in preparing the suppositories contained 10.25% w/w of anhydrous morphine, calculate the percent strength of anhydrous morphine in the suppositories.

ANSWERS TO "CASE IN POINT" AND PRACTICE PROBLEMS

Case in Point 19.1

By definition, a 400% extract represents four times the potency of the corresponding crude drug. Thus:

(a) 100 kg ÷ 4 = 25 kg extract
(b) 11% × 4 = 44% hydroxyanthracenes

Practice Problems

1. (a) 10 mL
   (b) 1 mL
   (c) 30 mL
2. (a) 100 mL
   (b) 400 mL
   (b) 200 mL
3. "157%" extract
4. 454 mL cascara sagrada fluidextract
5. 9.76 g powdered opium
6. 6250 mg sennosides
7. 51 mg sennosides
8. 9.6 mg ginkgo heterosides
9. 70 mg silymarin
10. 2.7 mg hypericin
11. 2.4 mg valeric acid
12. 10×
13. 0.02 mL Asian ginseng fluidextract
14. 625%
15. 6.4 mg black cohosh extract
16. 33.3% hydrastine
17. 47 to 120 mg lycopene

AUTHORS' EXTRA POINT

ALTERNATIVE/COMPLEMENTARY MEDICINE

Alternative medicine refers to healing practices that are *not* based on the scientific method of conventional medicine. It includes *traditional medicine* practices such as homeopathy, herbal medicine, naturopathy, traditional Chinese medicine, techniques as acupuncture, qigong, tai chi, yoga, and other physical, mental, spiritual, and mind–body therapies.[a,b] *Complementary or integrative medicine* is alternative medicine used together with conventional medicine.

In the United States, the National Center for Complementary and Alternative Medicine (NCCAM), part of the National Institutes of Health within the U.S. Department of Health and Human Services, is the lead agency for scientific research and evidence-based information on the usefulness and safety of complementary and alternative medicine. Many other countries have similar agencies. To assist all countries, the World Health Organization has developed a strategic framework to make traditional or complementary/alternative medicine use safer, more accessible, and sustainable.[c]

The expanded use of herbal remedies in alternative and complementary medicine has made essential the need to establish quality standards. In 2013, the United States Pharmacopeial Convention (USP) introduced the online resource, the *Herbal Medicines Compendium (HMC)*, to provide standards of ingredient identity, strength, quality, and purity for the herbal ingredients used in herbal medicines.[d] And since the USP is accepted for its standards in over 140 countries, the impact of this effort is global. The USP also publishes the *USP Dietary Supplements Compendium (DSC)*, which contains nearly 800 monographs and specifications for dietary supplements, dietary ingredients, and other components of dietary supplements.[e,f]

To assist consumers and health professionals, MedlinePlus, a service of the U.S. National Library of Medicine National Institutes of Health, provides an online database of some 400 dietary supplements and herbal remedies, which contains for each item, information on the scientific basis for use, common side effects, important cautions, and a useful listing of cited references.[g]

[a] http://en.wikipedia.org/wiki/Alternative_medicine

[b] WHO Traditional Medicine Strategy for 2014–2023. Available at http: //www.who.int/medicines/publications/traditional/trm_strategy14_23/en/

[c] National Center for Complementary and Alternative Medicine (NCCAM). Available at http://nccam.nih.gov/

[d] *Herbal Medicines Compendium*. Available at https://hmc.usp.org/homepage?destination=homepage

[e] *USP Dietary Supplements Compendium*. Available at http://www.usp.org/dietary-supplements/compendium

[f] The "USP Verified Mark," the symbol awarded by USP to dietary supplement products that meet the stringent criteria of its voluntary Dietary Supplement Verification program, has appeared on more than 400 million supplement labels

[g] Herbs and Supplements. MedlinePlus. U.S. National Library of Medicine, National Institutes of Health. Available at http://www.nlm.nih.gov/medlineplus/druginfo/herb_All.html

References

1. U.S. Food and Drug Administration. What is a dietary supplement? Available at: http://www.fda.gov/AboutFDA/Transparency/Basics/ucm195635.htm. Accessed November 10, 2014.
2. *The United States Pharmacopeia–National Formulary (USP–NF)*. Available at: http://www.usp.org/usp-nf/official-text. Accessed November 6, 2014.
3. *Herbal Medicines Compendium*. Available at: https://hmc.usp.org/. Accessed November 6, 2014.
4. *USP Dietary Supplements Compendium*. Available at: http://www.usp.org/dietary-supplements/dietary-supplements-compendium. Accessed November 6, 2014.
5. Stockton SJ. Calculations. *International Journal of Pharmaceutical Compounding* 2010;14:230.

20

Calculation of Active Drug Moiety

OBJECTIVES

Upon successful completion of this chapter, the student will be able to:

- Calculate the active drug moiety portion of a chemical compound.
- Perform pharmaceutical calculations involving active drug moiety.

Pharmaceutical companies often create salt, ester, or other complex chemical forms of a drug substance in order to facilitate its solubility, biological absorption, or other desired physical–chemical or clinical characteristics. However, it is the active drug moiety portion of a drug compound that is responsible for its pharmacologic effects.

Some commercial drug products that are prepared into salt or other forms are labeled to indicate the equivalent content of active drug moiety, for example[1]:

PROAIR HFA Inhalation Aerosol: *Each actuation delivers120 mcg of albuterol sulfate, equivalent to 90 mcg of albuterol base.*

COSOPT PF Ophthalmic Solution: *Each mL contains 20 mg dorzolamide, equivalent to 22.26 mg of dorzolamide hydrochloride.*

BACTROBAN CREAM: *Contains 2.15% w/w mupirocin calcium, equivalent to 2.0% w/w mupirocin free acid.*

When not provided in product labeling, the content of active drug moiety may be calculated.

Example Calculations of Active Drug Moiety

To calculate the active drug moiety portion of a drug compound, the following equation may be used:

$$\frac{\text{Drug moiety (g/mole)}}{\text{Drug compound (g/mole)}} = \text{Drug moiety (fraction)}$$

NOTE: A Table of Atomic Weights is included at the back of this book for reference.

(1) *The chemical formula of fluoxetine HCl (PROZAC) is $C_{17}H_{18}F_3NO \cdot HCl$.*

(a) *Calculate the molecular weights of the base and salt forms.*

$$\begin{aligned} C_{17} &= (17 \times 12.01) = 204.17 \\ H_{18} &= (18 \times 1.00) = 18.00 \\ F_3 &= (3 \times 19.00) = 57.00 \\ N &= (1 \times 14.01) = 14.01 \\ O &= (1 \times 16.00) = \underline{16.00} \\ & \qquad \textbf{309.18, m.w., fluoxetine base} \end{aligned}$$

$$H = (1 \times 1.00) = 1.00$$
$$Cl = (1 \times 35.45) = \underline{35.45}$$
$$\mathbf{345.63, \text{ m.w., fluoxetine salt}}$$

(b) *Calculate the fraction of the fluoxetine base (active moiety) in the compound.*

$$\frac{309.18\ (\text{g/mole})}{345.63\ (\text{g/mole})} = \mathbf{0.895, \text{ fraction of fluoxetine base}}$$

(c) *Calculate the percent of fluoxetine base (active moiety) in the compound.*

$$0.895 \times 100\% = \mathbf{89.5\% \text{ fluoxetine base}}$$

(d) *Calculate the quantity of fluoxetine in a 10-mg dose of fluoxetine hydrochloride.*

$$10 \text{ mg} \times 89.5\% = \mathbf{8.95 \text{ mg fluoxetine}}$$

(e) *Calculate the quantity of fluoxetine hydrochloride needed to supply a 10-mg dose of fluoxetine.*

$$\frac{10 \text{ mg} \times 345.63\ (\text{g/mole})}{309.18\ (\text{g/mole})} = \mathbf{11.18 \text{ mg fluoxetine hydrochloride}}$$

(2) *Each "25-mg" tablet of JANUVIA contains 32.13 mg of sitagliptin phosphate monohydrate equivalent to 25 mg of sitagliptin base. If sitagliptin phosphate monohydrate has a molecular weight of 523.32, calculate the molecular weight of sitagliptin base.*

$$\frac{25 \text{ mg} \times 523.32}{32.13 \text{ mg}} = \mathbf{407.19, \text{ m.w., sitagliptin}}$$

(3) *What is the percentage strength of methadone (m.w. 309.4) in a solution containing 10 mg of methadone hydrochloride (m.w. 345.9) in each milliliter?*

$$\frac{10 \text{ mg} \times 309.4 \text{ g/mole}}{345.9 \text{ g/mole}} = 8.9 \text{ mg methadone}$$

$$8.9 \text{ mg} = 0.0089 \text{ g}$$

$$0.0089 \text{ g/1 mL} \times 100 = 0.89 \text{ g/100 mL} = \mathbf{0.89\% \text{ methadone}}$$

CASE IN POINT 20.1[a] A pediatrician wishes to prescribe the drug metronidazole (m.w. 171) for a pediatric patient in the oral treatment of amebiasis. The patient is unable to swallow solid dosage forms, and an oral suspension of the drug would be extremely bitter. An alternative would be for the pharmacist to compound an oral suspension using metronidazole benzoate (m.w. 275), which has a low water solubility and thus little taste.

If the pediatric dosage range of metronidazole in the treatment of amebiasis is 35 to 50 mg/kg/day, calculate the dosage range of metronidazole benzoate.

[a]Problem courtesy of Warren Beach, Pharmaceutical and Biomedical Sciences, College of Pharmacy, University of Georgia, Athens, GA.

PRACTICE PROBLEMS

1. If a prescription calls for the preparation of 30 mL of a 1% solution of lidocaine (m.w. 234), but for the purposes of solubility the pharmacist used lidocaine hydrochloride (m.w. 288), how many milligrams of the latter should be used?
2. Oral tablets of tofacitinib citrate (XELJANZ) are available, each containing the equivalent of 5 mg of tofacitinib. If the molecular weight of tofacitinib is 315.5 and that of tofacitinib citrate is 504.5, calculate its quantity in each tablet.
3. The molecular weight of mupirocin is 500.6. The product labeling for BACTROBAN CREAM states a content of 2.0% mupirocin (free acid), based on the actual content of mupirocin calcium. If there are two molecules of mupirocin for each calcium and two waters of hydration in the salt form, calculate the percent concentration of mupirocin calcium in the cream.
4. Each 0.5 mL of IMITREX injection contains 4 mg of sumatriptan base (m.w. 295.4) as the succinate salt (m.w. 413.5). Calculate the quantity of sumatriptan succinate per milliliter of injection.
5. LOTRISONE CREAM contains, in each gram, 0.643 mg of betamethasone dipropionate (m.w. 504.6) equivalent to 0.5 mg of betamethasone. Calculate the molecular weight of betamethasone base and its percent concentration in the cream.
6. How many grams of epinephrine bitartrate (m.w. 333) should be used in preparing 500 mL of an ophthalmic solution containing the equivalent of 2% of epinephrine (m.w. 183)?
7. From the molecular weight (385.8) of ciprofloxacin hydrochloride, $C_{17}H_{18}FN_3O_3 \cdot HCl \cdot H_2O$, calculate the molecular weight of ciprofloxacin base.
8. If 600 mg of glucosamine hydrochloride is equivalent to 500 mg of glucosamine (m.w. 179.2), calculate the molecular weight of glucosamine hydrochloride.
9. How many milligrams of betamethasone dipropionate (m.w. 504) should be used to prepare a 50-g tube of ointment labeled to contain the equivalent of 0.5 mg of betamethasone (m.w. 392) base per gram?
10. Sertraline hydrochloride capsules[2]:

℞	Sertraline hydrochloride (ZOLOFT tablets, 100 mg)	3 tablets
	Silica gel	6 g
	Calcium citrate	4 g
	M.ft. caps no. 40	
	Sig: Use as directed.	

Calculate the grams of calcium in the formula derived from calcium citrate, $C_{10}H_{10}Ca_3O_{14} \cdot 4H_2O$ (m.w. 570.5)

11. Fentanyl inhalation[3]:

℞	Fentanyl citrate	4.71 mg
	Sterile sodium chloride inhalation ad	60 mL
	Sig: Use as directed.	

Fentanyl citrate has a molecular weight of 528. Calculate the milligrams of the active drug moiety, fentanyl (m.w. 336), in the prescription.

12. A pediatric suspension of erythromycin ethylsuccinate (m.w. 862) contains the equivalent of 200 mg of erythromycin (m.w. 734) per 5-mL dose. Calculate the milligrams of erythromycin ethylsuccinate contained in 100 mL of the suspension.
13. A sterile ophthalmic suspension of BETOPTIC S contains 0.25% of betaxolol base (m.w. 307), present as the hydrochloride salt (m.w. 344). Calculate the percentage of betaxolol hydrochloride in the suspension.
14. If the molecular weight of the HIV protease inhibitor nelfinavir is 568 and that of nelfinavir mesylate is 664, calculate the milligrams of the latter in each tablet labeled to contain the equivalent of 250 mg of nelfinavir.
15. An ophthalmic solution is labeled to contain the equivalent of 0.3% of ciprofloxacin base (m.w. 332). How many milligrams of ciprofloxacin hydrochloride (m.w. 386) may be used to prepare each 5 mL of the solution?
16. The molecular weight of albuterol sulfate is 576, and the empirical formula is $(C_{13}H_{21}NO_3)_2 \cdot H_2SO_4$. If each actuation of an inhalation aerosol delivers 108 μg of albuterol sulfate, calculate the quantity of albuterol base delivered.
17. An injection contains 20 mg/mL of dolasetron mesylate monohydrate in 0.625-mL vials. The molecular weight of the drug is 438.5. Approximately 74% of dolasetron mesylate monohydrate is dolasetron base. Calculate the quantity of dolasetron base administered by 0.6 mL of injection.

CALCQUIZ

20.A. DIPROLENE ointment has a potency expressed as the equivalent of "0.05% betamethasone." Betamethasone dipropionate is actually used in the formulation. The molecular weight of betamethasone is 392.4 and that of betamethasone dipropionate is 504.6.

(a) Calculate the percent strength of betamethasone dipropionate in the ointment.
(b) Calculate the quantity of betamethasone dipropionate, in mg/g, in a 15-g tube of the ointment.
(c) If a pharmacist received an order to prepare an ointment containing 0.02% betamethasone, how many grams of ointment base would need to be mixed with a 15-g tube of DIPROLENE ointment?
(d) If the manufacturer decided to prepare ointments containing 0.075% betamethasone, how many *additional* milligrams of betamethasone dipropionate would be needed in each 15-g tube of DIPROLENE ointment?

20.B. AVELOX IV contains, in each 250-mL bag, moxifloxacin hydrochloride (equivalent to 400 mg of moxifloxacin) and 0.8% sodium chloride. The molecular weight of moxifloxacin hydrochloride is 437.9.

(a) Calculate the quantity, in mg/mL, of moxifloxacin hydrochloride in the injection.
(b) Calculate the milligrams and mEq of sodium in the IV solution.

ANSWERS TO "CASE IN POINT" AND PRACTICE PROBLEMS

Case in Point 20.1

$$\frac{171\ (\text{m.w.})}{275\ (\text{m.w.})} = \frac{35\ \text{mg/kg/day}}{x};$$
$$x = 56.29\ \text{mg/kg/day}$$
$$\frac{171\ (\text{m.w.})}{275\ (\text{m.w.})} = \frac{50\ \text{mg/kg/day}}{x};$$
$$x = 80.41\ \text{mg/kg/day}$$

Practice Problems

1. 369 mg lidocaine hydrochloride
2. 8 mg tofacitinib citrate
3. 2.15% mupirocin calcium
4. 11.2 mg sumatriptan succinate
5. 392.4 m.w. and 0.5% betamethasone
6. 18.2 g epinephrine bitartrate
7. 331.35 m.w. ciprofloxacin base
8. 215 m.w. glucosamine hydrochloride
9. 32.1 mg betamethasone dipropionate
10. 0.842 g calcium
11. 2.99 or 3 mg fentanyl
12. 4697.5 or 4698 mg erythromycin ethylsuccinate
13. 0.28%betaxolol hydrochloride
14. 292.3 mg nelfinavir mesylate
15. 17.4 mg ciprofloxacin hydrochloride
16. 89.6 μg albuterol base
17. 8.88 mg dolasetron base

References

1. *Physicians' Desk Reference*. 68th Ed. Montvale, NJ: PDR Network; 2014.
2. Allen LV Jr. Sertraline 7.5 mg capsules. *International Journal of Pharmaceutical Compounding* 1998;2:443.
3. Allen LV Jr. Fentanyl 300 mcg/6 mL inhalation. *International Journal of Pharmaceutical Compounding* 1998;2:153.

21

Selected Calculations Involving Radiopharmaceuticals

OBJECTIVES

Upon successful completion of this chapter, the student will be able to:

- Convert units of radioactivity within and between the *curie* and *becquerel* systems.
- Calculate radioactive decay and half-life.
- Perform dosage calculations of radiopharmaceuticals.

Radioisotopes

The atoms of a given element are not necessarily alike. In fact, certain elements actually consist of several components, called ***isotopes***, that are chemically identical but physically may differ slightly in mass. Isotopes, then, may be defined as atoms that have the same nuclear charge, and hence the same atomic number, but different masses. The mass number physically characterizes a particular isotope. As needed, the student may wish to review the area of isotope notation.

Isotopes can be classified as stable and unstable. Stable isotopes never change unless affected by some outside force; unstable isotopes are distinguishable by radioactive transformations and hence are said to be radioactive. The radioactive isotopes of the elements are called ***radioisotopes*** or ***radionuclides***. They can be divided into two types: naturally occurring and artificially produced radionuclides.

The branch of medicine that utilizes radioisotopes and radiation in the diagnosis and treatment of disease is ***nuclear medicine***. Pharmacists, who prepare radioactive pharmaceuticals or ***radiopharmaceuticals*** for use in patient care, practice ***nuclear pharmacy*** and are referred to as ***nuclear pharmacists***.[a]

The medical uses of nuclear materials may be described as:

(a) *Diagnostic*, as in body imaging and organ and tissue uptake of radiolabeled drugs to determine metabolic or other physiologic parameters

(b) *Therapeutic*, in the delivery of palliative or therapeutic doses of radiation to specific tissues or body areas, as in the treatment of cancer

(c) *Clinical research*, as in the study of a subject's response to a new radioactive drug or device

(d) *In vitro diagnostic testing* kits

[a]*Nuclear pharmacy* is a specialty area of pharmacy practice recognized by the Board of Pharmacy Specialties (BPS).[1] Pharmacists who are certified in this specialty may use the designation, "Board Certified Nuclear Pharmacist (BCNP)." Nuclear pharmacists are involved in the procurement, storage, handling, compounding, testing, quality assurance, dispensing, and documentation of radiopharmaceuticals used in nuclear medicine.[2,3] The cited references in this footnote may be used to explore detailed functions and opportunities in this practice specialty.

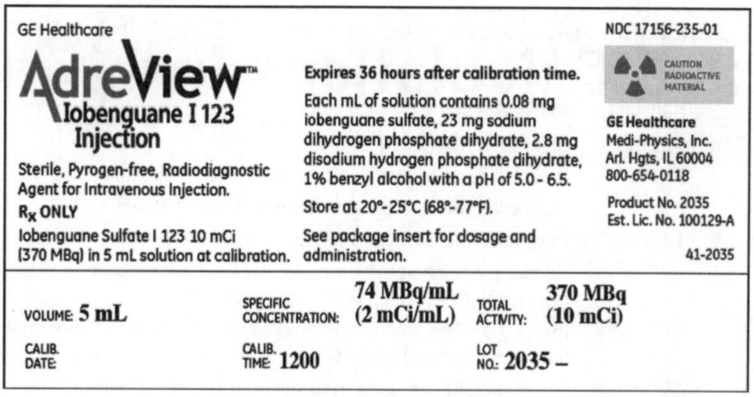

FIGURE 21.1 • Label of a radiodiagnostic agent administered by intravenous injection. *(Courtesy GE Healthcare. Source: DailyMed, U.S. National Library of Medicine. Available at http://dailymed.nlm.nih.gov/dailymed/index.cfm)*

Nuclear pharmacists most often utilize manufactured radiopharmaceuticals and nonradioactive *kit formulations* (Figs. 21.1 and 21.2) provided by suppliers. Less frequently, radiopharmaceuticals are produced in-house through generator systems.[2,3] The kit formulations are available in sterile vials containing all of the necessary components (e.g., stabilizers) for the desired preparation, except for the radioactive isotope. When a nuclear pharmacist adds the isotope, a chemical reaction occurs within the vial, which produces the final radiopharmaceutical. Guidelines for the compounding of radiopharmaceuticals may be found in the cited reference.[4]

The Unite States Pharmacopeia devotes chapter <823> to the compounding of radiopharmaceuticals for positron emission tomography (PET).[5] Radiopharmaceuticals administered for PET procedures typically incorporate radionuclides, which have very short half-lives. Technetium-99m (^{99m}Tc; the *m* standing for metastable), with a half-life of about 6 hours, is used in about 80 percent of nuclear diagnostic procedures.

Table 21.1 provides examples of radioisotopes used in nuclear medicine.

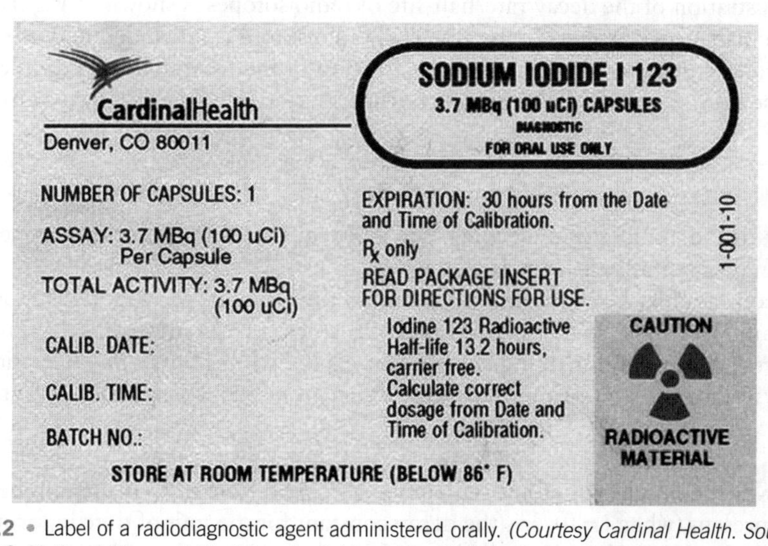

FIGURE 21.2 • Label of a radiodiagnostic agent administered orally. *(Courtesy Cardinal Health. Source: DailyMed, U.S. National Library of Medicine. Available at http://dailymed.nlm.nih.gov/dailymed/index.cfm)*

Table 21.1 • SELECTED RADIOISOTOPES USED IN NUCLEAR MEDICINE WITH THEIR HALF-LIVES AND APPLICATIONS[a]

Radioisotope	Half-Life	Applications
Fluorine-18	110 m	Diagnostic use in PET scans
Gallium-67	3.26 d	Diagnostic use in Hodgkin's disease, lymphoma, inflammation, and infection
Indium-111	2.8 d	Diagnostic use in brain and neuroendocrine studies
Iodine-123	13.2 h	Diagnostic use in thyroid function
Iodine-125	59.9 d	Cancer brachytherapy[b] (prostate and brain); evaluation of kidney filtration rate; diagnosis of deep vein thrombosis in the leg
Iodine-131	8.08 d	Imaging and treatment of thyroid cancer; diagnosis of abnormal liver function, renal (kidney) blood flow, and urinary tract obstruction
Samarium-153	46.3 h	Treatment of bone, lung, prostate, and breast cancers
Technetium 99m	6.02 h	Imaging of the skeleton, heart muscle, brain, thyroid, lungs, liver, spleen, kidney, and gall bladder
Thallium-201	73.1 h	Diagnostic use in coronary artery disease (nuclear cardiac stress test)
Yttrium-90	64 h	Cancer brachytherapy, particularly liver cancer; treatment of pain of arthritis in large synovial joints

[a]Half-lives and applications have been obtained from References[6–8]. Some half-lives have been rounded. Applications are representative, not all inclusive.

[b]*Brachytherapy* is radiation therapy delivered locally to a tumor, as opposed to the application of external radiation.

Radioactivity

The breakdown of an unstable isotope is characterized by radioactivity. In the process of radioactivity, an unstable isotope undergoes changes until a stable state is reached, and in the transformation, it emits energy in the form of radiation. This radiation may consist of *alpha particles*, *beta particles*, and *gamma rays*. The stable state is reached as a result of *radioactive decay*, which is characteristic of all types of radioactivity. Individual radioisotopes differ in the rate of radioactive decay, but in each case, a definite time is required for half the original atoms to decay. This time is called the ***half-life*** of the radioisotope. Each radioisotope, then, has a distinct half-life.

An illustration of the decay rate/half-life of radioisotopes is shown in Figure 21.3, and a list of the half-lives of some commonly used radioisotopes is included in Table 21.1.

The rate of decay is always a constant fraction of the total number of undecomposed atoms present. Mathematically, the rate of disintegration may be expressed as follows:

$$-\frac{dN}{dt} = \lambda N \qquad \text{(Equation 1)}$$

in which N is the number of undecomposed atoms at time t and λ is the decay constant or the fraction disintegrating per unit of time.

The constant may be expressed in any unit of time, such as reciprocal seconds, minutes, or hours, among others. The numeric value of the decay constant will be 24 times as great when expressed in days, for example, as when expressed in hours. This equation may be integrated to give the expression of the *exponential decay law*, which may be written:

$$N = N_0 e^{-\lambda t} \qquad \text{(Equation 2)}$$

in which N is the number of atoms remaining at elapsed time t, N_0 is the number of atoms originally present (when t = 0), λ is the decay constant for the unit of time in terms of which the interval t is expressed, and e is the base of the natural logarithm 2.71828.

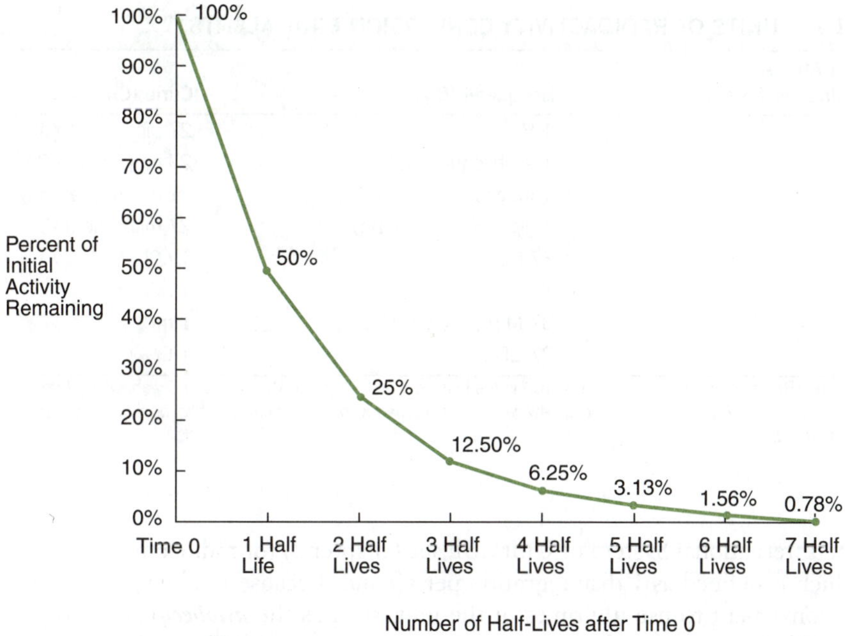

FIGURE 21.3 • Illustration of the decay rate/half-life of radioisotopes. *(Source: U.S. Department of Health and Human Services: Radiation Event Medical Management. Available at http://remm.nlm.gov/halflife.htm. Accessed February 15, 2015)*

Because the rate of decay can also be characterized by the half-life ($T_{1/2}$), the value of N in equation 2 at the end of a half period is $\frac{1}{2}N_0$. The equation then becomes:

$$\tfrac{1}{2}N_0 = N_0^{-\lambda T_{1/2}} \qquad \text{(Equation 3)}$$

Solving equation 3 by natural logarithms results in the following expression:

$$\ln \tfrac{1}{2} = -\lambda T_{1/2}$$

$$\text{or} \quad \lambda T_{1/2} = \ln 2$$

$$\text{then} \quad \lambda T_{1/2} = 2.303 \log 2$$

$$\text{and} \quad T_{1/2} = \frac{0.693}{\lambda} \qquad \text{(Equation 4)}$$

The half-life ($T_{1/2}$) is thus related to the disintegration constant λ by equation 4. Hence, if one value is known, the other can be readily calculated. The term "disintegration" is widely used; however, the alternative term "transformation" is used in some literature references.

Units of Radioactivity

The quantity of activity of a radioisotope is expressed in absolute units (total number of atoms disintegrating per unit time). The basic unit is the ***curie*** (Ci), which is defined as that quantity of a radioisotope in which 3.7×10^{10} (37 billion) atoms disintegrate per second. The ***millicurie*** (mCi) is one thousandth of a curie, and the ***microcurie*** (μCi) is one millionth of a curie. The ***nanocurie*** (nCi), also known as the ***millimicrocurie***, is one billionth of a curie (10^{-9} Ci).

Table 21.2 • UNITS OF RADIOACTIVITY CONVERSION EQUIVALENTS[a]

Number of Atoms Transforming per Second	Becquerel (Bq)	Curie (Ci)
1	1 Bq	27 picocurie (pCi)
1000	1 kilobecquerel (kBq)	27 nanocurie (nCi)
1×10^6	1 megabecquerel (MBq)	27 microcurie (μCi)
1×10^9	1 gigabecquerel (GBq)	27 millicurie (mCi)
37	37 Bq	1 nCi
37,000	37 kBq	1 μCi
3.7×10^7	37 MBq	1 mCi
3.7×10^{10}	37 GBq	1 Ci

[a]The becquerel (Bq) is the SI unit and the curie (Ci) is the historical unit. *(Source: World Health Organization. International Pharmacopeia, 2008. Radiopharmaceuticals. Available at http://www.who.int/medicines/publications/pharmacopoeia/Radgenmono.pdf)*

The International System of Units (SI; see Chapter 2) for radioactivity is the ***becquerel*** (Bq), which is defined as 1 disintegration per second. Because the becquerel is so small, it is more convenient to use multiples of the unit, such as the ***kilobecquerel*** (kBq), which is equal to 10^3 disintegrations per second; the ***megabecquerel*** (MBq), which is equal to 10^6 disintegrations per second; and the ***gigabecquerel*** (GBq), which is equal to 10^9 disintegrations per second.

The *United States Pharmacopeia* has adopted the becquerel to eventually replace the long-familiar curie as a matter of international agreement. For the present, both units are used to label radioactivity, and the doses of many radiopharmaceuticals are expressed in megabecquerels as well as in millicuries and/or microcuries (see Figs. 21.1 and 21.2).

Table 21.2 provides equivalents for conversion from the curie (and its subunits) to the becquerel (and its multiples), and vice versa.

Example Calculations of Radioactivity Unit Conversion

(1) *A thallous chloride Tl 201 injection has a labeled activity of 550 microcuries* (μCi). *Express this activity in terms of megabecquerels.*

$$550\ \mu\text{Ci} = 0.55\ \text{mCi}$$
$$1\ \text{mCi} = 37\ \text{MBq}$$
$$\frac{1\ (\text{mCi})}{0.55\ (\text{mCi})} = \frac{37\ (\text{MBq})}{\text{x}\ (\text{MBq})}$$
$$\text{x} = \mathbf{20.35\ MBq}$$

(2) *Sodium chromate Cr 51 injection is administered in a dose of 3.7 MBq for the determination of blood volume. Express this dose in terms of microcuries.*

$$1\ \text{MBq} = 0.027\ \text{mCi}$$
$$\frac{1\ (\text{MBq})}{3.7\ (\text{MBq})} = \frac{0.027\ (\text{mCi})}{\text{x}\ (\text{mCi})}$$
$$\text{x} = 0.1\ \text{mCi}$$
$$= \mathbf{100\ \mu Ci}$$

Example Calculations of Half-Life and Disintegration Constant

(1) *The disintegration constant of a radioisotope is 0.02496 day^{-1}. Calculate the half-life of the radioisotope.*

$$T_{1/2} = \frac{0.693}{\lambda}$$

$$\text{Substituting, } T_{1/2} = \frac{0.693}{0.02496 \text{ day}^{-1}}$$

$$T_{1/2} = 27.76 \text{ or } \mathbf{27.8 \text{ days}}$$

The half-life of ^{198}Au is 2.70 days. Calculate its disintegration constant.

$$T_{1/2} = \frac{0.693}{\lambda}$$

$$\text{Substituting, } 2.70 \text{ days} = \frac{0.693}{\lambda}$$

$$\lambda = \frac{0.693}{2.70 \text{ days}} = \mathbf{0.2567 \text{ day}^{-1}}$$

(2) *The original quantity of a radioisotope is given as 500 μCi (18.5 MBq)/mL. If the quantity remaining after 16 days is 125 μCi (4.625 MBq)/mL, calculate (a) the disintegration constant and (b) the half-life of the radioisotope.*

(a) Equation 2, written in logarithmic form, becomes:

$$\ln \frac{N}{N_0} = -\lambda t$$

or

$$\lambda = \frac{2.303}{t} \log \frac{N_0}{N}$$

Substituting:

$$\lambda = \frac{2.303}{16} \log \frac{500}{125} \text{ or, } \frac{2.303}{16} \log \frac{18.5 \text{ (MBq)}}{4.625 \text{ (MBq)}}$$

$$\lambda = \frac{2.303}{16} (0.6021)$$

$$\lambda = \mathbf{0.08666 \text{ day}^{-1}}$$

(b) Equation 4 may now be used to calculate the half-life.

$$T_{1/2} = \frac{0.693}{\lambda}$$

$$\text{Substituting, } T_{1/2} = \frac{0.693}{0.08666 \text{ day}^{-1}} = \mathbf{8.0 \text{ days}}$$

Pharmacists may find it useful to corroborate their complex calculations by referring to one of many Web sites that offer radioactive decay calculators, such as the one referenced.[9]

CALCULATIONS CAPSULE

Half-Life

The half-life equation is:

$$T_{1/2} = \frac{0.693}{\lambda}$$

λ = half-life coefficient or disintegration constant

Example Calculations of Remaining Activity Over Time

(1) *A sample of ^{131}I has an initial activity of 30 μCi (1.11 MBq). Its half-life is 8.08 days. Calculate its activity, in microcuries (megabecquerels), at the end of exactly 20 days.*

$$\text{By substituting } \lambda = \frac{0.693}{T_{1/2}} \text{ and } e^{-0.693} = ½$$

In Equation 2, the activity of a radioactive sample decreases with time according to the following expression:

$$N = N_0\left(2^{-t/T_{1/2}}\right) = N_0\left(\frac{1}{2^{t/T_{1/2}}}\right)$$

$$\text{Since} \quad t/T_{1/2} = \frac{20}{80.08} = 2.475$$

$$\text{then} \quad N = 30\left(\frac{1}{2^{2.475}}\right)$$

$$\begin{aligned} \text{Solving by logarithms, } \log N &= \log 30 - \log 2\,(2.475) \\ &= 1.4771 - 0.7450 \\ \log N &= 0.7321 \\ N &= 5.39 \text{ or } \mathbf{5.4\ \mu Ci} \end{aligned}$$

Or using megabecquerel units:

$$N = 1.11\left(\frac{1}{2^{2.475}}\right)$$

$$\begin{aligned} \text{Solving by logarithms, } \log N &= \log 1.11 - \log 2\,(2.475) \\ &= 0.0453 - 0.7450 \\ \log N &= -0.6997 \\ N &= 0.1997 \text{ or } \mathbf{0.2\ MBq} \end{aligned}$$

(2) *A vial of sodium phosphate P 32 solution has a labeled activity of 500 μCi (18.5 MBq)/mL. How many milliliters of this solution should be administered exactly 10 days after the original assay to provide an activity of 250 μCi (9.25 MBq)? The half-life of ^{32}P is 14.3 days.*

The activity exactly 10 days after the original assay is given by:

$$N = N_0\left(\frac{1}{2^{t/T_{1/2}}}\right)$$

$$\text{Since}\quad t/T_{1/2} = \frac{10}{14.3} = 0.6993$$

$$\text{then}\quad N = 500\left(\frac{1}{2^{0.6993}}\right)$$

$$\log N = \log 500 - \log 2\,(0.6993)$$
$$= 2.6990 - 0.2105$$
$$\log N = 2.4885$$
$$N = 308\ \mu\text{Ci/mL, activity after radioactive decay}$$

$$\frac{308\,(\mu\text{Ci})}{250\,(\mu\text{Ci})} = \frac{1\,(\text{mL})}{x\,(\text{mL})}$$

$$x = \mathbf{0.81\ mL}$$

Or using megabecquerel units:

$$N = 18.5\left(\frac{1}{2^{0.6993}}\right)$$
$$\log N = \log 18.5 - \log 2\,(0.6993)$$
$$= 1.2672 - 0.2105$$
$$\log N = 1.0567$$
$$= 11.39\ \text{MBq/mL, activity after radioactive decay}$$

$$\frac{11.39\,(\text{MBq})}{9.25\,(\text{MBq})} = \frac{1\,(\text{mL})}{x\,(\text{mL})}$$

$$x = \mathbf{0.81\ mL}$$

CASE IN POINT 21.1[a] The Nuclear Pharmacy receives an order for a 25-mCi technetium-99m MDP (bone scan dose) to be administered at 10:00 AM (1000 hours). The pharmacist has prepared an MDP bone kit with the concentration of 50 mCi/mL at 0600. What volume of the kit should be dispensed to provide the dose as ordered? The half-life of technetium-99m is 6.02 hours.

[a]Problem courtesy of Kenneth M. Duke, Clinical and Administrative Pharmacy, College of Pharmacy, University of Georgia, Athens, GA.

PRACTICE PROBLEMS

1. Cyanocobalamin Co 57 capsules are administered in doses of 0.5 to 1.0 μCi in a test for pernicious anemia. Express this dosage range in terms of becquerel units.
2. If 1 mCi of radioactivity is equivalent to 37 MBq in activity, how many becquerels of radioactivity would be the equivalent of 1 Ci?
3. A gallium citrate Ga 67 injection has a labeled activity of 366 MBq. Express this activity in terms of millicuries.
4. If 1.85 MBq of radioactivity is equivalent to 50 μCi, how many millicuries would be radioactivity would be the equivalent of 10 mCi?
5. If 50 μCi of radioactivity is equivalent to 1.85 MBq of activity, how many megabecquerels of radioactivity would be the equivalent of 10 mCi?
6. Express an administered dose of 5 mCi sodium phosphate P 32 solution in terms of megabecquerels.
7. Calculate the half-life of a radioisotope that has a disintegration constant of 0.00456 day^{-1}.
8. Calculate the half-life of ^{203}Hg, which has a disintegration constant of 0.0149 day^{-1}.
9. Calculate the disintegration constant of ^{64}Cu, which has a half-life of 12.8 hours.
10. Calculate the disintegration constant of ^{35}S, which has a half-life of 87.2 days.
11. The original quantity of a radioisotope is given as 100 mCi (3700 MBq). If the quantity remaining after 6 days is 75 mCi (2775 MBq), calculate the disintegration constant and the half-life of the radioisotope.
12. A series of measurements on a sample of a radioisotope gave the following data:

Days	*Counts per Minute*
0	5600
4	2000

Calculate the disintegration constant and the half-life of the radioisotope.

13. The original activity of a radioisotope is given as 10 mCi (370 MBq) per 10 mL. If the quantity remaining after exactly 15 days is 850 μCi (31.45 MBq)/mL, calculate the disintegration constant and the half-life of the radioisotope.
14. If the half-life of a radioisotope is 12 hours, what will be the activity after 4 days of a sample that has an original activity of 1 Ci (37,000 MBq)? Express the activity in terms of microcuries (megabecquerels).
15. Sodium iodide I 131 capsules have a labeled potency of 100 μCi (3.7 MBq). What will be their activity exactly 3 days after the stated assay date? The half-life of ^{131}I is 8.08 days.
16. A sodium chromate Cr 51 injection has a labeled activity of 50 mCi (1850 MBq) at 5:00 PM on April 19. Calculate its activity at 5:00 PM on May 1. The half-life of ^{51}Cr is 27.8 days.
17. Iodinated I 125 albumin injection contains 0.5 mCi (18.5 MBq) of radioactivity per milliliter. How many milliliters of the solution should be administered exactly 30 days after the original assay to provide an activity of 60 μCi (2.22 MBq)? The half-life of I 125 is 60 days.
18. An ytterbium Yb 169 pentetate injection has a labeled radioactivity of 5 mCi (185 MBq)/mL. How many milliliters of the injection should be administered 10 days after the original assay to provide an activity of 100 μCi (3.7 MBq)/kg of body weight for a person weighing 110 lb? The half-life of ^{169}Yb is 32.0 days.

19. A sodium pertechnetate ^{99m}Tc injection has a labeled activity of 15 mCi (555 MBq)/mL. If the injection is administered 10 hours after the time of calibration, (a) what will be its activity and (b) how many milliliters of the injection will be required to provide a dose of 15 mCi (555 MBq)? The half-life of ^{99m}Tc is 6.0 hours.
20. A sodium phosphate P 32 solution contains 1 mCi (37 MBq)/mL at the time of calibration. How many milliliters of the solution will provide an activity of 500 μCi (18.5 MBq) 1 week after the original assay? The half-life of ^{32}P is 14.3 days.
21. Convert:
    (a) 3.7 Bq to kBq
    (b) 1 mCi to kBq
    (c) 1 nCi to kBq
    (d) 1 μCi to nCi
    (e) 1 mCi to Ci
22. Using the information in Fig. 21.2, convert the quantity of sodium iodide I 123 in each capsule to (a) mCi and (b) nCi.
23. Using the information in Fig. 21.1, convert the quantity of iobenguane I 123 to Ci/5 mL.
24. Radium Ra 223 dichloride (XOFIGO) is a radiopharmaceutical approved for the treatment of castration-resistant prostate cancer. It is available as a 27-µCi/mL (1000 kBq/mL) injection and the dosage is 1.35 µCi/kg (50 kBq/kg) given intravenously at 4-week intervals for six injections.[10]
    (a) What would be the dose, in kBq, for a 75-year-old male patient weighing 187 lb?
    (b) The product information supplies a decay correction factor table to account for the change in radioactivity of the drug over time, and each vial of the drug is labeled with a reference date. The volume of solution to be administered is divided by the correction factor to determine the actual amount of solution to use. If this patient is to receive the dose on February 28, and the reference date on the vial is February 20 (of the same year), how many milliliters of the injection should be used for the dose? According to the table, 8 days from the reference date should have a correction factor of 0.605.[10]
    (c) The actual quantitative concentration of radium 223 in the injection at the reference date is 0.53 ng/mL. What is this concentration expressed as a ratio strength?
    (d) The injectable solution also contains 6.3 mg/mL sodium chloride to adjust tonicity and 7.2 mg/mL sodium citrate to adjust pH. How many milliequivalents of sodium would the patient receive from the dose calculated in part B? (NaCl, m.w., 58.5; $Na_3C_6H_5O_7$, m.w., 258).

CALCQUIZ

21.A.[a] An iodine I 131 capsule has been ordered for administration on Tuesday, November 11, at 12 noon. The requested dose is 25 mCi. If the patient is unable to make the appointment on November 11, what dose remains for a 12 noon appointment on Thursday, November 13? The half-life of iodine I 131 is 8 days.

21.B.[a] An order is received for a 100-mCi vial of technetium-99m pertechnetate calibrated for 8:00 AM (0800 hours) to be used as a linearity source for dose calibrator testing at one of the nuclear medicine accounts. The pharmacy must prepare the dose for delivery at 0500. What activity should be dispensed at 0500 to deliver the desired activity? The half-life of technetium-99m pertechnetate is 6.02 hours.

21.C.[11] A pharmacist receives an order for an 8-μCi dose of ^{99m}Tc-mertiatide for a study to be performed at 10:30 AM. At 6:00 AM, the morning of the study, the pharmacist prepares the dose. The standard decay equation yields a fraction of 0.596 of the initial activity remaining after 4.5 hours. How many μCi are needed at 6:00 AM to obtain the correct dose at 10:30 AM?

[a]Problem courtesy of Kenneth M. Duke, Clinical and Administrative Pharmacy, College of Pharmacy, University of Georgia, Athens, GA.

ANSWERS TO "CASE IN POINT" AND PRACTICE PROBLEMS

Case in Point 21.1

Solving first for the half-life coefficient, lambda (λ), for ^{99m}Tc:

$\lambda = 0.693/T_{1/2}$

$\lambda = 0.693/6$ (hours)

$\lambda = 0.1155$ hours^{-1}

Since the stock solution was compounded to contain 50 mCi/mL at 0600, we can decay this concentration to the 1000 dosage time and solve as a proportion problem.

Using the decay formula: $A = A_0e^{-\lambda t}$

A = Final activity

A_0 = Initial activity

t = Decay time

$A = 50\ e^{-(0.1155)4}$

$A = 50\ (0.63)$

A = 31.5 mCi/mL

Required dose = 25 mCi

Volume to dispense = 25 mCi/31.5 mCi/mL = 0.79 mL

Practice Problems

1. 18,500 to 37,000 Bq
2. 3.7×10^{10} Bq
3. 9.9 mCi
4. 0.2 mCi
5. 370 MBq
6. 185 MBq
7. 152 days
8. 46.5 days
9. 0.0541 $hour^{-1}$
10. 0.00795 $hour^{-1}$
11. $\lambda = 0.04794\ day^{-1}$
    $T_{1/2} = 14.5$ days
12. $\lambda = 0.2574\ day^{-1}$
    $T_{1/2} = 2.7$ days
13. $\lambda = 0.01084\ day^{-1}$
    $T_{1/2} = 64$ days
14. 3907 μCi (144.5 MBq)
15. 77.3 μCi (2.86 MBq)
16. 37.1 mCi (1372.7 MBq)
17. 0.17 mL
18. 1.24 mL
19. (a) 4.7 mCi (174.8 MBq)
    (b) 3.2 mL
20. 0.7 mL
21. (a) 0.0037 kBq
    (b) 37,000 kBq
    (c) 0.037 kBq
    (d) 1000 nCi
    (e) 0.001 Ci
22. (a) 0.1 mCi
    (b) 100,000 nCi
23. 0.01 Ci/5 mL
24. (a) 4250 kBq
    (b) 7.02 mL
    (c) 1:1,886,792,452.83 w/v
    (d) 1.34 mEq sodium

References

1. Board of Pharmacy Specialties. Available at: http://www.bpsweb.org/specialties/specialties.cfm. Accessed February 15, 2015.
2. What is nuclear pharmacy? Available at: http://nuclear.pharmacy.purdue.edu/what.php. Accessed February 15, 2015.
3. Patidar AK, Patidar P, Tandel TS, et al. Current trends in nuclear pharmacy practice. *International Journal of Pharmaceutical Sciences Review and Research* 2010;5:145–150. Available at: http://globalresearchonline.net/journalcontents/volume5issue2/Article-026.pdf. Accessed February 15, 2015.
4. American Pharmaceutical Association. Nuclear Pharmacy Guidelines for the Compounding of Radiopharmaceuticals. Available at: http://nuclearpharmacy.uams.edu/Compounding.PDF. Accessed February 15, 2015.
5. *United States Pharmacopeia*. Rockville, MD: United States Pharmacopeial Convention. Chapter <823>. Available at: http://www.usp.org/support-home/frequently-asked-questions/general-chapter-823. Accessed February 15, 2015.
6. Vargas J. List of radiopharmaceuticals used in nuclear medicine. Available at: http://www.slideshare.net/hikikomorijcv18/list-of-radiopharmaceuticals-used-in-nuclear-medicine. Accessed February 15, 2015.
7. World Nuclear Association. Radioisotopes in medicine. Available at: http://www.world-nuclear.org/info/Non-Power-Nuclear-Applications/Radioisotopes/Radioisotopes-in-Medicine/. Accessed February 15, 2015.
8. National Isotope Development Center. Medical radioisotopes. Available at: https://www.isotopes.gov/outreach/med_isotopes.html. Accessed February 15, 2015.
9. *Radioactive Decay Calculator*. University of Washington, Environmental Health & Safety. Available at: http://www.ehs.washington.edu/rso/calculator/activity_calc.shtm. Accessed February 15, 2015.
10. U.S. Food and Drug Administration. *XOFIGO (radium Ra 223 dichloride) Injection*. Department of Health and Human Services. Available at: http://www.accessdata.fda.gov/drugsatfda_docs/label/2013/203971lbl.pdf. Accessed January 5, 2015.
11. Basmadjian N. Prescription preparation in nuclear pharmacy: three case studies. *International Journal of Pharmaceutical Compounding* 1998;2:429–431.

22

Selected Bioavailability and Pharmacokinetic Calculations

OBJECTIVES

Upon successful completion of this chapter, the student will be able to:

- Perform basic calculations of bioavailability and bioequivalence.
- Perform basic calculations of elimination half-life and volume of distribution.

The availability to the biologic system of a drug substance formulated into a pharmaceutical product is integral to the goals of dosage form design and paramount to the effectiveness of the medication.

Before a drug substance can be absorbed by the biologic system, it must be released from its dosage form (e.g., tablet) or drug delivery system (e.g., transdermal patch) and dissolved in the physiologic fluids. Several factors play a role in a drug's biologic availability, including the physical and chemical characteristics of the drug itself, such as its particle size and solubility, and the features of the dosage form or delivery system, such as the nature of the formulative ingredients and the method of manufacture. The area of study that deals with the properties of drug substances and dosage forms that influence the release of the drug for biologic activity is termed ***biopharmaceutics***. The term ***bioavailability*** is defined as "the rate and extent to which the active ingredient or active moiety is absorbed from a drug product and becomes available at the site of action."[1]

Pharmacokinetics is the study and characterization of the time course of the absorption, distribution, metabolism, and excretion (ADME) of drugs. ***Drug absorption*** is the process of uptake of the compound from the site of administration into the systemic circulation. ***Drug distribution*** refers to the transfer of the drug from the blood to extravascular fluids and tissues. ***Drug metabolism*** is the enzymatic or biochemical transformation of the drug substance to (usually less toxic) metabolic products, which may be eliminated more readily from the body. ***Drug excretion*** is the removal of the drug substance or its metabolites from the body, such as through the kidney (urine), intestines (feces), skin (sweat), and/or saliva.

The relationship among the processes of ADME influences the therapeutic and toxicologic effects of drugs. The application of pharmacokinetic principles in the treatment of individual patients in optimizing drug therapy is referred to as ***clinical pharmacokinetics***.

Drug Availability from Dosage Forms and Delivery Systems

The availability of a drug from a dosage form or delivery system is determined by measuring its dissolution characteristics *in vitro* (outside the biologic system) and/or its absorption patterns *in vivo* (within the biologic system). Generally, data are collected that provide information on both *rate* and *extent* of drug dissolution and/or absorption. The data collected may be plotted as a graph to depict concentration versus time curves for the drug's dissolution and/or absorption.

Plotting and Interpreting Drug Dissolution Data

Drug dissolution data are obtained in vitro for tablets or capsules using the USP Dissolution Test, which defines the apparatus and methods to be used.[2] The data obtained may be presented in tabular form and depicted graphically, as in the following example.

The following dissolution data were obtained from a 250-mg capsule of ampicillin. Create a graph from the data and determine the approximate percentage of ampicillin dissolved following 15, 30, and 45 minutes of the study.

Period (minutes)	*Ampicillin Dissolved (mg)*
5	12
10	30
20	75
40	120
60	150

Plotting the data:

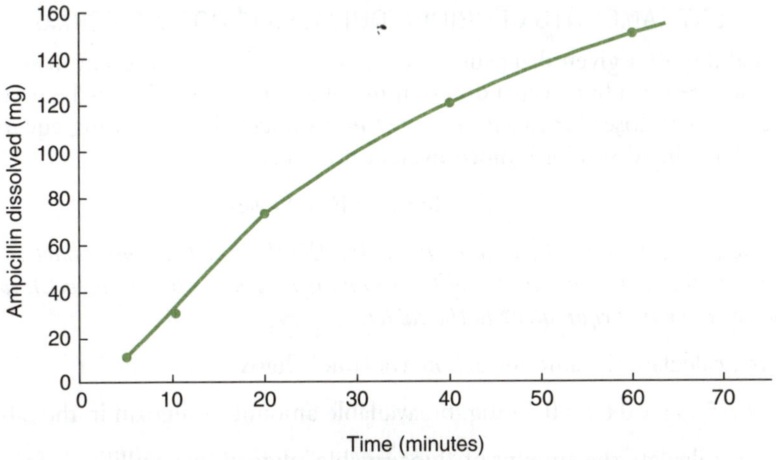

Determining the intercepts at 15, 30, and 45 minutes:

At 15 minutes, approximately 50 mg or **20%** of the ampicillin
At 30 minutes, approximately 100 mg or **40%** of the ampicillin
At 45 minutes, approximately 125 mg or **50%** of the ampicillin

Example Calculations of Bioavailability and Bioequivalence

AMOUNT OF DRUG BIOAVAILABLE FROM A DOSAGE FORM

If drug dissolution or drug absorption studies demonstrate consistently that only a portion of a drug substance in a dosage form is "available" for biologic absorption, the drug's bioavailability factor (F), which represents the decimal percentage of a drug substance available, may be used to calculate bioavailability. The value of F may be zero, indicating no absorption, to a maximum of a value of 1, indicating complete absorption, such as an intravenous infusion. *Absolute* bioavailability is used most commonly and refers to the comparison of the amount of drug absorbed from a dosage form to the amount delivered in an intravenous dose. *Relative* bioavailability refers to the comparison of amounts absorbed from two different dosage forms such as an oral tablet and transdermal patch or two different routes of administration such as oral and intramuscular. The administration of a medication with food can also affect bioavailability.

(1) *If the bioavailability factor (F) for a drug substance in a dosage form is 0.60, how many milligrams of drug would be available for absorption from a 100-mg tablet of the drug?*

The bioavailability factor (F) indicates that only 60% of the drug present in the dosage form is available for absorption. Thus:

$$100 \text{ mg} \times 0.60 = \mathbf{60 \text{ mg}}$$

(2) *The oral bioavailability of 10-mg alendronate (FOSAMAX) tablets is stated as 0.59%. Concomitant administration with coffee or orange juice reduces the bioavailability by approximately 60%. Calculate the quantity of alendronate bioavailable, in milligrams, following a 10-mg dose swallowed with orange juice.*

$$10 \text{ mg} \times 0.59\% = 0.059 \text{ mg}$$
$$0.059 \text{ mg} \times 40\% = \mathbf{0.0236 \text{ mg}}$$

"BIOEQUIVALENT" AMOUNTS OF "BIOINEQUIVALENT" DOSAGE FORMS

The bioavailability of a given drug substance may vary when in different dosage forms or in the same dosage form but from a different manufacturer. Thus, it may be desired to calculate the equivalent doses for two *bioinequivalent* products. The following equation can be used when calculating doses for bioinequivalent products:

$$F_1 \times \text{Dose}_1 = F_2 \times \text{Dose}_2$$

(1) *If the bioavailability (F) of digoxin (LANOXIN) in a 0.25-mg tablet is 0.60 compared to the bioavailability (F) of 0.75 in a digoxin elixir (0.05 mg/mL), calculate the dose of the elixir equivalent to the tablet.*

First, calculate the amount of "bioavailable" digoxin in the tablet:

$0.25 \text{ mg} \times 0.60 = 0.15 \text{ mg}$, bioavailable amount of digoxin in the tablet

Next, calculate the amount of "bioavailable" digoxin per milliliter of the elixir:

$0.05 \text{ mg} \times 0.75 = 0.0375 \text{ mg}$, bioavailable amount of digoxin per milliliter of the elixir

Finally, determine the quantity of elixir that will provide 0.15 mg of "bioavailable" digoxin: By proportion:

$$\frac{0.0375 \text{ (mg)}}{0.15 \text{ (mg)}} = \frac{1 \text{ (mL)}}{x \text{ (mL)}}$$
$$x = \mathbf{4 \text{ mL}}$$

Or utilizing the equation:

$$0.6 \times 0.25 \text{ mg} = 0.75 \times \text{Dose}_{\text{elixir}}$$
$$\text{Dose}_{\text{elixir}} = 0.2 \text{ mg}$$
$$0.2 \text{ mg} \times 1 \text{ mL}/0.05 \text{ mg} = \mathbf{4 \text{ mL}}$$

(2) *A newly admitted hospital patient has been taking a brand of digoxin tablets, 250 μg, that are 60% bioavailable. The physician wishes to administer a comparable IV dose (F = 1) using an injection containing digoxin, 0.5 mg/2 mL. What is the comparable dose?*

$$250\ \mu g \times 60\% = 150\ \mu g \text{ (effective or absorbed dose)}$$

$$\text{Injection} = 0.5\ mg/2\ mL = 500\ \mu g/2\ mL$$

$$150\ \mu g \times \frac{2\ mL}{500\ \mu g} = \mathbf{0.6\ mL\ digoxin\ injection}$$

Plotting and Interpreting a Blood Level–Time Curve

Following the administration of a medication, if blood samples are drawn from the patient at specific time intervals and analyzed for drug content, the resulting data may be plotted as a graph to prepare a blood level–time curve. The vertical axis of this type of plot characteristically presents the concentration of drug present in the blood, serum, or plasma, and the horizontal axis presents the times the samples were obtained after administration of the drug. When the drug is first administered (time zero), the blood concentration of the drug should also be zero. As an orally administered drug passes into the stomach and/or intestine, it is released from the dosage form, fully or partially dissolves, and is absorbed. As the sampling and analysis continue, the blood samples reveal increasing concentrations of drug, until the maximum (peak) concentration (C_{max}) is reached. Then the blood level of the drug decreases progressively due to distribution to the tissues and elimination, and if no additional dose is given, eventually falls back to zero.

For conventional dosage forms, such as tablets and capsules, the C_{max} will usually occur at only a single time point, referred to as T_{max}. The amount of drug is usually expressed in terms of its concentration in relation to a specific volume of blood, serum, or plasma. For example, the concentration may be expressed as g/100 mL, μg/mL, mg/dL, or mg% (mg/100 mL). The quantity of a dose administered and its bioavailability, dissolution, and absorption characteristics influence the blood concentration for a drug substance. The rate or speed of drug absorption determines the T_{max}, the time of greatest blood drug concentration after administration; the faster the rate of absorption, the sooner the T_{max}.

In a blood level–time curve, the area under the curve (AUC) is considered representative of the *total* amount of drug absorbed into systemic circulation. The AUC may be measured mathematically, using a technique known as the trapezoidal rule. The procedure may be found in other textbooks, references, and at various Web sites.[3]

From the following data, plot a serum concentration–time curve and determine (a) the peak height concentration (C_{max}) and (b) the time of the peak height concentration (T_{max}).

Time Period (hours)	*Serum Drug Concentration (mcg/mL)*
0.5	1.0
1.0	2.0
2.0	4.0
3.0	3.8
4.0	2.9
6.0	1.9
8.0	1.0
10.0	0.3
12.0	0.2

Plotting the data and interpretation of the curve:

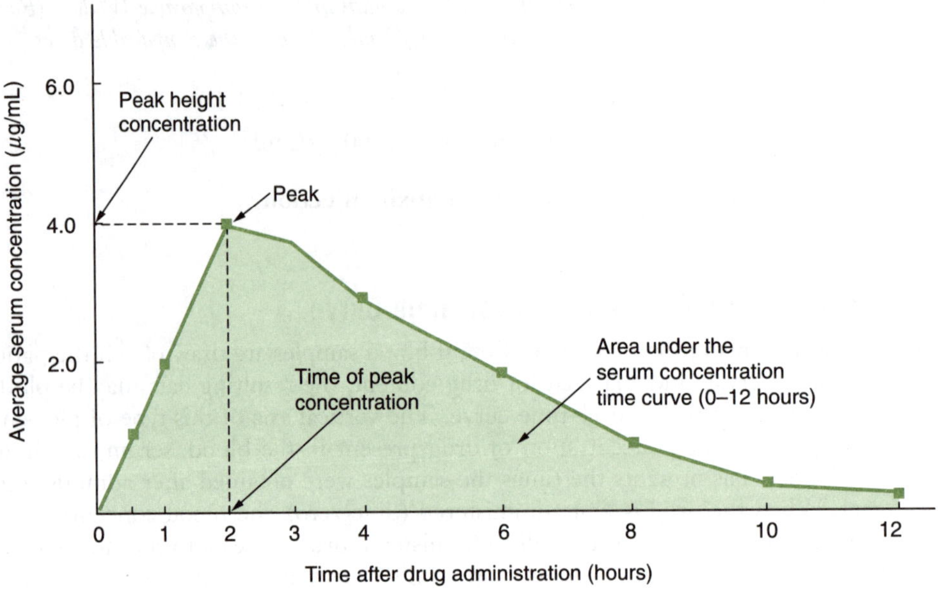

Determining the intercept for C_{max} and T_{max}:

$$C_{max} = \mathbf{4.0\,\mu g/mL}$$

$$T_{max} = \mathbf{2\ hours}$$

Calculation of the absolute bioavailability (F) of a drug may be determined by comparison of the AUC data for the particular dosage form against the intravenous form[4]:

$$F = \frac{AUC_{\text{dosage form}}}{AUC_{\text{intravenous}}}$$

It is recalled that the value F is the fraction of an administered dose that enters the systemic circulation. The intravenous route is the reference standard for comparison since the quantity of drug administered intravenously is considered to enter completely into the systemic circulation.

If the AUC for an oral dose of a drug administered by tablet is 4.5 mcg h/mL and the intravenous dose is 11.2 mcg h/mL, calculate the bioavailability of the oral dose of the drug.[4]

$$F = \frac{AUC_{\text{oral tablet}}}{AUC_{IV}}$$

$$F = \frac{4.5\text{ mcg h/mL}}{11.2\text{ mcg h/mL}} = \mathbf{0.4\ or\ 40\%}$$

CASE IN POINT 22.1[4] A hospitalized patient has been receiving ranitidine (ZANTAC) 50 mg by intravenous injection every 8 hours. After discharge, the patient's physician wishes to continue treatment with a bioequivalent dose of the oral liquid form of ranitidine. From the literature, the community pharmacist determines that the oral liquid is 50% bioavailable. The product is available in a concentration of 75 mg/5 mL, to be taken twice a day. How many milliliters of the oral liquid should be indicated per dose on the prescription label?

Introductory Concepts and Calculations Involved in Pharmacokinetics

As defined previously, pharmacokinetics is the study and characterization of the time course of absorption, distribution, metabolism, and excretion of drugs. Many of the calculations involved in pharmacokinetics are complex and the subject of advanced textbooks devoted to this important field. The intention in the following discussion is to define and describe some of the more introductory concepts and calculations.

Example Calculations of Selected Pharmacokinetic Parameters

PLASMA CONCENTRATION OF UNBOUND VERSUS BOUND DRUGS

Once absorbed into the circulation, a portion of the total drug plasma concentration (C_T) is bound to plasma proteins (usually albumin), and a portion remains unbound, or free. It is the unbound drug (C_U) that is available for further transport to its site of action in the body. The fraction of unbound drug compared with bound drug (C_B) is primarily a function of the affinity of the drug molecules for binding to the plasma proteins and the concentration of the latter (some patients may have a reduced or elevated serum albumin concentration). Some drug molecules may be more than 90% bound to plasma proteins, whereas others may be bound only slightly. Any change in the degree of binding of a given drug substance can alter its distribution and elimination and thus its clinical effects.

The fraction of unbound drug in the plasma compared with the total plasma drug concentration, bound and unbound, is termed ***alpha*** (or α).

Thus,

$$\alpha = \frac{C_U}{C_U + C_B} = \frac{C_U}{C_T}$$

If one knows the value of α for a drug and the total plasma concentration (C_T), the concentration of free drug in the plasma may be determined by a rearranged equation:

$$C_U = \alpha \times (C_T)$$

If the alpha (α) value for the drug digoxin is 0.70, what would be the concentration of free drug in the plasma if the total plasma concentration of the drug were determined to be 0.7 ng/mL?

$$C_U = (0.70) \times (0.7 \text{ ng/mL})$$
$$= \mathbf{0.49\ ng/mL}$$

APPARENT VOLUME OF DISTRIBUTION OF A DRUG SUBSTANCE

The apparent volume of distribution for a drug is not a "real" volume but rather a hypothetical volume of body fluid that would be required to dissolve the total amount of drug at the same concentration as that found in the blood. The volume of distribution is an indicator of the extent of a drug's distribution throughout the body fluids and tissues. The information is useful in understanding how the body processes and distributes a given drug substance. After a dose of a drug is administered intravenously, a change in the concentration of the drug in the blood means a corresponding change in the drug's concentration in another body fluid or tissue. This sequence allows an understanding of the pattern of the drug's distribution.

It may be useful in understanding the concept of volume of distribution to imagine a 100-mg amount of a drug substance dissolved in an undetermined volume of water. If the analysis of a sample of the resultant solution revealed a drug concentration of 20 mg/L, it can be seen that the total volume of water in which the drug was dissolved equaled 5 L; that is:

$$\frac{20\ (\text{mg})}{100\ (\text{mg})} = \frac{1\ (\text{L})}{x\ (\text{L})}$$
$$x = 5\ \text{L}$$

Different drugs administered in the same amount will show different volumes of distribution because of different distribution characteristics. For example, drugs that remain in the blood after intravenous administration because of the drug binding to plasma proteins or to blood cells show high blood concentrations and low volumes of distribution. Conversely, drugs that exit the circulation rapidly and diffuse into other body fluids and tissues show low blood concentrations and high volumes of distribution.

If the volume of distribution in an adult is 5 L, the drug is considered confined to the circulatory system, as it would be immediately after a rapid intravenous injection (IV bolus). If the volume of distribution is between 10 and 20 L, or between 15% and 27% of the body weight, it is assumed that the drug has been distributed into the extracellular fluids; if it is between 25 and 30 L, or between 35% and 42% of body weight, it is assumed that the drug has been distributed into the intracellular fluid; if it is about 40 L, or 60% of the body weight, the assumption is that the drug has been distributed in the whole body fluid.[5] If the apparent volume of distribution actually exceeds the body weight, it is assumed that the drug is being stored in body fat, bound to body tissues, or is distributed in peripheral compartments.

The equation for determining the volume of distribution (Vd) is:

$$\text{Vd} = \frac{\text{D}}{\text{C}_\text{p}}$$

in which D is the total amount of drug in the body and C_p is the drug's plasma concentration at any given time. The apparent volume of distribution may be expressed as a simple volume or as a percentage of body weight.

A patient received a single intravenous dose of 300 mg of a drug substance that produced an immediate blood concentration of 8.2 μg of drug per milliliter. Calculate the apparent volume of distribution.

$$\text{Vd} = \frac{\text{D}}{\text{C}_\text{p}}$$
$$= \frac{300\ \text{mg}}{8.2\ \mu\text{g/mL}} = \frac{300\ \text{mg}}{8.2\ \text{mg/L}}$$
$$= \mathbf{36.6\ L}$$

TOTAL AMOUNT OF DRUG BASED ON VOLUME OF DISTRIBUTION AND PLASMA CONCENTRATION

Calculating the total amount of drug in a body, given the volume of distribution and the plasma drug concentration, involves the following:

Four hours following the intravenous administration of a drug, a patient weighing 70 kg was found to have a drug blood level concentration of 10 μg/mL. Assuming the apparent volume of distribution is 10% of body weight, calculate the total amount of drug present in body fluids 4 hours after the drug was administered.

$$Vd = \frac{D}{C_P} \quad D = (Vd) \times (C_P)$$

$$Vd = 10\% \text{ of } 70 \text{ kg} = 7 \text{ kg} = 7 \text{ L}$$

$$C_P = 10\ \mu g/mL = 10 \text{ mg/L}$$

$$7 \text{ L} = \frac{D}{10 \text{ mg/L}}$$

$$D = (7 \text{ L}) \times (10 \text{ mg/L})$$

$$= \mathbf{70\ mg}$$

ELIMINATION HALF-LIFE AND ELIMINATION RATE CONSTANT

The elimination phase of a drug from the body is reflected by a decline in the drug's plasma concentration. The ***elimination half-life*** ($t_{½}$) is the time it takes for the plasma drug concentration (as well as the amount of drug in the body) to fall by one-half. For example, if it takes 3 hours for the plasma concentration of a drug to fall from 6 to 3 mg/L, its half-life would be 3 hours. It would take the same period of time (3 hours) for the concentration to fall from 3 to 1.5 mg/L or from 1.5 to 0.75 mg/L. Most drug substances follow first-order kinetics in their elimination from the body, meaning that the rate of drug elimination per unit of time is proportional to the amount present at that time, as shown in the following equation:

$$C_t = C_0 e^{-Kt}$$

where C_t is the amount of drug in the blood at time t, C_0 is the amount of drug given intravenously, and K, or K_{el}, is the elimination rate constant. Relatively few drugs follow zero order or other types of elimination kinetics, and their discussion is beyond the scope of this chapter. For all equations and problems discussed in this chapter, first-order elimination will be assumed.

As demonstrated previously, the elimination half-life is independent of the amount of drug in the body, and the amount of drug eliminated is less in each succeeding half-life. After five elimination half-lives, it may be expected that virtually all of a drug (97%) originally present will have been eliminated. The student might wish to examine this point, starting with a 100-mg dose of a drug (after first half-life, 50 mg, etc.).

Blood level data from a drug may be plotted against time as a regular graph to obtain an exponential curve, or it may be plotted as a semilogarithmic graph to obtain a straight line. From the latter, the elimination half-life may be determined, as shown in the example that follows in this section.

The elimination rate constant (K_{el}) characterizes the elimination process and may simply be regarded as the *fractional rate of drug removal per unit time, expressed as a decimal fraction* (e.g., 0.01 min^{-1}, meaning 1% per minute). The elimination rate constant for a first-order process may be calculated using the equation:

$$K_{el} = \frac{0.693}{t_{1/2}}$$

The derivation of this equation is described for the exponential decay of radioisotopes (see Chapter 21, p. 377).

(1) *A patient received 12 mg of a drug intravenously, and blood samples were drawn and analyzed at specific time intervals, resulting in the following data. Plot the data as a semilogarithmic graph and determine the elimination half-life of the drug.*

Time (hours)	*Plasma Drug Level Concentration (μg/100 mL)*
1	26.5
2	17.5
3	11.5
4	7.6
5	5.0
6	3.3

Plotting the data:

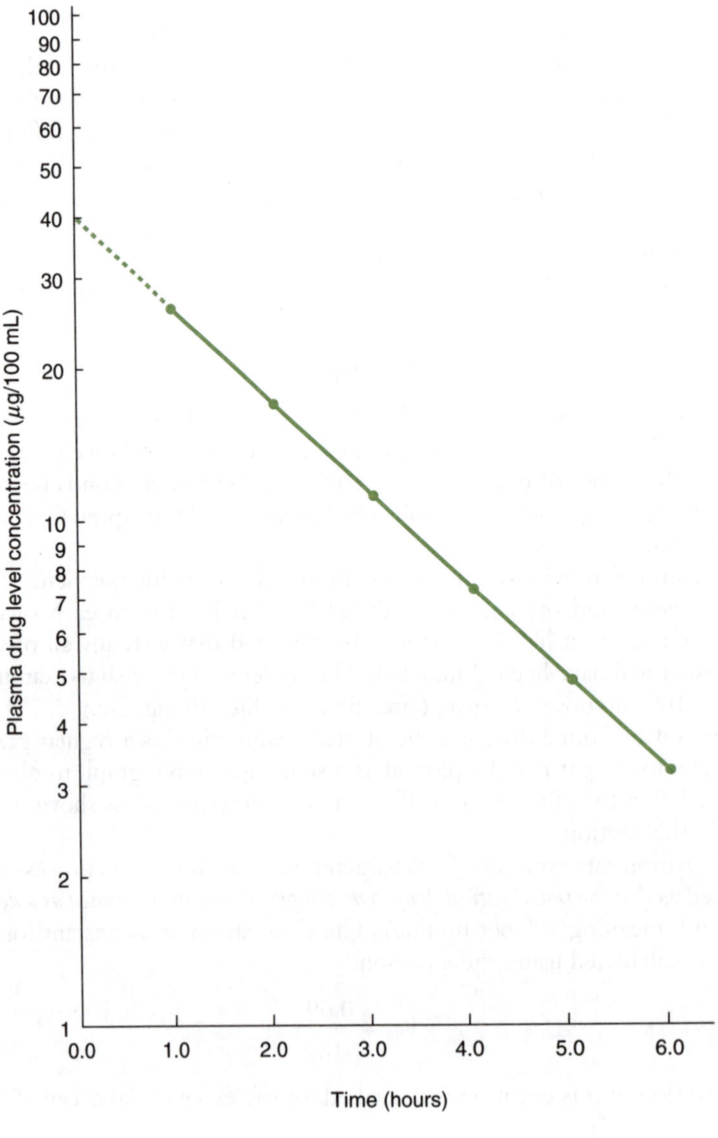

From the plotted data, the straight line may be extrapolated to time zero to determine the initial plasma drug concentration, which is found to be 40 μg/100 mL. The time it takes to reduce that level to one-half, or 20 μg/100 mL, is the elimination half-life. The 20 μg/100 mL concentration intersects the straight line at 1.7 hours.

Therefore, the elimination half-life is **1.7 hours.**

NOTE: the same answer may be obtained by selecting any plasma drug concentration (e.g., 10 μg/100 mL), determining the time of that plasma level from the intercept, repeating the process for one-half of that drug level (5 μg/100 mL), and determining the elapsed time by subtraction to obtain the elimination half-life.

(2) *Calculate the elimination rate constant for a drug that has an elimination half-life of 50 minutes.*

$$K_{el} = \frac{0.693}{t_{1/2}}$$

$$= \frac{0.693}{50 \text{ min}}$$

$$= \mathbf{0.0139 \text{ min}^{-1}}$$

Additional related calculations, such as drug dosage based on creatinine clearance, may be found in Chapter 10.

CALCULATIONS CAPSULE

Selected Bioavailability and Pharmacokinetics

Comparative dose calculation based on bioavailability (F):

$$F_1 \times Dose_1 = F_2 \times Dose_2$$

Volume of distribution (Vd):

$$Vd = \frac{D}{C_P}$$

D = total administered (IV) amount of drug

C_P = blood/plasma concentration of drug

First-order elimination rate constant (K_{el}):

$$K_{el} = \frac{0.693}{t_{1/2}}$$

PRACTICE PROBLEMS

Calculations of Bioavailability and Bioequivalence

1. If the bioavailability factor (F) for a 100-mg tablet of a drug is 0.70 compared with the bioavailability factor of 1.0 for an injection of the same drug, how many milliliters of the injection containing 40 mg/mL would be considered bioequivalent to the tablet?
2. If 5 mL of an elixir containing 2 mg/mL of a drug is bioequivalent to a 15-mg tablet having a bioavailability factor of 0.60, what is the bioavailability factor (F) of the elixir?
3. If 500 mg of a drug are administered orally and 300 mg are absorbed into the circulation, calculate the bioavailability factor (F).
4.[4] A drug is 40% bioavailable by the oral route and 58% bioavailable by the transdermal route. If a patient is taking a 2.5-mg oral dose twice a day and is switched to the counterpart 2% ointment, how many grams of the ointment should be administered each day to provide the equivalent dose of the drug?
5.[4] A drug used to treat asthma is 55% bioavailable as 5-mg tablets to be taken once daily. If a patient is switched to the inhalant form of the drug, which is 87% bioavailable, how many metered 500-μg sprays should the patient administer every 12 hours to receive an equivalent drug dose?

Calculations of Bound Drug, Elimination Half-Life, and Volume of Distribution

6.[4] If a 6-mg dose of a drug is administered intravenously and produces a blood concentration of 0.4 mcg/mL, calculate its apparent volume of distribution.
7. If at equilibrium, two-thirds of the amount of a drug substance in the blood is bound to protein, what would be the alpha (α) value of the drug?
8. The alpha (α) value for a drug in the blood is 0.90, equating to 0.55 ng/mL. What is the concentration of total drug in the blood?
9. A patient received an intravenous dose of 10 mg of a drug. A blood sample was drawn immediately after administration, and it contained 40 μg/100 mL. Calculate the apparent volume of distribution for the drug.
10. The volume of distribution for a drug was found to be 10 L with a blood level concentration of 2 μg/mL. Calculate the total amount of drug present in the patient.
11. Calculate the elimination rate constant for a drug having an elimination half-life of 1.7 hours.
12. Plot the following data as a semilogarithmic graph and determine (a) the elimination half-life of the drug and (b) the elimination rate constant.

Time (hours)	*Plasma Drug Concentration (mg/100 mL)*
0.5	8.5
1.0	6.8
1.5	5.4
2.0	4.0
2.5	3.2
3.0	2.5

13. What percentage of an originally administered intravenous dose of a drug remains in the body following three half-lives?

14. If the half-life of a drug is 4 hours, approximately what percentage of the drug administered would remain in the body 15 hours after administration?
15. The elimination half-life of dapagliflozin propanediol (FARXIGA) is 12.9 hours. What is the elimination rate constant?
16. If 100 mg of a drug are administered intravenously, and the resultant drug plasma concentration is determined to be 2.5 μg/mL, calculate the apparent volume of distribution.
17. If a dose of 1 g of a drug is administered intravenously to a patient and the drug plasma concentration is determined to be 65 μg/mL, calculate the apparent volume of distribution.
18. The volume of distribution for a drug has been determined to be 34 L. Calculate the expected drug plasma concentration of the drug, in micrograms per deciliter, immediately after an intravenous dose of 5 mg.
19. In normal subjects, blood makes up about 7% of the body weight.
    (a) Calculate the approximate blood volume, in liters, for a man weighing 70 kg.
    (b) If the drug ranitidine (ZANTAC) reached peak blood levels of about 500 ng/mL 2 to 3 hours after an oral dose, calculate the total amount of the drug, in milligrams, in the blood of the patient described in (a) when peak blood levels are achieved.
20. Hydromorphone (DILAUDID) has a bioavailability of 24% when given as an immediate-release tablet and produces a C_{max} of 5.5 ng/mL at approximately 45 minutes following administration. The volume of distribution is 2.9 L/kg, and elimination half-life is 2.6 hours and is approximately 14% protein bound. Calculate (a) the amount of drug absorbed from an 8-mg tablet based on the bioavailability, (b) the amount of unbound drug based on the amount absorbed in (a), (c) the total amount of drug present in a patient weighing 160 lb at C_{max} based on the Vd, and (d) the amount of time necessary to eliminate virtually all of the drug from the body.

CALCQUIZ

22.A. A package insert for cefdinir capsules and oral suspension states that following oral administration, the bioavailability of cefdinir suspension is 120% relative to the capsules. The bioavailability of cefdinir capsules is stated as 21% following the administration of a 300-mg capsule dose and 16% following the administration of a 600-mg capsule dose. Calculate the bioavailable quantity of cefdinir, in milligrams, following the administration of a dose of the oral suspension containing 300 mg of cefdinir.

22.B.[a] The drug aminophylline is 80% theophylline. A patient to be discharged from the hospital has been receiving aminophylline 40 mg/h by IV infusion. Upon discharge, the physician orders oral theophylline tablets. The pharmacist recognizes that the prescribed tablets have 85% bioavailability. What oral daily dose, in milligrams of theophylline, should the patient receive by tablets?

22.C. Directly following a 7.5-mg intravenous injection of the drug alefacept (AMEVIVE) for a patient weighing 65 kg, a peak plasma concentration of 1.23 mcg/mL is reached. Calculate the apparent volume of distribution as milliliters per kilogram of body weight. If the drug's half-life is stated in the literature as 270 hours, calculate the elimination rate constant.

[a]Problem courtesy of Flynn Warren, Bishop, GA.

ANSWERS TO "CASE IN POINT" AND PRACTICE PROBLEMS

Case in Point 22.1

$$\text{IV daily dose} = \frac{50\text{ mg}}{1\text{ dose}} \times \frac{3\text{ doses}}{1\text{ day}} = 150\text{ mg/day}$$

F for the IV route = 1 or 100%

$$100\% \times 150\text{ mg/day} = 50\% \times \text{Dose}_{oral}$$

$\text{Dose}_{oral} = 300$ mg/day

$$\frac{300\text{ mg}}{1\text{ day}} \times \frac{1\text{ day}}{2\text{ doses}} = 150\text{ mg/dose}$$

$$\frac{150\text{ mg}}{1\text{ dose}} \times \frac{5\text{ mL}}{75\text{ mg}} = 10\text{ mL/dose}$$

Practice Problems

1. 1.75-mL injection
2. 0.9
3. 0.6
4. 0.17 g ointment
5. 3.16 or 3 sprays
6. 15 L
7. 0.33
8. 0.61 ng/mL
9. 25 L
10. 20 mg
11. 0.408 hour^{-1}
12. $t_{1/2} = 1.4$ hours
    $K_{el} = 0.5\ \text{hour}^{-1}$
13. 12.5%
14. 7.44%
15. 0.054 hour^{-1}
16. 40 L
17. 15.38 L
18. 14.71 μg/dL
19. (a) 4.9 L
    (b) 2.45 mg ranitidine
20. (a) 1.92 mg
    (b) 1.65 mg
    (c) 1.16 mg
    (d) 13 hours

References

1. U.S. Food and Drug Administration. Part 320. Bioavailability and Bioequivalence Requirements. *Code of Federal Regulations*. Title 21, Volume 5, Chapter I, Subchapter D [book online]. Department of Health and Human Services. [U.S. Food and Drug Administration Website.] Available at: http://www.accessdata.fda.gov/scripts/cdrh/cfdocs/cfcfr/CFRSearch.cfm?fr=320.1. Accessed April 17, 2015.
2. Dissolution. U.S. Pharmacopeial Convention, Inc. *United States Pharmacopeia 37 National Formulary 32 [book online]*. Rockville, MD: U.S. Pharmacopeial Convention, Inc.; 2014.
3. Shargel L, Wu-Pong S, Yu ABC. Mathematical fundamentals in pharmacokinetics. In: *Applied Biopharmaceutics and Pharmacokinetics*. 6th Ed. New York, NY: McGraw-Hill Co.; 2012:24–26.
4. Prince SJ. In: Ansel HC, Prince SJ. *Pharmaceutical Calculations: The Pharmacist's Handbook*. 6th Ed. Baltimore, MD: Lippincott Williams & Wilkins; 2004:150–164.
5. Ritschel WA, Kearns GL. *Handbook of Basic Pharmacokinetics…Including Clinical Applications*. 7th Ed. Washington, DC: American Pharmacists Association; 2009:156.

23

Cost Differential Calculations in Drug Therapy

OBJECTIVES

Upon successful completion of this chapter, the student will be able to:

- Perform cost differential calculations between drugs within a therapeutic category.
- Perform cost differential calculations between branded and generic drug products.
- Perform cost differential calculations between dosage forms and routes of administration.
- Perform cost differential calculations based on dosing regimens.
- Perform cost differential calculations between utilizing split versus whole tablets.
- Perform cost differential calculations based on alternative treatment plans.

In drug therapy, among the many considerations in the selection of a drug and drug product is the cost differential between the proposed drug and drug product and acceptable alternatives. Examples of such considerations follow.

Calculations Based on Drug and Drug Product Selection

Cost Differential of Drugs within a Therapeutic Category

Often, there is a substantial cost differential between drugs, even within a single therapeutic category. If the therapeutic outcomes among the drug choices are expected to be comparable, the least expensive drug may be prescribed. However, if one drug is considered to be therapeutically advantageous over others, even though it may be more expensive, it would likely be selected for use.

Calculate the cost differential between the thrombolytic agents streptokinase (250,000 IU; $96.41) and the biotechnology derived drug alteplase (50 mg; $1100) if the total amount proposed to be administered to a patient is either 1,500,000 IU of streptokinase or 90 mg of alteplase.

Cost of streptokinase: $\frac{250{,}000\ \text{IU}}{1{,}500{,}000\ \text{IU}} = \frac{\$96.41}{x}$; $x = \$578.46$

Cost of alteplase: $\frac{50\ \text{mg}}{90\ \text{mg}} = \frac{\$1100}{x}$; $x = \$1980$

Cost differential: $1980 − $578.46 = **$1401.54**

Cost Differential between Branded Drug Products and Generic Equivalents

Drug entities that are protected by patents are typically first available as brand-name products from a single source, the innovator (or originator) company. When the patent protection expires, the now *off-patent drug* usually becomes available as *generic products*,[a] manufactured and/or distributed by multiple sources (*multisource products*). Sometimes, a noninnovator company will provide a brand name to their version of a generic drug product, a type of product referred to as a *branded generic*.

Generic drugs are lower in price than innovator products since they do not bear the original costs of drug discovery research and product development. For economic reasons, prescribers and individual patients may request the dispensing of generic products, and insurance companies and other third-party payers may require their use for reimbursement.

The generic equivalent of a drug costs $12.40/100 tablets, whereas the innovator product costs $46.20/100 tablets. Calculate the drug cost differential for a 30-day supply if two tablets are taken daily.

Tablets required: 2 tablets (daily) × 30 (days) = 60 tablets

Cost of generic drug: $\frac{100 \text{ tablets}}{60 \text{ tablets}} = \frac{\$12.40}{x}$; x = $7.44

Cost of innovator drug: $\frac{100 \text{ tablets}}{60 \text{ tablets}} = \frac{\$46.20}{x}$; x = $27.72

Cost differential: $27.72 – $7.44 = **$20.28**

Cost Differential between Dosage Forms and Routes of Administration

There is often a cost differential between different dosage forms of the same drug due to dissimilar costs of product development and production. Solid dosage forms, as tablets and capsules, are among the least expensive to develop and manufacture, whereas injectable products and transdermal patches are among the most expensive.

There is also a cost factor with regard to route of administration. The oral route is simple and routine for most patients and caregivers. However, medications administered by injection require special supplies and technique. For patients receiving intravenous fluids, the associated costs are further expanded by the additional skilled personnel and equipment required. In fact, many hospital cost containment programs encourage the conversion from parenteral medications to oral therapy as soon as feasible, providing that the desired therapeutic outcomes are not compromised.

(1) *Verapamil 80-mg tablets are taken three times a day and cost $7.52/100 tablets. Extended-release capsules containing 240 mg of verapamil are taken once daily and cost $15.52/100 capsules. Calculate the treatment cost differential over a 30-day period.*

80-mg tablets: $7.52 ÷ 100 (tablets) = $0.0752 (per tablet)
3 tablets (per day) × 30 (days) = 90 tablets
$0.0752 × 90 (tablets) = $6.768 or $6.77

240-mg capsules: $15.52 ÷ 100 (capsules) = $0.1552 (per capsule)
1 capsule (per day) × 30 (days) = 30 capsules
$0.01552 × 30 (capsules) = $4.656 or $4.66

Cost differential: $6.77 – $4.66 = **$2.11**

---

[a]According to the FDA, a generic drug is a drug product that is comparable to a brand/reference listed drug product in dosage form, strength, route of administration, quality and performance characteristics, and intended use.[1]

(2) *A hospitalized patient was switched from intravenous ciprofloxacin (400 mg q12h) to oral ciprofloxacin (500 mg q12h). Calculate the daily drug cost savings if the intravenous product cost is $12.00 per 200 mg and the oral product cost is $2.95 per 250-mg capsule.*

Intravenous ciprofloxacin:	400 mg × 2 (times per day) = 800 mg
	800 mg × $12.00/200 mg = $48.00
Oral ciprofloxacin:	500 mg × 2 (times per day) = 1000 mg
	1000 mg × $2.95/250 mg = $11.80
Cost differential:	$48.00 – $11.80 = **$36.20**

Cost Differential of Dosing Regimens

On a case-by-case basis, a dosing regimen may be changed to be more cost effective without affecting the desired therapeutic outcome.

A dosage interval adjustment was made in the intravenous administration of the drug ranitidine in a group of 23 hospitalized patients such that the number of doses per patient per treatment day was reduced from an average of 2.33 to 1.51 without sacrificing therapeutic outcomes. If the cost of each dose of ranitidine was $4.02, calculate the daily cost savings to the hospital.

Reduction in doses per patient per day:	2.33–1.51 = 0.82 doses
Reduction in doses in patient group:	0.82 dose × 23 (patients) = 18.86 doses
Cost savings:	$4.02 × 18.86 (doses) = **$75.82**

Cost Differential of Utilizing Split versus Whole Tablets

Splitting whole tablets is a practice undertaken through the agreement of both prescriber and patient. In these instances, whole tablets are prescribed and dispensed at twice the dosing strength but in half the quantity, thereby reducing drug cost. The patient (or when requested, the pharmacist) splits the whole tablets using an appropriate device to obtain relatively even portions.

It should be noted, and the patient advised, that some tablets should never be split or otherwise broken due to the presence of special tablet coatings and/or disintegration and absorption features inherent in the tablet's design.

A physician prescribed fifteen 80-mg tablets of simvastatin tablets and instructed the patient to split the tablets in half for a 30-day supply at a 40-mg daily dose. One hundred 80-mg tablets cost $12.50 and an equal number of 40-mg tablets cost $10.50. Calculate the patient's savings on a month's supply.

80-mg tablets: 15 tablets × $12.50/100 tablets = $1.88

40-mg tablets: 30 tablets × $10.50/100 tablets = $3.15

$3.15 – $1.88 = **$1.27 savings**

Cost Differential of Alternative Treatment

Drug therapy is extremely cost effective when it reduces or eliminates the need for patient hospitalization.

If the daily treatment of an ulcer patient with cimetidine prevents readmission to a hospital, calculate the potential savings over reoccurrence of hospitalization if the daily drug costs are $1.38 and the prior 5-day hospital bill was $4056.

Drug cost:	$1.38 × 5 (days) = $6.90
Potential savings:	$4056 – $6.90 = **$4049.10**

CASE IN POINT 23.1 A hospital's Pharmacy and Therapeutics Committee is determining the most economical of three drugs considered to be therapeutically equivalent. The least expensive drug, per patient treatment day, is to be added to the hospital's drug formulary.

Drug A: 0.5 g/mL, 5-mL vial; dose, 1 mL q6h; cost, $16.50/vial
Drug B: 1 g/mL, 10-mL vial; dose, 0.75 mL q8h; cost, $57.42/vial
Drug C: 1.5 g/mL, 1-mL ampul; dose, 1 mL q12h; cost, $15.94/ampul

Which drug is most economical, per patient treatment day, not taking into consideration any material or personnel costs?

PRACTICE PROBLEMS

1. An antianginal drug is available in a three-times-a-day tablet at $42.50/100 tablets, in a twice-a-day tablet at $64.00/100 tablets, and in a once-a-day tablet at $80.20/100 tablets. Which form would be most economical to a compliant patient and at what cost?
2. A physician inquires a pharmacist regarding the most economical of the following antihypertensive therapies: drug A, 30-mg tablets taken q.i.d. costing $0.33/tablet; drug B, 10-mg tablets taken t.i.d. costing $0.20/tablet; or drug C, 2.5-mg tablets taken b.i.d, costing $0.38/tablet. Indicate the most economical drug and the drug cost for a 30-day supply.
3. A physician offers a patient the option of prescribing 30 scored sertraline (ZOLOFT) 100-mg tablets (for the patient to break in half with a dose of one-half tablet) or 60 tablets containing 50 mg of the drug. Calculate the cost differential and indicate the most economical option for the patient if the 100-mg tablets cost $126.78 per 100 tablets and the 50-mg tablets cost $115.00 per 100 tablets.
4. Calculate the daily drug cost differential between a dose of a drug administered q8h and costing $6.25/dose and a counterpart drug administered once daily and costing $26.50/dose.
5. If 100 tablets of an innovator drug cost $114.50 and 60 tablets of a generic equivalent cost $27.75, calculate the cost differential for a 30-day supply with one tablet per day dosing.
6. A pharmacist can purchase 5-mg tablets of a drug at (a) $16.21 for a bottle of 100 tablets, (b) $73.41 for a bottle of 500 tablets, or (c) $124.25 for a bottle of 1000 tablets. Calculate the drug costs for each of the package sizes to fill a prescription for 60 tablets.
7. A hospital pharmacy recommended parenteral cefazolin (dose: 0.5 g q8h; cost: $1.80/g) over parenteral cefoxitin (dose: 1 g q6h; cost: $6.48/g) to balance therapeutic outcomes with cost containment. Calculate the difference in drug cost between these two treatments per patient day.
8. An anti-AIDS compound is commonly taken at an adult daily dose of 600 mg, in two or more divided doses. If 300-mg tablets cost $265 per 60, calculate the drug cost per year.
9. The drug hydralazine may be administered intravenously when needed to control hypertension at 20-mg doses in D5W every 12 hours for 48 hours, after which the patient is converted to oral dosage, 10-mg tablets four times per day for 2 days, and then 25-mg tablets four times per day for the next 5 days. If the 20-mg IV ampul costs

$6.00; 10-mg tablets, $18.00/100 tablets; 25-mg tablets, $26.00/100 tablets; and D5W, $10.00 per bottle, calculate the *average daily* costs of intravenous and oral therapy.

10. A physician has a choice of prescribing the following ACE inhibitor drugs to treat hypertension, with the pharmacist's cost of each, per 100 tablets, given in parentheses: drug A, 10 mg ($63.00); drug B, 25 mg ($59.00); drug C, 5 mg ($84.00); and drug D, 10 mg ($70.00). Each drug is once-a-day dosing except for drug B tablets, which are taken twice a day. Calculate the 30-day medication cost for each drug.
11. The cost to a hospital of a drug is $16.97 per 10-mg vial. If the drug is administered by intermittent injection at 0.15 mg/kg/h for 24 hours, calculate the daily cost of the drug used for a 70-kg patient.
12. If the drug in the preceding problem may be administered to the same patient by continuous infusion (rather than by intermittent injection) with a 0.1 mg/kg loading dose and subsequent doses of 0.05 mg/kg for the next 23 hours, calculate the daily cost of the drug by this route of administration.
13. The intravenous dosing schedules and costs of the following cephalosporin antimicrobial agents are cefazolin, 1 g every 8 hours ($3.00); cefoxitin, 1 g every 6 hours ($6.24); and cefotetan, 1 g every 24 hours ($31.39). Calculate the daily cost of each drug.
14. A patient is converted from taking 20-mg atorvastatin calcium tablets once daily, to splitting 40-mg tablets and taking one split tablet every other night at bedtime. If the cost to the patient is $15 for 30 tablets as a co-pay with insurance benefits, irrespective of tablet strength, calculate the cost savings to the patient over a 12-week period.
15. The cost of an anticancer drug is $5,425 for 400 mg. The drug is administered by IV infusion at a dose of 5 mg/kg every 2 weeks for six treatments. An alternative drug would cost $11,000 for the entire course of treatment. Calculate the cost differential between the two drugs if administered to a 152-lb patient.

CALCQUIZ

23.A.[a] Colchicine and nonsteroidal anti-inflammatory drugs (NSAIDs) are included among the treatments of gout. Treatment with colchicine results in fewer adverse effects than does treatment with NSAIDs. The average monthly drug-only cost of colchicine may run 10 times the approximate $30 per month cost for NSAIDs. On the other hand, for the 1.8% to 1.9% of gout patients receiving NSAIDs who require hospitalization due to a serious adverse event, the cost of hospitalization at $____ per day for an average of 5 days is a serious factor to consider in drug selection.

Student research: obtain, and utilize in the calculations, information on the average daily hospitalization cost in the local community, region, or nation.

Calculate: the comparative monthly treatment costs for two hypothetical 100-patient treatment groups, one (NSAID) with average incidence of adverse effects, and the other group taking colchicine.

23.B. A pharmacist-member of a hospital formulary committee compared the cost of 10 days of IV therapy with moxifloxacin hydrochloride (400 mg/250 mL IV once daily) against 4 days of IV therapy (400 mg/250 mL IV once daily) followed by 6 days of oral moxifloxacin hydrochloride therapy (400-mg tablets PO once daily).

Student research: obtain information on the usual pharmacy acquisition costs of the medications-dosage forms in the problem.

Calculate: the difference in the cost of 10 days of medication for the two treatments.

[a]Problem derived from data from Wertheimer et al.[2]

ANSWERS TO "CASE IN POINT" AND PRACTICE PROBLEMS

Case in Point 23.1

Drug A dose, in mL/day:

$$1 \text{ mL/dose} \times 4 \text{ doses/day} = 4 \text{ mL/day}$$

Cost/day:

$$\frac{5 \text{ mL}}{\$16.50} = \frac{4 \text{ mL}}{x}\; x = \$13.20\text{/day}$$

Drug B dose, in mL/day:

$$0.75 \text{ mL/dose} \times 3 \text{ doses/day} = 2.25 \text{ mL/day}$$

Cost/day:

$$\frac{10 \text{ mL}}{\$57.42} = \frac{2.25}{x}\; x = \$12.92\text{/day}$$

Drug C dose, in mL/day:

$$1 \text{ mL/dose} \times 2 \text{ doses/day} = 2 \text{ mL/day}$$

Cost/day:

$$\frac{1 \text{ mL}}{\$15.94} = \frac{2 \text{ mL}}{x}\; x = \$31.84\text{/day}$$

Therefore, drug B is the least expensive per day.

Practice Problems

1. Once-a-day tablet, $0.80/day
2. Drug B, $18.00
3. $30.97, 100-mg tablets
4. $7.75
5. $20.47
6. (a) $9.73
   (b) $8.81
   (c) $7.46
7. $23.22
8. $3224.17
9. IV therapy, $32.00 per day, average oral therapy, $0.74 per day, average
10. Drug A, $18.90
    Drug B, $35.40
    Drug C, $25.20
    Drug D, $21.00
11. $427.64
12. $148.49
13. Cefazolin, $9.00
    Cefoxitin, $24.96
    Cefotetan, $31.39
14. $31.50
15. $17,111

References

1. U.S. Food and Drug Administration Center for Drug Evaluation and Research. Generic drugs. Available at: http://www.fda.gov/downloads/Drugs/DevelopmentApprovalProcess/SmallBusinessAssistance/ucm127615.pdf. Accessed November 22, 2014.
2. Wertheimer AI, Davis MW, Lauterio TJ. A new perspective of the pharmacoeconomics of colchicine. *Current Medical Research and Opinion* 2011;27:931–937.

A

Common Systems of Measurement and Intersystem Conversion

The International System of Units (SI) is the *official* system for weights and measures in the *United States Pharmacopeia—National Formulary*. However, other so-called *common systems of measurement* are encountered in pharmacy and thus must be learned. The ***Apothecaries' System of Measurement*** is the traditional system of pharmacy, and although it is now largely of historic significance, components of this system are occasionally used on prescriptions. The ***avoirdupois system*** is the common system of commerce, employed along with the SI in the United States. It is through this system that items are purchased and sold by the ounce and pound. This appendix defines these common systems, expresses their quantitative relationship to one another and to the SI, and provides the means for intersystem conversion. Conversion of temperature between the Fahrenheit and Celsius (or centigrade) scales is also included in this appendix.

Apothecaries' Fluid Measure

60 minims (♏)	=	1 fluidrachm or fluidram (fʒ or ʒ)[a]
8 fluidrachm (480 minims)	=	1 fluidounce (f℥ or ℥)[a]
16 fluidounces	=	1 pint (pt)
2 pints (32 fluidounces)	=	1 quart (qt)
4 quarts (8 pints)	=	1 gallon (gal)

Apothecaries' Measure of Weight

20 grains (gr)	=	1 scruple (℈)
3 scruples (60 grains)	=	1 drachm or dram (ʒ)
8 drachms (480 grains)	=	1 ounce (℥)
12 ounces (5760 grains)	=	1 pound (℔)

[a]When it is apparent on a prescription or in a formula that the symbol refers to a liquid rather than a solid, the "f" may be absent.

Typical Format of a Prescription in the Apothecaries' System

When prescriptions were commonly written in the apothecaries' system, the following format was used.

℞	Codeine Sulfate	gr iv
	Ammonium Chloride	ʒ iss
	Cherry Syrup ad	f℥ iv
	Sig. ʒi as directed	

Avoirdupois Measure of Weight

437½ or 437.5 grain (gr)	=	1 ounce (oz)
16 ounces (7000 grains)	=	1 pound (lb)

Relationship between Avoirdupois and Apothecaries' Systems of Weight

The *grain* represents the same weight in both the avoirdupois and apothecaries' systems; other units, even though they bear the same name (i.e., *ounce* and *pound*) in the two systems, differ in weight as demonstrated in the tables above. If there is need to convert a quantity from one system to the other, the given quantity should be reduced to grains and then converted to units of weight in the other system.

Intersystem Conversion

To convert a given weight or volume from units of one system to equivalent units of another system, *conversion factors* or *conversion equivalents* are used.

Table A.1 presents both practical and precise conversion equivalents. In most pharmacy practice applications, the practical equivalents generally suffice. The most direct equivalent to use in a conversion is one that contains both the given and the desired units. For example, to convert a number of fluidounces to milliliters, the equivalent "1 f℥ = 29.57 mL" is the most direct.

Conversions may be accomplished by basic arithmetic, ratio and proportion, or dimensional analysis.

(1) *How many milliliters are equivalent to 8 fluidounces of a cough syrup?*

$$1 \text{ f℥} = 29.57 \text{ mL}$$

$$8 \text{ f℥} = 8 \times 29.57 \text{ mL} = \mathbf{236.56\ mL}$$

(2) *A tumor measures 6.35 mm. Express the dimension in inches.*

$$6.35 \text{ mm} \times \frac{1 \text{ cm}}{10 \text{ mm}} \times \frac{1 \text{ inch}}{2.54 \text{ cm}} = \mathbf{0.25\ inch}$$

Table A.1 • PRACTICAL AND PRECISE CONVERSION EQUIVALENTS

Unit	Practical Pharmacy Equivalent	Precise Equivalent[a]
Conversion Equivalents of Length		
1 m	39.37 in	39.37008 in
1 in	2.54 cm (exact)	
Conversion Equivalents of Volume		
1 mL	16.23 ♏	16.23073 ♏
1♏	0.06 mL	0.06161152 mL
1 fʒ	3.69 mL	3.696691 mL
1f℥	29.57 mL	29.57353 mL
1 pt	473 mL	473.1765 mL
1 gal. (US)[b]	3785 mL	3785.412 mL
Conversion Equivalents of Weight		
1 g	15.432 gr	15.43236 gr
1 kg	2.20 lb (avoir.)	2.204623 lb (avoir.)
1 gr	0.065 g (65 mg)	0.06479891 g
1 oz. (avoir.)	28.35 g	28.349523125 g
1℥	31.1 g	31.1034768 g
1 lb (avoir.)	454 g	453.59237 g
1 lb (apoth.)	373 g	373.2417216 g
Other Useful Equivalents		
1 oz. (avoir.)	437.5 gr (exact)	
1℥	480 gr (exact)	
1 gal. (US)	128 f℥ (exact)	

[a]Precise equivalents from the National Institute of Standards and Technology. Available at: http://ts.nist.gOv/WelghtsAndMeasures/Publlcatlons/appxc.cfm#1. Accessed March 15, 2011.

[b]The US gallon is specified because the British imperial gallon and other counterpart measures differ substantially, as follows: British imperial gallon, 4545 mL; pint, 568.25 mL; f℥, 28.412 mL: fʒ, 3.55 mL; and ♏, 0.059 mL. Note, however, that the SI unit is used in both the U.S. Pharmacopeia and British Pharmacopeia.

(3) *An archived prescription calls for ʒii of calcium carbonate. Convert this quantity to grams.*

$$ʒii = 2 \times 60 \text{ gr} = 120 \text{ gr}$$

$$1 \text{ gr} = 0.065 \text{ g}$$

$$120 \text{ gr} \times 0.065 \text{ g/gr} = \mathbf{7.8\ g}$$

(4) *A low-dose aspirin tablet contains 81 mg of aspirin. Convert this quantity to grains.*

$$1 \text{ gr} = 65 \text{ mg}$$

$$\frac{81 \text{ mg}}{x \text{ gr}} = \frac{65 \text{ mg}}{1 \text{ gr}} = \mathbf{1.25\ gr\ or\ 1\tfrac{1}{4}\ gr}$$

Or,

$$81 \text{ mg} \times \frac{1 \text{ gr}}{65 \text{ mg}} = \mathbf{1.25\ gr\ or\ 1\tfrac{1}{4}\ gr}$$

"Consumer Approximate" Measures

A consumer may ask for a quantity of a product that differs from the system of measurement on the desired product's label. It is a simple matter to find a "consumer approximate" equivalent. For example, a requested "pint" of a mouthwash may be satisfied by a product labeled "500 mL." Similarly, a request for an "ounce" of a product would be satisfied with a 30-g size package if a solid or a 30-mL size package if a liquid. *"Consumer approximate" measures may not substitute for equivalent measures used in pharmaceutical calculations.*

Conversion of Temperatures

There are a number of different arithmetic methods for the conversion of temperatures from the centigrade scale to the Fahrenheit scale and vice versa, including[1]:

$$°F = \frac{9}{5}°C + 32, \quad \text{and}$$

$$°C = \frac{5}{9} \times (°F - 32)$$

Example Calculations of Temperature Conversions

(1) *Convert 26°C to corresponding degrees Fahrenheit.*

$$°F = \frac{9}{5}(26°C) + 32 = \mathbf{78.8°F}$$

(2) *Convert 98.6°F to corresponding degrees centigrade.*

$$°C = \frac{5}{9} \times (98.6°F - 32) = \mathbf{37°C}$$

Clinical Aspects of Thermometry

The instrument used to measure body temperature is termed a *clinical* or *fever thermometer*. Traditional clinical thermometers include the (1) *oral thermometer*, slender in the design of stem and bulb reservoir; (2) *rectal thermometer*, having a blunt, pear-shaped, thick-bulb reservoir for both safety and to ensure retention in the rectum; and (3) *universal or security thermometer*, which is stubby in design, for oral or rectal use. Upon body contact, heat is absorbed causing an expansion and rise of mercury or other liquid in the thermometer, which is then read on the instrument's scale. Oral *electronic digital fever thermometers* are also commonly available (Fig. A.1).

Of particular application in pediatrics are *infrared emission detection ear thermometers*. When aimed into the ear, they measure heat radiated from the tympanic membrane without touching the membrane. Along the same lines, noncontact handheld infrared and laser thermometers are widely used at certain airports and other ports of entry to screen passengers for fever/illness. These devices are held at about 6 inches from the subject and, when pointed directly at the forehead, display a digital readout of body temperature in about 1 second.

Other specialized thermometers include *basal thermometers* and *low-reading thermometers*. The *basal temperature* is the body's normal resting temperature, generally taken immediately on awakening in the morning. In women, body temperature normally rises slightly

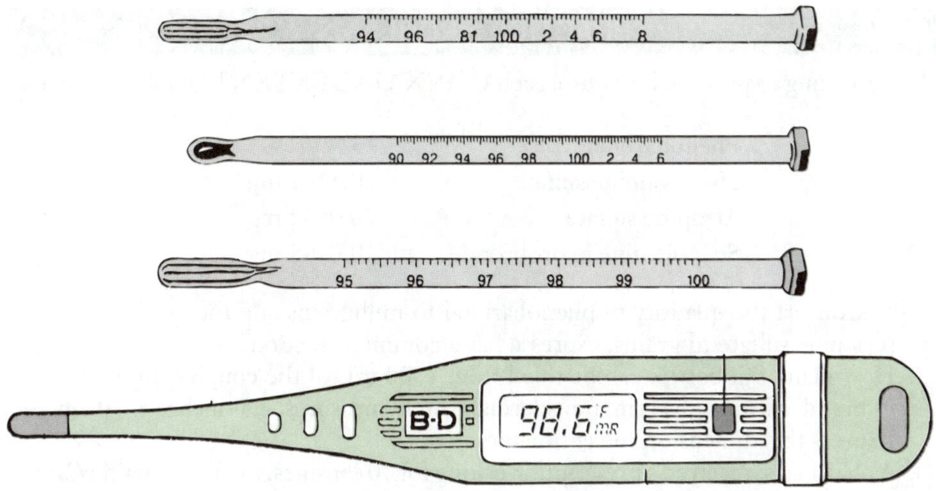

FIGURE A.1 • Examples of various clinical thermometers. From top to bottom: oral fever thermometer, rectal thermometer, basal thermometer, oral digital fever thermometer. (Courtesy of Becton Dickinson and Company.)

because of hormonal changes associated with ovulation. *Basal thermometers*, calibrated in tenths of a degree, are designed to measure these slight changes in temperature. When charted over the course of a month, these changes are useful in assessing optimal times for conception.

Low-reading thermometers are used in diagnosing hypothermia. The standard clinical thermometer reads from 34.4°C (94°F) to 42.2°C (108°F), which is not fully satisfactory for measuring hypothermia, which may involve body temperatures of 35°C (95°F) or lower. A low-reading thermometer registers temperatures between 28.9°C (84°F) and 42.2°C (108°F).

Normal adult temperature may vary widely between individuals, with lowest body temperatures generally occurring in the early morning and peak high temperatures in the late afternoon.

Pharmaceutical Aspects of Temperature

Temperature control is an important consideration in the manufacture, shipping, and storage of pharmaceutical products. Excessive temperature can result in chemical or physical degradation of a therapeutic agent or its dosage form. For this reason, the labeling of pharmaceutical products contains information on the appropriate temperature range under which the product should be maintained. The *United States Pharmacopeia* provides the following definitions for the storage of pharmaceuticals[2]:

Freezer—between −25°C and −10°C (−13°F and 14°F)
Cold—not exceeding 8°C (46°F)
Controlled cold—between 2°C and 8°C (36°F and 46°F)
Cool—between 8°C and 15°C (46°F and 59°F)
Controlled room temperature—between 20°C and 25°C (68°F and 77°F)
Warm—between 30°C and 40°C (86°F and 104°F)
Excessive heat—above 40°C (104°F)

PRACTICE PROBLEMS

1. According to product literature, each DONNATAL EXTENTAB tablet contains:

Phenobarbital	3/4 gr
Hyoscyamine sulfate	0.3111 mg
Atropine sulfate	0.0582 mg
Scopolamine hydrobromide	0.0195 mg

Convert the quantity of phenobarbital to milligrams and the quantity of hyoscyamine sulfate to grains, expressed as a common fraction.

2. How many f℥ii bottles can be filled from 1000 mL of the cough syrup?
3. A brand of nitroglycerin transdermal patch measures 2.5 inches in diameter. Express this dimension in centimeters.
4. A pharmacist received a prescription calling for 30 capsules, each to contain 1/200 gr of nitroglycerin. How many 0.4-mg nitroglycerin tablets would supply the amount required?
5. If a child accidentally swallowed 2 fluidounces of FEOSOL Elixir, containing 2/3 gr of ferrous sulfate per 5 mL, how many milligrams of ferrous sulfate did the child ingest?
6. The usual dose of colchicine for an acute gout attack is 1/120 gr every hour for 8 doses. How many milligrams of colchicine are represented in the usual dose?
7. A formula for a cough syrup contains 1/8 gr of codeine phosphate per teaspoonful (5 mL). How many grams of codeine phosphate should be used in preparing 1 pint of the cough syrup?
8. Convert the following from centigrade to Fahrenheit:
   (a) 10°C
   (b) −30°C
   (c) 4°C
   (d) −173°C
9. Convert the following from Fahrenheit to centigrade:
   (a) 77°F
   (b) 240°F
   (c) 98.9°F
   (d) 227.1°F
10. A woman charting her basal temperature finds that her body temperature on day 14 is 97.7°F and on day 18 is 98.6°F. Express this temperature range and the difference in degrees centigrade.

ANSWERS TO PRACTICE PROBLEMS

1. 48.75 mg phenobarbital and ≈1/209 gr hyoscyamine sulfate
2. 16 bottles
3. 6.35 cm
4. 24+ nitroglycerin tablets
5. 512.55 mg ferrous sulfate
6. 0.54 mg colchicine
7. 0.769 g codeine phosphate
8. (a) 50°F
   (b) −22°F
   (c) 39.2°F
   (d) −279.4°F
9. (a) 25°C
   (b) 115.6°C
   (c) 37.2°C
   (d) 108.4°C
10. 36.5° to 37°C
    0.5°C

References

1. United States Pharmacopeial Convention. *United States Pharmacopeia 31–National Formulary 26*. Vol. 1(8). Rockville, MD: United States Pharmacopeial Convention, 2008:905–906.
2. United States Pharmacopeia. General notices and requirements. Available at: http://www.usp.org/sites/default/files/usp_pdf/EN/USPNF/USP34-NF29General%20Notices.pdf. Accessed December 3, 2014.

B

Glossary of Pharmaceutical Dosage Forms and Drug Delivery Systems[a]

Aerosols. Pharmaceutical aerosols are products packaged under pressure that contain therapeutically active ingredients that are released as a fine mist, spray, or foam on actuation of the valve assembly. Some aerosol emissions are intended to be inhaled deep into the lungs (*inhalation aerosol*), whereas others are intended for topical application to the skin or to mucous membranes. Aerosols with metered valve assemblies permit a specific quantity of emission for dosage regulation.

Boluses. Boluses are large elongated tablets intended for administration to animals.

Caplet. Caplets are tablets manufactured in the shape of a capsule.

Capsules. Capsules are solid dosage forms in which one or more medicinal and/or inert substances are enclosed within small shells of gelatin. Capsule shells are produced in varying sizes, shapes, color, and hardness. *Hard-shell* capsules, which have two telescoping parts, are used in the manufacture of most commercial capsule products and in the extemporaneous filling of prescriptions. They are filled with powder mixtures or granules.

Soft-shell gelatin capsules, sometimes called *softgels*, are formed, filled, and sealed in a continuous process by specialized large-scale equipment. They may be filled with powders, semisolids, or liquids.

Capsules contain a specific quantity of fill, with the capsule size selected to accommodate that quantity. In addition to their medication content, capsules usually contain inert substances, such as fillers. When swallowed, the gelatin capsule shell is dissolved by gastrointestinal fluids, releasing the contents.

Delayed-release capsules are prepared in such a manner as to resist the release of the contents until the capsules have passed through the stomach and into the intestines.

Extended-release capsules are prepared in such a manner as to release the medication from the capsules over an extended period following ingestion.

Creams. Creams are semisolid preparations containing one or more drug substances dissolved or dispersed in a suitable base. Many creams are either oil-in-water emulsions or aqueous microcrystalline dispersions in a water-washable base. Compared to ointments, creams are easier to spread and remove. Creams are used for administering drugs to the skin and, to a lesser extent, to mucous membranes.

Drug Delivery Systems. Drug delivery systems are physical carriers used to deliver medications to site-specific areas. They include transdermal, ocular, and intrauterine systems. See Table B.1 for more information.

Transdermal drug delivery systems support the passage of drug substances from the surface of the skin, through its various layers, and into the systemic circulation. These

[a]*Some portions of this glossary have been abstracted from USP34-NF29, <1151>. Copyright 2010 The United States Pharmacopeial Convention. Permission Granted.*

Table B.1 • ROUTES OF DRUG ADMINISTRATION AND PRIMARY DOSAGE FORMS AND DRUG DELIVERY SYSTEMS

Route	Site	Dosage Forms/Drug Delivery Systems
Oral	Mouth	Tablets, capsules, oral solutions, drops, syrups, elixirs, suspensions, magmas, gels, powders, troches, lozenges
Sublingual	Under the tongue	Tablets
Parenteral		Solutions, suspensions
Intravenous	Vein	
Intra-arterial	Artery	
Intracardiac	Heart	
Intraspinal/Intrathecal	Spine	
Intraosseous	Bone	
Intra-articular	Joint	
Intrasynovial	Joint fluid	
Intracutaneous/Intradermal/ Subcutaneous	Skin	
Intramuscular	Muscle	
Epicutaneous	Skin surface	Ointments, creams, pastes, plasters, powders, aerosols, lotions, transdermal patches, solutions (topical)
Conjunctival	Eye conjunctiva	Ointments
Intraocular	Eye	Solutions, suspensions
Intranasal	Nose	Solutions, ointments
Aural	Ear	Solutions, suspensions (drops)
Intrarespiratory	Lung	Solutions (aerosols)
Rectal	Rectum	Solutions, ointments, suppositories
Vaginal	Vagina	Solutions, ointments, emulsion foams, gels, tablets/inserts
Urethral	Urethra	Solutions, suppositories, inserts

systems are sophisticated skin patches containing a drug formulation within a reservoir for the controlled delivery of drug.

Ocular drug delivery systems consist of drug-impregnated membranes that, when placed in the lower conjunctival sac, release medication at a constant rate over an extended period.

Intrauterine drug delivery systems consist of a drug-containing intrauterine device that releases medication over an extended period after insertion into the uterus.

Elixirs. Elixirs are sweetened, flavored, hydroalcoholic solutions intended for oral administration. They may be medicated or nonmedicated. Compared to syrups, elixirs are usually less sweet and less viscous because they contain a lesser amount of sugar. Because of their hydroalcoholic character, elixirs are better able than are syrups to maintain both water-soluble and alcohol-soluble components in solution.

Emulsions. An emulsion is a type of system in which one liquid is dispersed throughout another liquid in the form of fine droplets. The two liquids, generally an oil and water, are immiscible and constitute two phases that would separate into layers without the presence of a third agent, an *emulsifier* or *emulsifying agent*. The latter facilitates the emulsification process and provides physical stability to the system.

If oil is the internal phase, then the emulsion is termed an oil-in-water, or o/w, emulsion. If water is the internal phase, then the emulsion is termed a water-in-oil, or w/o, emulsion. The type of emulsion produced is largely determined by the emulsifying agent, with hydrophilic agents generally producing oil-in-water emulsions and lipophilic agents generally producing water-in-oil emulsions. Emulsifying agents may have both hydrophilic and lipophilic characteristics, hence the term hydrophilic–lipophilic balance (HLB). Some emulsions, packaged in a pressurized aerosol container, are released as a foam.

Depending on their formulation, emulsions may be administered orally, topically, or by intravenous injection.

Extracts. Extracts are concentrated preparations of vegetable or animal drugs prepared by extracting the constituents from the natural source and drying the extractive to the desired pilular or powdered form.

Fluidextracts. Fluidextracts are liquid extractives of vegetable drugs generally prepared such that 1 mL represents the active constituents from 1 g of the vegetable drug.

Gels. Gels are semisolid systems consisting of either suspensions of small inorganic particles or large organic molecules interpenetrated by a liquid.

Implants or Pellets. Implants or pellets are small, sterile, solid dosage forms containing a concentrated drug for subcutaneous implantation in the body where they continuously release their medication over prolonged periods.

Inhalations. Inhalations are finely powdered drug substances, solutions, or suspensions of drug substances administered by the nasal or oral respiratory route for local or systemic effects. Special devices are used to facilitate their administration. *Metered-dose inhalers (MDIs)* are propellant-driven drug suspensions or solutions in liquefied gas propellant, intended to deliver metered doses of drug to the respiratory tract. MDIs are packaged to contain multiple doses (often several hundred) with each valve actuation delivering controlled volumes ranging from 25 to 100 μL.

Injections. Injections are sterile preparations intended for parenteral administration by needle or pressure syringe. Drugs may be injected into most any vessel or tissue of the body, but the most common routes are intravenous (IV), intramuscular (IM), and subcutaneous (SC). Injections may be solutions or suspensions of a drug substance in an aqueous or nonaqueous vehicle. They may be small-volume injections, packaged in ampules for single-dose administration, or vials for multiple-dose injections. Large-volume parenterals, containing 100 mL to 1 L of fluid, are intended for the slow intravenous administration (or infusion) of medications and/or nutrients in the institutional or home care setting.

Inserts. Inserts are solid medicated dosage forms intended for insertion into the vagina or urethra.

Irrigations. Irrigations are sterile solutions intended to bathe or flush open wounds or body cavities.

Liniments. Liniments are alcoholic or oleaginous solutions, suspensions, or emulsions of medicinal agents intended for external application to the skin, generally by rubbing. Liniments have application both in human and veterinary medicine.

Lotions. Lotions are liquid preparations intended for external application to the skin. They are generally suspensions or emulsions of dispersed solid or liquid materials in an aqueous vehicle. Their fluidity allows rapid and uniform application over a wide skin surface. Lotions are intended to soften the skin and leave a thin coat of their components on the skin's surface as they dry.

Lozenges. Lozenges are solid preparations containing one or more medicinal agents in a flavored, sweetened base intended to dissolve or disintegrate slowly in the mouth, releasing medication generally for localized effects.

Ointments. Ointments are semisolid preparations intended for topical application to the skin, eye, ear, or various mucous membranes. With some exceptions, ointments are applied for their local effects on the tissue membrane rather than for systemic effects. *Ophthalmic ointments* are sterile preparations intended for application to the eye.

Nonmedicated ointments serve as vehicles, or as *ointment bases*, in the preparation of medicated ointments. Because ointments are semisolid preparations, they are prepared and dispensed on a weight basis.

Pastes. Pastes are semisolid dosage forms that contain one or more drug substances intended for topical application to the skin. Generally, pastes contain a higher proportion of solid materials than do ointments and thus are more stiff, less greasy, and more absorptive of serous secretions.

Plasters. Plasters are solid or semisolid adhesive masses spread across a suitable backing material and intended for external application to a part of the body for protection or for the medicinal benefit of added agents.

Powders. Powders are dry mixtures of finely divided medicinal and nonmedicinal agents intended for internal or external use. Powders may be dispensed in bulk form, or they may be divided into single-dosage units and packaged in folded papers or unit-of-use envelopes.

Premixes. Premixes are mixtures of one or more drug substances with suitable vehicles intended for admixture to animal feedstuffs before administration. They are generally in powdered, pelletized, or granulated form.

Solutions. Solutions are liquid preparations that contain one or more chemical substances (*solutes*) dissolved in a solvent or mixture of solvents. The most common solvent used in pharmaceuticals is water; however, alcohol, glycerin, and propylene glycol also are widely used as solvents or cosolvents.

Depending upon their purpose, solutions are formulated and labeled for use by various routes, including oral, topical, inhalation, ophthalmic, otic, nasal, rectal, urethral, and parenteral. The concentration of active ingredients in solutions varies widely depending on the nature of the therapeutic agent and its intended use. The concentration of a given solution may be expressed in molar strength, milliequivalent strength, percentage strength, ratio strength, milligrams per milliliter, or another expression describing the amount of active ingredient per unit of volume.

Suppositories. Suppositories are solid dosage forms intended for insertion into body orifices. They are used rectally, vaginally, and, occasionally, urethrally. Suppositories are of various weights, sizes, and shapes, depending on their intended use. Various types of *suppository bases* are used as vehicles for the medication, including cocoa butter (theobroma oil), glycerinated gelatin, polyethylene glycols, hydrogenated vegetable oils, and fatty acid esters of polyethylene glycol. Depending on the base used, the suppository softens, melts, or dissolves after insertion, releasing its medication for the intended local action or for absorption and systemic effects.

Suspensions. Suspensions are preparations containing finely divided, undissolved drug particles dispersed throughout a liquid vehicle. Because the drug particles are not dissolved, suspensions assume a degree of opacity depending on the concentration and size of the suspended particles. Because particles tend to settle when left standing, suspensions should be shaken to redistribute any settled particles before use to ensure uniform dosing. Depending on their formulation, suspensions are administered orally, by intramuscular injection, and topically to the eye.

Syrups. Syrups are concentrated aqueous solutions of a sugar or sugar substitute. Syrups may be medicated or nonmedicated. *Nonmedicated syrups* are used as vehicles for medicinal substances to be added later, either in the extemporaneous compounding of prescriptions or in the preparation of a formula for a medicated syrup. In addition to the sugar or sweetener, syrups also contain flavoring agents, colorants, cosolvents, and antimicrobial preservatives to prevent microbial growth. Medicated syrups are administered orally for the therapeutic value of the medicinal agent(s).

Tablets. Tablets are solid dosage forms containing one or more medicinal substances. Most tablets also contain added pharmaceutical ingredients, as diluents, disintegrants, colorants, binders, solubilizers, and coatings. Tablets may be coated for appearance, for stability, to mask the taste of the medication, or to provide controlled drug release. Most tablets are manufactured on an industrial scale by compression, using highly sophisticated machinery. Punches and dies of various shapes and sizes enable the preparation of a wide variety of tablets of distinctive shapes, sizes, and surface markings.

Most tablets are intended to be swallowed whole. However, some are prepared to be chewable, others to be dissolved in the mouth (*buccal tablets*) or under the tongue (*sublingual tablets*), and still others to be dissolved in water before taking (*effervescent tablets*). Tablets are formulated to contain a specific quantity of medication. To enable flexibility in dosing, manufacturers commonly make available various tablet strengths of a given medication. Some tablets are scored, or grooved, to permit breaking into portions for dosing flexibility. Tablets may be formulated for *immediate release (oral disintegrating)*, *delayed release*, or *extended release* of the active therapeutic ingredient(s).

Tinctures. Tinctures are alcoholic or hydroalcoholic solutions of either pure chemical substances or of plant extractives. Most chemical tinctures are applied topically (e.g., iodine tincture). Plant extractives are used for their content of active pharmacologic agents.

Comprehensive Review Problems*

1. Translate the prescription notations and calculate as directed:

   (a) ℞ E.E.S Filmtabs 400 mg
   Sig: Tabs i stat p.o., i q.i.d. q6h × 10 days.

   Each E.E.S Filmtab contains 400 mg of erythromycin ethylsuccinate. If the patient taking the medication weighs 160 lb, calculate the daily dose on the basis of mg/kg.

   (b) ℞ RESTASIS 0.4 mL
   Sig: gtt i o.u. b.i.d. q12h.

   RESTASIS contains 0.05% cyclosporine. If the dropper used delivers 16 drops/mL, how many micrograms of cyclosporine are delivered daily?

   (c) ℞ BIAXIN 250 mg/5 mL
   Sig: ʒss t.i.d. q8h × 10 days.

   BIAXIN contains clarithromycin in suspension. How many milliliters of the medication will the patient require during the course of therapy?

   (d) ℞ TUSSIONEX PENNKINETIC
   Disp: 60 mL
   Sig: 1 teaspoonful. NMT 2 teaspoonfuls/day.

   TUSSIONEX PENNKINETIC contains the equivalent of 2 mg/mL of hydrocodone bitartrate and 1.6 mg/mL of chlorpheniramine maleate. Calculate the maximum daily dose of each in milligrams.

   (e) ℞ Benzoyl peroxide 5.5%
   Cream base ad 15 g
   M.ft. cream

   If the patient applies 0.5 g for each use, how many milligrams of benzoyl peroxide will have been applied?

Solutions:

(a) Swallow one (1) tablet to start, and then swallow one (1) tablet four (4) times a day every six (6) hours for ten (10) days.
160 lb × 1 kg/2.2 lb = 72.7 kg
4 × 400 mg = 1600 mg
1600 mg/72.2 kg = **22.16 mg/kg of erythromycin succinate**

(b) Instill one (1) drop into each eye two (2) times a day every 12 hours.
0.4 mL × 0.05% = 0.0002 g = 0.2 mg = 200 μg
0.4 mL × 16 drops/mL = 6.4 drops
200 μg/6.4 drops = 31.25 μg/drop

*Some formulas and problems in this section are credited and referenced as the contributions of other authors.

Gtt i o.u. b.i.d. = 1 drop into each eye 2 times a day = 4 drops/day.
4 drops/day × 31.25 μg/drop = **125 μg/day of cyclosporine**
Or,
4 drops × 0.05 g/100 mL × 1000 mg/1 g × 1000 μg/1 mg × 1 mL/16 drops = **125 μg of cyclosporine**

(c) Take one-half (1/2) teaspoonful three (3) times a day every eight (8) hours for 10 days.
ʒss = ½ teaspoonful
5 mL/teaspoonful × ½ = 2.5 mL
2.5 mL × 3 times/day × 10 days = **75 mL BIAXIN suspension**

(d) Take one (1) teaspoonful. Do not take more than two (2) teaspoonfuls a day.
5 mL/teaspoonful × 2 teaspoonfuls = 10 mL
Hydrocodone bitartrate: 2 mg/mL × 10 mL = **20 mg**
Chlorpheniramine maleate: 1.6 mg × 10 mL = **16 mg**

(e) Mix and make a cream.
15 g × 5.5% = 0.825 g = 825 mg
825 mg × 0.5 g/15 g = **27.5 mg benzoyl peroxide**
Or,
0.5 g × 5.5% = 0.0275 g = **27.5 mg benzoyl peroxide**

2. Calculate the following hospital medication orders as directed:
(a) Medication Order: sirolimus oral solution (RAPAMUNE), 1 mg/m²/day.
Preparation Administered: 1 mg/mL sirolimus oral solution.
Calculate: daily dose, in milliliters, for a 5-feet 8-inch patient weighing 149 lb.
(b) Medication Order: cefixime, 8 mg/kg/day in two divided doses.
Preparation Administered: cefixime oral suspension 200 mg/5 mL.
Calculate: dose, in milliliters, for a 36-lb child.
(c) Medication Order: heparin 15 units/kg/h.
Preparation Administered: 25,000 heparin units in 500 mL normal saline solution.
Calculate: infusion rate, in mL/h, for a 187-lb patient.
(d) Medication Order: lidocaine, 2 μg/kg/min.
Preparation Administered: lidocaine, 1 g/500-mL infusion with an infusion set delivering 15 drops/mL.
Calculate: flow rate, in drops/min for a 142-lb patient.
(e) Medication Order: potassium bolus of 40 mEq of KCl in 200 mL of 0.9% sodium chloride injection to be administered at a rate of 10 mEq/h.
Calculate: drip rate in microdrops/min.

Solutions:
(a) 5 feet 8 inches = 68 inches × 2.54 cm/inch = 172.72 cm
149 lb × 1 kg/2.2 lb = 67.73 kg

$$\text{BSA, m}^2 = \sqrt{\frac{172.72\,(\text{cm}) \times 67.73\,(\text{kg})}{3600}} = \sqrt{3.25} = 1.80\ \text{m}^2$$

1 mg/m²/day × 1.80 m² = 1.8 mg/day
1.8 mg/day × 1 mL/1 mg = **1.8 mL/day, sirolimus oral solution**

(b) 36 lb × 1 kg/2.2 lb = 16.36 kg
8 mg/kg/day × 16.36 (kg) = 130.88 mg/day
130.88 mg/2 doses = 65.44 mg/dose
65.44 mg × 5 mL/200 mg = 1.636 or **1.6 mL cefixime oral suspension**

(c) 187 lb × 1 kg/2.2 lb = 85 kg
15 units/kg/h × 85 kg = 1275 units/h
1275 units/h × 500 mL/25,000 units = **25.5 mL/h heparin in NSS**

(d) 142 lb × 1 kg/2.2 lb = 64.55 kg
2 μg/kg/min × 64.55 kg = 129.1 μg/min
129.1 μg/min × 500 mL/1 g × 1 g/1,000,000 μg = 0.06455 mL/min
0.06455 mL/min × 15 drops/mL = 0.968 or **1 drop/min lidocaine infusion**

(e) NOTE: unless otherwise indicated, microdrop infusion sets deliver 60 drops/mL. Also, although not recommended, the abbreviation "mcgtts" for microdrops occasionally is encountered.
60 microdrops/1 mL × 200 mL/40 mEq × 10 mEq/1 h × 1 h/60 min = **50 microdrops/min**

3. Identify any errors in the calculations for each of the following prescriptions.

(a) ℞

Allopurinol	20 mg/mL
Cherry syrup	60 mL
Methylcellulose suspension ad	120 mL

Sig. Take one teaspoonful daily in AM.

Having no allopurinol powder, six 300-mg tablets of allopurinol are used in compounding this prescription.

(b) ℞

Triamcinolone acetonide cream	0.1%
Aquaphor Unibase aa	30 g

M. ft. ungt.
Sig. Apply to affected area on skin t.i.d.

Fifteen grams each of a 0.1% triamcinolone acetonide cream and Aquaphor Unibase are used in compounding this prescription.

(c) ℞

Ephedrine sulfate	0.4% w/v
Benzocaine	1:1000 w/v
Cocoa butter ad	2 g
M. ft. suppos. DTD no.	24

Sig. Insert one rectal suppository each night at bedtime.

In compounding this prescription, it is acceptable to calculate for two extra suppositories to account for unavoidable loss. If a 10% w/w benzocaine ointment is used as the source of the benzocaine, 0.052 g of the ointment would supply the proper amount.

(d) ℞ Patient: weight 132 lb
LEUKERAN 0.1 mg/kg/day
Disp: 2 mg tabs
Sig: Take ______ tablets every day × 21 days.

The pharmacist calculates the dose to be 3 tablets daily and dispenses 63 tablets.

(e) ℞ Patient: height, 5 feet 2 inches; weight 108 lb
Dexamethasone
Dose @ 20 mg/m²/day
Disp: 5-mg tablets
Sig: Take _____ tablets daily for treatment cycle on days 1, 2, 3, 4, 9, 10, 11.

The pharmacist calculates the dose to be 6 tablets daily for treatment cycle on days 1, 2, 3, 4, 9, 10, and 11.

Solutions:

(a) 20 mg/mL × 120 mL = 2400 mg allopurinol needed

$$2400 \text{ mg} \times \frac{1 \text{ tablet}}{300 \text{ mg}} = \mathbf{8 \text{ tablets}}$$

Eight tablets should have been used

(b) "aa" means "of each;" thus, **30 g** of each component should be used.

(c) 2 g/1 suppos. × 26 suppos. = 52 g
52 g × 1 g (benzocaine)/1000 g = 0.052 g benzocaine needed

$$0.052 \text{ g (benzocaine)} \times \frac{100 \text{ g (benzocaine ointment)}}{10 \text{ g (benzocaine)}} = \mathbf{0.52 g \text{ benzocaine ointment}}$$

0.52 g of benzocaine ointment should be used.

(d) 132 lb × 1 kg/2.2 lb = 60 kg
60 kg × 0.1 mg/kg/day = 6 mg/day
6 mg/day × 1 tab/2 mg = 3 tablets/day
There are no errors in the calculations

(e) 5 feet 2 inches = 62 inches = 157.48 cm (62 inches × 2.54 cm/inch)
108 lb × 1 kg/2.2 lb = 49.09 kg

$$\text{BSA, m}^2 = \sqrt{\frac{157.48 \text{ cm} \times 49.09 \text{ kg}}{3600}} = \sqrt{2.15} = 1.47 \text{ m}^2$$

20 mg/m²/day × 1.47 m² = 29.4 mg/day
29.4 mg/day × 1 tablet/5 mg = 5.88 or 6 tablets/day
There are no errors in the calculations.

4. Calculate as indicated for each of the following prescriptions:

(a) ℞[a]

Noscapine	0.72 g
Guaifenesin	4.8 g
Alcohol	15 mL
Cherry syrup ad	120 mL

Sig. ʒi t.i.d. p.r.n. cough.

How many milligrams each of noscapine and guaifenesin would be contained in each dose?

(b) ℞[a] Clotrimazole 1 g
Gentamicin sulfate 300 mg
Polyethylene glycol ad 100 mL
Sig: Two drops in each ear t.i.d.

Calculate the amount of gentamicin sulfate, in micrograms, present in each dose from a dropper service that delivers 20 drops/mL.

(c) ℞[a] Miconazole 2% w/v
Tolnaftate 1 g
Polyethylene glycol 300 qs ad 100 mL
Sig: Apply to skin b.i.d.

How many grams each of miconazole and tolnaftate are needed to prepare 8 fl. oz. of the prescription?

(d) ℞[a] Interferon alpha-2a 100 million units
Ammonium acetate 7.7 mg
Benzyl alcohol 100 mg
Human albumin 10 mg
Sterile water for injection ad 10 mL

Interferon alpha-2a is available in syringes containing 9 million units or 33.3 μg in 0.5 mL of solution. Calculate the (i) milliliters of this solution required to prepare the prescription, (ii) the number of micrograms, and (iii) the number of units of interferon alpha-2a in each 0.05 mL of the filled prescription.

Solutions:

(a) A "ʒ" in the Signa portion of a prescription may be interpreted as a teaspoonful and thus 5 mL.
120 mL/5 mL = 24 doses
0.72 g = 720 mg noscapine
720 mg/24 doses = **30 mg noscapine/dose**
4.8 g = 4800 mg guaifenesin
4800 mg/24 doses = 200 mg **guaifenesin/dose**

(b) $2 \text{ drops} \times \frac{300 \text{ mg}}{100 \text{ mL}} \times \frac{1000\ \mu\text{g}}{1 \text{ mg}} \times \frac{1 \text{ mL}}{20 \text{ drops}} = 300 \text{ mg gentamicin sulfate}$

(c) 8 (fl. oz.) × 29.57 mL = 236.56 mL
Miconazole: 2% (w/v) × 236.56 mL = **4.73 g**
Tolnaftate: 1% (w/v) × 236.56 mL = **2.36 g**

(d) 100 million units × 0.5 mL/9 million units = 5.56 mL of solution

$$0.05 \text{ mL} \times \frac{100 \text{ million units}}{10 \text{ mL}} = \mathbf{0.5 \text{ million units interferon alpha-2a}}$$

$$0.05 \text{ mL} \times \frac{100 \text{ million units}}{10 \text{ mL}} \times \frac{33.3\ \mu\text{g}}{9 \text{ million units}} = \mathbf{1.85\ \mu g \text{ interferon alpha-2a}}$$

5. ℞ Entecavir 0.5 mg
Lactose ad 300 mg
M. ft. such caps # 12
Sig: i cap q.i.d.

(a) Explain how you would obtain the correct quantity of entecavir using a prescription balance with a sensitivity requirement of 6 mg and an acceptable weighing error of not greater than 5%.

(b) Rather than weighing the required quantity of entecavir powder, a pharmacist uses 1-mg entecavir tablets (crushed and powdered) to compound the prescription. If each tablet weighs 92 mg, how many milligrams of lactose would be needed to fill the prescription?

Solutions:

(a) The least amount that should be weighed on this prescription balance is calculated by: 6 mg × 100%/5% = 120 mg.
Thus, 120 mg or greater of entecavir must be weighed.
The prescription requires 0.5 mg × 12 (capsules) = 6 mg of entecavir.
Using an arbitrary multiple of 20, the amount of entecavir that can be weighed is 120 mg (20 × 6 mg).

Weigh 120 mg of entecavir, add 2280 mg of lactose (20 × 120 mg = 2400 mg – 120 mg entecavir), and weigh 1/20th of the 2400 mg mixture, 120 mg, which will contain the required 6 mg of entecavir (proof: 1/20th of the 120 mg = 6 mg entecavir).

(b) Number of tablets required = 6 mg/1 mg per tablet = 6 tablets
6 (tablets) × 92 mg per tablet = 552 mg
300 mg per capsule × 12 capsules = 3600 mg total
3600 mg – 552 mg (powdered entecavir tablets) = **3048 mg lactose**

6. A periodontist inquires as to how you would calculate 120 mL of a prescription for a concentrated solution of chlorhexidine gluconate from which a patient could take a medicinal tablespoonful, add it to a pint of water, and produce a 0.12% solution that may be used as a dental rinse.

(a) How many milliliters of chlorhexidine gluconate (a liquid chemical) are needed to prepare the prescription?

(b) Prove that the resultant solution as prepared by the patient is indeed 0.12% v/v.

(c) Calculate the percent concentration of chlorhexidine gluconate, v/v, in the prescription.

(d) If chlorhexidine gluconate has a specific gravity of 1.07, calculate its percent concentration, w/v, in the prescription.

Solutions:

(a) A tablespoonful (15 mL) of the prescription plus a pint (473 mL) of water = 488 mL.
488 mL × 0.12% (v/v) = 0.5856 or 0.59 mL chlorhexidine gluconate.

So, if there is 0.59 mL of chlorhexidine gluconate in the 488 mL of dental rinse prepared by the patient, it came from the one tablespoonful of the concentrated prescription. And, since there are 8 tablespoonfuls available in the prescription (120 mL/15 mL), 8 (tablespoons) × 0.59 mL chlorhexidine gluconate = **4.72 mL chlorhexidine gluconate needed to fill the prescription.**

(b) 0.59 mL/488 mL × 100% = **0.12%**

(c) 4.72 mL/120 mL × 100% = **3.93% v/v**

(d) 4.72 mL × 1.07 g/mL = 5.05 g
5.05 g/120 mL × 100% = **4.2% w/v**

7. ASTELIN nasal spray contains 0.1% azelastine hydrochloride and 125 μg/mL of benzalkonium chloride as a preservative. A container is capable of delivering 200 metered sprays of 0.137 mL each.
   (a) Calculate the quantity, in micrograms, of azelastine hydrochloride in each spray.
   (b) Calculate the percentage strength and ratio strength of benzalkonium chloride in the preparation.
   (c) The molecular weight of azelastine hydrochloride is 418.4. Calculate the quantity, in milligrams, of azelastine (base), in a 30-mL container.

Solutions:

(a) 0.137 mL × 0.1% = 0.000137 g = 0.137 mg = **137 μg**

(b) 125 μg/mL = 0.0125 g/100 mL = **0.0125%**
100 (mL)/0.0125 (g) = **1:8000 w/v ratio strength**

(c) Molecular weight azelastine hydrochloride: 418.4.
Molecular weight azelastine (base): 418.4 − 36.5 (HCl) = 381.9
381.9/418.4 = 91.3% (percent of azelastine hydrochloride that is azelastine base)
30 mL × 0.1% = 0.03 g = 30 mg (azelastine hydrochloride)
30 mg (azelastine hydrochloride) × 91.3% = **27.39 mg azelastine (base)**

8. Refer to ASTELIN nasal spray in the previous problem.
   (a) If ASTELIN nasal spray is packaged in 30-mL spray containers, how many milliliters would remain after 200 metered sprays?
   (b) The recommended dose of the spray for allergic rhinitis is one spray in each nostril twice daily. At this dose, how many days will the package last a patient?
   (c) In a clinical trial of 391 patients, using two sprays in each nostril twice daily, the most common adverse effects were a bitter taste among 77 patients and a headache in 57 patients. Calculate the percent occurrence of each of these adverse effects.

Solutions:

(a) 0.137 mL/spray × 200 sprays = 27.4 mL
30 mL − 27.4 mL = **2.6 mL**

(b) 200 sprays/4 sprays per day = **50 days**

(c) Bitter taste: 77/391 × 100% = **19.69%**
Headache: 57/391 × 100% = **14.58%**

9.[1] A patient is prescribed DURAGESIC 75 μg/h patches with one patch to be worn and replaced every 72 hours. The size of the patch is 30 cm^2 and contains 7.5 mg of fentanyl.

(a) What is the size of the patch in square inches?

(b) If the patch is worn for 72 hours, how much fentanyl is remaining in the patch when it is removed?

(c) Assuming that the drug release rate from the patch remains constant, how long will it take for all of the fentanyl to be released from the patch?

(d) If the patient is running a fever of 40°C, the amount of fentanyl released from the patch could increase by approximately one-third. How much drug is being released from the patch at this elevated body temperature, and how long will it take for all of the drug to be released from the patch?

(e) Express the body temperature of 40°C as Fahrenheit.

Solutions:

(a) $30\ cm^2 \times (1\ inch/2.54\ cm)^2 =$ **4.65 inches²**

(b) 75 μg/h × 1 mg/1000 μg × 72 h = 5.4 mg released
7.5 mg − 5.4 mg = **2.1 mg remaining**

(c) 7.5 mg × 1000 μg/mg × 1 h/75 μg = 100 h × 1 day/24 h = **4.17 days or 4 days 4 hours**
75 μg/h × 1/3 = 25 μg/h

(d) 75 μg/h + 25 μg/h = **100 mg/h released from the patch at elevated body temperature**
7.5 mg × 1000 μg/mg × 1 h/100 μg = 75 h × 1 day/24 h = **3.13 days or 3 days 3 hours**

(e) F = 1.8(40°C) + 32 = **104°F**

10. REGLAN injection contains in each milliliter 5 mg metoclopramide and 8.5 mg sodium chloride in water for injection. It is available in 2-mL, 10-mL, and 30-mL vials. The drug is used as an antiemetic. The usual adult dose is 10 mg. For doses greater than 10 mg, the injection should be diluted in 50 mL of sodium chloride injection and administered as an intravenous infusion.

(a) If metoclopramide has an E-value of 0.10, calculate the tonicity of REGLAN injection.

(b) For highly emetogenic drugs, as used in cancer chemotherapy, the initial dose of metoclopramide is generally 2 mg/kg. Calculate the volume of REGLAN injection at this dose for a 132-lb patient.

(c) If the dose in (b) is added to a 50-mL bag of sodium chloride injection and totally infused over a period of 30 minutes, calculate the flow rate in mL/min.

Solutions:

(a) 5 mg metoclopramide × 0.10 (E-value) = 0.5 mg
8.5 mg (NaCl) + 0.5 mg = 9 mg
9 mg/1 mL = 900 mg/100 mL = 0.9 g/100 mL = **0.9% sodium chloride = isotonic**

(b) 132 lb × 1 kg/2.2 lb = 60 kg
60 kg × 2 mg/kg = 120 mg (dose)
120 mg × 1 mL/5 mg = **24 mL REGLAN injection**

(c) 24 mL (REGLAN injection) + 50 mL (sodium chloride injection) = 74 mL
74 mL/30 min = **2.47 mL/min**

11.[b] ℞ Indomethacin 0.05%
Boric acid qs
Purified water ad 15 mL
Ft. isotonic ophthalmic solution

(a) How many milligrams of boric acid are needed to render the product isotonic (E-values: boric acid = 0.52, indomethacin = 0.16).

(b) How many milliliters of a 5.5% boric acid stock solution may be used to obtain the needed amount of boric acid?

(c) Indomethacin is available in vials, each containing 1 mg of indomethacin powder for reconstitution with sterile water for injection to prepare 1 mL of solution. Explain how you could obtain the indomethacin required.

Solutions:

(a) For isotonicity: 0.9% × 15 mL = 0.135 g or 135 mg NaCl (or equivalent) needed.
Indomethacin in ℞ = 0.05% × 15 mL = 0.0075 g = 7.5 mg
7.5 mg × 0.16 (E-value) = 1.2 mg
135 mg − 1.2 mg = 133.8 mg NaCl (or equivalent) needed
133.8 mg/0.52 (boric acid E-value) = **257.3 mg of boric acid**

(b) 5.5% boric acid = 5.5 g/100 mL = 5500 mg/100 mL
257.3 mg × 100 mL/5500 mg = **4.68 mL boric acid solution**

(c) Indomethacin required = 0.05% × 15 mL = 0.0075 g = 7.5 mg
7.5 mg × 1 (vial)/1 mg = 7.5 vials
Use 8 vials; add purified water to make 1 mL in each; draw out a total of 7.5 mL

12.[2] The following is a formula for a testosterone nasal spray:

Testosterone	1 g
Alcohol	10 mL
Propylene glycol	20 mL
Benzalkonium chloride	15 mg
Purified water qs ad	100 mL

(a) Calculate the quantity of each ingredient needed to fill twelve 15-mL nasal spray bottles of the formula.

(b) Benzalkonium chloride is available as a 1:750 w/v stock solution. How many milliliters would provide the amount determined in (a)?

(c) If the propylene glycol is found to be contaminated with 1.7 ppm of a solid foreign substance, how many micrograms of that substance would be contained in each bottle of the nasal spray?

(d) If the pharmacist checked the weighing of testosterone using a highly sensitive electronic balance and found that 2.13 g were actually weighed rather than the calculated quantity in (a), what was the percent error in the weighing?
(e) If the pharmacist had decided to use testosterone cipionate injection, 200 mg/mL, as a source of the testosterone, calculate the quantity needed for the amount determined in (a) if the molecular weight of testosterone is 288.4 and that of testosterone cipionate is 412.6.
(f) The normal blood level of testosterone in males is 270 to 1070 ng/dL. If a 5-mL blood sample is found to contain 32.6 ng of testosterone, would the patient's testosterone level fall within the normal range?

Solutions:

(a) 12 bottles × 15 mL/bottle = 180 mL
Formula conversion factor = 180 mL/100 mL = 1.8
Testosterone: 1 g × 1.8 = **1.8 g**
Alcohol: 10 mL × 1.8 = **18 mL**
Propylene glycol: 20 mL × 1.8 = **36 mL**
Benzalkonium chloride: 15 mg × 1.8 = **27 mg**
Purified water: **qs ad 180 mL**

(b) 27 mg × 1 g/1000 mg × 750 mL/1 g = **20.25 mL**

(c) 36 mL/12 bottles = 3 mL propylene glycol/bottle
3 mL (propylene glycol) × 1.7 g (foreign substance)/1,000,000 mL = 0.0000051 g
= 0.0051 mg
= 5.1 μg

(d) Error = 2.13 g − 1.8 g = 0.33 g
% error = 0.33 g/1.8 g × 100% = **18.33%**

(e) 288.4/412.6 = 0.6989 or 0.7 (fraction of testosterone cipionate that is testosterone base)
1.8 g (testosterone)/0.7 = 2.57 g (testosterone cipionate equivalent)
2.57 g × 1 mL/200 mg × 1000 mg/1 g = **12.85 mL**

(f) 32.6 ng/5 mL × 1000 mL/L × 1 L/10 dL = **652 ng/dL and within the normal range**

13.[a,3] The following is a formula for the compounding of an oral suspension of carvedilol, a beta-blocker, used in the treatment of hypertension and congestive heart failure in patients unable to swallow oral solid dosage forms.

Carvedilol	(Calculate)
Xanthan gum	200 mg
Sodium carboxymethylcellulose	25 mg
Glycerin	2 mL
Sorbitol 70% solution	5 mL
Saccharin sodium	200 mg
Methylparaben	100 mg
Citric acid	100 mg
Sodium phosphate, dibasic	60 mg
Potassium sorbate	150 mg
Simethicone	100 mg
Purified water, ad	100 mL

(a) If the initial starting dose for carvedilol is 6.25 mg twice a day, how many milligrams of the drug should be used in the formula to provide each dose in a teaspoonful?

(b) How many milliliters of the formula should be prepared to last the patient the initial 14 days of treatment?

(c) If 25-mg carvedilol tablets are used as the source of drug, how many are required to provide the medication for the initial 2-week period?

(d) If sorbitol powder is available, how many grams would be required for quantity in (b)?

Solutions:

(a) 100 mL/5 mL (dose) = 20 doses
20 doses × 6.25 mg/dose = **125 mg**

(b) 5 mL/dose × 2 doses/day = 10 mL
10 mL/day × 14 days = **140 mL**

(c) 6.25 mg/dose × 2 doses/day = 12.5 mg/day
12.5 mg/day × 14 days = 175 mg
175 mg/25 mg/tablet = **7 tablets**

(d) 5 mL × 1.4 (formulation factor) = 7 mL
7 mL × 70% = **4.9 g**

14.[a,4] ℞

Amitriptyline hydrochloride	10 mg
Bentonite or silica gel	200 mg
Polyethylene glycol 1000	1.35 g
Polyethylene glycol 3350	0.44 g
M.ft. suppos. DTD # xxiv	

(a) Calculate the total weight of each suppository.

(b) Calculate the quantity of each ingredient for the preparation of the prescription plus two extra suppositories to assure complete fill of the mold.

(c) Polyethylene glycol 3350 is a solid with a melting point of between 48 and 54°C. What are the corresponding temperatures on the Fahrenheit scale?

(d) Silica gel particles are between 2 and 7 μm in size. Convert this range to centimeters.

Solutions:

(a) 0.01 g (10 mg) + 0.2 g (200 mg) + 1.35 g + 0.44 g = **2 g**

(b) Prescription is for 24 suppositories, plus 2 extra = 26
Amitriptyline hydrochloride: 10 mg × 26 = **260 mg**
Bentonite or silica gel: 200 mg × 26 = **5200 mg**
Polyethylene glycol 1000: 1.35 g × 26 = **35.1 g**
Polyethylene glycol 3350: 0.44 g × 26 = **11.44 g**

(c) Temperature conversion formula: F° = 9/5°C + 32°
9/5 × 48°C + 32° = **118.4°F**
9/5 × 54°C + 32° = **129.2°F**

(d) 2 μm = **0.0002 cm**
7 μm = **0.0007 cm**

15. A pharmacist has prepared stock creams containing 0.1% and 5% hydrocortisone from hydrocortisone powder and a cream base in order to facilitate compounding requests for intermediate strengths of hydrocortisone cream.
   (a) How many grams each of the 0.1% and 5% hydrocortisone creams should be mixed to compound 1 ounce (Apothecary) of a 0.75% cream?
   (b) How many grams of hydrocortisone powder could be added to 30 g of the 0.1% cream to prepare one containing 1% hydrocortisone?
   (c) If the pharmacist mixed equal quantities of hydrocortisone powder, the cream base, and each of the 0.1% and 5% creams, what would be the resultant strength of the mixture?

Solutions:

(a) One Apothecary ounce = 31.1 g
By alligation alternate, the proportions to mix are 4.25 parts of the 0.1% cream and 0.65 parts of the 5% cream for a total of 4.9 parts
Each part = 31.1 g/4.9 = 6.35 g (rounded)
Quantity of the 0.1% cream = 4.25 (parts) × 6.35 = 26.98 = **27 g (rounded)**
Quantity of the 5% cream = 0.65 (parts) × 6.41 g = **4.1 g (rounded)**

(b) By alligation alternate, the proportions to mix are 0.9 part of the powder (100% hydrocortisone) and 99 parts of the 0.1% cream
Since the 99 parts (0.1% cream) = 30 g, the 0.9 part (powder) = 30 g × 0.9/99 = **0.27 g hydrocortisone powder**

(c) Arbitrarily use 100 g of each, therefore:

Hydrocortisone powder:	100 g × 100%	=	100 g hydrocortisone
Cream base:	100 g × 0%	=	0 g hydrocortisone
Hydrocortisone cream (0.1%):	100 g × 0.1%	=	0.1 g hydrocortisone
Hydrocortisone cream (5%):	100 g × 5%	=	5 g hydrocortisone
	400 g		105.1 g hydrocortisone

105.1 g (hydrocortisone)/400 g (mixture) × 100% = **26.28% hydrocortisone**

16.[5] The package insert information for a 500-mg vial of ceftriaxone sodium states that 1 mL of diluent should be added to produce a final concentration of 350 mg/mL.
   (a) What is the volume of fluid in the vial after reconstitution?
   (b) How much volume is displaced by the powder after reconstitution?
   (c) How much solution will have to be injected to administer a 500-mg dose?
   (d) If a pharmacist adds 3 mL of diluent to the vial, what would be the resulting concentration in mg/mL?
   (e) To what final volume should the 500-mg vial be diluted with normal saline (NS) to reach a concentration of 10 mg/mL?
   (f) If the diluted solution in part (e) is to be administered over a 30-minute period using an administration set with a drop factor of 20 drops/mL, what would be the flow rate in drops/min?
   (g) ROCEPHIN contains approximately 83 mg (3.6 mEq) of sodium per gram of ceftriaxone activity. How many milliequivalents of sodium would a patient receive from the infusion solution in part (e)? (m.w. NaCl = 58.5).

Solutions:

(a) 500 mg × 1 mL/350 mg = **1.43 mL**

(b) 1.43 mL – 1 mL = **0.43 mL displaced**

(c) 500 mg × 1 mL/350 mg = **1.43 mL**

(d) 3 mL diluent + 0.43 mL displacement = 3.43 mL final volume
500 mg/3.43 mL = **145.83 mg/mL**

(e) 500 mg × 1 mL/10 mg = **50 mL**

(f) 50 mL/30 min × 20 drops/mL = 33.33 drops/min ≈ **33 drops/min**

(g) 3.6 mEq Na/g ceftriaxone × 1 g/1000 mg × 500 mg ceftriaxone = 1.8 mEq Na
50 mL NS × 0.9 g NaCl/100 mL × 1000 mg/g = 450 mg NaCl
450 mg NaCl × 1 mEq/58.5 mg = 7.69 mEq Na
Total = 1.8 mEq + 7.69 mEq = **9.49 mEq Na**

17. ℞ Clarithromycin oral suspension 100 mL
Dose: 7.5 mg/kg
Sig: 2.5 mL q12h.

(a) To prepare 100 mL of a clarithromycin suspension containing 125 mg/5 mL, a pharmacist adds 55 mL of purified water to the granules contained in the commercial package. Calculate the content of clarithromycin in the package, in milligrams.

(b) At the dose prescribed (7.5 mg/kg), how many milliliters of the oral suspension should be administered (rather than the 2.5 mL indicated) to a 28-lb child?

(c) Rather than change the Signa directions, how many milliliters of purified water may be added to the package to prepare a suspension containing the prescribed dose of 7.5 mg/kg/2.5 mL for the 28-lb child in (b)?

(d) Prove your answer to (c).

Solutions:

(a) 125 mg (clarithromycin) × 100 mL/5 mL = **2500 mg clarithromycin**

(b) Dose for child: 7.5 mg × 28 lb/2.2 lb/kg = 95.45 mg clarithromycin
95.45 mg × 5 mL/125 mg = **3.82 ≈ 3.8 mL oral suspension** (rounded)

(c) 2.5 mL × 2500 mg/95.45 mg = 65.48 mL (volume that can be prepared to deliver 95.45 mg/2.5 mL)
100 mL – 55 mL (purified water) = 45 mL (volume occupied by suspended granules)
65.48 mL – 45 mL = **20.48 mL of purified water to add**

(d) 45 mL (granule volume) + 20.48 mL (purified water) = 65.48 mL
2500 mg (clarithromycin)/65.48 mL × 2.5 mL = **95.45 mg clarithromycin**
NOTE: A calibrated oral syringe should be dispensed to assure administration of the correct dose.

18. A hospital pharmacist in a critical care unit receives a medication order for a 210-lb patient calling for a continuous infusion of isoproterenol hydrochloride, 5 μg/min. The pharmacist prepares the infusion by adding the contents of a 5-mL ampule of isoproterenol hydrochloride, 0.2 mg/mL to 250 mL of sodium chloride injection. The critical care nurse programs the automated infusion set to deliver 12 drops per milliliter.
    (a) The label of the ampule of isoproterenol hydrochloride indicates the strength in both mg/mL and as a ratio strength. Calculate the latter.
    (b) Calculate the dose of isoproterenol hydrochloride for this patient, based on μg/kg.
    (c) Calculate the infusion rate, in drops/min.
    (d) Calculate the infusion time, in minutes.

Solutions:
(a) 0.2 mg/mL = 0.0002 g/1 mL = 1 g/x mL; x = **1:5000 isoproterenol hydrochloride**
(b) 210 lb × 1 kg/2.2 lb = 95.5 kg
0.2 mg/mL × 5 mL = 1 mg or 1000 μg isoproterenol hydrochloride
1000 μg/95.5 kg = **10.47 μg/kg**
(c) 5 μg/min × 255 mL/1000 μg = 1.275 mL/min
1.275 mL/min × 12 drops/mL = **15.3 drops/min**
(d) 255 mL × 1 min/1.275 mL = **200 minutes infusion time**

19.[b] A 176-lb cardiology patient received an initial heparin bolus dose of 60 units/kg followed by a heparin drip at 15 units/kg/h. The heparin concentration was 10,000 units per 100 mL and the intravenous set delivered 15 drops per milliliter. The last partial thromboplastin time (PTT) indicated that the patient was being underdosed, and according to the hospital's weight-based heparin protocol, the heparin rate should be increased by 30%.
    (a) Calculate the patient's initial heparin bolus dose in units and milliliters, if the product administered contained 5000 units/mL.
    (b) Calculate the revised dosage in units per kilogram per hour.
    (c) Calculate the revised flow rate in drops per minute.

Solutions:
(a) 176 lb/2.2 lb/kg = 80 kg
80 kg × 60 units/kg = **4800 units heparin bolus dose**
4800 units/5000 units/mL = 0.96 mL ≈ **1 mL heparin bolus dose**
(b) 15 units/kg/h × 30% = 4.5 units/kg/h (increase)
15 units/kg/h + 4.5 units/kg/h = **19.5 units/kg/h**
(c) 19.5 units × 80 kg = 1560 units (dose/h)
1560 units/h × 100 mL/10,000 units = 15.6 mL/h
15.6 mL/h × 15 drops/mL = 234 drops/h
234 drops/h × 1 h/60 min = **3.9 or 4 drops/min**

20.[b] The following is a TPN to be administered 80 mL/h for 24 hours.

Dextrose	200	g
HepatAmine	60	g
Sodium chloride	50	mEq
Potassium chloride	40	mEq
Sodium acetate	20	mEq
Magnesium sulfate	10	mEq
Sodium phosphate	9	mmol
Potassium acetate	15	mEq
Calcium chloride	2	mEq
Multivitamins-12	5	mL
Trace elements-5	1	mL
Vitamin K1	0.5	mg
Pepcid	10	mg
Regular insulin	20	units
Sterile water qs ad	960	mL

(a) How many calories will the dextrose (3.4 kcal/g) provide over 24 hours of administration?

(b) If dextrose is available as a 70% solution, how many milliliters would be needed to prepare the above formula?

(c) If magnesium sulfate ($M_2SO_4 \cdot 7H_2O$) is available as a 50% solution, how many milliliters would be needed to prepare the above formula?

(d) If Pepcid is available as an injection, 40 mg/4 mL, how many milliliters would be needed to prepare the above formula?

(e) If sodium chloride is available as a 23.4% injection, how many milliliters would be needed to prepare the above formula?

(f) How many mEq of sodium would be added as a result of the sodium phosphate?

Solutions:

(a) 960 mL (total volume)/80 mL/h = 12 hours of fluid per bag.
200 g × 3.4 kcal/g = 680 kcal in 12 h × 2 = **1360 kcal in 24 h**

(b) 200 g × 100 mL/70 g = **285.7 mL dextrose solution**

(c) $MgSO_4 \cdot 7\ H_2O$ (m.w. – 246)
Mg is divalent; 246 mg = 2 mEq or 123 mg/mEq
123 mg/mEq × 10 mEq = 1230 mg needed
1230 mg × 100 mL/50 g × 1 g/1000 mg = **2.46 mL magnesium sulfate solution**

(d) 10 mg × 4 mL/40 mg = **1 mL Pepcid injection**

(e) NaCl (m.w. = 58.5)
Na is monovalent; 58.5 mg = 1 mEq
58.5 mg/mEq × 50 mEq = 2925 mg needed
2925 mg × 100 mL/23.4 g × 1 g/1000 mg = **12.5 mL sodium chloride injection**

(f) Na_3PO_4 (m.w. = 164)
164 mg = 3 mmol of Na per mmol Na_3PO_4
9 mmol of Na_3PO_4 × 3 = 27 mmol of sodium
1 mmol of Na = 1 mEq of Na (Na is monovalent)
Thus, 27 mmol = **27 mEq of sodium added**

21.[b] A physician orders the following formula for an intravenous fluid described as "TPN Lite." A flow rate of 1 mL/kg/h is ordered.

Dextrose	15%
Amino acids	4%
Sodium chloride	0.75%
Potassium chloride	0.2%
MVI-12	10 mL
Sterile water for injection ad	1000 mL

How many milliliters of each of the following will be required?

(a) Dextrose injection, 700 mg/mL
(b) Amino acids injection, 10%
(c) Sodium chloride injection, 4 mEq/mL
(d) Potassium chloride injection, 2 mEq/mL
(e) Sterile water for injection.

Solutions:

(a) 1000 mL × 15% = 150 g dextrose needed
Dextrose injection = 700 mg or 0.7 g/mL
150 g/0.7 g/mL = **214.3 mL dextrose injection**

(b) 1000 mL × 4% = 40 g amino acids needed
Amino acids injection = 10 g/100 mL
Thus, 40 g in **400 mL amino acids injection**

(c) 1000 mL × 0.75% = 7.5 g or 7500 mg sodium chloride needed
Sodium chloride (m.w. 58.5) = 58.5 mg/mEq
7500 mg/58.5 mg/mEq = 128.2 mEq needed
128.2 mEq/4 mEq/mL = 32.05 or **32 mL sodium chloride injection**

(d) 1000 mL × 0.2% = 2 g or 2000 mg potassium chloride needed
Potassium chloride (m.w. 74.5) = 74.5 mg/mEq
2000 mg/74.5 mg/mEq = 26.85 mEq needed
26.85/2 mEq/mL = **13.4 mL potassium chloride injection**

(e) 214.3 mL + 400 mL + 32 mL + 13.4 mL + 10 mL (MVI-12) = 669.7 mL
1000 mL − 669.7 = **330.3 mL sterile water for injection**

22.[6] Normosol-R injection contains the following in each 100 mL:

Magnesium chloride (m.w. 95)	30 mg
Potassium chloride (m.w. 74.5)	37 mg
Sodium acetate (m.w. 82)	222 mg
Sodium chloride (m.w. 58.5)	526 mg
Sodium gluconate (m.w. 218)	502 mg

(a) What would be the calculated osmolarity of this solution in mOsmol/L?
(b) What would be the concentration of chloride in this solution in mmol/L?
(c) If a patient receives this solution as an intravenous infusion at a rate of 65 mL/h, how many milliequivalents of sodium will be administered in 1 day?

Solutions:

(a) Magnesium chloride:

30 mg/100 mL × 1000 mL/L × 3 mOsmol/95 mg = 9.47 mOsmol/L

Potassium chloride:

37 mg/100 mL × 1000 mL/L × 2 mOsmol/74.5 mg = 9.93 mOsmol/L

Sodium acetate:

222 mg/100 mL × 1000 mL/L × 2 mOsmol/82 mg = 54.15 mOsmol/L

Sodium chloride:

526 mg/100 mL × 1000 mL/L × 2 mOsmol/58.5 mg = 179.83 mOsmol/L

Sodium gluconate:

502 mg/100 mL × 1000 mL/L × 2 mOsmol/218 mg = 46.06 mOsmol/L

Total osmolarity = **299.44 mOsmol/L**

(b) Magnesium chloride:

30 mg/100 mL × 1000 mL/L × 1 mmol/95 mg = 3.16 mmol/L

Potassium chloride:

37 mg/100 mL × 1000 mL/L × 1 mmol/74.5 mg = 4.97 mmol/L

Sodium chloride:

526 mg/100 mL × 1000 mL/L × 1 mmol/58.5 mg = 89.91 mmol/L

Total chloride = **98.04 mmol/L**

(c) 65 mL/h × 24 h/day = 1560 mL/day infused.

Sodium acetate:

222 mg/100 mL × 1560 mL/day × 1 mEq/82 mg = 42.23 mEq/day

Sodium chloride:

526 mg/100 mL × 1560 mL/day × 1 mEq/58.5 mg = 140.27 mEq/day

Sodium gluconate:

502 mg/100 mL × 1560 mL/day × 1 mEq/218 mg = 35.92 mEq/day

Total sodium = **218.42 mEq/day**

23.[b,7] ENSURE PLUS liquid contains 54.2 g of protein, 197.1 g of carbohydrate, and 53 g of fat in each liter. ENSURE PLUS also supplies 1.5 kcal in each milliliter.

(a) If a patient consumes four 240-mL cans of ENSURE PLUS each day, how many grams of each nutrient is she receiving?

(b) If the patient is a 68-year-old woman who is 5′3″ and moderately active, what weight, in lb, will she maintain by consuming four 240-mL cans of ENSURE PLUS each day?

Solutions:

(a) 240 mL/can × 4 cans/day × 1 L/1000 mL × 54.2 g protein/L = **52.03 g protein/day**

240 mL/can × 4 cans/day × 1 L/1000 mL × 197.1 g carbohydrate/L = **189.22 g carbohydrate/day**

240 mL/can × 4 cans/day × 1 L/1000 mL × 53 g fat/L = **50.88 g fat/day**

(b) 240 mL/can × 4 cans/day × 1.5 kcal/mL = 1440 kcal/day from the ENSURE PLUS

The resting metabolic energy (RME) or basal energy expenditure (BEE) for women can be calculated using the equation below:

$$\text{RME} = 655 + (9.6 \times W) + (1.8 \times H) - (4.7 \times A)$$

Furthermore, the patient's RME should be multiplied by an activity factor of approximately 1.25 to calculate the amount of calories she will need daily to maintain her weight at her current activity level.
RME × 1.25 = 1440 kcal/day
RME = 1152 kcal/day = 655 + (9.6 × W) + (1.8 × H) − (4.7 × A)
W = weight in kilograms
H = height in centimeters = 5′3″ = 63 inches × 2.54 cm/inch = 160.02 cm
A = age in years = 68
1152 kcal/day = 655 + (9.6 × W) + (1.8 × 160.02) − (4.7 × 68)
1152 kcal/day = 623.44 + (9.6 × W)
528.56 kcal/day = 9.6 × W
W = 55.06 kg × 2.2 lb/kg = **121.13 lb**

24. The dose of entecavir is adjusted based on the patient's renal status as determined by creatinine clearance:

Creatinine Clearance (mL/min)	Usual Dose Entecavir
≥50	0.5 mg once daily
30 to <50	0.25 mg once daily, or 0.5 mg every 48 hours
10 to <30	0.15 mg once daily, or 0.5 mg every 72 hours
<10	0.05 mg daily, or 0.5 mg every 7 days

(a) Calculate the creatinine clearance, using the Cockcroft-Gault equation, for a 35-year-old male patient, 68 inches tall, weighing180 lb, and with a serum creatinine of 2.6 mg/dL.
(b) Based on the answer to (a), determine the dose of entecavir as given in the table.
(c) Convert the daily dose of entecavir, as determined in (b), to μg/kg and mg/m² for the patient described in (a).

Solutions:
(a) Cockcroft-Gault equation for males:

$$\text{CrCl (mL/min)} = \frac{[(140 - \text{patient's age}) \times \text{patient's body weight (kg)}]}{[72 \times \text{serum Cr (mg/dL)}]}$$

$$\text{CrCl (mL/min)} = \frac{[(140 - 35) \times 81.8 \text{ kg}]}{[72 \times 2.6 \text{ (mg/dL)}]}$$

$$= \frac{105 \times 81.8}{187.2} = \frac{8589}{187.2} = \mathbf{45.9 \text{ mL/min}}$$

(b) Dose = **0.25 mg once daily or 0.5 mg every 48 hours**

(c) 0.25 mg/81.8 kg = 250 μg/81.8 kg = **3.06 μg/kg**
Using the BSA equation:

$$\text{BSA}\left(\text{m}^2\right)=\sqrt{\frac{\text{Height (cm)}\times\text{Weight (kg)}}{3600}}=\sqrt{\frac{68\text{ inches}\times 2.54\,\frac{\text{cm}}{\text{inches}}\times 81.8\text{ kg}}{3600}}$$

$$=\sqrt{\frac{14128.5}{3600}}=\sqrt{3.92}=1.98\text{ m}^2$$

0.25 mg/1.98 m² = **0.13 mg/m²**

25.[b] A physician prescribes lamivudine for a 35-year-old male patient who stands 5 ft 8 inches tall and weighs 180 lb. The drug dose must be adjusted based on a patient's renal function. The patient's serum creatinine is 2.6 mg/dL.

(a) Calculate the patient's creatinine clearance (CrCl) using the Cockcroft-Gault equation and the patient's ideal body weight (IBW).

(b) If the literature for lamivudine states the following, what is the appropriate dose for the patient? Available are scored 150-mg tablets and 300-mg film-coated tablets.

(c) If the patient is unable to swallow tablets, how many milliliters of an oral liquid containing 10 mg lamivudine per milliliter could be administered as the initial dose?

(d) Calculate the initial dose for this patient on the basis of mg/kg of body weight.

(e) Calculate the patient's body mass index (BMI) and interpret the result, that is, underweight, normal, overweight, or obese.

Creatinine Clearance (mL/min)	Initial Dose (mg)	Maintenance Dose
<5	50	25 mg once daily
5–14	150	50 mg once daily
15–29	150	100 mg once daily
30–49	150	150 mg once daily

Solutions:

(a) The Cockcroft-Gault equation (for males) and IBW calculation (for males):

$$\text{CrCl}\left(\text{mL/min}\right)=\frac{\left[\left(140-\text{patient's age}\right)\times\text{patient's body weight}\left(\text{kg}\right)\right]}{\left[72\times\text{serum Cr}\left(\text{mg/dL}\right)\right.}$$

1BW = 50 kg + 2.3 kg for each inch in height over 5 ft
1BW = 50 kg + 2.3 kg × 8 = 50 kg + 18.4 kg = **68.4 kg**

$$\text{CrCl}\left(\text{mL/min}\right)=\frac{\left[\left(140-35\right)\times 68.4\text{ kg}\right]}{72\times 2.6\text{ mg/dL}}=\frac{7182}{187.2}=\mathbf{38.3654\ mL/min}$$

(b) From the dosing table, **150 mg initially, then 150 mg once daily**

(c) 150 mg dose × 1 mL/10 mg = **15 mL per dose**

(d) 180 lb × 1 kg/2.2 lb = 81.8 kg
150 mg/81.8 kg = **1.8 mg/kg**

(e) $$\text{BMI} = \frac{\text{Weight (lb)}}{\text{Height (inches)}^2} \times 704.5 = \frac{180}{4624} \times 704.5$$
= **27.4 and "overweight"** (re: Table 14.1)

26. The drug mitoxantrone hydrochloride is used in veterinary medicine in the treatment of leukemia. Cats are administered the drug by 30-minute intravenous infusion at 6.5 mg/m^2.
(a) Calculate the dose for a 3.1-lb cat.
(b) How many milliliters should be used from a vial containing mitoxantrone hydrochloride, 20 mg/10 mL, to provide the dose calculated in (a)?
(c) For the administration of the 30-minute infusion at a rate of 10 mL/kg/h, how many milliliters of infusion should be prepared?

Solutions:
(a) By using literature sources, or the table in Chapter 17, the relationship between body weight and body surface area of cats and dogs may be found
In this case, a cat weighing 3.1 lb or 1.4 kg (3.1 lb × 1 kg/2.2 lb) is shown by the table to have a BSA of about 1.2 m^2.
Thus, 6.5 mg/m^2 × 1.2 m^2 = **7.8 mg, dose of mitoxantrone hydrochloride**
(b) 7.8 mg × 10 mL/20 mg = **3.9 mL mitoxantrone hydrochloride injection**
(c) 1.4 kg × 10 mL/kg/h = 14 mL/h
14 mL/h × 0.5 h = **7 mL**

27. The biotechnology drug bortezomib is available in vials each containing 3.5 mg of powdered drug. When reconstituted with 3.5 mL of 0.9% sodium chloride injection, a concentration of bortezomib, 1 mg/mL results (the volume of the powdered drug when dissolved is negligible). The drug is used in the treatment of patients with multiple myeloma.
(a) The dose of bortezomib is 1.3 mg/m^2. Calculate the dose, in milligrams, for a patient who weighs 165 lb and measures 70 inches in height.
(b) The drug is coadministered with melphalan and prednisone according to the schedule:
bortezomib (1.3 mg/m^2): D-1, D-4, D-8, D-11, D-22, D-25, D-29, D-32
melphalan (9 mg/m^2) and prednisone (60 mg/m^2): D-1-4
How many milligrams of each drug would be administered to the above patient on the first day of the protocol?
(c) Calculate the total volume of bortezomib administered during the treatment schedule.

Solutions:

(a) By the nomogram in Chapter 8, the patient's BSA is determined to be 1.92 m². Confirmed by calculation:

$$\text{BSA, m}^2 = \sqrt{\frac{75\text{ kg} \times 177.8\text{ cm}}{3600}} = 1.92\text{ m}^2$$

1.3 mg × 1.92 (m²) = 2.496 mg or **2.5 mg**

(b) bortezomib: **2.5 mg**
melphalan: 9 mg × 1.92 (m²) = 1.728 or **1.7 mg**
prednisone: 60 mg × 1.92 (m²) = **115.2 mg**

(c) 2.5 mL/treatment × 8 treatments = **20 mL**

28.[b] A patient with a "superinfection" is judged to require antibiotic therapy at dosage levels greater than usual. The patient has normal kidney function, and the drug selected is eliminated entirely by the kidney. The intravenous bolus dose administered is 0.5 g, which resulted in a drug plasma level of 12 μg/mL.

(a) Calculate the apparent volume of distribution.

(b) If the half-life of the drug is 3 hours and the desired drug plasma level should be maintained at, or above, 3 μg/mL for effectiveness, when should the second dose be administered?

Solutions:

(a) $$\text{Vd} = \frac{\text{D (total amount of drug in the body)}}{\text{Cp (drug plasma concentration)}} = \frac{0.5\text{ g}}{12\text{ mg/mL}} = \frac{0.5\text{ g}}{0.012\text{ g/L}} = \mathbf{41.67\text{ L}}$$

(b) One half-life, or 3 hours, reduces the drug's plasma level to ½ of 12 μg/mL, or to 6 μg/mL.

A second half-life, or 6 hours total, reduces the drug's plasma level to ½ of 6 μg/mL, or to 3 μg/mL.

Thus, to maintain the plasma level at or above 3 μg/mL, the second dose should be administered **approximately 6 hours after the first dose.**

29.[8] A medication order calls for a patient to receive 200 μCi of sodium iodide I-123 for a thyroid function test. Sodium iodide I-123 is available in 3.7-MBq capsules and can be used up to 30 hours after measurement using a radioactivity calibration system.

(a) How many capsules should be dispensed to provide the prescribed dose?

(b) How many μCi of radioactivity will be available at the 30-hour cutoff time if the half-life of I-123 is 13.2 hours?

Solutions:

(a) 200 μCi/dose × 0.037 MBq/μCi × 1 capsule/3.7 MBq = **2 capsules**

(b) $N = N_0 e^{-\lambda t}$
$t_{1/2} = 0.693\lambda$

Where N is the amount of activity at elapsed time t, N_0 is the amount of activity initially present, e is the base of the natural logarithm (2.718), λ is the disintegration constant, and $t_{1/2}$ is the half-life.

$13.2 \text{ hours} = 0.693/\lambda$

$= 0.0525 \text{ h}^{-1}$

$N = 200\ \mu\text{Ci}\ e^{-(0.0525\ \text{h}^{-1})t}$

$N = 200\ \mu\text{Ci}\ e^{-(0.0525\ \text{h}^{-1})(30\ \text{hours})} = \mathbf{41.39\ \mu Ci}$

30. COLCRYS tablets contain 0.6 mg of the active constituent colchicine for use in the treatment of gout.
   (a) Colchicine is an "old" drug, having been approved for use in the United States over five decades ago. Prior to the "metrification" of units in the pharmaceutical industry, labels indicating the strengths of colchicine tablets were expressed in fractions of a grain. Refer to Table A.1 in Appendix A and convert 0.6 mg to the approximate fraction of a grain equivalent.
   (b) Referring once again to Table A.1, how many 0.6-mg colchicine tablets can be manufactured from 1 oz (Avoirdupois) of colchicine?
   (c) The recommended dose of colchicine for the prophylaxis of gout flares is 0.6 mg once or twice daily in adults with a maximum dose 1.2 mg/day. In the treatment of gout flares, the dose is 1.2 mg at the first sign of a gout flare followed by 0.6 mg one hour later. The dose generally is not to be repeated earlier than 3 days later. The dose requires downward adjustment in the elderly, in those with compromised hepatic and renal conditions, and when coadministered with certain interacting drugs. Colchicine is a highly toxic drug. The literature advises that fatalities have been reported in adults and children who have ingested colchicine. For the above dosage recommendations, how many 0.6-mg tablets might be dispensed as a maximum for two treatments?

Solutions:

(a) According to Table A.1, the practical equivalent is 1 gr = 65 mg (the precise equivalent is 1 gr = 64.798891 mg)

Since the question asks for the "approximate fraction of a grain equivalent," we may use the practical equivalent and do some rounding in our calculations.

0.6 mg × 1 grain/65 mg = 0.0092 or 0.009 grain

0.009 grain = **9/1000 or approximately 1/111 gr**

(b) 1 oz = 28.35 g or 28,350 mg

28,350 mg × 1 tablet/0.6 mg = **47,250 tablets**

(c) First day, 2 tablets (1.2 mg, first dose) + 1 tablet (0.6 mg, 1 hour later) = 3 tablets

3 days later = 2 tablets + 1 tablet = 3 tablets

Total, maximum = **6 tablets**

31.[9] The CetIri chemotherapy regimen to treat colorectal cancer in a 42-week cycle is as follows:

Cetuximab 400 mg/m² IV, day 1 of first cycle only (loading dose).

Cetuximab 250 mg/m² IV weekly, days 1, 8, 15, 22, 29, and 36, except for day 1 of first cycle.

Irinotecan 125 mg/m² IV, weekly for 4 weeks, followed by 2 weeks of rest; administer on days 1, 8, 15, and 22.

(a) Calculate the dose of each drug, including the loading and maintenance dose of cetuximab, for a patient who is 5'6" tall and weighs 138 pounds.

(b) Cetuximab is available as a solution with a concentration of 2 mg/mL to be infused via an infusion pump or a syringe pump without dilution. The first dose should be administered over 120 minutes with subsequent doses administered over 60 minutes, and the maximum infusion rate is 5 mL/min. Calculate the infusion rates for the cetuximab doses calculated in (a).

(c) Irinotecan is available as a solution with a concentration of 20 mg/mL and must be diluted with 5% dextrose injection prior to infusion to a final concentration range of 0.12 to 2.8 mg/mL. The solution should be infused over 90 minutes. Determine the amount of irinotecan solution to be used and the final volume range for the infusion solution that can be used for the irinotecan dose calculated in (a).

(d) The irinotecan dose is diluted in 5% dextrose solution to a final volume of 250 mL. What would be the infusion rate for the solution in (b)?

(e) If the patient begins the CetIri regimen on September 26, list the infusion schedule for the first two cycles.

Solutions:

(a) 5'6" = 66 in × 2.54 cm/in = 167.64 cm
138 lb × 1 kg/2.2 lb = 62.73 kg

$$\text{BSA} = \sqrt{\frac{167.64\ \text{cm} \times 62.73\ \text{kg}}{3600}} = 1.71\ \text{m}^2$$

Cetuximab (loading dose): 400 mg/m^2 × 1.71 m^2 = **683.64 mg**
Cetuximab: 250 mg/m^2 × 1.71 m^2 = **427.27 mg**
Irinotecan: 125 mg/m^2 × 1.71 m^2 = **213.64 mg**

(b) Loading dose: 683.64 mg × 1 mL/2 mg = 341.82 mL
341.82 mL/120 min = **2.85 mL/min**
Maintenance dose: 427.27 mg × 1 mL/2 mg = 213.64 mL
213.64 mL/60 min = **3.56 mL/min**

(c) 213.64 mg × 1 mL/20 mg = **10.68 mL of irinotecan solution**
213.64 mg × 1 mL/0.12 mg = 1780.31 mL
213.64 mg × 1 mL/2.8 mg = 76.299 mL
The dose should be diluted to 76.299 – 1780.31 mL with 5% dextrose solution before infusion.

(d) 250 mL/90 min = **2.78 mL/min**

(e) Cycle #1
September 26
Cetuximab: 2.85 mL/min over 120 minutes (683.64 mg dose)
Irinotecan: 213.64 mg diluted to 250 mL with D5W infused at 2.78 mL/min
October 3, 10, and 17
Cetuximab: 3.56 mL/min over 60 minutes (427.27 mg dose)
Irinotecan: 213.64 mg diluted to 250 mL with D5W infused at 2.78 mL/min
October 24 and 31
Cetuximab: 3.56 mL/min over 60 minutes (427.27 mg dose)
No irinotecan

Cycle #2
November 7, 14, 21, and 28
Cetuximab: 3.56 mL/min over 60 minutes (427.27 mg dose)
Irinotecan: 213.64 mg diluted to 250 mL with D5W infused at 2.78 mL/min
December 5 and 12
Cetuximab: 3.56 mL/min over 60 minutes (427.27 mg dose)
No irinotecan

32. An order for an IV admixture is as follows:
Calcium gluconate 15 mEq in 500 mL D5½NS
 (a) How many milliliters of a calcium gluconate 10% w/v injection should be used in preparing this IV admixture?
 (b) What would be the osmolarity of the IV admixture solution? (Assume volumes are additive and complete dissociation.)
 (c) If the flow rate of this solution is 45 mL/h, how many milliequivalents of calcium would the patient receive daily? (Assume volumes are additive and continuous infusion.)
 (d) A patient begins receiving the IV admixture at 7:00 AM at the rate in (c). At 11:30 AM, an order is received to increase the flow rate to 60 mL/h. At what time should the next container of solution be started, assuming that the rate on the existing container was changed at 11:30 AM?

Solutions:
(a) m.w. $Ca(C_6H_{11}O_7)_2$ = 40 + 2(195) = 430
 15 mEq × 430 mg/2 mEq × 1 g/1000 mg × 100 mL/10 g = **32.25 mL**
(b) Total volume = 500 mL (D5½NS) + 32.25 mL ($Ca(C_6H_{11}O_7)_2$) = 532.25 mL
 $Ca(C_6H_{11}O_7)_2$:
 15 mEq/532.25 mL × 430 mg/2 mEq × 3 mOsmol/430 mg × 1000 mL/L = 42.27 mOsmol/L
 Dextrose (m.w. = 180):
 5 g/100 mL × 500 mL = 25 g
 25 g/532.25 mL × 1000 mg/g × 1 mOsmol/180 mg × 1000 mL/L = 260.95 mOsmol/L
 NaCl (m.w. = 23 + 35.5 = 58.5):
 0.45 g/100 mL × 500 mL = 2.25 g
 2.25 g/532.25 mL × 1000 mg/g × 2 mOsmol/58.5 mg × 1000 mL/L = 144.52 mOsmol/L
 Total = 42.27 mOsmol/L + 260.95 mOsmol/L + 144.52 mOsmol/L = **447.74 mOsmol/L**
(c) 15 mEq/532.25 mL × 45 mL/h × 24 h/day = **30.44 mEq/day**
(d) 7 AM to 11:30 AM = 4.5 hours
 45 mL/h × 4.5 h = 202.5 mL infused
 532.25 mL − 202.5 mL = 329.75 mL remaining
 329.75 mL × 1 h/60 mL = 5.495 h ≈ 5 h 30 min
 11:30 AM + 5 h 30 min = **5:00 PM**

33. Concentrated glycolic acid consists of 70% w/w glycolic acid and has a specific gravity of 1.27.
    (a) How many milliliters of the concentrated acid would be needed to prepare 3 fl.oz. of a 10% w/v solution?
    (b) If the strength of the concentrated acid were mistakenly read as 70% w/v, how much of the concentrated acid would be used to prepare the solution in (a)?
    (c) What would be the percent error in the amount of concentrated glycolic acid measured in (b)?
    (d) What would be the resulting percent strength of the diluted acid solution in (b) due to the mistake?

Solutions:

(a) 3 fl.oz. × 29.57 mL/fl.oz. = 88.71 mL solution to prepare
88.71 mL × 10 g/100 mL = 8.87 g glycolic acid needed
8.87 g glycolic acid × 100 g conc. acid/70 g glycolic acid = 12.67 g conc. acid.
12.67 g × 1 mL/1.27 g = **9.98 mL concentrated acid needed**

(b) 8.87 g glycolic acid × 100 mL conc. acid/70 g glycolic acid = **12.67 mL conc. acid**

(c) Error = 12.67 mL – 9.98 mL = 2.69 mL

$$\% \text{ error} = \frac{2.69 \text{ mL} \times 100}{9.98 \text{ mL}} = \mathbf{27\%}$$

(d) 12.67 mL conc. acid × 1.27 g/mL = 16.09 g conc. acid
16.09 g conc. acid × 70 g glycolic acid/100 g conc. acid = 11.27 g glycolic acid
11.27 g glycolic acid/88.71 mL soln × 100 = **12.7% w/v**

34. The formula for Tolu balsam syrup NF is as follows[10]:

℞	Tolu balsam tincture	10 mL
	Magnesium carbonate	2 g
	Sucrose	164 g
	Purified water qs	200 mL

(a) How much of each ingredient would be needed to prepare 4 fl.oz. of this syrup?
(b) Tolu balsam tincture contains 80% v/v ethyl alcohol. What is the percent strength of ethyl alcohol in the syrup mixture?
(c) What is the ratio strength of magnesium carbonate in the syrup mixture?
(d) What is the percent strength of sucrose in the syrup mixture?
(e) An empty 25-mL specific gravity bottle weighs 21.04 g, 46.05 g when filled with water, and 52.93 g when filled with the syrup mixture. What is the specific gravity of the syrup?

Solutions:

(a) 4 fl.oz. × 29.57 mL/fl.oz. = 118.28 mL syrup to prepare
Formula conversion factor = 118.28 mL/200 mL = 0.5914
Tolu balsam tincture: 10 mL × 0.5914 = **5.91 mL**
Magnesium carbonate: 2 g × 0.5914 = **1.18 g**
Sucrose: 164 g × 0.5914 = **96.99 g**
Purified water: **qs 118.28 mL**

(b) 10 mL tincture × 80 mL EtOH/100 mL tincture = 8 mL EtOH
8 mL EtOH/200 mL syrup × 100 = **4% v/v**

(c) 200 mL syrup/2 g $MgCO_3$ = 100 mL syrup/1 g $MgCO_3$ = **1:100 w/v**

(d) 164 g sucrose/200 mL syrup × 100 = **82% w/v**

(e) 46.05 g – 21.04 g = 25.01 g water
52.93 g – 21.04 g = 31.89 g syrup
Specific gravity = 31.89 g/25.01 g = **1.275**

35. K-PHOS NEUTRAL tablets contain 852 mg dibasic sodium phosphate anhydrous, 155 mg monobasic potassium phosphate, and 130 mg monobasic sodium phosphate monohydrate in each tablet.

(a) How many milliosmoles of sodium phosphate dibasic are contained in each tablet?

(b) How many millimoles of potassium phosphate monobasic are contained in a dose of two tablets?

(c) If a patient takes two tablets four times daily, how many total milliequivalents of sodium is she ingesting each day?

(d) The normal blood level for phosphate is 2.5 to 5 mg%. Calculate the phosphate amount range contained in a 4-mL blood sample to fall within the normal range.

Solutions:

(a) m.w. Na_2HPO_4 = 2(23) + 96 = 142
852 mg/tablet × 3 mOsmol/142 mg = **18 mOsmol/tablet**

(b) m.w. KH_2PO_4 = 39 + 97 = 136
155 mg/tablet × 1 mmol/136 mg × 2 tablets/dose = **2.28 mmol/dose**

(c) Na_2HPO_4:
852 mg/tablet × 2 tablets/dose × 4 doses/day = 6816 mg/day
6816 mg/day × 2 mEq/142 mg = 96 mEq sodium/day
$NaH_2PO_4 \cdot H_2O$:
m.w. = 23 + 97 + 18 = 138
130 mg/tablet × 2 tablets/dose × 4 doses/day = 1040 mg/day
1040 mg/day × 1 mEq/138 mg = 7.54 mEq sodium/day
Total sodium = 96 mEq/day + 7.54 mEq/day = **103.54 mEq/day**

(d) 2.5 mg/100 mL × 4 mL × 1000 mcg/mg = 100 mcg
5 mg/100 mL × 4 mL × 1000 mcg/mg = 200 mcg
Range = **100 – 200 mcg**

Credits

[a]Formulas and methods of preparation courtesy of Loyd V. Allen, Jr., Editor-in-Chief, *International Journal of Pharmaceutical Compounding*, Edmond, OK.
[b]Problem courtesy of Flynn Warren, Bishop, GA.

References

1. Prince SJ. Calculations. *International Journal of Pharmaceutical Compounding* 2004;8:294.
2. Stockton SJ. Calculations. *International Journal of Pharmaceutical Compounding* 2010;14:140.
3. Anonymous. Carvedilol 1-mg/mL oral suspension. *International Journal of Pharmaceutical Compounding* 2010;14:423.
4. Anonymous. Amitriptyline hydrochloride suppositories. *International Journal of Pharmaceutical Compounding* 2010;14:334.
5. Stockton SJ. Calculations. *International Journal of Pharmaceutical Compounding* 2010;14:327.
6. Stockton SJ. Calculations. *International Journal of Pharmaceutical Compounding* 2011;15:416.
7. Prince SJ. Calculations. *International Journal of Pharmaceutical Compounding* 2005;9:146.
8. Prince SJ. Calculations. *International Journal of Pharmaceutical Compounding* 1998;2:453.
9. Stockton SJ, Saluja HS. Calculations. *International Journal of Pharmaceutical Compounding* 2012;16:498.
10. Tolu Balsam Syrup NF. US Pharmacopeial Convention, Inc. *United States Pharmacopeia 37-National Formulary 32* [book online]. Rockville, MD: US Pharmacopeial Convention, Inc.; 2014.

Index

Note: Page numbers in *italic* denote figures; those followed by *t* denote tables.

TABLE OF ATOMIC WEIGHTS[a]

Name	Symbol	Atomic Number	Atomic Weight (Accurate to 4 Figures[b])	Approximate Atomic Weight
Actinium	Ac	89	*	227
Aluminum	Al	13	26.98	27
Americium	Am	95	*	243
Antimony	Sb	51	121.8	122
Argon	Ar	18	39.95	40
Arsenic	As	33	74.92	75
Astatine	At	85	*	210
Barium	Ba	56	137.3	137
Berkelium	Bk	97	*	247
Beryllium	Be	4	9.012	9
Bismuth	Bi	83	209.0	209
Bohrium	Bh	107	*	272
Boron	B	5	10.81	11
Bromine	Br	35	79.90	80
Cadmium	Cd	48	112.4	112
Calcium	Ca	20	40.08	40
Californium	Cf	98	*	251
Carbon	C	6	12.01	12
Cerium	Ce	58	140.1	140
Cesium	Cs	55	132.9	133
Chlorine	Cl	17	35.45	35
Chromium	Cr	24	52.00	52
Cobalt	Co	27	58.93	59
Copper	Cu	29	63.55	64
Curium	Cm	96	*	247
Darmstadtium	Ds	110	*	281
Dubnium	Db	105	*	268
Dysprosium	Dy	66	162.5	163
Einsteinium	Es	99	*	252
Erbium	Er	68	167.3	167
Europium	Eu	63	152.0	152
Fermium	Fm	100	*	257
Fluorine	F	9	19.00	19
Francium	Fr	87	*	223
Gadolinium	Gd	64	157.3	157
Gallium	Ga	31	69.72	70
Germanium	Ge	32	72.64	73
Gold	Au	79	197.0	197

[a]Table derived from Weiser ME. Pure and Applied Chemistry 2006; 78:2051–2066. Available at http://old.iupac.org/publications/pac/2006/pdf/7811x2051.pdf. Accessed October 1, 2011.

[b]When rounded off to 4-figure accuracy, these weights are practically identical to the similarly rounded-off weights in the older table based on oxygen = 16.0000.

(*Continued*)

TABLE OF ATOMIC WEIGHTS[a] (*Continued*)

Name	Symbol	Atomic Number	Atomic Weight (Accurate to 4 Figures[b])	Approximate Atomic Weight
Hafnium	Hf	72	178.5	179
Hassium	Hs	108	*	277
Helium	He	2	4.003	4
Holmium	Ho	67	164.9	165
Hydrogen	H	1	1.008	1
Indium	In	49	114.8	115
Iodine	I	53	126.9	127
Iridium	Ir	77	192.2	192
Iron	Fe	26	55.85	56
Krypton	Kr	36	83.80	84
Lanthanum	La	57	138.9	139
Lawrencium	Lr	103	*	260
Lead	Pb	82	207.2	207
Lithium	Li	3	6.941	7
Lutetium	Lu	71	175.0	175
Magnesium	Mg	12	24.31	24
Manganese	Mn	25	54.94	55
Meitnerium	Mt	109	*	276
Mendelevium	Md	101	*	258
Mercury	Hg	80	200.6	201
Molybdenum	Mo	42	95.94	96
Neodymium	Nd	60	144.2	144
Neon	Ne	20	20.18	20
Neptunium	Np	93	*	237
Nickel	Ni	28	58.69	59
Niobium	Nb	41	92.91	93
Nitrogen	N	7	14.01	14
Nobelium	No	102	*	259
Osmium	Os	76	190.2	190
Oxygen	O	8	16.00	16
Palladium	Pd	46	106.4	106
Phosphorus	P	15	30.97	31
Platinum	Pt	78	195.1	195
Plutonium	Pu	94	*	244
Polonium	Po	84	*	209
Potassium	K	19	39.10	39
Praseodymium	Pr	59	140.9	141
Promethium	Pm	61	*	145
Protactinium	Pa	91	231.0	231
Radium	Ra	88	226.0	226
Radon	Rn	86	*	222
Rhenium	Re	75	186.2	186

TABLE OF ATOMIC WEIGHTS[a] (*Continued*)

Name	Symbol	Atomic Number	Atomic Weight (Accurate to 4 Figures[b])	Approximate Atomic Weight
Rhodium	Rh	45	102.9	103
Roentgenium	Rg	111	*	280
Rubidium	Rb	37	85.47	85
Ruthenium	Ru	44	101.1	101
Rutherfordium	Rf	104	*	267
Samarium	Sm	62	150.4	150
Scandium	Sc	21	44.96	45
Seaborgium	Sg	106	*	271
Selenium	Se	34	78.96	79
Silicon	Si	14	28.09	28
Silver	Ag	47	107.9	108
Sodium	Na	11	22.99	23
Strontium	Sr	38	87.62	88
Sulfur	S	16	32.07	32
Tentalum	Ta	73	180.9	181
Technetium	Tc	43	*	98
Tellurium	Te	52	127.6	128
Terbium	Tb	65	158.9	159
Thallium	Tl	81	204.4	204
Thorium	Th	90	232.0	232
Thulium	Tm	69	168.9	169
Tin	Sn	50	118.7	119
Titanium	Ti	22	47.87	48
Tungsten	W	74	183.8	184
Unnilhexium	Unh	116	*	263
Unnilpentium	Unp	115	*	262
Unnilquadium	Unq	114	*	261
Ununbium	Uub	112	*	285
Ununoctium	Uuo	118	*	294
Ununtrium	Uut	113	*	284
Uranium	U	92	238.0	238
Vanadium	V	23	50.94	51
Xenon	Xe	54	131.3	131
Ytterbium	Yb	70	173.0	173
Yttrium	Y	39	88.91	89
Zinc	Zn	30	65.38	65
Zirconium	Zr	40	91.22	91

*The isotopic composition of natural or artificial radioactive elements usually varies in specific samples, depending upon their origin.